ADULT-GERONTOLOGY ACUTE CARE NURSE PRACTITIONER

CERTIFICATION REVIEW

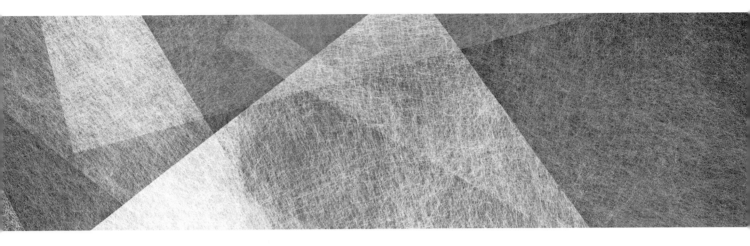

ADULT-GERONTOLOGY ACUTE CARE NURSE PRACTITIONER

CERTIFICATION REVIEW

Jill Beavers-Kirby, DNP, MS, ACNP-BC
Nurse Practitioner
Bicycle Health
Redwood City, California

ELSEVIER

ELSEVIER

3251 Riverport Lane
St. Louis, Missouri 63043

ADULT-GERONTOLOGY ACUTE CARE NURSE PRACTITIONER
CERTIFICATION REVIEW

ISBN: 978-0-323-55606-4

Library of Congress Control Number: 2020943168

Senior Content Strategist: Sandra Clark
Senior Content Development Manager: Lisa P. Newton
Senior Content Development Specialist: Tina Kaemmerer
Publishing Services Manager: Julie Eddy
Project Manager: Andrew Schubert
Design Direction: Brian Salisbury

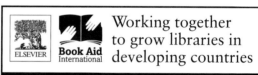

Printer in the United States of America
Last digit is the print number: 9   8   7   6   5   4   3   2   1

This book is dedicated to all the Adult-Gerontology Acute Care Nurse Practitioner students. My hope is that this book will help you achieve your dream of becoming the best nurse practitioner that you can be.

Contributors

THOMAS LAWSON, MS
Nurse Practitioner
Neurocritical Care
The Ohio State University Wexner Medical Center
Columbus, Ohio

JOEL RICE, MS
Nurse Practitioner
Madison Health
London, Ohio

Reviewers

DANIELLE WILLIAMS, MSN, AGACNP-BC
Acute Care Nurse Practitioner
St. Vincent Evansville
Evansville, Indiana

JENNIFER J. YEAGER, PHD, RN, APRN
Assistant Professor
Tarleton State University
Stephenville, Texas

Preface and Acknowledgments

The inspiration for this book came from necessity – like so many nursing ideas. As an educator, I wanted to recommend a test preparation book for students who were studying to become an Adult-Gerontology Acute Care Nurse Practitioner (AGACNP). The book had to contain the latest information and needed to mirror the certification exam. I searched high and low but could not find what I was looking for, so I decided to create it myself. This book is the result of that search.

I would like to acknowledge my contributors who helped me with this book. Without their involvement, this project would not have been possible.

I would also like to acknowledge my husband James for being my rock and helping me keep my sanity when I burn the candle at both ends.

Jill R. Beavers-Kirby

Contents

Test-Taking Strategies

Congratulations! You have graduated from your nurse practitioner (NP) program and now it is time to take your board certification exam. So where do you begin?

There are essentially six steps to becoming a certified, employed NP. These steps are graduation, certification, licensure, obtaining a National Provider Identifier (NPI) number, obtaining a Drug Enforcement Administration (DEA) number, and credentialing.

Certification

Passing the Adult-Gerontology Acute Care Nurse Practitioner (AGACNP) certification exam is the key to entering practice after you graduate from your ACAGNP program. It is the only thing standing between you and employment as an NP. You may be wondering which exam to take and whether you will pass.

Adult Gerontology Acute Care NPs must choose between two certifying bodies:

1. American Nurses Credentialing Center (ANCC): Awards the Adult-Gerontology Acute Care Nurse Practitioner-Board Certified credential (AGACNP-BC; https://www.nursingworld.org/our-certifications/).
2. American Association of Critical Care Nurses (AACN): Awards the Acute Care Nurse Practitioner Certified–Adult Gerontology credential (ACNPC-AG; https://www.aacn.org/certification/get-certified/acnpc-ag).

In practice and as far as employment is concerned, it does not make a difference which exam you take. Once you pass your exam, you will be an AGACNP-BC ready to apply for your license to practice. The initials behind your name may be a bit different depending on the certifying organization, but this difference simply reflects the board through which you are certified, not a difference in scope of practice or ability.

So how do these two acute care certification exams compare, and which exam are AGACNPs more likely to pass?

Eligibility

To be eligible to take the exam through AACN, you need an active unencumbered license and completion of a graduate-level advanced practice education program with a minimum of 500 hours of faculty-supervised clinical hours. You can find more about the educational requirements at https://www.aacn.org/~/media/aacn-website/certification/get-certified/handbooks/acnpcagexamhandbook.pdf.

To be eligible to take the exam through the ANCC, you need to hold a current, active registered nurse (RN) license in a state or territory of the United States or hold the professional, legally recognized equivalent in another country and hold a master's, postgraduate, or doctoral degree from an adult-gerontology acute care NP program accredited by the Commission on Collegiate Nursing Education (CCNE) or the Accreditation Commission for Education in Nursing (ACEN). A minimum of 500 faculty-supervised clinical hours must be included in the adult-gerontology acute care NP role and population. You can find more about the educational requirements at https://www.nursingworld.org/our-certifications/adult-gerontology-acute-care-nurse-practitioner/.

Advanced Practice Registered Nurse (APRN) certification candidates may be authorized to sit for the exam after all coursework is complete, before degree conferral. ANCC will retain your exam result and will issue certification on the date the requested documents are received, all eligibility requirements are met, and a passing result is on file. All fees must be paid at the time your application is submitted to the ANCC. Applications received with insufficient funds or missing documentation will delay the review of your application for eligibility and delay your ability to schedule and take the certification exam.

Cost

For the AACN exam, candidates who are also members of the AACN can take the test for $255; however, nonmembers must pay $360 to take the test.

The cost to take the exam through the ANCC also depends on the candidate's membership status. For nonmembers, the cost is $395, but for members of the ANCC or other recognized organizations, the cost ranges from $290 to $340.

Test Content and Length

The ACNPC-AG exam through the AACN consists of 175 multiple-choice questions of which only 150 are scored. Seventy-three percent of the questions are based on clinical judgment related to nursing care of the adult-gerontology patient population. The remaining questions test candidates on nonclinical judgment knowledge with three major content dimensions including patient care problems, skills and procedures, and validated competencies. Candidates have 3 {1/2} hours to complete the ACNPC-AG exam.

The AGACNP-BC certification exam through the ANCC is a bit lengthier and is comprised of 175 scored questions and 25 pretest questions. Candidates have 4 hours to answer all 200 questions. Only 46% of the ANCC exam is based on clinical practice. In addition, candidates also are tested on three other domains of practice like APRN core competencies, role-professional responsibility, and health care systems.

How to Apply to Take the Exam

Both exams give you the option to register online. The AACN also allows you to register through the mail by sending your original, final transcripts for all graduate-level coursework required; proof of your conferred degree; the completed eligibility form; application honor statement; and the application fee. This information should be sent, in one envelope, to AACN Certification Corporation, 27071 Aliso Creek Road, Aliso Viejo, CA 92656-3399.

Renewal Requirements

Both certifications are valid for 5 years; however, their renewal requirements differ slightly. The ANCC requires all renewal candidates to complete a mandatory 75 continuing education hours (CHs) in your certification specialty, plus one or more of the eight ANCC renewal categories. The eight categories are CHs, academic credits, presentations, evidence-based quality improvement project (such as a publication or research project), preceptor hours, professional service (such as volunteering), practice hours, and assessment/exam. All APRNs also are required to complete 25 CHs of pharmacotherapeutics as a portion of the mandatory 75 CHs in the NP certification held.

ACNPC-AGs have the option to renew in one of three ways: through 1000 practice hours and continuing education (CE) including pharmacology CE; through 1000 practice hours, pharmacology CE, and passing the certification exam; and through 150 CEs including pharmacology CEs and passing the certification exam.

Test-Taking Strategies

It is important to create a study strategy for passing your certification exam. First, you need to establish a routine for reviewing and studying. This means setting aside a small amount of time every day to study; shorter study sessions are more effective than long cram sessions. Study in a quiet, distraction-free environment. You also should start your study strategy 6 months before you plan to take your exam. Gather your review materials and consider signing up for a review course.

Six months before the completion of your NP program, establish the schedule and procedure for your certification studies. Research available study materials and review the courses. Purchase or enroll for those you wish to take. It is also a good idea to take a practice exam. This will help you pinpoint those areas in which you are weaker and need to really focus your study efforts. You can find practice exams on the ANCC site at https://www.nursingworld.org/certification/our-certifications/study-aids-ce/sample-test-questions/stq-agacutecarenp/ or on the Mometrix test site at https://www.mometrix.com/academy/adult-gerontology-acute-care-nurse-practitioner-practice-test/.

Three to 6 months before graduation is when you need to create your study calendar. Make a list of body systems that need to be studied and then divide each according to the process you need to study according to the test blueprint, for example, Monday 7:00 to 9:00 p.m.: cardiac: heart failure–types of heart failure and how to diagnose and appropriate pharmacological treatment of all types of heart failure.

Six to 8 weeks before graduation consider taking another practice exam. How does this one compare with the one you took months before? Review and study those areas that need improvement.

Four weeks before graduation order three to four copies of your transcripts. Remember that official copies should be *unopened in the original envelope.*

The night before the big day it is important to have a good dinner and a good night's rest. Read and understand the instructions regarding what to do and what to bring to the testing center. Make sure that you bring the required forms of identification to the exam and any other required documents.

How to Break Down the Questions

There are different types of questions that you will encounter on your exam. If the question is in the form of multiple choice, try to change the question to a true/false form as it applies to the question. Eliminate incorrect statements immediately. Narrow the answer choices down to the best two possible answers then come up with the rationale why each one would be the correct answer.

If the words "never," "all," "always," "best," or "worst" are in the answer, then you can eliminate that answer choice because there are no absolutes in the practice of medicine.

When answering "Select all that apply" questions remember to look at each response as an individual answer and then formulate them as a true/false question like you would for a regular multiple-choice question.

Identify the concept that is being tested. Reframe, critique, and evaluate the stem of each questions. Ask yourself: "What is the question really asking?"

Read the stem slowly and carefully before looking at the answer options. Do NOT add information from you own mind. Look for the key words in the stem: "not," "except," "contraindicated," "unacceptable," and "avoid."

As you study, keep in mind that the NP certification exam is testing your ability to know the following:

- The patient is at risk for a problem. Why?
- The development of a clinical problem.
- What is the most likely clinical presentation of the condition?
- Effective interventions.
- How that intervention works.
- What is the most likely clinical outcome?
- Why this clinical problem is of significance to the overall health care system?

Licensure

After you have passed your certification exam, you will need to apply for licensure in your state. Go to your state's Board of Nursing website and search for "licensure." Read through the instructions thoroughly and then start assembling your documents. Follow the instructions precisely to delay obtaining your license. It can take up to 16 weeks to process your license.

National Provider Identifier

The NPI is an administrative simplification standard under the Health Insurance Portability and Accountability Act (HIPAA). The NPI is a unique identification number for insured health care providers. Insured service providers and all health insurance companies, and health care clearinghouses must use the NPI in administrative and financial transactions under HIPAA. The NPI is a 10-digit numeric identifier (10-digit number). This means that the numbers do not contain any other information about the health care providers, such as the state in which they live or their medical specialty. The NPI must be used in the standard HIPAA transactions in place of identifiers from older health care providers.

Health care providers can apply for NPIs in one of three ways:

- The quickest way to apply is by going online. Simply log onto the National Plan and Provider Enumeration System (NPPES) and apply online.
- Health care providers can agree to have an Electronic File Interchange (EFI) Organization (EFIO) submit application data on their behalf (i.e., through a bulk enumeration process) if an EFIO requests their permission to do so.
- Health care providers can apply by submitting a copy of the paper NPI Application/Update Form (CMS-10114) and mail the completed, signed application to the NPI Enumerator located in Fargo, North Dakota. This form is now available for download from the Centers for Medicare & Medicaid Services (CMS) website. Health care providers who require assistance with this form from the NPI Enumerator may contact the enumerator in any of these ways:
  - Phone: 1-800-465-3203 or TTY 1-800-692-2326
  - Email: customerservice@npienumerator.com
  - Mail:
    NPI Enumerator
    P.O. Box 6059
    Fargo, ND 58108-6059

U.S. Drug Enforcement Administration Number

NPs must register with the DEA and receive a DEA number to prescribe controlled medications. Some states also require their own license, which allows nurses to prescribe. This is a relatively straightforward process and can be done online. It will take 4 to 6 weeks after you have completed your online application to obtain your DEA license.

To apply for your DEA number, you will need to go to the U.S. Department of Justice Drug Enforcement Administration Diversion Control Division website and fill out the form.

Credentialing

Once you have accepted a job, a process called *credentialing* takes place. This is where your employer works with insurance companies to verify your eligibility so that your employer is paid for the services you provide to patients. You do not have to worry about that. This process is usually coordinated by your employer and only requires the NP to sign a few forms. While you do not have to manage the logistics for issuing authorizations yourself, the process can delay your start date after acceptance of a position.

I know this seems like a lot but just remember to take it step by step and before you know it, you will be a credentialed and licensed NP!

2

Cardiovascular

1. A 45-year-old man presented to the emergency department after he suffered from syncope. He has no significant history except for an upper respiratory tract infection 1 week ago. Physical exam revealed temperature 98.9°F, pulse 90 beats/min, blood pressure 100/60 mmHg, and respiratory rate 13 breaths/min. His neck veins are distended, and his heart sounds are muffled and distant. Auscultation of the lungs reveals bilateral vesicular breathing with no added sounds and chest x-ray showed small bilateral pleural effusion with enlarged cardiac silhouette. Electrocardiography was done and it showed varied QRS complex from beat to beat. Which of the following complications is obviously developing in this patient?

    1. Cardiac tamponade.

    2. Cardiomyopathy.

    3. Pulmonary embolism.

    4. Myocardial infarction.

2. Which of the following are the main components of the Beck triad in cardiac tamponade?

    1. Hypotension, electrical alternans, prominent x-descent in neck veins.

    2. Muffled heart sounds, friction rub, hypotension.

    3. Jugular venous distension, Kussmaul sign, electrical alternans.

    4. Hypotension, muffled heart sounds, jugular venous distension.

3. A 66-year-old man, known to have melanoma, presents to the emergency department with dizziness and shortness of breath for that last 3 days. On exam his blood pressure is 80/50 mmHg. He has muffled heart sounds and pedal edema. Chest x-ray revealed an enlarged cardiac silhouette. Which of the following is most likely true of his physical exam?

    1. Clear lungs with decreased jugular venous pressure (JVP).

    2. Increased JVP with inspiration.

    3. A greater than 10 mmHg drop in his systolic blood pressure with inspiration.

    4. Pericardial knock.

4. A 70-year-old woman, known to have breast cancer, presents to the emergency department with a sudden attack of syncope. On exam she is hypotensive, blood pressure (BP) is 75/50 mmHg, bilateral vesicular breathing with no added sounds are heard on auscultation of the chest, distant heart sounds, and more than 10 mmHg drop of systolic BP with inspiration. Which of the following findings is most probably seen on electrocardiogram when requested?

    1. Prolonged PR interval with dropped P-wave.

    2. Widespread ST elevation.

    3. Varied QRS complex from beat to beat.

    4. Delta wave in almost all leads.

5. All of the following physical findings could be found in cardiac tamponade, *except*:

    1. Sinus bradycardia.

    2. Sinus tachycardia.

    3. Increased jugular venous pressure.

    4. None of the above.

6. All of the following sentences are true about cardiac tamponade, *except*:

    1. Acute cardiac tamponade occurs within minutes and it can be caused by trauma.

    2. Subacute cardiac tamponade occurs within days to weeks and it can be caused by neoplasm.

    3. Beck triad (hypotension, increased jugular venous pressure, muffled heart sounds) is present in almost all patients with cardiac tamponade.

    4. Cardiomegaly associated with acute cardiac tamponade is not usually seen on a chest x-ray until 200 mL fluid accumulates in the pericardial sac.

7. Which of the following drugs is involved in cardiac tamponade formation?

    1. Corticosteroids.

    2. Ranitidine.

    3. Amiodarone.

    4. Procainamide.

8. A 69-year-old man presents to the emergency department with a sudden attack of syncope. On exam, his blood pressure is 70/45 mmHg. He has muffled heart sounds, pulsus paradoxus, and peripheral edema. The chest x-ray reveals an enlarged cardiac silhouette. He was diagnosed with lung cancer 3 years ago. Which of the following is most correct management step for this patient?

    1. Giving streptokinase immediately.

    2. Urgent catheter pericardiocentesis.

    3. Percutaneous coronary intervention within minutes.

    4. Immediate open cardiac surgery.

9. A 70-year-old man presented to the emergency department with a sudden attack of syncope after experiencing severe chest pain that radiated to his back. He described the pain as like being stabbed with a knife. He is known to have type 2 diabetes and hypertension. He has been a heavy smoker since he was young. On exam, his blood pressure is 70/40 mmHg. He has muffled heart sounds, pulsus paradoxus, and increased jugular venous pressure. Which of the following is the most correct next step for the management of this patient?

    1. Giving streptokinase immediately.

    2. Urgent catheter pericardiocentesis.

    3. Percutaneous coronary intervention within minutes.

    4. Immediate open cardiac surgery.

10. A 32-year-old male patient developed viral pericarditis 1 month ago. He was relatively asymptomatic and just complaining of mild chest pain. He was treated with ibuprofen as an outpatient. He now presents to the emergency department with new-onset dizziness and dyspnea. His blood pressure is 90/50 mmHg. He has muffled heart sounds and elevated jugular venous pressure. Which of the following statements is false?

    1. Echocardiogram is unlikely to show a thickened pericardium.

    2. He is likely to demonstrate Kussmaul sign.

    3. His electrocardiogram is likely to show reduced voltage or electrical alternans.

    4. He is likely to have a pulsus paradoxus.

11. Which of the following is the most sensitive sign in patients with cardiac tamponade?

    1. Drop in systolic blood pressure (BP) more than 10 mmHg during inspiration.

    2. Drop in systolic BP more than 20 mmHg during changing the position of the patient.

    3. Distant heart sounds.

    4. Absent radial pulse during inspiration.

12. A 72-year-old man presents to the emergency department with a sudden attack of shortness of breath and dizziness. On exam his blood pressure is 75/35 mmHg. He has distant heart sounds, pulsus paradoxus, and peripheral edema. Chest x-ray revealed an enlarged cardiac silhouette. He was diagnosed with lung cancer 5 years ago. While awaiting pericardiocentesis, what does immediate supportive care for this patient with cardiac tamponade include?

    1. Diuresis with furosemide.

    2. Nitrates to lower venous congestion.

    3. Morphine to relieve dyspnea.

    4. Intravenous fluids.

13. A 60-year-old man presents to the emergency department complaining of dyspnea and weakness over the last 3 days. He has a history of upper respiratory tract infection 3 weeks ago. His blood pressure is 87/55 mmHg and pulse is 120 beats/min. Oxygen saturation is 95% on room air. Internal jugular venous pressure is 11 cm H_2O. Lungs are clear to auscultation. Heart sounds are muffled and distant. Which of the following is the most likely cause of the patient's complaints?

    1. Decreased left ventricular preload.

    2. Decreased cardiac contractility.

    3. Increased right ventricular compliance.

    4. Absent radial pulse during inspiration.

14. A 70-year-old woman presents to the emergency department with sudden onset of syncope. She has hypertension. On exam, she is confused and agitated, blood pressure is 90/50 mmHg and heart rate is 110 beats/min. The jugular veins are distended. The lungs are clear for auscultation. An intraarterial catheter in the radial artery shows significant variation of systolic blood pressure related to the respiratory cycle. Chest x-ray shows widening of the mediastinum. Which of the following is the most likely cause of the patient's syncope?

    1. Aortic stenosis.

    2. Cardiac tachyarrhythmia.

    3. Hypovolemia.

    4. Pericardial fluid accumulation.

15. A 25-year-old male patient is brought to the emergency department after a motor vehicle accident. At the scene of the accident he was unresponsive and intubated by paramedics. His blood pressure is 70/40 mmHg and pulse is 120 beats/min. His pupils are equal and reactive to light. His neck veins are distended. There are multiple bruises involving the anterior chest and upper abdomen. His chest x-ray shows a small, left-sided pleural effusion and normal cardiac contours. Which of the following is the most likely diagnosis?

    1. Aortic rupture.

    2. Bronchial rupture.

    3. Esophageal rupture.

    4. Cardiac tamponade.

16. A 60-year-old man, with no significant past medical history presents to the office because of 4 months of dyspnea that was exertional initially but now he becomes breathless at rest. There is no chest pain, palpitations, syncope, or ankle swelling. He has been smoking a pack of cigarettes daily for the last 30 years and has been drinking alcohol heavily for the last 5 years. Temperature is 98°F, blood pressure is 113/76 mmHg, and pulse is 86 beats/min. An S3 is heard on cardiac auscultation. On chest auscultation there are bibasilar crackles. His abdomen is soft with no evidence of ascites. Chest x-ray reveals cardiac silhouette enlargement and signs of pulmonary venous congestion. Echocardiography shows a dilated left ventricle with an estimated left ventricular ejection fraction of 24%. Angiography is done with no abnormalities. Complete blood count shows macrocytic anemia, aspartate transaminase is 180 units/L, alanine transaminase is 66 units/L, and alkaline phosphatase is 44 units/L. Which of the following measures is most likely to reverse this patient's heart function?

    1. Abstinence from alcohol.

    2. Cessation of cigarette smoking.

    3. Initiation of digoxin therapy.

    4. Initiation of an angiotensin-converting enzyme inhibitor.

17. A 30-year-old woman, with no significant past medical or drug history, presents to the clinic because of progressive dyspnea 3 weeks after returning from a vacation in Texas. The dyspnea started on exertion only, but she progressed to it happening at rest. There is no chest pain, skin rash, or joint pain. There is no family history of coronary artery disease, heart failure, or sudden cardiac death. Temperature is 99.6°F, blood pressure is 110/70 mmHg, pulse is 100 beats/min, respiratory rate is 14 breaths/min. Bilateral ankle edema is present. Chest auscultation reveals bibasilar decreased breath sounds. Cardiac auscultation reveals the presence of a third heart sound. Electrocardiogram shows nonspecific ST segment changes. Which of the following is the most likely cause of this patient's symptoms?

    1. Coccidioidomycosis.

    2. Atherosclerosis.

    3. Hypothyroidism.

    4. Viral infection.

18. A 30-year-old female patient with a history of a cold 2 weeks ago presents to the emergency department with shortness of breath, fatigue, and swelling of the feet for the last several days. She has no significant past medical or surgical history. Temperature is 100.4°F, blood pressure is 110/65 mmHg, pulse is 90 beats/min, respiratory rate is 20 breaths/min. Physical exam reveals bilateral basal crackles of the lungs, bilateral pitting edema extending above the ankles, and elevated jugular venous pressure. Complete blood count shows no abnormalities. Which of the following will most likely be shown on an echocardiogram of her heart?

    1. Asymmetrical septal hypertrophy.

    2. Eccentric hypertrophy of the heart.

    3. Dilated ventricles with diffuse hypokinesia.

    4. Hypokinesia of the inferior wall.

19. A 20-year-old man is brought to the emergency department after he passed out while playing soccer. The episode lasted only 3 minutes and was not associated with postevent confusion, sleepiness, or weakness. There is no significant past medical or drug history. His grandfather died suddenly at age 39 from a heart attack. Blood pressure is 130/75 mmHg and heart rate is 67 beats/min and regular. A fourth heart sound is heard at the cardiac apex. A faint midsystolic murmur is heard along the lower left sternal border when the patient is supine. When the patient is asked to stand, a 3/6 systolic crescendo-decrescendo murmur is heard in the same location. What is the likeliest cause for this patient's presentation?

    1. Dilated cardiomyopathy.

    2. Hypertrophic cardiomyopathy.

    3. Restrictive cardiomyopathy.

    4. Myocardial infarction.

20. A 20-year-old man is brought to the emergency department after he passed out while playing soccer. The episode lasted only 3 minutes and was not associated with postevent confusion, sleepiness, or weakness. There is no significant past medical or drug history. His grandfather died suddenly at age 39 from a heart attack. Blood pressure is 130/75 mmHg and heart rate is 67 beats/min and regular. A fourth heart sound is heard at the cardiac apex. A faint midsystolic murmur is heard along the lower left sternal border when the patient is supine. When the patient is asked to stand, a 3/6 systolic crescendo-decrescendo murmur is heard in the same location. What is the mode of inheritance of the diagnosis of the scenario?

    1. Autosomal recessive.

    2. Autosomal dominant.

    3. X-linked dominant.

    4. X-linked recessive.

21. A 20-year-old man is brought to the emergency department after he passed out while playing soccer. The episode lasted only 3 minutes and was not associated with postevent confusion, sleepiness, or weakness. There is no significant past medical or drug history. His grandfather died suddenly at age 39 from a heart attack. Blood pressure is 130/75 mmHg and heart rate is 67 beats/min and regular. A fourth heart sound is heard at the cardiac apex. A faint midsystolic murmur is heard along the lower left sternal border when the patient is supine. When the patient is asked to stand, a 3/6 systolic crescendo-decrescendo murmur is heard in the same location. The patient will most likely benefit from which of the following medications?

    1. Amiodarone.

    2. Amlodipine.

    3. Atorvastatin.

    4. Metoprolol.

22. A 20-year-old man is brought to the emergency department after he passed out while playing soccer. The episode lasted only 3 minutes and was not associated with postevent confusion, sleepiness, or weakness. There is no significant past medical or drug history. His grandfather died suddenly at age 39 from a heart attack. Blood pressure is 130/75 mmHg and heart rate is 67 beats/min and regular. A fourth heart sound is heard at the cardiac apex. A faint midsystolic murmur is heard along the lower left sternal border when the patient is supine. When the patient is asked to stand, a 3/6 systolic crescendo-decrescendo murmur is heard in the same location. Which of the following is the most likely mitral valve abnormality in this patient?

    1. Rupture of chordae tendineae.

    2. Dilated mitral valve annulus.

    3. Mitral annulus calcifications.

    4. Prolapse of the mitral valve leaflet.

23. A 20-year-old man is brought to the emergency department after he passed out while playing soccer. The episode lasted only 3 minutes and was not associated with postevent confusion, sleepiness, or weakness. There is no significant past medical or drug history. His grandfather died suddenly at age 39 from a heart attack. Blood pressure is 130/75 mmHg and heart rate is 67 beats/min and regular. A fourth heart sound is heard at the cardiac apex. A faint midsystolic murmur is heard along the lower left sternal border when the patient is supine. When the patient is asked to stand, a 3/6 systolic crescendo-decrescendo murmur is heard in the same location. Which of the following maneuvers would increase the intensity of the murmur?

    1. Standing.

    2. Valsalva maneuver.

    3. Handgrip exercise.

    4. Standing and Valsalva maneuver.

24. A 69-year-old woman comes to the clinic because of progressive lower limb edema over the last 8 weeks. She becomes tried and short of breath with daily activities. Her stomach feels full and her appetite has been decreased. Blood pressure is 140/75 mmHg and pulse is 70 beats/min and regular. Jugular veins are distended. No heart murmurs are present. Breath sounds are decreased bilaterally at the bases of the lungs. The abdomen is distended with flank dullness on percussion. There is +3 peripheral edema. Urine protein excretion is 1 g/24 h. Echocardiogram reveals left atrial enlargement, marked concentric left ventricular hypertrophy, and left ventricular ejection fraction of 70%. Hemoglobin is 11.2 g/dL and electrolyte panel is within normal range. Which of the following is the most likely cause for this patient's presentation?

    1. Dilated cardiomyopathy.

    2. Hypertrophic cardiomyopathy.

    3. Restrictive cardiomyopathy.

    4. Myocardial infarction.

25. A 17-year-old man was brought to the emergency department after a syncopal episode while playing basketball. His older brother had experienced a similar event 3 years ago. Which of the following is the physical exam most likely to reveal?

    1. Rapid carotid upstroke.

    2. Outflow murmur that increases with the Valsalva maneuver.

    3. Delayed carotid upstroke.

    4. A and B.

26. Which of the following maneuvers will enhance the murmur of hypertrophic cardiomyopathy?

    1. Valsalva maneuver.

    2. Leaning forward while sitting.

    3. Squatting.

    4. Hand grip.

27. A 40-year-old man with a strong family history of dilated cardiomyopathy presents to the clinic with shortness of breath, pulmonary crackles, distended jugular veins, finger clubbing, and peripheral edema. An S3 is heard on cardiac auscultation. Which of the following investigations would not be useful in dilated cardiomyopathy?

    1. Chest x-ray.

    2. Electrocardiogram.

    3. Echocardiography.

    4. Biopsy.

28. A 55-year-old man, with no significant past medical or drug history, is admitted to the hospital with a 6-week history of fatigue, lower limb edema, and dyspnea on exertion. He has had occasional palpitations for months but no chest pain. Blood pressure is 150/90 mmHg and pulse is 130 beats/min and irregular. Lungs are clear on auscultation. Electrocardiogram does not show clear P-waves. Echocardiography shows an ejection fraction of 35% and left atrial and left ventricular dilatation with global hypokinesia. Which of the following interventions is most likely to restore left ventricular function in this patient?

    1. Inotropic medications.

    2. Decreasing afterload.

    3. Coronary revascularization.

    4. Preload optimization.

29. Which of the following trace elements is implicated as a cause of cardiomyopathy when it is deficient?

    1. Zinc.

    2. Selenium.

    3. Copper.

    4. Iron.

30. Which main feature of hypertrophic cardiomyopathy is responsible for its signs and symptoms?

    1. Asymmetrical septal hypertrophy.

    2. Symmetrical septal hypertrophy.

    3. Left ventricular wall hypertrophy.

    4. Right ventricular wall hypertrophy.

31. A 22-year-old man with hypertrophic cardiomyopathy presents to the clinic with complaints of being dizzy but has not had syncopal episodes. Which of the following would indicate an increased risk of sudden cardiac death if present in this patient?

    1. Systolic anterior movement of the mitral valve on echocardiography.

    2. Worsening exertional angina.

    3. Left ventricular outflow tract gradient of 80 mmHg.

    4. Significant blood pressure drop during exercise.

32. A 25-year-old woman, with no significant past medical or drug history, has worsening fatigue with dyspnea, palpitations, chest pain, and fever over the last few days. Temperature is 102°F, respiratory rate is 30 breaths/min, pulse is 105 beats/min, and blood pressure is 95/65 mmHg. Heart rate is irregular. Electrocardiogram shows diffuse ST-T segment changes. Chest x-ray shows mild cardiomegaly. Slight mitral and tricuspid regurgitation is shown on echocardiography, but there are no valvular vegetations. Her troponin I is 12 ng/mL (normal is less than 0.04). She recovers over the next 2 weeks with no apparent sequels. If the patient's condition deteriorates and does not improve, she will most likely develop:

    1. Hypertrophic cardiomyopathy.

    2. Dilated cardiomyopathy.

    3. Infective endocarditis.

    4. Restrictive cardiomyopathy.

33. A 25-year-old woman, with no significant past medical or drug history, has worsening fatigue with dyspnea, palpitations, chest pain, and fever over the last few days. Temperature is 102°F, respiratory rate is 30 breaths/min, pulse is 105 beats/min, and blood pressure is 95/65 mmHg. Heart rate is irregular. Electrocardiogram shows diffuse ST-T segment changes. Chest x-ray shows mild cardiomegaly. Slight mitral and tricuspid regurgitation is shown on echocardiography, but there are no valvular vegetations. Her troponin I is 12 ng/mL (normal is less than 0.04). She recovers over the next 2 weeks with no apparent sequels. Which of the following laboratory test findings best explains the underlying etiology for these events?

    1. Antistreptolysin O titer of 1:512.

    2. Coxsackie B serological titer of 1:160.

    3. Sodium electrolyte level about 150 mEq/L.

    4. Blood culture positive for streptococcus, viridans group.

34. A 40-year-old man with no past medical history other than arthritis presents with complaints of worsening orthopnea and ankle edema over the past 6 months. He denies chest pain. Chest x-ray shows cardiomegaly with both enlarged left and right heart borders with pulmonary edema. Electrolyte and chemistry panels are normal except for hyperglycemia. Which of the following further investigations would you request for this patient?

    1. Anticyclic citrullinated peptide antibody level.

    2. Antinuclear antibody test level.

    3. Ferritin level.

    4. Antimitochondrial antibody level.

35. Which of the following hereditary diseases causes reversible dilated cardiomyopathy?

    1. Wilson disease.

    2. Alpha-1 antitrypsin deficiency.

    3. Hereditary hemochromatosis.

    4. Gilbert disease.

36. A 55-year-old woman comes to the clinic with dyspnea over the last few months. She has received trastuzumab and doxorubicin for breast cancer and completed her course of chemotherapy a few months earlier. Blood pressure is 120/80 mmHg and pulse is 90 beats/min and regular. Bilateral pitting peripheral edema is present on exam of lower limbs and crackles are heard at the bases on auscultation of the lungs. Which of the following is the most likely cause for her cardiac failure?

    1. Ischemic cardiomyopathy.

    2. Dilated cardiomyopathy.

    3. Pleural effusion.

    4. Multiple pulmonary embolism.

37. A 66-year-old alcoholic man had an enlarging abdomen for several months. There is no abdominal pain or chest pain. He has a nontender abdomen with no palpable mass, but there is a fluid thrill. Abdominal ultrasound shows large abdominal fluid collection with a small cirrhotic liver. Chest x-ray shows a globally enlarged heart. S3 sound is heard on cardiac auscultation. Which of the following conditions is most likely to be present?

    1. Nonbacterial thrombotic endocarditis.

    2. Dilated cardiomyopathy.

    3. Lymphocytic myocarditis.

    4. Myocardial amyloid deposition.

38. On physical exam, a 40-year-old male patient is found to have a jerky pulse. Which of the following conditions is associated with a jerky pulse?

    1. Hypertrophic cardiomyopathy.

    2. Dilated cardiomyopathy.

    3. Aortic stenosis.

    4. Cardiac tamponade.

39. A 38-year-old male patient attends a consultation after his brother is diagnosed with a familial hypertrophic cardiomyopathy. What is the best screening method for familial hypertrophic cardiomyopathy?

    1. Genetic testing.

    2. Exercise electrocardiogram.

    3. Transthoracic echocardiogram.

    4. Transesophageal echocardiogram.

40. A 30-year-old man who is known to have hypertrophic cardiomyopathy has an out-of-hospital cardiac arrest. Fortunately, he is successfully resuscitated. What is the most appropriate next step in the management of this patient?

    1. Beta-blocker.

    2. Calcium channel blocker.

    3. Amiodarone.

    4. Implantable defibrillator.

41. What is the most common electrocardiogram (ECG) abnormality in patients with pulmonary embolism?

    1. Sinus arrhythmia.

    2. Sinus bradycardia.

    3. Sinus tachycardia.

    4. Normal ECG.

42. All of the following sentences are true about second-degree heart block Mobitz II, *except*:

    1. PR interval is usually normal in duration and fixed in length.

    2. The duration of prolongation is fixed if the PR interval is prolonged.

    3. Blocked beats occur suddenly without progressive lengthening of the PR interval.

    4. Atropine is used as first-line management because it increases atrioventricular conduction.

43. What is the most common cause of third-degree heart block in adults?

    1. Myocardial infarction.

    2. Infectious causes.

    3. Ankylosing spondylitis.

    4. Simple fibrous degenerative changes.

44. All of the following are true about multifocal atrial tachycardia, *except*:

    1. Characterized by regular supraventricular rhythm at rates 100 to 200 beats/min.

    2. At least three different P-wave forms that vary from beat to beat, as does the PR interval.

    3. Generally seen in elderly patients or those with chronic lung disease who are experiencing respiratory failure.

    4. Beta-blockers are the preferred drug for treatment.

45. A 55-year-old patient presents to the clinic after recent hospitalization of congestive heart failure. He has no known lung disease. The patient inquires about the results of his pulmonary function that was preformed recently. The testing was most likely done before the initiation of which of the following drugs?

    1. Metoprolol.

    2. Nitroglycerin.

    3. Digoxin.

    4. Amiodarone.

46. A 70-year-old man with controlled type 2 diabetes mellitus and hypertension maintained on lisinopril and hydrochlorothiazide presents to the clinic for generalized malaise and palpitations for the last 3 weeks. Last year, an echocardiogram for the patient showed mild atrial dilation and left ventricular hypertrophy. Electrocardiogram is done and it illustrates an irregularly irregular pulse with narrow-complex tachycardia and no organized P-waves. Which of the following is the most appropriate next step in the management of this patient?

    1. Adenosine.

    2. Cardioversion.

    3. Diltiazem.

    4. Lidocaine.

47. A 70-year-old man with controlled type 2 diabetes mellitus and hypertension maintained on lisinopril and hydrochlorothiazide presents to the clinic for generalized malaise and palpitations for the last 3 weeks. Last year, an echocardiogram for the patient showed mild atrial dilation and left ventricular hypertrophy. Electrocardiogram is done and it illustrates an irregularly irregular pulse with narrow-complex tachycardia and no organized P-waves. What should the patient receive to prevent systemic embolization?

    1. Aspirin.

    2. Aspirin or warfarin.

    3. Warfarin.

    4. No need for any medication to prevent systemic embolization.

48. A 40-year-old man presents to the clinic with palpitations. An electrocardiogram is done and shows supraventricular tachycardia. Blood pressure is 125/80 mmHg. Which of the following is the best next step in the management of this patient?

    1. Carotid massage and adenosine.

    2. Cardioversion and epinephrine.

    3. Carotid sinus massage and metoprolol.

    4. Lidocaine only is enough for this patient.

49. Adenosine is the novel drug for which of the following abnormal electrocardiogram rhythms?

    1. Multifocal atrial tachycardia.

    2. Supraventricular tachycardia.

    3. Third-degree atrioventricular block.

    4. Atrial flutter.

50. Which of the following cases of atrial fibrillation needs an oral anticoagulant?

    1. 60-year-old male patient with hypertension and colon cancer.

    2. 55-year-old female patient with breast cancer and rheumatoid arthritis.

    3. 68-year-old female patient with ovarian cancer and diabetes mellitus.

    4. 62-year-old male patient with diabetes mellitus and lung cancer.

51. In a patient with atrial fibrillation, which of the following has the highest risk for systemic embolization?

    1. Female gender.

    2. Age greater than 75 years.

    3. Hypertension.

    4. Congestive heart failure.

52. Patients with atrial fibrillation will not need digoxin for their treatment, unless they have:

    1. Hypertension.

    2. Diabetes mellitus.

    3. Vascular disease.

    4. Congestive heart failure.

53. A 45-year-old athlete presents to the clinic for routine workup. An electrocardiogram is done and shows normal and evenly spaced ventricular complexes. The heart rate is 55 beats/min. He is generally well and does not have any complaints. Blood pressure is 120/80 mmHg and temperature is 98.6°F. Which of the following is the best next step in the management of this patient?

    1. Carotid massage and adenosine.

    2. Atropine with pacing.

    3. Pacing directly and right now.

    4. There is nothing to do for this patient.

54. A 72-year-old man with a medical history of hypertension, coronary artery disease, and aortic stenosis undergoes coronary artery bypass surgery and aortic valve replacement surgery. The surgery is uncomplicated, and the patient is extubated and transferred to the step-down unit on postoperative day 2. That evening, he suddenly experiences chest tightness, weakness, and shortness of breath. Blood pressure is 60/30 mmHg, pulse is 155 beats/min, and respiratory rate is 30 breaths/min. Bilateral basal crackles are heard on lung auscultation. The electrocardiogram rhythm was irregularly irregular with absent P-waves. Which of the following is the best next step in the management of this patient?

    1. Direct current cardioversion.

    2. Percutaneous transcutaneous pacing.

    3. Metoprolol.

    4. Diltiazem.

55. A 55-year-old male patient with a 5-week history of fatigue, dyspnea on exertion, and decreased exercise tolerance is admitted to the hospital. He has had occasional palpitations for 2 months. He has no significant past medical or drug history. He usually drinks alcohol in moderate amounts, but he had two binge-drinking episodes last month. Blood pressure is 140/90 mmHg and pulse is 130 beats/min and irregular. Chest auscultation is clear. Electrocardiogram shows an irregularly irregular rhythm with absent P-waves. Echocardiogram shows an ejection fraction of 35%, moderate central mitral regurgitation, and left atrial and left ventricular dilation with global hypokinesis. Which of the following interventions is most likely to restore left ventricular function in this patient?

    1. Rate or rhythm control.

    2. Decreasing afterload.

    3. Preload optimization.

    4. Valve surgery.

56. An 80-year-old man with progressively worsening fatigue, decreased exercise tolerance, and lower limb edema over the last 4 months presents to the clinic. No history of cough or chest pain. He has diabetes and hypertension controlled with metformin and lisinopril. He has a 50 pack-year smoking history. Blood pressure is 135/85 mmHg and pulse is 130 beats/min and irregularly irregular. Complete blood count and electrolytes are within normal range. Lung auscultation reveals bilateral basal crepitation. Electrocardiogram shows absent P-waves with an irregularly irregular rhythm. Ejection fraction is 30% on echocardiogram. What is the CHADS2 score for this patient?

    1. 4.

    2. 3.

    3. 2.

    4. 1.

57. An 80-year-old man with progressively worsening fatigue, decreased exercise tolerance, and lower limb edema over the last 4 months presents to the clinic. No history of cough or chest pain. He has diabetes and hypertension controlled with metformin and lisinopril. He has a 50 pack-year smoking history. Blood pressure is 135/85 mmHg and pulse is 130 beats/min and irregularly irregular. Complete blood count and electrolytes are within normal range. Lung auscultation reveals bilateral basal crepitation. Electrocardiogram shows absent P-waves with an irregularly irregular rhythm. Ejection fraction is 30% on echocardiogram. What is the most likely cause for systolic dysfunction in this patient?

    1. Atrial flutter.

    2. Supraventricular tachycardia.

    3. Atrial fibrillation.

    4. Valve surgery.

58. An 80-year-old man with progressively worsening fatigue, decreased exercise tolerance, and lower limb edema over the last 4 months presents to the clinic. No history of cough or chest pain. He has diabetes and hypertension controlled with metformin and lisinopril. He has a 50 pack-year smoking history. Blood pressure is 135/85 mmHg and pulse is 130 beats/min and irregularly irregular. Complete blood count and electrolytes are within normal range. Lung auscultation reveals bilateral basal crepitation. Electrocardiogram shows absent P-waves with an irregularly irregular rhythm. Ejection fraction is 30% on echocardiogram. Which of the following is the best treatment to prevent long-term complications in this patient?

    1. Amiodarone.

    2. Warfarin.

    3. Spironolactone.

    4. Hydrochlorothiazide.

59. An 80-year-old man with progressively worsening fatigue, decreased exercise tolerance, and lower limb edema over the last 4 months presents to the clinic. No history of cough or chest pain. He has diabetes and hypertension controlled with metformin and lisinopril. He has a 50 pack-year smoking history. Blood pressure is 135/85 mmHg and pulse is 130 beats/min and irregularly irregular. Complete blood count and electrolytes are within normal range. Lung auscultation reveals bilateral basal crepitation. Electrocardiogram shows absent P-waves with an irregularly irregular rhythm. Ejection fraction is 30% on echocardiogram. Which of the following treatments is the best to normalize left ventricular dysfunction in this patient?

    1. Rate or rhythm control.

    2. Decreasing afterload.

    3. Preload optimization.

    4. Open cardiac surgery.

60. An 80-year-old man with progressively worsening fatigue, decreased exercise tolerance, and lower limb edema over the last 4 months presents to the clinic. No history of cough or chest pain. He has diabetes and hypertension controlled with metformin and lisinopril. He has a 50 pack-year smoking history. Blood pressure is 135/85 mmHg and pulse is 130 beats/min and irregularly irregular. Complete blood count and electrolytes are within normal range. Lung auscultation reveals bilateral basal crepitation. Electrocardiogram shows absent P-waves with an irregularly irregular rhythm. Ejection fraction is 30% on echocardiogram. Which of the following part of this patient's history has the strongest effect on systemic embolization?

    1. History of hypertension.

    2. History of diabetes mellitus.

    3. Age.

    4. Congestive heart failure.

61. A 50-year-old male patient with no significant medical history comes to the clinic for follow-up. He went to the emergency department 3 weeks ago complaining of palpitations. He was found to have atrial fibrillation with rapid ventricular response, but he spontaneously converted to normal sinus rhythm overnight and was discharged home the next day. He does not use tobacco or alcohol. Blood pressure is 130/70 mmHg and pulse is 80 beats/min and regular. Jugular venous pressure is estimated at 5 cm H_2O. No abnormalities are found on physical exam and laboratory investigations. Echocardiogram shows mildly dilated left atrium, normal left and right ventricular function, and no valvular abnormalities. What is the best treatment for this patient?

    1. Aspirin and warfarin.

    2. Aspirin and clopidogrel.

    3. Amiodarone.

    4. No additional dug is needed.

62. A 50-year-old man with no past medical or drug history comes to the emergency department complaining of weakness and palpitations on and off over the last 24 hours. He does not use tobacco or alcohol. His mother has myasthenia gravis and the patient's father had a myocardial infarction at age 68. An electrocardiogram is performed and shows irregularly irregular rhythm with absent P-waves. The patient should be evaluated for which of the following?

    1. Cushing syndrome.

    2. Hyperthyroidism.

    3. Aortic dissection.

    4. Polycystic kidney disease.

63. Which of the following conditions is the most common risk factor and associated condition for atrial fibrillation?

    1. Congestive heart failure.

    2. Hyperthyroidism.

    3. Hypertension.

    4. Polycystic kidney disease.

64. A 70-year-old man has a sudden attack of syncope. He came to the emergency department because he injured his forehead when he collapsed. An electrocardiogram is done and shows sinus rhythm with a heart rate of 60 beats/min. Three-blocked P-waves are observed and the PR interval appears constant on all other beats. He remains asymptomatic in the hospital. Which of the following is the most appropriate next step in the management of this patient?

    1. Refer for electrophysiological study.

    2. Refer for pacemaker implantation.

    3. Discharge to home after 24 hours of monitoring.

    4. Adenosine.

65. A 75-year-old patient is brought to the emergency department after a sudden attack of syncope. She has a history of breast cancer, hypertension, and diabetes. An electrocardiogram is done and shows the loss of relationship between P-waves and QRS complexes (complete dissociation). After stabilizing the patient, what is the best next step of management?

    1. Refer for electrophysiological study.

    2. Refer for pacemaker implantation.

    3. Discharge to home after 24 hours of monitoring.

    4. Adenosine.

66. Which of the following antiarrhythmic drugs is known to cause hypothyroidism and hyperthyroidism?

    1. Procainamide.

    2. Amiodarone.

    3. Lidocaine.

    4. Flecainide.

67. A 55-year-old male patient comes to the clinic for follow-up. He has a history of hypertension and diabetes mellitus. He complains of constipation for 1 week. On exam, his blood pressure is 130/80 mmHg, temperature is 98.6°F, respiratory rate is 13 breaths/min, SaO_2 is 97%, and there is bilateral lower limb edema. Which of the following medications is most likely the cause for this patient complaint?

    1. Procainamide.

    2. Amiodarone.

    3. Amlodipine.

    4. Lidocaine.

68. Which of the following antiarrhythmic medications can cause a lupus-like syndrome?

    1. Procainamide.

    2. Metoprolol.

    3. Amlodipine.

    4. Lidocaine.

69. Which of the following medications can cause heart block if administered via rapid intravenous push?

    1. Metoprolol.

    2. Phenytoin.

    3. Amiodarone.

    4. Lidocaine.

70. Which of the following antiarrhythmic medications can cause heart block, hypoglycemia, hypotension, asthma, lethargy, impotence, and hyperkalemia?

    1. Procainamide.

    2. Beta-blockers.

    3. Calcium channel blockers.

    4. Amiodarone.

71. A 70-year-old man comes to the clinic complaining of heart palpitations for the last 3 weeks. He has a history of hypertension, type 2 diabetes mellitus, and coronary artery disease. Irregularly irregular pulse is present during physical exam and electrocardiogram. Which of the following anatomic sites is the most likely origin for this patient's arrhythmia?

    1. Atrioventricular node.

    2. Pulmonary veins.

    3. Sinoatrial node.

    4. Tricuspid annulus.

72. A 38-year-old man comes to the clinic for routine checkup of premature atrial complexes found on electrocardiogram. He has had no chest pain, shortness of breath, or lightheadedness. He has smoked 2 packs of cigarettes daily and consumed one to two beers a day for the last 15 years. His mother had a history of myocardial infarction at age 66, and his father had a history of stroke at age 72. Vital signs are normal. What is the best next step in the management of this patient?

    1. Order 24-hour Holter monitoring.

    2. Stop alcohol and tobacco.

    3. Perform transthoracic echocardiogram.

    4. Start beta-blocker therapy.

73. An 80-year-old male patient with a history of hypertension, stable coronary artery disease, hyperlipidemia, and type 2 diabetes mellitus is brought to the emergency department after a brief episode of syncope. Since yesterday he is lightheaded and fatigued. There is no chest pain or palpitations. Blood pressure is 80/40 mmHg. He appears mildly confused but answers questions correctly. Chest auscultation is clear and electrocardiogram shows sinus bradycardia. Which of the following is the best next step in the management of this patient?

    1. Adenosine.

    2. Amiodarone.

    3. Atropine.

    4. Glucagon.

74. A 45-year-old male patient comes to the clinic after suffering from left-sided chest pain for 1 day. The pain was sudden in its onset, constant in its character, and increases with left hand movement. There is no nausea, dyspnea, or diaphoresis. He has a 25 pack-year smoking history. Vital signs are normal. On exam, there is tenderness on palpation of the left-sided chest wall muscles. Electrocardiogram shows a normal sinus rhythm of 90 beats/min and QRS complexes are normal. PR interval is constant with a duration of 280 ms. There is no significant ST segment or T-wave abnormality. What is the best next step in treatment?

    1. Electrophysiological study.

    2. Observation.

    3. Permanent pacemaker.

    4. Vagal maneuver.

75. A 26-year-old male patient is brought to the emergency department after he suddenly starts to suffer from dizziness and palpitations. He has had similar episodes provoked by stressful life events and fatigue. He usually stops these similar episodes by squatting and taking a deep breath, but these actions did not help him during this attack. Blood pressure is 65/40 mmHg and pulse is 240 beats/min. He is diaphoretic and his extremities are cold. Electrocardiogram shows a regular, narrow-complex tachycardia. What is the best next step in the management of this patient?

    1. Synchronized cardioversion.

    2. Unsynchronized cardioversion.

    3. Intravenous (IV) procainamide.

    4. IV amiodarone.

76. A 70-year-old woman comes to the emergency department because of intermittent chest pain for the last 3 days. There is no cough or wheeze, but there is shortness of breath. She describes the pain as chest pressure. No history of past similar attacks. She has a history of hypertension and hyperlipidemia. No heart murmurs are present on exam. Electrocardiogram shows normal sinus rhythm with T-wave inversion in leads V4 to V6. Initial troponin I is undetectable. Three hours after the initial evaluation, she becomes unresponsive. Her telemetry strip shows ventricular fibrillation. Which of the following is the most appropriate next step in the management of this patient?

    1. Synchronized cardioversion.

    2. Unsynchronized cardioversion.

    3. Intravenous (IV) procainamide.

    4. IV amiodarone.

77. A special form of polymorphic ventricular tachycardia (PVT) is called torsade de pointes. It occurs in the setting of a congenital or acquired prolonged QT interval. What is the first line of management for this special form of PVT in stable patients?

    1. Synchronized cardioversion.

    2. Unsynchronized cardioversion.

    3. Intravenous (IV) magnesium.

    4. IV amiodarone.

78. A 36-year-old male patient, a known case of Wolff-Parkinson-White syndrome, presents to the emergency department with palpitations for the last 3 hours. There is no associated chest pain, shortness of breath, or dizziness. He has a history of three prior episodes of supraventricular tachycardia. No history of drug intake, but he drinks alcohol occasionally. He had four cans of beer at a party the previous night. Blood pressure is 120/80 mmHg and pulse is irregular. What is the best next step in the management of this patient?

    1. Synchronized cardioversion.

    2. Unsynchronized cardioversion.

    3. Intravenous (IV) procainamide.

    4. IV amiodarone.

79. A 36-year-old male patient, a known case of Wolff-Parkinson-White syndrome, presents to the emergency department with palpitations for the last 3 hours. There is no associated chest pain, shortness of breath, or dizziness. He has a history of three prior episodes of supraventricular tachycardia. No history of drug intake, but he drinks alcohol occasionally. He had four cans of beer at a party the previous night. Blood pressure is 120/80 mmHg and pulse is irregularly irregular. If the blood pressure is 70/30 mmHg and the patient presents with syncope, what is the best next step in the management of this patient?

    1. Synchronized cardioversion.

    2. Unsynchronized cardioversion.

    3. Intravenous (IV) procainamide.

    4. IV amiodarone.

80. A 36-year-old male patient, a known case of Wolff-Parkinson-White syndrome, presents to the emergency department with palpitations for the last 3 hours. There is no associated chest pain, shortness of breath, or dizziness. He has a history of three prior episodes of supraventricular tachycardia. No history of drug intake, but he drinks alcohol occasionally. He had four cans of beer at a party the previous night. Blood pressure is 120/80 mmHg and pulse is irregularly irregular. What is the main pathophysiology of palpitations in this patient?

    1. Accessory pathway.

    2. Atrioventricular block.

    3. Sinoatrial block.

    4. Left bundle branch block.

81. A 66-year-old female patient with a known history of hypertension was admitted yesterday to the coronary care unit because of repetitive chest pain, which was diagnosed as stable angina. On discharge, the cardiologist prescribes nitroglycerin to take when the pain happens. How does this drug cause pain relief?

    1. Increases heart contractility.

    2. Decreases coronary blood flow.

    3. Dilates systemic veins.

    4. Increases ventricular afterload.

82. A 60-year-old female patient presents to the outpatient clinic because of bilateral leg swelling, which started 1 month ago. The patient also complains of dyspnea and orthopnea. Six months ago, the patient was admitted with an inferior myocardial infarction and was discharged on aspirin, atorvastatin, and Plavix. Which of the following investigations can diagnose the cause of patient's symptoms?

    1. Abdominal computed tomography scan.

    2. Echocardiography.

    3. Urinalysis.

    4. Abdominal ultrasound.

83. A 50-year-old male patient recently diagnosed with hypertension had a blood pressure average over the last 2 weeks of 150/95 mmHg. His body mass index is 35 kg/m^2, he is a smoker, and he drinks five glasses of alcohol daily. What is the first step of his management?

    1. Lifestyle modifications.

    2. Bisoprolol.

    3. Enalapril.

    4. Amlodipine.

84. A 60-year-old female patient comes to the emergency department complaining of retrosternal chest pain, which radiated to the left arm and neck. In addition, the patient complains of shortness of breath. These symptoms started only half an hour ago. Electrocardiogram showed ST elevation in leads II and III. She is given 325 mg of aspirin and 80 mg of atorvastatin. What is the next step in the management in this patient?

    1. Digoxin.

    2. Normal saline.

    3. Clopidogrel.

    4. Amlodipine.

85. A 40-year-old male patient with no remarkable past history comes to the outpatient clinic for evaluation of high blood pressure. His blood pressure last week was around 160/95 mmHg. The patient had no complaints, does not take any drugs, and does not smoke or drink. He has a family history of hypertension. His physical exam was normal. In addition to a complete blood count and chemistry panel, what else should be done?

    1. Abdominal ultrasound.

    2. Thyroid stimulating hormone.

    3. 24-hour collection urine.

    4. Electrocardiogram.

86. A 66-year-old male patient presented to the emergency department with retrosternal chest pain that started 1 hour ago. The pain radiated to the left arm, left jaw, and was associated with severe shortness of breath and diaphoresis. On physical exam, the patient's blood pressure is 80/50 mmHg, pulse is 40 beats/min, and respiratory rate is 14 breaths/min. Lung auscultation reveals bilateral crackles. Electrocardiogram shows ST elevation in the inferior leads. Which of the following drugs is contraindicated in this patient?

    1. Furosemide.

    2. Metoprolol.

    3. Amlodipine.

    4. Verapamil.

87. A 50-year-old African American male patient with newly diagnosed hypertension, which is uncontrolled, presented to the clinic for evaluation. His blood pressure is 155/95 mmHg. What is the drug of choice for this patient?

    1. Bisoprolol.

    2. Verapamil.

    3. Furosemide.

    4. Spironolactone.

88. A 25-year-old male patient presented to the emergency department with complaints of stabbing pain in his chest. On physical exam, blood pressure is 90/45 mmHg, pulse is 140 beats/min with distended jugular vein, and there are muffled heart sounds. After stabilizing the patient, what is the next step in his management?

    1. Electrocardiogram.

    2. High-resolution computed tomography scan.

    3. Echocardiography.

    4. Chest tube.

89. A 50-year-old male patient with a history of type 2 diabetes mellitus, taking metformin, presented to the emergency department after a feeling of crushing retrosternal chest pain began 50 minutes ago and radiated to his left arm. The patient is complaining of diaphoresis and nausea. On physical exam, his blood pressure is 80/50 mmHg and pulse is 50 beats/min. The chest exam is clear. Electrocardiogram showed ST elevation in the inferior leads. What is the next step in management?

    1. Furosemide.

    2. Heparin.

    3. Fluid.

    4. Metoprolol.

90. A 60-year-old female patient with a history of hypertension presents to the emergency department with retrosternal chest pain, which started 1 hour ago. The pain radiates to her left arm and jaw. On physical exam, her blood pressure is 110/80 mmHg, pulse is 120 beats/minute, and the chest is clear. Electrocardiogram shows Q wave in the inferior leads with no ST elevation. What is the next step of management?

    1. Heparin.

    2. Furosemide.

    3. Thrombolysis.

    4. Digoxin.

91. A 40-year-old male patient who smokes a half-pack of cigarettes a day for the last 10 years presents for a routine checkup. The patient drinks one glass of wine every day. He works as a programmer, and his body mass index is 32 kg/m². On physical exam, his blood pressure is 145/95 mmHg and his pulse is 90 beats/min. Which of the following has a significant effect on reducing his blood pressure?

    1. Exercise 30 minutes every week.

    2. Weight loss.

    3. Stop smoking.

    4. Stop drinking.

92. A 60-year-old female patient suffered from a right-sided headache and decrease of visual field in the right eye and jaw claudication. Which of the following investigations can be used to discover the complications of this patient's disease?

    1. Abdominal computed tomography scan.

    2. Colonoscopy.

    3. Doppler ultrasound.

    4. Serial chest x-ray.

93. A 50-year-old male patient complains of recurrent chest pain that radiates to the left arm. It happens mainly during heavy lifting and lasts for 10 minutes then improves. He has no history of dyspnea or cough. He has a history of hypertension. On physical exam, his blood pressure is 120/80 mmHg and pulse is 80 beats/min. Heart and lung exams are normal. Electrocardiogram (ECG) is normal. What is the next step in management?

    1. Echocardiogram.

    2. Chest x-ray.

    3. Exercise ECG.

    4. Abdominal computed tomography scan.

94. A 60-year-old male patient with newly diagnosed hypertension was started on enalapril 3 weeks ago. Now the patient complains of dry cough, which started a couple of weeks. The patient denied any history of upper respiratory tract infection, fever, dyspnea, or weight loss. On physical exam, his blood pressure is 130/80 mmHg, pulse is 80 beats/min, and his chest was clear. What is your next step in management?

    1. High-resolution chest computed tomography scan.

    2. Stop enalapril and switch to valsartan.

    3. Start antibiotics.

    4. Start omeprazole.

95. A 50-year-old female patient has an anterior myocardial infarction that is complicated by heart failure. In which of the following circumstances can nitroglycerin be given and be effective as a first medication?

    1. Patient with clear lungs and blood pressure of 120/80 mmHg.

    2. Patient with bibasilar crackles and blood pressure of 90/40 mmHg.

    3. Patient with clear lungs and blood pressure of 90/50 mmHg.

    4. Patient with bibasilar crackles and blood pressure of 130/85 mmHg.

96. A 50-year-old male patient presents to the clinic for his routine follow-up. His nurse practitioner orders a serum lipid profile. Which of the following results is associated with an increased risk of coronary artery disease?

    1. High-density lipoprotein (HDL) is 30 and total cholesterol is 300.

    2. HDL is 50 and total cholesterol is 200.

    3. HDL is 60 and total cholesterol is 250.

    4. HDL is 45 and total cholesterol is 140.

97. A 17-year-old male patient presented to the outpatient clinic with complaints of a chronic headache. The patient denies any history of blurred vision, fever, or vomiting. On exam, blood pressure is 150/95 mmHg. Pulse is 120 beats/minute in both arms, but it is weak in the femoral arteries. Cardiac auscultation revealed continuous murmur. What is your next step in management?

    1. Electrocardiogram.

    2. Urinalysis.

    3. Brain computed tomography.

    4. Echocardiograph.

98. A 15-year-old male patient presented to the outpatient clinic with newly discovered hypertension. He complains of a chronic headache. The patient denied any history of blurred vision, fever, or vomiting. On exam, his blood pressure is 150/95 mmHg. Pulse 120 beats/minute in both arms, but it is weak in the femoral arteries. Cardiac auscultation revealed continuous murmur. What is your diagnosis?

    1. Coarctation of aorta.

    2. Primary hypertension.

    3. Cushing syndrome.

    4. Hyperaldosteronism.

99. An 80-year-old male patient with long-standing hypertension for 40 years visits the clinic for routine follow-up. His chest x-ray revealed cardiomegaly. Which of the following findings can be present on the electrocardiogram and support your diagnosis?

    1. ST elevation in whole leads.

    2. Right axis deviation.

    3. High QRS voltage in V5 and V6.

    4. Prolonged QT interval.

100. A 70-year-old male patient with long-standing hypertension for 25 years visits the clinic for routine follow-up. His chest x-ray revealed cardiomegaly, Electrocardiogram shows left axis deviation with high-voltage QRS. What is your diagnosis?

    1. Left ventricular hypertrophy.

    2. Dilated cardiomyopathy.

    3. Calcified aortic stenosis.

    4. Aortic root dilatation.

101. A 51-year-old male patient with a known history of uncontrolled hypertension, presented to the emergency department after complaining of a headache. He denied any history of vomiting, loss of consciousness, or any muscle weakness. On physical exam, his blood pressure is 220/120 mmHg, pulse is 120 beats/min, and chest and heart exam are clear. Funduscopic exam was done. Which of the following funduscopic results may be present in this patient?

    1. Retinal detachment.

    2. Optic atrophy.

    3. Cotton wool spot.

    4. Retinitis obliterans.

102. A 60-year-old female patient with type 2 diabetes mellitus and dyslipidemia presented to the emergency department with complaints of chest pain that began 30 minutes ago. She also complains of diaphoresis and nausea. On physical exam, blood pressure is 110/80 mmHg, pulse is 120 beats/min, and the chest is clear. What is your next step in management?

    1. Echocardiograph.

    2. Electrocardiogram.

    3. Calcium score.

    4. Coronary angiography.

103. A 70-year-old female patient with type 2 diabetes mellitus and dyslipidemia presented to the emergency department after she started complaining of epigastric pain that began 2 hours ago and is not relieved by antacid. She also complains of shortness of breath and nausea. The patient denied cough, hemoptysis, or chest pain. Physical exam was unremarkable. Electrocardiogram shows Q change in inferior leads with no ST elevation. Which of the following is your diagnosis?

    1. Pulmonary embolism.

    2. Myocardial infarction.

    3. Aortic dissection.

    4. Gastroesophageal reflux disease.

104. A 60-year-old female patient with type 2 diabetes mellitus and dyslipidemia presented to the emergency department complaining of chest pain that began 30 minutes ago. She also complains of diaphoresis and nausea. On physical exam, blood pressure is 110/80 mmHg, pulse is 120 beats/min, and the chest is clear. What is the mechanism behind the patient's condition?

    1. Vasculitis.

    2. Aortic root dilatation.

    3. Rupture of atherosclerotic plaque.

    4. Calcified aortic valve.

105. A 51-year-old male patient with a history of uncontrolled hypertension presented to the emergency department after complaining of a headache. He denies any history of vomiting, loss of consciousness, or muscle weakness. On physical exam, his blood pressure is 220/120 mmHg, pulse is 120 beats/min, and chest and heart exam are unremarkable. Which of the following is the next step of management?

    1. Brain computed tomography.

    2. Chest x-ray.

    3. Abdominal ultrasound.

    4. Echocardiograph.

106. A 70-year-old female patient with a history of type 2 diabetes mellitus and dyslipidemia presented to the emergency department after she started complaining of epigastric pain that began 2 hours ago and is not relieved by antacid. She also has shortness of breath and nausea. The patient denies cough, hemoptysis, or chest pain. Physical exam was unremarkable. Which of the following will be your next step of management?

    1. Give patient intravenous omeprazole.

    2. Electrocardiogram.

    3. Computed tomography angiography.

    4. Chest x-ray.

107. A 40-year-old male patient visits his nurse practitioner for routine follow-up. His blood pressure average for the last week is 150/96 mmHg. His lab work is sodium 140 mEq/L, potassium 3.5 mEq/L, glucose 100 mg, and creatinine 0.9 mg. What is his diagnosis?

    1. Conn syndrome.

    2. Cushing syndrome.

    3. Renal artery stenosis.

    4. Essential hypertension.

108. A 50-year-old male patient was admitted to the hospital 3 days ago after diagnosis of inferior wall myocardial infarction. Today he complains of new chest pain and shortness of breath. On physical exam, blood pressure is 90/50 mmHg and pulse is 130 beats/min. Cardiac exam revealed a new holosystolic murmur. What happened in this patient?

    1. Right heart failure.

    2. Interventricular septum rupture.

    3. Free wall rupture.

    4. Pericarditis.

109. A 60-year-old male patient was admitted to the hospital 5 days ago after he was diagnosed with an inferior wall myocardial infarction. Today he complains of new chest pain and shortness of breath. On physical exam, blood pressure is 60/50 mmHg and pulse is 130 beats/min with jugular venous distention and muffled heart sounds. What is the most common artery typically involved?

    1. Right coronary artery.

    2. Left circumflex artery.

    3. Left anterior descending.

    4. Right marginal artery.

110. A 50-year-old male patient was admitted to the hospital 7 days ago after a diagnosis of inferior wall myocardial infarction. Today he complains of new pleuritic chest pain that is relieved by leaning forward. The patient's physical exam was unremarkable. What is your next step in management?

    1. Echocardiograph.

    2. Chest x-ray.

    3. Electrocardiogram.

    4. Sputum culture.

111. A 55-year-old male patient was admitted to the hospital after diagnosis of unstable angina; he underwent percutaneous transcutaneous angiography 1 day ago. Now the plan for this patient is discharge. When can this patient drive his car?

    1. After 2 weeks.

    2. Immediately after discharge.

    3. After 1 week.

    4. After 1 month.

112. A 50-year-old female patient was admitted to the coronary care unit 3 days ago because of inferior wall myocardial infarction. She is now discharged on clopidogrel. What is the mechanism of action of this drug?

    1. Antiinflammatory effect.

    2. Inhibit cyclooxygenase pathway.

    3. Glycoprotein IIB/IIIa receptor antagonist.

    4. Adenosine diphosphate receptor antagonist.

113. A 60-year-old male patient presented to the emergency department with chest pain radiating to his left arm. On physical exam, blood pressure is 120/85 mmHg and pulse is 54 beats/min. Lung and cardiac exams are clear. Electrocardiogram shows type 2 heart block. Which of the following arteries is occluded?

    1. Left coronary artery.

    2. Right coronary artery.

    3. Circumflex artery.

    4. Left anterior descending.

114. A 66-year-old male patient with a history of hypertension and dyslipidemia was diagnosed with myocardial infarction 1 week ago. Today he starts feeling short of breath and is having palpitations. On physical exam, blood pressure is 110/75 mmHg and pulse is 120 beats/min and is irregularly irregular. Cardiac exam revealed holosystolic murmur. Which is the cause of this murmur and the patient's symptoms?

    1. Aortic valve stenosis.

    2. Mitral valve stenosis.

    3. Tricuspid regurgitation.

    4. Mitral valve regurgitation.

115. A 61-year-old male patient with a known history of hypertension visits his nurse practitioner for routine follow-up. On physical exam, his blood pressure is 180/100 mmHg and pulse is 80 beats/min. Lung auscultation revealed bibasilar crackles. Which of the following is the pathology for this patient?

    1. Left ventricular hypertrophy.

    2. Aortic valve stenosis.

    3. Pulmonary hypertension.

    4. Mitral valve regurgitation.

116. An 80-year-old male patient with no past medical history presents to his nurse practitioner for a routine exam. On physical exam, his blood pressure is 180/80 mmHg and pulse is 80 beats/min. The other exams are unremarkable. Which of the following is the drug of choice for this patient?

    1. Enalapril.

    2. Thiazide diuretic.

    3. Bisoprolol.

    4. Furosemide.

117. A 60-year-old woman with a history of hypertension and dyslipidemia presented to the emergency department because of chest pain that radiated to her left arm one hour ago. She also has nausea and diaphoresis. On physical exam, her blood pressure is 120/80 mmHg and her pulse is 90 beats/min; otherwise her exam is unremarkable. Which of the following is most specific for the patient's diagnosis?

    1. ST elevation in electrocardiogram.

    2. Change in Q wave.

    3. Akinesia in echocardiograph.

    4. Elevated cardiac enzymes.

118. A 50-year-old female patient presented with chest pain that began 30 minutes ago not relieved by rest and associated with diaphoresis. On exam, her blood pressure is 120/80 mmHg and pulse is 120 beats/min; otherwise her exam is unremarkable. Electrocardiogram (ECG) shows ST elevation. What is the next step of management?

    1. Echocardiograph.

    2. Cardiac enzymes.

    3. Exercise ECG.

    4. Percutaneous coronary intervention.

119. A 60-year-old male patient with previous history of myocardial infarction (MI) 3 years ago is on aspirin (81 mg) and enalapril. His cholesterol level is 6 mmol/L. Which of the following can reduce the risk of a second MI?

    1. Warfarin.

    2. Increase dose of aspirin.

    3. Atorvastatin.

    4. Furosemide.

120. A-60-year-old male patient with a history hypertension was admitted to the coronary care unit 4 days ago because of inferior wall myocardial infarction. Today, the patient suffered from new-onset chest pain with moderate shortness of breath that increases when the patient is lying down. On physical exam, his blood pressure is 80/50 mmHg and his pulse is 150 beats/min. Chest x-ray is normal. Which of the following will be found on his physical exam?

    1. Jugular vein distention.

    2. Distant heart sound.

    3. Holosystolic murmur.

    4. Leg swelling.

121. A 62-year-old male patient who smokes and has a history of uncontrolled hypertension presented to the emergency department because of complaints of chest pain. The pain radiates to his back and began 1 hour ago. On physical exam, his blood pressure is 160/90 mmHg and his pulse is 120 beats/min. Electrocardiogram (ECG) shows inferior myocardial infarction. Which of the following is the next step in management?

    1. Surgery.

    2. Exercise ECG.

    3. Thrombolysis.

    4. Abdominal ultrasound.

122. A 60-year-old female patient with a previous history of ischemic heart disease began rosuvastatin (40 mg), clopidogrel, and aspirin 2 months ago. She now complains of muscle aches and pains. What is the next step in management?

    1. Stop rosuvastatin and start cholestyramine.

    2. Decrease dose of rosuvastatin to 10 mg.

    3. Stop rosuvastatin and start gemfibrozil.

    4. Stop rosuvastatin.

123. A 55-year-old male patient with a history of type 2 diabetes mellitus presented with severe retrosternal chest pain that began 40 minutes ago and is associated with nausea. This pain radiates to his left arm and jaw. If the patient was diagnosed with a myocardial infarction (MI), which of the following is a contraindication to thrombolysis?

    1. The patient had an ischemic stroke 1 month ago.

    2. Elevation of ST in leads I, II, and aVF.

    3. Blood pressure of 120/80 mmHg.

    4. Head trauma within the past 3 months.

124. An 18-year-old male patient, visited his nurse practitioner because of back pain. On physical exam, the nurse practitioner performs bimanual palpation of the supraumbilical area. What is most likely to show on an echocardiogram?

    1. Mitral stenosis.

    2. Aortic aneurysm.

    3. Pericardial effusion.

    4. Coarctation of aorta.

125. A 70-year-old female patient with a history of type 2 diabetes mellitus presented to the emergency department with crushing retrosternal chest pain that radiated to the left arm. If percutaneous coronary intervention (PCI) is not available, what is the indication to perform thrombolysis?

    1. ST elevation 2 mm in leads V1 to V4.

    2. ST depression in leads I and II.

    3. Q-wave change in leads II and aVF.

    4. Right bundle branch block.

126. A 55-year-old male patient with a history of hypertension and dyslipidemia presented to the emergency department with retrosternal chest pain that radiated to his left arm and started an hour ago. Electrocardiogram shows Q-wave change in V1 to V3 and left bundle branch block. What is the next step of management?

    1. Percutaneous coronary intervention.

    2. Thrombolysis.

    3. Warfarin.

    4. Heparin.

127. A 50-year-old female patient underwent percutaneous coronary intervention; two stents were put in the left anterior descending artery and she is scheduled for discharge today. Which of the following drugs should be prescribed for this patient?

    1. Heparin.

    2. Atorvastatin.

    3. Warfarin.

    4. Digoxin.

128. A 60-year-old man is brought to the emergency department because of severe chest pain that started suddenly nearly 1 hour ago. He states that the pain is sharp and is the worst pain he ever felt. He feels the pain anteriorly and in his upper back. The patient has had type 2 diabetes mellitus for the last 15 years, and he is not compliant with his medications. Electrocardiogram shows sinus tachycardia with nonspecific T-wave changes. Chest x-ray shows widening of the superior mediastinum. Which of these conditions most likely accounts for this patient's condition?

    1. Diabetes mellitus.

    2. Atherosclerosis.

    3. Systemic hypertension.

    4. Pulmonary hypertension.

129. A 40-year-old male patient, presents to the outpatient clinic for a routine checkup. His blood pressure is 150/85 mmHg. He is slightly obese, he is a heavy smoker, consumes two glasses of alcohol every day, and drinks two cups of espresso coffee every day. Lab studies show no abnormalities in electrolytes, creatinine, or serum glucose. He has a normal urinalysis and normal electrocardiogram. He returns for follow-up after 1 month, and his blood pressure is 155/91 mmHg. He prefers to not take any medications right now, so which of the following is the most beneficial for his blood pressure?

    1. To quit smoking.

    2. To stop alcohol use.

    3. Weight loss and exercise.

    4. Reduction of daily coffee intake.

130. A 40-year-old man presents to his nurse practitioner for evaluation of elevated blood pressure. On his previous two visits, his blood pressure has been 150/85 and 155/90 mmHg. He has no other complaints. He does not smoke or drink alcohol. His brother was diagnosed with hypertension when he was 45. He follows an exercise routine and a low-salt diet. His body mass index is 28 kg/m². His cardiovascular and respiratory exams were normal. No vascular bruits are heard, and peripheral pulses are normal and symmetrical. Electrocardiogram shows normal sinus rhythm. Complete blood count and chemistry panel are normal. His blood pressure today is 160/95 mmHg. Which of the following is the most appropriate next step in management?

    1. Lipid profile and urinalysis.

    2. Thyroid-stimulating hormone.

    3. Plasma renin activity.

    4. Renal ultrasound.

131. A thin-appearing 18-year-old female patient comes to the clinic for a routine visit. She reports intermittent shortness of breath with activity. She reports that she has been trying to gain weight but is having trouble doing this. She also reports frequent upper respiratory infections. Her vital signs are within normal limits. Exam shows grade III harsh holosystolic murmur in the left lower sternal area. No thrill over the pericardial region on palpation. Brachial and femoral pulses are +2 and equal. Her nail beds are pale, and capillary refill is >3 seconds. Electrocardiogram is normal. What is the most likely diagnosis in this patient?

    1. Atrial septal defect.

    2. Ventricular septal defect.

    3. Truncus arteriosus.

    4. Tricuspid atresia.

132. A thin-appearing 18-year-old female patient comes to the clinic for a routine visit. She reports intermittent shortness of breath with activity. She reports that she has been trying to gain weight but is having trouble doing this. She also reports frequent upper respiratory infections. Her vital signs are within normal limits. Exam shows grade III harsh holosystolic murmur in the left lower sternal area. No thrill over the pericardial region on palpation. Brachial and femoral pulses are +2 and equal. Her nail beds are pale, and capillary refill is >3 seconds. Electrocardiogram is normal. What is the best next step for this patient?

    1. Echocardiography.

    2. Supplemental oxygen delivery.

    3. Admission to the hospital.

    4. Referral to a dietician.

133. A thin-appearing 18-year-old female patient comes to the clinic for a routine visit. She reports intermittent shortness of breath with activity. She reports that she has been trying to gain weight but is having trouble doing this. She also reports frequent upper respiratory infections. Her vital signs are within normal limits. Exam shows grade III harsh holosystolic murmur in the left lower sternal area. No thrill over the pericardial region on palpation. Brachial and femoral pulses are +2 and equal. Her nail beds are pale, and capillary refill is >3 seconds. Electrocardiogram is normal. What is the most common type of this congenital abnormality?

    1. Muscular.

    2. Membranous.

    3. Perimembranous.

    4. Inlet-type ventricular septal defect.

134. A 19-year-old male patient goes to the clinic after he noticed blue discoloration of his fingernails. He reports that he does not have enough energy to get through the day. No history of trauma or surgery is present. Exam shows perioral cyanosis, clubbing of his fingers, and a systolic murmur along the left upper sternal border. When he squats down, the loudness of the murmur increases and the cyanosis improves. What is the most likely diagnosis in this patient?

    1. Atrial septal defect.

    2. Tetralogy of Fallot.

    3. Truncus arteriosus.

    4. Tricuspid atresia.

135. A 19-year-old male patient goes to the clinic after he noticed blue discoloration of his fingernails. He reports that he does not have enough energy to get through the day. No history of trauma or surgery is present. Exam shows perioral cyanosis, clubbing of his fingers, and a systolic murmur along the left upper sternal border. When he squats down, the loudness of the murmur increases and the cyanosis improves. What would be the most common valvular abnormality in this patient?

    1. Mitral stenosis.

    2. Pulmonary stenosis.

    3. Tricuspid stenosis.

    4. Mitral regurgitation.

136. A 19-year-old male patient goes to the clinic after he noticed blue discoloration of his fingernails. He reports that he does not have enough energy to get through the day. No history of trauma or surgery is present. Exam shows perioral cyanosis, clubbing of his fingers, and a systolic murmur along the left upper sternal border. When he squats down, the loudness of the murmur increases and the cyanosis improves. Why does squatting relieve the cyanosis of this patient?

    1. Decreased pulmonary vascular resistance.

    2. Increased pulmonary vascular resistance.

    3. Decreased systemic vascular resistance.

    4. Increased systemic vascular resistance.

137. On exam of a 15-year-old female patient, a systolic ejection murmur is present at the left upper sternal border with wide fixed splitting of the S2 sound. Otherwise she looks well, and her vital signs are within normal limits. What is the most likely diagnosis?

    1. Atrial septal defect.

    2. Tetralogy of Fallot.

    3. Truncus arteriosus.

    4. Tricuspid atresia.

138. What is the most common type of atrial septal defect found in most patients?

    1. Ostium primum.

    2. Ostium secundum.

    3. Sinus venosus.

    4. Coronary sinus.

139. All of the following items represent cyanotic heart disease, *except*:

    1. Tetralogy of Fallot.

    2. Tricuspid atresia.

    3. Transposition of great vessels.

    4. Atrial septal defect.

140. What is the most common congenital cardiac abnormality in patients with Down syndrome?

    1. Endocardial cushion defect.

    2. Patent ductus arteriosus.

    3. Ventricular septal defect.

    4. Atrial septal defect.

141. Which of the following is the least likely condition associated with infective endocarditis?

    1. Atrial septal defect.

    2. Prosthetic valves.

    3. Coarctation of the aorta.

    4. Previous infective endocarditis.

142. Which of the following organisms is the most common cause for acute bacterial endocarditis?

    1. *Staphylococcus aureus*

    2. *Streptococcus viridians*

    3. Fungal infection

    4. *Streptococcus pyogenes*

143. Which of the following is the most common cause of death in patients with infective endocarditis?

    1. Glomerulonephritis.

    2. Congestive heart failure.

    3. Septic pulmonary infarction.

    4. Hemorrhagic stroke.

144. Which of the following represents the two major criteria for infective endocarditis?

    1. Abnormal echocardiography and fever.

    2. Positive blood cultures and intravenous (IV) drug use.

    3. Abnormal echocardiography and positive blood cultures.

    4. Fever and IV drug use.

145. A 28-year-old female patient, with a history of right arm cellulitis 6 months ago, presents to the emergency department with fever, chills, and generalized weakness. Vital signs are blood pressure 110/65 mmHg, pulse 110 beats/min, respiratory rate 18 breaths/min, and temperature 103°F. On exam, the oropharynx is normal and lungs are clear to auscultation. Cardiac auscultation shows holosystolic murmur at the lower sternal area that increases in intensity with inspiration. There are multiple puncture sites (track marks) in the patient's right arm. What is the most probable diagnosis in this patient?

    1. Infectious mononucleosis.

    2. Lyme disease.

    3. Syphilis.

    4. Infective endocarditis.

146. A 28-year-old female patient, with a history of right arm cellulitis 6 months ago, presents to the emergency department with fever, chills, and generalized weakness. Vital signs are blood pressure 110/65 mmHg, pulse 110 beats/min, respiratory rate 18 breaths/min, and temperature 103°F. On exam, the oropharynx is normal and lungs are clear to auscultation. Cardiac auscultation shows holosystolic murmur at the lower sternal area that increases in intensity with inspiration. There are multiple puncture sites (track marks) in the patient's right arm. What is the most likely cause for this patient's murmur?

    1. Mitral stenosis.

    2. Pulmonary stenosis.

    3. Tricuspid regurgitation.

    4. Tricuspid stenosis.

147. A 28-year-old female patient, with a history of right arm cellulitis 6 months ago, presents to the emergency department with fever, chills, and generalized weakness. Vital signs are blood pressure 110/65 mmHg, pulse 110 beats/min, respiratory rate 18 breaths/min, and temperature 103°F. On exam, the oropharynx is normal and lungs are clear to auscultation. Cardiac auscultation shows holosystolic murmur at the lower sternal area that increases in intensity with inspiration. There are multiple puncture sites (track marks) in the patient's right arm. What is the most likely organism involved in this patient's clinical picture?

    1. *Streptococcus pneumoniae.*

    2. *Staphylococcus aureus.*

    3. *Hemophilus influenza.*

    4. *Moraxella catarrhalis.*

148. A 28-year-old female patient, with a history of right arm cellulitis 6 months ago, presents to the emergency department with fever, chills, and generalized weakness. Vital signs are blood pressure 110/65 mmHg, pulse 110 beats/min, respiratory rate 18 breaths/min, and temperature 103°F. On exam, the oropharynx is normal and lungs are clear to auscultation. Cardiac auscultation shows holosystolic murmur at the lower sternal area that increases in intensity with inspiration. There are multiple puncture sites (track marks) in the patient's right arm. What is the most likely predisposing factor for this patient?

    1. Congenital cardiac anomaly.

    2. Underlying autoimmune disease.

    3. Intravenous drug use.

    4. Underlying malignancy.

149. A 28-year-old female patient, with a history of right arm cellulitis 6 months ago, presents to the emergency department with fever, chills, and generalized weakness. Vital signs are blood pressure 110/65 mmHg, pulse 110 beats/min, respiratory rate 18 breaths/min, and temperature 103°F. On exam, the oropharynx is normal and lungs are clear to auscultation. Cardiac auscultation shows holosystolic murmur at the lower sternal area that increases in intensity with inspiration. There are multiple puncture sites (track marks) in the patient's right arm. What is the best next step in the management of this patient?

    1. Ampicillin-sulbactam.

    2. Oxacillin.

    3. Vancomycin.

    4. Clindamycin.

150. Which of the following is the most common clinical finding in patients with infective endocarditis?

    1. Petechiae.

    2. Heart murmur.

    3. Fever.

    4. Osler nodes.

151. Which of the following is the least common clinical finding in patients with infective endocarditis?

    1. Petechiae.

    2. Roth spots.

    3. Fever.

    4. Osler nodes.

152. A 27-year-old male patient, with no significant medical history, presents to the clinic with generalized weakness and anorexia for the last week. He has no cough, chest pain, arthralgia, or diarrhea. He underwent an uncomplicated root canal procedure 5 weeks ago. Temperature is 100.3°F, blood pressure is 135/76 mmHg, pulse is 90 beats/min, and respiratory rate is 18 breaths/min. Early diastolic murmur is heard on cardiac auscultation. Electrocardiogram and chest x-ray exams are normal, and urinalysis shows microscopic hematuria. What is the most probable diagnosis in this patient?

    1. Infectious mononucleosis.

    2. Lyme disease.

    3. Syphilis.

    4. Infective endocarditis.

153. A 27-year-old male patient, with no significant medical history, presents to the clinic with generalized weakness and anorexia for the last week. He has no cough, chest pain, arthralgia, or diarrhea. He underwent an uncomplicated root canal procedure 5 weeks ago. Temperature is 100.3°F, blood pressure is 135/76 mmHg, pulse is 90 beats/min, and respiratory rate is 18 breaths/min. Early diastolic murmur is heard on cardiac auscultation. Electrocardiogram and chest x-ray exams are normal, and urinalysis shows microscopic hematuria. What is the best next step to confirm the diagnosis of this patient?

    1. Transesophageal echocardiography.

    2. Transthoracic echocardiography.

    3. Start antibiotic immediately.

    4. Bacterial blood culture.

154. A 27-year-old male patient, with no significant medical history, presents to the clinic with generalized weakness and anorexia for the last week. He has no cough, chest pain, arthralgia, or diarrhea. He underwent an uncomplicated root canal procedure 5 weeks ago. Temperature is 100.3°F, blood pressure is 135/76 mmHg, pulse is 90 beats/min, and respiratory rate is 18 breaths/min. Early diastolic murmur is heard on cardiac auscultation. Electrocardiogram and chest x-ray exams are normal, and urinalysis shows microscopic hematuria. What is the cause for this patient's murmur?

    1. Mitral stenosis.

    2. Pulmonary stenosis.

    3. Tricuspid regurgitation.

    4. Aortic regurgitation.

155. A 27-year-old male patient, with no significant medical history, presents to the clinic with generalized weakness and anorexia for the last week. He has no cough, chest pain, arthralgia, or diarrhea. He underwent an uncomplicated root canal procedure 5 weeks ago. Temperature is 100.3°F, blood pressure is 135/76 mmHg, pulse is 90 beats/min, and respiratory rate is 18 breaths/min. Early diastolic murmur is heard on cardiac auscultation. Electrocardiogram and chest x-ray exams are normal, and urinalysis shows microscopic hematuria. What is the most likely causative organism for this clinical presentation?

    1. *Streptococcus viridians.*

    2. *Staphylococcus aureus.*

    3. *Hemophilus influenza.*

    4. *Moraxella catarrhalis.*

156. Which of the following is the most common valvular abnormality detected in patients with infective endocarditis?

    1. Mitral regurgitation.

    2. Pulmonary stenosis.

    3. Tricuspid regurgitation.

    4. Aortic regurgitation.

157. Which of the following is the most common cause for infective endocarditis in patients with nosocomial urinary tract infections?

    1. *Streptococcus viridians.*

    2. *Staphylococcus aureus.*

    3. Enterococci.

    4. *Moraxella catarrhalis.*

158. A 55-year-old man goes to see his nurse practitioner with complaints of a 4-week history of anorexia, fever, muscle aches, and weight loss. There is no cough or dyspnea. He has a 20 pack-year smoking history. Temperature is 101.0°F, blood pressure is 120/76 mmHg, pulse is 90 beats/min, and respiratory rate is 16 breaths/min. Lung auscultation is normal. Echocardiogram shows mitral valve vegetation. Blood cultures grow *Streptococcus bovis* biotype 1. Other than antibiotic treatment, what additional treatment is recommended in this patient?

    1. Bronchoscopy.

    2. Cystoscopy.

    3. Colonoscopy.

    4. Fecal occult blood test.

159. A 35-year-old male patient with no significant past medical history presents to the hospital with acute renal failure secondary to post-streptococcal glomerulonephritis. On the fourth day of hospitalization, he suddenly starts to suffer from retrosternal, nonradiating chest pain that is relieved by leaning forward. Temperature is 99.6°F, blood pressure is 140/95 mmHg, pulse is 80 beats/min, and respiratory rate is 20 breaths/min. Electrocardiogram shows nonspecific T-wave changes. Echocardiography is normal except for trivial pericardial effusion. Hematuria, mild proteinuria, and red cell casts are found on urinalysis. Blood urea nitrogen is 62 mg/dL and serum creatinine is 3.8 mg/dL. What is the most likely diagnosis in this clinical scenario?

    1. Myocarditis.

    2. Uremic pericarditis.

    3. Infective endocarditis.

    4. Myocardial infarction.

160. A 35-year-old male patient with no significant past medical history presents to the hospital with acute renal failure secondary to post-streptococcal glomerulonephritis. On the fourth day of hospitalization, he suddenly starts to suffer from retrosternal, nonradiating chest pain that is relieved by leaning forward. Temperature is 99.6°F, blood pressure is 140/95 mmHg, pulse is 80 beats/min, and respiratory rate is 20 breaths/min. Electrocardiogram shows nonspecific T-wave changes. Echocardiography is normal except for trivial pericardial effusion. Hematuria, mild proteinuria, and red cell casts are found on urinalysis. Blood urea nitrogen is 62 mg/dL and serum creatinine is 3.8 mg/dL. What is the most appropriate next step in the management of this patient?

    1. Broad-spectrum antibiotics.

    2. Hemodialysis.

    3. Indomethacin.

    4. Intravenous corticosteroids.

161. A 35-year-old male patient with no significant past medical history presents to the hospital with acute renal failure secondary to post-streptococcal glomerulonephritis. On the fourth day of hospitalization, he suddenly starts to suffer from retrosternal, nonradiating chest pain that is relieved by leaning forward. Temperature is 99.6°F, blood pressure is 140/95 mmHg, pulse is 80 beats/min, and respiratory rate is 20 breaths/min. Electrocardiogram shows nonspecific T-wave changes. Echocardiography is normal except for trivial pericardial effusion. Hematuria, mild proteinuria, and red cell casts are found on urinalysis. Blood urea nitrogen is 62 mg/dL and serum creatinine is 3.8 mg/dL. What is the typical finding on electrocardiogram for this diagnosis?

    1. Diffuse ST elevation with typical PR depression.

    2. Diffuse ST depression with typical PR depression.

    3. S1 Q3 T3 in leads II, III, and aVF.

    4. Third-degree heart block.

162. A 45-year-old male patient who recently emigrated from China to the United States presents to the nurse practitioner complaining of shortness of breath, abdominal distension, and fatigue for the last 2 months. He has no significant medical history. He worked as a farmer his entire life. Temperature is 98.4°F, blood pressure is 110/60 mmHg, pulse is 80 beats/min, and respiratory rate is 16 breaths/min. On exam, there is pedal edema, increased abdominal girth with free fluid, and elevated jugular venous pressure with inspiration. Cardiac auscultation reveals decreased heart sounds and accentuated sound directly after the second heart sound in early diastole. A chest x-ray demonstrates a ring of calcification around the heart. What is the most likely diagnosis in this patient?

    1. Myocarditis.

    2. Constrictive pericarditis.

    3. Infective endocarditis.

    4. Myocardial infarction.

163. A 45-year-old male patient who recently emigrated from China to the United States presents to the nurse practitioner complaining of shortness of breath, abdominal distension, and fatigue for the last 2 months. He has no significant medical history. He worked as a farmer his entire life. Temperature is 98.4°F, blood pressure is 110/60 mmHg, pulse is 80 beats/min, and respiratory rate is 16 breaths/min. On exam, there is pedal edema, increased abdominal girth with free fluid, and elevated jugular venous pressure with inspiration. Cardiac auscultation reveals decreased heart sounds and accentuated sound directly after the second heart sound in early diastole. A chest x-ray demonstrates a ring of calcification around the heart. What is the most likely cause for the diagnosis in this patient?

    1. Pneumoconiosis.

    2. Cor pulmonale.

    3. Tuberculosis.

    4. Psittacosis.

164. A 45-year-old male patient who recently emigrated from China to the United States presents to the nurse practitioner complaining of shortness of breath, abdominal distension, and fatigue for the last 2 months. He has no significant medical history. He worked as a farmer his entire life. Temperature is 98.4°F, blood pressure is 110/60 mmHg, pulse is 80 beats/min, and respiratory rate is 16 breaths/min. On exam, there is pedal edema, increased abdominal girth with free fluid, and elevated jugular venous pressure with inspiration. Cardiac auscultation reveals decreased heart sounds and accentuated sound directly after the second heart sound in early diastole. A chest x-ray demonstrates a ring of calcification around the heart. What is the sound heard on cardiac auscultation?

    1. Pericardial friction rub.

    2. Pericardial knock.

    3. Holosystolic murmur.

    4. Systolic ejection murmur.

165. A 45-year-old male patient who recently emigrated from China to the United States presents to the nurse practitioner complaining of shortness of breath, abdominal distension, and fatigue for the last 2 months. He has no significant medical history. He worked as a farmer his entire life. Temperature is 98.4°F, blood pressure is 110/60 mmHg, pulse is 80 beats/min, and respiratory rate is 16 breaths/min. On exam, there is pedal edema, increased abdominal girth with free fluid, and elevated jugular venous pressure with inspiration. Cardiac auscultation reveals decreased heart sounds and accentuated sound directly after the second heart sound in early diastole. A chest x-ray demonstrates a ring of calcification around the heart. What will the jugular venous pulse tracing for this patient show?

    1. Prominent a wave.

    2. Cannon wave.

    3. Absent a wave.

    4. Prominent x and y descent.

166. A 45-year-old male patient who recently emigrated from China to the United States presents to the nurse practitioner complaining of shortness of breath, abdominal distension, and fatigue for the last 2 months. He has no significant medical history. He worked as a farmer his entire life. Temperature is 98.4°F, blood pressure is 110/60 mmHg, pulse is 80 beats/min, and respiratory rate is 16 breaths/min. On exam, there is pedal edema, increased abdominal girth with free fluid, and elevated jugular venous pressure with inspiration. Cardiac auscultation reveals decreased heart sounds and accentuated sound directly after the second heart sound in early diastole. A chest x-ray demonstrates a ring of calcification around the heart. What does "elevated jugular venous pressure on inspiration" typically describe?

    1. Pulsus paradoxus.

    2. Kussmaul sign.

    3. Water hammer pulse.

    4. Pulsus parvus et tardus.

167. A 45-year-old male patient who recently emigrated from China to the United States presents to the nurse practitioner complaining of shortness of breath, abdominal distension, and fatigue for the last 2 months. He has no significant medical history. He worked as a farmer his entire life. Temperature is 98.4°F, blood pressure is 110/60 mmHg, pulse is 80 beats/min, and respiratory rate is 16 breaths/min. On exam, there is pedal edema, increased abdominal girth with free fluid, and elevated jugular venous pressure with inspiration. Cardiac auscultation reveals decreased heart sounds and an accentuated sound directly after the second heart sound in early diastole. A chest x-ray demonstrates a ring of calcification around the heart. Which of the following will be found on physical exam of this patient?

    1. Pulsus paradoxus.

    2. Holosystolic murmur.

    3. Water hammer pulse.

    4. Pulsus parvus tardus.

168. A 19-year-old male patient with a history of runny nose and nasal congestion for the last week arrives in the emergency department with complaints of fever and dyspnea. His daily fever began 6 days ago, and he has been increasingly tired with muscle aches and worsening dyspnea. Albuterol is given with no benefit. Temperature is 101.3°F, blood pressure is 100/60 mmHg, pulse is 150 beats/min, respiratory rate is 32 breaths/min, and pulse oximetry is 95% on room air. He has nasal flaring and subcostal retractions. Despite bronchodilator treatment, scattered wheezes are heard at the lung bases. Scattered mobile lymph nodes are palpable in the anterior cervical chain. A grade III/VI

holosystolic murmur is best heard at the cardiac apex. Chest x-ray shows cardiomegaly. Which of the followings is the most likely diagnosis?

    1. Acute rheumatic fever.

    2. Asthma exacerbation.

    3. Community acquired pneumonia.

    4. Viral myocarditis.

169. A 19-year-old male patient with a history of runny nose and nasal congestion for the last week arrives in the emergency department with complaints of fever and dyspnea. His daily fever began 6 days ago, and he has been increasingly tired with muscle aches and worsening dyspnea. Albuterol is given with no benefit. Temperature is 101.3°F, blood pressure is 100/60 mmHg, pulse is 150 beats/min, respiratory rate is 32 breaths/min, and pulse oximetry is 95% on room air. He has nasal flaring and subcostal retractions. Despite bronchodilator treatment, scattered wheezes are heard at the lung bases. Scattered mobile lymph nodes are palpable in the anterior cervical chain. A grade III/VI holosystolic murmur is best heard at the cardiac apex. Chest x-ray shows cardiomegaly. Which of the following represents the most causative organisms for the diagnosis of the patient?

    1. Coxsackievirus B and adenovirus.

    2. Coxsackievirus A and rhinovirus.

    3. Respiratory syncytial virus and parainfluenza.

    4. Influenza virus and adenovirus.

170. A 19-year-old male patient with a history of runny nose and nasal congestion for the last week arrives in the emergency department with complaints of fever and dyspnea. His daily fever began 6 days ago, and he has been increasingly tired with muscle aches and worsening dyspnea. Albuterol is given with no benefit. Temperature is 101.3°F, blood pressure is 100/60 mmHg, pulse is 150 beats/min, respiratory rate is 32 breaths/min, and pulse oximetry is 95% on room air. He has nasal flaring and subcostal retractions. Despite bronchodilator treatment, scattered wheezes are heard at the lung bases. Scattered mobile lymph nodes are palpable in the anterior cervical chain. A grade III/VI holosystolic murmur is best heard at the cardiac apex. Chest x-ray shows cardiomegaly. What is the most likely cause for the murmur heard on physical exam?

    1. Functional pulmonic stenosis.

    2. Functional mitral stenosis.

    3. Innocent murmur.

    4. Functional mitral regurgitation.

171. A 19-year-old male patient with a history of runny nose and nasal congestion for the last week arrives in the emergency department with complaints of fever and dyspnea. His daily fever began 6 days ago, and he has been increasingly tired with muscle aches and worsening dyspnea. Albuterol is given with no benefit. Temperature is 101.3°F, blood pressure is 100/60 mmHg, pulse is 150 beats/min, respiratory rate is 32 breaths/min, and pulse oximetry is 95% on room air. He has nasal flaring and subcostal retractions. Despite bronchodilator treatment, scattered wheezes are heard at the lung bases. Scattered mobile lymph nodes are palpable in the anterior cervical chain. A grade III/VI holosystolic murmur is best heard at the cardiac apex. Chest x-ray shows cardiomegaly. What is the gold standard for the diagnosis of this patient?

    1. Electrocardiograph.

    2. Electroencephalogram.

    3. Magnetic resonance imaging.

    4. Myocardial biopsy.

172. A 68-year-old man, with a history of hypertension, type 2 diabetes mellitus, and congestive heart failure, presents to the emergency department with a 2-week history of progressive shortness of breath, orthopnea, and lower limb edema. He has a history of myocardial infarction 8 years ago. Current medications include digoxin, metoprolol, enalapril, furosemide, spironolactone, and aspirin. Blood pressure is 135/80 mmHg and pulse is 75 beats/min and regular. Symmetrical +2 bilateral pitting edema of the lower limbs is present. Point of maximal impulse is displaced to the left, and a soft holosystolic murmur is heard at the apex. Bilateral crackles are present over the lower lobes. His hemoglobin is 11 g/dL and his sodium is 128 mEq/L. Electrocardiogram shows normal sinus rhythm and no acute ischemic changes. Which of the following is the most likely diagnosis for this patient?

    1. Chronic obstructive pulmonary disease exacerbation.

    2. Asthma exacerbation.

    3. Decompensated heart failure.

    4. Pericarditis.

173. A 68-year-old man, with a history of hypertension, type 2 diabetes mellitus, and congestive heart failure, presents to the emergency department with a 2-week history of progressive shortness of breath, orthopnea, and lower limb edema. He has a history of myocardial infarction 8 years ago. Current medications include digoxin, metoprolol, enalapril, furosemide, spironolactone, and aspirin. Blood pressure is 135/80 mmHg and pulse is 75 beats/min and regular. Symmetrical +2 bilateral pitting edema of the lower limbs is present. Point of maximal impulse is displaced to the left, and a soft holosystolic murmur is heard at the apex. Bilateral crackles are present over the lower lobes. His hemoglobin is 11 g/dL and his sodium is 128 mEq/L. Electrocardiogram shows normal sinus rhythm and no acute ischemic changes. Which of the following is most likely correct regarding this patient's condition?

    1. Increasing sodium intake will control the electrolyte abnormalities.

    2. Serum norepinephrine is low.

    3. Hyponatremia indicates severe heart failure.

    4. Increasing the dose of digoxin may be indicated.

174. A 68-year-old man, with a history of hypertension, type 2 diabetes mellitus, and congestive heart failure, presents to the emergency department with a 2-week history of progressive shortness of breath, orthopnea, and lower limb edema. He has a history of myocardial infarction 8 years ago. Current medications include digoxin, metoprolol, enalapril, furosemide, spironolactone, and aspirin. Blood pressure is 135/80 mmHg and pulse is 75 beats/min and regular. Symmetrical +2 bilateral pitting edema of the lower limbs is present. Point of maximal impulse is displaced to the left, and a soft holosystolic murmur is heard at the apex. Bilateral crackles are present over the lower lobes. His hemoglobin is 11 g/dL and his sodium is 128 mEq/L. Electrocardiogram shows normal sinus rhythm and no acute ischemic changes. Which of the following clinical signs would best correlate with this patient?

    1. Cyanosis.

    2. Extremity edema.

    3. Third heart sounds.

    4. Wheezing.

175. In patients with congestive heart failure, which of the following abnormalities is found?

    1. Decreased renal venous pressure.

    2. Decreased intraglomerular pressure.

    3. Decreased renal venous pressure.

    4. Constriction of the efferent renal arteriole.

176. A 70-year-old woman with a history of hypertension presents to the emergency department with complaints of progressive dyspnea over the last 5 days. She is non-compliant with her antihypertensive medications. She has a history of deep vein thrombosis 10 years ago and received 8 months of anticoagulation. She is a 40 pack-year smoker. Blood pressure is 182/109 mmHg and pulse is 109 beats/min and regular. Oxygen saturation is 90% on room air. Lung auscultation reveals bibasilar crepitations and scattered wheezes. Which of the following is the most appropriate next step in the management of this patient?

    1. Intravenous (IV) amiodarone.

    2. IV furosemide.

    3. IV metoprolol.

    4. IV digoxin.

177. A 60-year-old male patient with left ventricular systolic dysfunction suffered from shortness of breath on climbing stairs. There is no shortness of breath at rest. Which of the following drugs would improve the patient's prognosis?

    1. Amiodarone.

    2. Bisoprolol.

    3. Amlodipine.

    4. Digoxin.

178. Which of the following blood test results suggests a worse prognosis in heart failure?

    1. Hypokalemia.

    2. Decreased pro-brain natriuretic peptide levels.

    3. Anemia.

    4. Hypernatremia.

179. A 77-year-old female patient has type 2 diabetes mellitus that is poorly controlled. She also has heart failure that is controlled with enalapril, bisoprolol, and furosemide. Which of the following hypoglycemic agents is contraindicated in patients with congestive heart failure?

    1. Acarbose.

    2. Glipizide.

    3. Nateglinide.

    4. Pioglitazone.

180. A 60-year-old male patient presents with gynecomastia. He is receiving treatment for heart failure and gastro-esophageal reflux. Which of the following drugs is most likely to be responsible for his gynecomastia?

    1. Spironolactone.

    2. Aspirin.

    3. Ramipril.

    4. Furosemide.

181. A 70-year-old male patient comes to the emergency department with intermittent, burning midline chest pain radiating to his shoulder over the last 3 hours. Electrocardiogram is done and shows ST elevation in leads II, III, and aVF. He is given sublingual nitroglycerin. Three minutes later, he experiences extreme weakness and lightheadedness. Temperature is 100°F, blood pressure is 70/40 mmHg, and pulse is 60 beats/min. the patient is diaphoretic, and his extremities are cold. Chest auscultation reveals bilateral vesicular breathing with no added sounds. Which of the following is the most appropriate next step in the management of this patient?

    1. Administer intramuscular epinephrine.

    2. Prepare for immediate pericardiocentesis.

    3. Prepare for temporary cardiac pacemaker.

    4. Administer normal saline bolus.

182. If you suspect inferior myocardial infarction in a 55-year-old patient who presents with typical cardiac chest pain, and who has a history of uncontrolled hypertension for the last 15 years, which of the following is the *incorrect* treatment to be given to this patient at the moment?

    1. Oxygen.

    2. Aspirin.

    3. Nitroglycerin.

    4. Intravenous fluid.

183. If a patient has ST elevation in leads II, III, and aVF on standard electrocardiogram (ECG) leads, which of the following investigations should be ordered?

    1. Echocardiography.

    2. Chest x-ray.

    3. Right-sided ECG.

    4. Arterial blood gas.

184. All of the following parameters are found in patients with cardiogenic shock, *except*:

    1. Decreased cardiac index.

    2. Decreased cardiac preload.

    3. Decreased pulmonary capillary wedge pressure.

    4. Increased systemic vascular resistance.

185. All of the following can cause high-output cardiac failure, *except*:

    1. Dilated cardiomyopathy.

    2. Morbid obesity.

    3. Beriberi disease.

    4. Sepsis.

186. A 60-year-old male patient presents with acute respiratory failure after a blood transfusion and was thought to have developed acute respiratory distress syndrome. Which of the following is not true regarding this condition?

    1. It is also called "noncardiogenic pulmonary edema."

    2. It is characterized by high-protein pulmonary edema.

    3. Bilateral infiltration on the chest radiography.

    4. Increased pulmonary capillary wedge pressure.

187. A 45-year-old patient is admitted to the intensive care unit for ventilator support several hours after being admitted to the emergency department following a motor vehicle accident. He is extremely hypoxic, and chest x-ray shows bilateral infiltrates. He is diagnosed with acute respiratory distress syndrome (ARDS; noncardiogenic pulmonary edema). Which of the following is a direct cause for ARDS?

    1. Burns.

    2. Anaphylaxis.

    3. Pulmonary trauma.

    4. Sepsis.

188. A 44-year-old male patient comes to the emergency department with fever, chills, productive cough, and dyspnea. He drinks alcohol every day. He has a history of multiple episodes of alcohol-withdrawal seizures in the last year. He has no other medical problems and takes no medications. Temperature is 102°F, blood pressure is 100/70 mmHg, pulse is 120 beats/min, and respiratory rate is 20 breaths/min. His mucus membranes are dry. Chest auscultation reveals bilateral crackles and bronchial breath sounds. Cardiac exam is unremarkable. Chest x-ray reveals right lower lobe consolidation. He is started on intravenous antibiotics. Twelve hours later, he develops significant shortness of breath. SaO_2 is 80% on nonrebreather mask. He is intubated emergently. Repeated chest x-ray reveals bilateral white lungs. Which of the following is most likely to be present in this patient before intubation?

    1. Increased left-ventricular end-diastolic pressure.

    2. Normal alveolar-arterial oxygen gradient.

    3. Normal pulmonary arterial pressure.

    4. Decreased lung compliance.

189. The mainstay of the treatment of acute respiratory distress syndrome (ARDS) is to treat the underlying cause in addition to the mechanical ventilation of the patient. Which of the following parameters on a mechanical ventilation device is not correct regarding the management of this syndrome?

    1. High positive-end expiratory pressure (PEEP).

    2. Low tidal volume.

    3. Permissive hypercapnia.

    4. Low PEEP.

190. A 50-year-old male patient was admitted to the coronary care unit because of inferior wall myocardial infarction. He received the appropriate management and his chest pain has subsided. Three hours later, his blood pressure is 70/50 mmHg and his pulse is 35 beats/min. What is the next step in treatment?

    1. Temporary pacemaker.

    2. Atropine.

    3. Digoxin.

    4. Bolus of normal saline.

191. A 45-year-old female patient with a history of uncontrolled hypertension is on a thiazide diuretic. She arrives at the clinic for routine follow-up. Her blood pressure is 150/90 mmHg and her pulse is 75 beats/min. The nurse practitioner adds enalapril to get her blood pressure under control. Which of the following is a contraindication to enalapril?

    1. Bilateral renal artery stenosis.

    2. Patient with microalbuminuria.

    3. Patient with chronic obstructive pulmonary disease.

    4. Patient with diastolic heart failure.

192. A 60-year-old man with long-standing uncontrolled hypertension presents to the outpatient clinic with shortness of breath, which happens with minimal effort. On physical exam, his blood pressure is 160/100 mmHg; otherwise his exam is unremarkable. Chest x-ray shows prominent left heart border and echocardiogram shows left ventricular hypertrophy. Which of the following is the first line of management?

    1. Captopril.

    2. Metoprolol.

    3. Thiazide.

    4. Furosemide.

193. A 50-year-old male patient underwent percutaneous transluminal coronary angioplasty 3 months ago because of severe anginal symptoms that were not controlled by medications. Over the last week he has started to complain of retrosternal chest pain that is aggravated by exercise and relieved by rest. What is the cause of the patient's symptoms?

    1. Dislocation of stent.

    2. Restenosis over the stent.

    3. New stenosis in another branch of the coronary artery.

    4. Embolus closes small branch of the coronary artery.

194. A 60-year-old man who is a heavy smoker with long-standing uncontrolled hypertension, diabetes mellitus, chronic kidney disease, and dyslipidemia presents to the outpatient clinic with shortness of breath, which happens with minimal effort. On physical exam, his blood pressure is 160/100 mmHg; otherwise his exam is unremarkable. Chest x-ray shows prominent left heart border and echocardiogram shows left ventricular hypertrophy. Which of the following risk factors is the main cause for this patient's symptoms?

    1. Uncontrolled hypertension.

    2. Smoking.

    3. Diabetes mellitus.

    4. Chronic kidney disease.

195. A 65-year-old male patient with a history of diabetes mellitus type 2 presented to the emergency department with retrosternal chest pain that radiated to the left arm and began 50 minutes ago. On physical exam, his blood pressure is 85/54 mmHg and his pulse is 40 beats/min. Lungs are clear and there is distension in jugular veins. Which of the following best describes this patient's electrocardiogram?

    1. ST elevation in leads II, III, and aVF.

    2. ST depression in lead V1.

    3. ST elevation in lead V4.

    4. ST elevation in V5 and V6.

196. A 50-year-old man with long-standing uncontrolled hypertension presents to the outpatient clinic with shortness of breath with minimal effort. On physical exam, his blood pressure is 160/100 mmHg and his pulse is 100 beats/min; otherwise his exam is unremarkable. Chest x-ray shows prominent left heart border. Which of the following will be found in echocardiograph?

    1. Akinetic movement of septal wall.

    2. Aortic valve stenosis.

    3. Foramen ovale.

    4. Left ventricular hypertrophy.

197. A 40-year-old previously healthy male patient visited his nurse practitioner for routine follow-up. On physical exam, his blood pressure is 120/75 mmHg and his pulse is 70 beats/min. Chest is clear with systolic ejection murmur. Echocardiograph shows right ventricular overload. Which of the following will be present in his electrocardiogram?

    1. Left bundle branch block.

    2. Right axis deviation.

    3. ST elevation in all leads.

    4. Short PR interval.

198. A 60-year-old man with a history of uncontrolled hypertension presented to the emergency department with a headache that started 2 hours ago and is associated with nausea, vomiting, and altered level of consciousness. On physical exam, he looks confused, his blood pressure is 240/130 mmHg, his pulse is 90 beats/min, and his lungs are clear; otherwise his exam is unremarkable. A computed tomography scan of his head shows no hemorrhage or mass. Which of the following is the next step of management?

    1. Order a magnetic resonance imaging of his brain.

    2. Give him nitroprusside.

    3. Give furosemide.

    4. Perform a lumbar puncture.

199. A 50-year-old female patient with uncontrolled hypertension presented with a pulsating mass in her abdomen. Abdominal ultrasound revealed a 5-cm aortic aneurysm. Which of the following is a contraindication for elective repair of an aortic aneurysm?

    1. Aneurysm size is less than 6 cm.

    2. Patient has history of metastatic pancreatic cancer.

    3. Patient with history of myocardial infarction 2 years ago.

    4. Aneurysm expansion of 0.5 cm per year.

200. A 55-year-old male patient, with uncontrolled hypertension, presented to the outpatient clinic with abdominal pain for the last 2 weeks. On exam, his blood pressure is 150/95 mmHg, his pulse is 90 beats/min, and there is a pulsating mass in the periumbilical region; otherwise his exam is unremarkable. Abdominal ultrasound shows a 6-cm aortic aneurysm. Which of the following is true about an aortic aneurysm?

    1. Most aortic aneurysms are in the thoracic region.

    2. The main cause of aortic aneurysm is atherosclerosis.

    3. Any aortic aneurysm more than 3 cm needs emergent repair.

    4. Mortality rate of aneurysm larger than 6 cm is only 10% per year.

201. A 60-year-old man who is a heavy smoker was diagnosed with chronic obstructive pulmonary disease 1 year ago. Recently, he has been diagnosed with hypertension, but he has not started medication for this yet. On exam, his blood pressure is 150/95 mmHg and his pulse is 80 beats/min. Which of the following is the first line of management for this patient?

    1. Metoprolol.

    2. Hydrochlorothiazide.

    3. Doxazosin.

    4. Furosemide.

202. A 67-year-old man with a history of hypertension is on one medication for this. He presented to the emergency department with swelling in the right big toe, which began a few hours ago. It is associated with hotness, redness, and limited joint movement. Which of the following has contributed to this patient's condition?

    1. Enalapril.

    2. Metoprolol.

    3. Hydrochlorothiazide.

    4. Doxazosin.

203. A 19-year-old female patient visited her nurse practitioner for routine follow-up. On physical exam, she is tall and thin with disproportionately long arms, legs, and fingers. Her blood pressure is 130/80 mmHg and her pulse is 80 beats/min. Cardiac exam revealed a systolic murmur with an S3 sound. Which of the following findings will be seen in his echocardiograph?

    1. Aortic stenosis.

    2. Tricuspid regurgitation.

    3. Ventricular-septal defect.

    4. Mitral regurgitation.

204. A 45-year-old male patient presented to the outpatient clinic with shortness of breath that has become significantly worse over the last couple of days. He has a history of stroke 6 months ago. On physical exam, his blood pressure is 120/80 mmHg and his pulse is 140 beats/min. Cardiac auscultation reveals a middiastolic rumble with an increasing intensity of S1. Chest x-ray shows a demarcated left border cardiac silhouette sign. Which of the following findings will be seen in the patient's electrocardiogram?

    1. Atrial fibrillation.

    2. ST elevation in leads II and III.

    3. Increase the amplitude of R wave in lead V5.

    4. PR depression in lead V1.

205. A 45-year-old male patient presented to the outpatient clinic with shortness of breath, which has become significantly worse over the last couple of days. He has a history of stroke 6 months ago. On the physical exam, his blood pressure is 120/80 mmHg and his pulse is 140 beats/min. Cardiac auscultation reveals a middiastolic rumble with an increasing intensity of S1. Chest x-ray shows a demarcated left border cardiac silhouette sign. Electrocardiogram shows atrial fibrillation. Which of the following is the pathological cause of the patient's condition?

    1. Senile aortic stenosis.

    2. Rheumatic mitral stenosis.

    3. Aortic aneurysm.

    4. Atrial septal defect.

206. A 67-year-old man with a history of hypertension, who is on hydrochlorothiazide, presented to the emergency department with swelling in the right big toe that began a few hours ago. It is associated with hotness, redness, and limited joint movement. Which of the following laboratory results will be seen with this patient?

    1. Elevation of liver enzymes.

    2. Increased uric acid level in the blood.

    3. Impaired kidney function.

    4. Decreased albumin level in serum.

207. A 55-year-old woman with a history of uncontrolled diabetes mellitus, neuropathy, uncontrolled hypertension, and dyslipidemia suddenly collapsed and died in her kitchen. Which of the following is the most likely cause of death?

    1. Pulmonary embolism.

    2. Septic shock.

    3. Myocardial infarction.

    4. Stroke.

208. A 55-year-old woman with a history of diabetes mellitus and hypertension presents to her nurse practitioner for routine follow-up. On physical exam, her blood pressure is 135/75 mmHg and her pulse is 80 beats/min; otherwise her exam is unremarkable. Urinalysis shows 3+ protein and 2+ glucose. Which of the following drugs is the best choice for this patient?

    1. Metoprolol.

    2. Hydrochlorothiazide.

    3. Enalapril.

    4. Doxazosin.

209. A 60-year-old male patient presented to the emergency department with retrosternal chest pain that started 2 hours ago. He has a history of diabetes mellitus. On physical exam, his blood pressure is 100/60 mmHg and his pulse is 130 beats/min. Electrocardiogram shows ST elevation in leads II, III, and aVF. He was admitted to the coronary care unit and he received alteplase. Two hours later, he died suddenly. Which of the following is the most likely cause of death after myocardial infarction?

    1. Rupture of the free ventricular wall.

    2. Arrhythmia.

    3. Pulmonary embolism.

    4. Pericardial tamponade.

210. A 45-year-old male patient visited his nurse practitioner for routine follow-up. On physical exam, his blood

pressure is 140/90 mmHg and his pulse is 80 beats/min. The nurse practitioner decides to prescribe atorvastatin. Which of the following is true regarding the pharmacological treatment of dyslipidemia?

    1. Pharmacological treatment should be prescribed for a diabetic patient with a low-density lipoprotein (LDL) level greater than 200 mg/dL.

    2. Pharmacological treatment should be prescribed for a patient with coronary artery disease with an LDL level greater than 130 mg/dL.

    3. Statin drugs are the only choice that leads to a decrease in cardiological mortality.

    4. Statin drugs do not decrease the mortality rate in a patient with coronary artery disease.

211. A 60-year-old man with diabetes mellitus and hypertension presented to the outpatient clinic with increased shortness of breath over the last 4 months associated with orthopnea. On physical exam, his blood pressure is 150/95 mmHg and his pulse is 80 beats/min. Chest auscultation revealed bilateral basal crackles. Chest x-ray shows cardiomegaly and pulmonary congestion. Which of the following is the next step of management?

    1. Coronary angiography.

    2. Exercise electrocardiogram.

    3. Computed tomography of the chest.

    4. Sleep study.

212. A 60-year-old man presented to the emergency department with retrosternal chest pain that started 30 minutes ago. Electrocardiogram showed ST elevation in V1 to V4, so the patient underwent percutaneous coronary intervention. Two days later, the patient was discharged on prasugrel. Which of the following is a contraindication for this drug?

    1. Patient with a history of unstable angina.

    2. Patient weight more than 60 kg.

    3. Patient with thrombocytopenia.

    4. Female patient.

213. A 50-year-old male patient with a history of severe angina underwent coronary angiography, which revealed that three main arteries were occluded. Ejection fraction is 35% according to his last echocardiography. Which of the following is the next step of management for this patient?

    1. Medical therapy.

    2. Antithrombolytic therapy.

    3. Coronary artery bypass graft.

    4. Percutaneous coronary intervention.

214. A 60-year-old Caucasian man, with a history of uncontrolled hypertension on amlodipine, visits his nurse practitioner for routine follow-up. On physical exam, his blood pressure is 150/95 mmHg and his pulse is 100 beats/min. He needs a second hypertensive drug. Which of the following is the best choice for this patient?

    1. Metoprolol.

    2. Enalapril.

    3. Hydrochlorothiazide.

    4. Diltiazem.

215. A 55-year-old man with a history of diabetes mellitus and hypertension was admitted to the coronary care unit with an inferior wall myocardial infarction. Today the patient was discharged on aspirin, atorvastatin, metformin, and clopidogrel. Which of the following medications will lead to reduction of mortality for this patient?

    1. Bisoprolol.

    2. Furosemide.

    3. Enalapril.

    4. Amlodipine.

216. A 55-year-old man presented to the emergency department with chest pain that started 30 minutes ago and nausea and diaphoresis. Electrocardiogram showed ST elevation in leads V1 to V4. Management of myocardial infarction was begun in this patient, which includes 300 mg aspirin, morphine, and oxygen. Which of the following is a contraindication for aspirin?

    1. Patient with a history of peptic ulcer.

    2. Patient with a history of allergy to aspirin.

    3. Patient with a history of upper gastrointestinal bleeding.

    4. Patient with a history of gastroesophageal reflux disease.

217. A 60-year-old man with a history of anterolateral myocardial infarction 6 weeks ago was discharged from hospital after 5 days. Today he visits his nurse practitioner because of increasing shortness of breath, especially after exercise. Electrocardiogram showed ST elevation in leads V1 to V4. Which of the following is the next step in management for this patient?

    1. Alteplase.

    2. Cardiac enzyme.

    3. Echocardiography.

    4. Coronary angiography.

218. A 60-year-old man has a history of anterolateral myocardial infarction (MI) 6 weeks ago and was discharged from hospital after 5 days. Today he visits his nurse practitioner because of increasing shortness of breath, especially after exercise. Electrocardiogram showed ST elevation in leads V1 to V4. Cardiac enzymes were normal. What is the patient's diagnosis?

    1. Pericarditis.

    2. New MI.

    3. Normal change after MI.

    4. Left ventricular aneurysm.

219. A 70-year-old male patient who is a heavy smoker with a history of hypertension is found dead in his home. The postmortem report revealed that the cause of death is rupture of an aortic aneurysm. What is the main cause of developing aortic aneurysm in this patient?

    1. Giant cell arteritis.

    2. Atherosclerosis.

    3. Thromboangiitis obliterans.

    4. Traumatic injury.

220. A 70-year-old male patient who is a heavy smoker with a history of hypertension, diabetes mellitus, and dyslipidemia is found dead in his home. The postmortem report revealed that the cause of death is rupture of an aortic aneurysm. Which of the following is not a risk factor for aortic aneurysm?

    1. Hypertension.

    2. Hypercholesterolemia.

    3. Diabetes mellitus.

    4. Aging.

221. A 60-year-old male patient presented to the outpatient clinic complaining of chest pain that happens when he lies down. In addition, he has a history of heart failure with an ejection fraction of 25%. On physical exam, his blood pressure is 120/80 mmHg and his pulse is 70 beats/min. What is the main diagnosis for the patient?

    1. Unstable angina.

    2. Decubitus angina.

    3. Aortic dissection.

    4. Muscle spasm.

222. A 55-year-old man with a history of uncontrolled hypertension for a long time presents to the emergency department with sudden severe chest pain radiating to his back that began 1 hour ago. He also complains of numbness in his right arm. On physical exam, his blood pressure is 190/105 mmHg and his pulse is 130 beats/min. Chest x-ray shows a widened mediastinum. What is the treatment of choice for this patient?

    1. Angiotensin-converting enzyme inhibitor.

    2. Beta-blocker.

    3. Amlodipine.

    4. Thiazide.

223. A 40-year-old man presented to the emergency department complaining of left leg pain that started 2 hours ago. He noticed that he has become progressively short of breath over the last week. He has a previous history of rheumatic heart disease. On exam, his blood pressure is 120/80 mmHg and his pulse is 140 beats/min. His leg appears pale with no pulse palpable in the posterior tibial artery. What is the main cause of the patient's symptoms?

    1. Embolus.

    2. Atherosclerosis.

    3. Deep venous thrombosis.

    4. Arteritis.

224. A 40-year-old man presented to the emergency department complaining of left leg pain that began 2 hours ago. He noticed that he has become progressively short of breath over the last week. He has a history of rheumatic heart disease. On exam, his blood pressure is 120/80 mmHg and his pulse is irregularly irregular. Cardiac auscultation revealed a systolic ejection murmur. His leg appears pale with no pulse palpable in the posterior tibial artery. What is the underlying cause of the patient's symptoms?

    1. Atrial fibrillation.

    2. Atrial septal defect.

    3. Aortic aneurysm.

    4. Deep vein thrombosis.

225. A 40-year-old man presented to the emergency department complaining of left leg pain that started 2 hours ago. He noticed that he has become progressively short of breath over the last week. On exam, his blood pressure is 120/80 mmHg and his pulse is irregularly irregular. Cardiac auscultation revealed a systolic ejection murmur. His leg appears pale with no pulse palpable in the posterior tibial artery. Which of the following is *not* considered a part of management choices?

    1. Aspirin.

    2. Heparin.

    3. Embolectomy.

    4. Catheter-directed thrombolysis.

226. A 66-year-old male patient presented to the emergency department with chest pain that started 1 hour ago. The pain radiates to his left arm and left jaw. He also has severe shortness of breath and diaphoresis. On physical exam, the patient's blood pressure is 80/50 mmHg, pulse is 40 beats/min, and the respiratory rate is 14 breaths/min. Which electrocardiographic change does not happen with a myocardial infarction?

    1. Left bundle branch block.

    2. Pathological Q wave.

    3. ST-elevation.

    4. Right bundle branch block.

227. A 50-year-old woman with a history of hypertension visits her nurse practitioner for routine follow-up. On physical exam, her blood pressure is 130/85 mmHg and her pulse is 80 beats/min. Her blood tests reveal sodium 135 mEq/L, potassium 2.9 mEq/L, creatinine 0.7 mg/dL, and glucose 100 mg/dL. Which medication would be first-line treatment for the patient?

    1. Enalapril.

    2. Amlodipine.

    3. Hydrochlorothiazide.

    4. Bisoprolol.

228. A 55-year-old man was discharged from a coronary care unit 2 weeks ago after a myocardial infarction. Today he presents to the emergency department with chest pain relieved by leaning forward. On physical exam, his blood pressure is 130/80 mmHg and his pulse is 90 beats/min. Cardiac exam revealed a friction rub. What is the next step of management?

    1. Echocardiography.

    2. Cardiac marker.

    3. Electrocardiogram.

    4. Chest x-ray.

229. A 55-year-old man was discharged from a coronary care unit 2 weeks ago after a myocardial infarction. Today he presents to the emergency department with chest pain that is relieved by leaning forward. On physical exam, his blood pressure is 130/80 mmHg and his pulse is 90 beats/min. Cardiac exam revealed a friction rub. Electrocardiogram showed ST elevation in all leads. Which is the next step of management?

    1. Nonsteroidal antiinflammatory drugs.

    2. Heparin.

    3. Paracetamol.

    4. Alteplase.

230. A 55-year-old Caucasian man was newly diagnosed with hypertension so he was placed on Norvasc. He presented to the outpatient clinic with bilateral ankle swelling. The patient does not have any history of trauma, dyspnea, or orthopnea. On physical exam, his blood pressure is 130/80 mmHg and his pulse is 80 beats/min. There is bilateral mild ankle swelling. The cardiac exam was normal. What is the cause of the leg swelling?

    1. Heart failure.

    2. Medication side effect.

    3. Deep vein thrombosis.

    4. Nephrotic syndrome.

231. A 55-year-old Caucasian man was newly diagnosed with hypertension and placed on single-drug therapy. He presented to the outpatient clinic with bilateral ankle swelling. The patient does not have any history of trauma. On physical exam, his blood pressure is 130/80 mmHg and his pulse is 80 beats/min. There is bilateral mild ankle swelling. Which of these drugs is the cause of the patients' symptoms?

    1. Thiazide.

    2. Amlodipine.

    3. Enalapril.

    4. Metoprolol.

232. A 55-year-old man with uncontrolled hypertension is on metolazone 5 mg. He visited his physician for routine follow-up. On physical exam, his blood pressure is 160/95 mmHg and his pulse is 90 beats/min. Which is the next step of management?

    1. Increase dose of thiazide.

    2. Switch from thiazide to enalapril.

    3. Add enalapril.

    4. Continue the same treatment.

233. A 21-year-old male patient presented to the emergency department after he was stabbed in his chest. He appeared confused, hypotensive, and had jugular venous distension. Cardiac auscultation revealed muffled heart sounds. Which of the following abnormalities will be found in his chest x-ray?

    1. Kerley B lines.

    2. Globular heart shape.

    3. Pulmonary congestion.

    4. Widening mediastinum.

234. A 55-year-old man with a history of hypertension presented to the emergency department with fatigue and weakness. On physical exam, his blood pressure is 130/80 mmHg and his pulse is 80 beats/min. His lab results are sodium 135 mEq/L, potassium 6 mEq/L, and creatinine 2 mg/dL. Which of these drugs is the cause of hyperkalemia in this patient?

    1. Bisoprolol.

    2. Hydrochlorothiazide.

    3. Aspirin.

    4. Lisinopril.

235. A 33-year-old man who has no past medical history visits his nurse practitioner for his annual physical. On exam, his blood pressure is 170/100 mmHg and his pulse is 90 beats/min; otherwise his exam is unremarkable. His father died from kidney problems at age 50. His creatinine is 2 mg/dL and potassium is 5.5 mEq/L. Which of the following investigations will help you to diagnose this patient's disease?

    1. Abdominal ultrasound.

    2. Arterial angiography.

    3. Echocardiography.

    4. 24-hour urine collection.

236. A 33-year-old man who has no past medical history visits his nurse practitioner for his annual physical. On exam, his blood pressure is 170/100 mmHg and his pulse is 90 beats/min; otherwise his exam is unremarkable. His father died from kidney problems at age 50. His creatinine is 2 mg/dL and potassium is 5.0 mEq/L. Which is the drug of choice for this patient?

    1. Captopril.

    2. Indapamide.

    3. Doxazosin.

    4. Metoprolol.

237. A 55-year-old man with a long-standing history of uncontrolled hypertension presents to the emergency department with sudden severe chest pain that radiated to his back and began 1 hour ago. He also complains of numbness in his right arm. On physical exam, his blood pressure is 190/105 mmHg and his pulse is 130 beats/min. Chest x-ray shows widened mediastinum. What is the definitive diagnostic test for this patient?

    1. Echocardiography.

    2. Electrocardiogram.

    3. Chest computed tomography scan with contrast.

    4. Pulmonary angiography.

238. A 60-year-old male patient presented to the outpatient clinic complaining of chest pain that happens when he lies down. In addition, he has a history of heart failure with an ejection fraction of 25%. On physical exam, his blood pressure is 120/80 mmHg and his pulse is 70 beats/min. Other exams are unremarkable. What will be the next step of management?

    1. Echocardiography.

    2. Chest computed tomography.

    3. Coronary angiography.

    4. Exercise electrocardiogram.

239. A 66-year-old man who has diabetes mellitus on metformin, aspirin, and atorvastatin visits his nurse practitioner for a routine follow-up. On physical exam, his blood pressure is 130/85 mmHg and his pulse is 80 beats/min. His laboratory results show creatinine is 0.9 mg/dL, fasting blood glucose is 200 mg/dL, triglyceride is 300 mg/dL, and high-density lipoprotein is 30 mg/dL. Which of the following will be needed to identify the cause of the patient's results?

    1. Hemoglobin A1c.

    2. Liver enzyme tests.

    3. Electrocardiogram.

    4. Sedimentation rate.

240. A 66-year-old man who has diabetes mellitus on metformin, aspirin, and 40 mg atorvastatin visited his physician for a routine follow-up. On physical exam, his blood pressure is 130/85 mmHg and his pulse is 80 beats/min. The other exam is unremarkable. His laboratory results show creatinine 0.9 mg/dL, fasting blood glucose 200 mg/dL, triglyceride 300 mg/dL, and high-density lipoprotein 30 mg/dL. What is the next step of his management?

    1. Add ezetimibe.

    2. Increase dose of atorvastatin.

    3. Add fenofibrate.

    4. Add cholestyramine.

241. A 50-year-old man arrives in the emergency department via ambulance after he lost consciousness during exercise. He regained consciousness immediately but reports some chest pain right before he "passed out." He also reports that this has happened before and that lately, he feels very tired after routine exertion. When asked if he has any palpitations, he says, "It feels like my heart beat jumps around in my chest sometimes." He also reports that he feels short of breath after walking three blocks. On physical exam, his blood pressure is 130/85 mmHg and his pulse is 100 beats/min. The cardiac exam revealed a systolic ejection murmur with a narrow pulse. Which of the following is appropriate management for this patient?

    1. Heparin.

    2. Aortic valve replacement.

    3. Aspirin, clopidogrel, and statin.

    4. Aortic valvuloplasty.

242. A 60-year-old man was admitted to the coronary artery unit 4 days ago because of an inferior wall myocardial infarction, and he received appropriate management. Today he is discharged on aspirin, bisoprolol, clopidogrel, and simvastatin. What is the mechanism of action of simvastatin?

    1. Sequestration of bile acid.

    2. Decrease absorption of cholesterol.

    3. Decrease synthesis of cholesterol.

    4. Decrease oxidation of fatty acid.

243. An 85-year-old man with hypertension on a thiazide diuretic and aliskiren visited his nurse practitioner for routine follow-up. On physical exam, his blood pressure is 130/85 mmHg and his pulse is 80 beats/min. What is the mechanism of action of aliskiren?

    1. Inhibition of the angiotensin-converting enzyme.

    2. Direct aldosterone receptor blocker.

    3. Decrease absorption of sodium from proximal convoluted tubule.

    4. Renin inhibitor.

244. A 50-year-old man presented to the emergency department with right-sided weakness that began 1 hour ago. On physical exam, his blood pressure is 140/90 mmHg and his pulse is 100 beats/min. Neurological exam revealed right-sided weakness with muscle power of 1/5. Ten minutes later, his symptoms resolved and muscle power returned to normal (5/5). Brain computed tomography was normal. What is your next step in management of this patient?

    1. Brain magnetic resonance imaging.

    2. Carotid ultrasound.

    3. Echocardiograph.

    4. Electrocardiogram.

245. A 50-year-old man presented with right-sided weakness that began 1 hour ago. On physical exam, his blood pressure is 140/90 mmHg and his pulse is 100 beats/min. Neurological exam revealed right-sided weakness with muscle power of 1/5. Ten minutes later, his symptoms resolved and muscle power returned to normal (5/5). Brain computed tomography was unremarkable. Carotid ultrasound shows 80% stenosis in the left carotid artery. What is the next step in management of this patient?

    1. Aspirin.

    2. Left carotid endarterectomy.

    3. Warfarin.

    4. Clopidogrel.

246. A 60-year-old male patient with a history of pancreatic cancer has just recovered from Whipple surgery. He presented to the emergency department with retrosternal chest pain that started 45 minutes ago. On physical exam, his blood pressure is 120/90 mmHg and his pulse is 120 beats/min. Electrocardiogram showed ST elevation in leads V1 to V4. What is the most appropriate management of this patient?

    1. Alteplase.

    2. Coronary artery bypass graft.

    3. Angioplasty.

    4. Aspirin.

247. A 35-year-old female patient with a history of hypertension and currently 10 weeks' pregnant visits her nurse practitioner for routine follow-up. On physical exam, her blood pressure is 140/90 mmHg and her pulse is 90 beats/min. Her urine dipstick and funduscopy were standard. Electrocardiogram shows normal sinus rhythm. What is the target blood pressure level in this patient?

    1. 120/80 mmHg.

    2. 150/100 mmHg.

    3. 140/90 mmHg.

    4. 100/70 mmHg.

248. An 80-year-old man with no past medical history is seen by his nurse practitioner for his annual exam. His blood pressure is 160/100 mmHg and his pulse is 80 beats/min. He reports that he checks his blood pressure at those machines in the drug store and his "blood pressure is always that high." He quit smoking 10 years ago. His body mass index is 25 kg/m^2. What is your next step in management of this patient?

    1. Prescribe antihypertensive for him.

    2. Ambulatory 24-hour blood pressure.

    3. Aspirin.

    4. 24-hour urine collection

249. A 55-year-old man presents with recurrent retrosternal chest pain that happens during exercise and is relieved by rest within 5 minutes. He also has a history of hypertension and diabetes mellitus. His electrocardiogram was normal and cardiac enzymes are within the normal range. Later, the patient underwent coronary artery angiography. Which is considered significant coronary artery disease?

    1. Stenosis is more than 50% in one of the epicardial arteries.

    2. Stenosis is more than 30% in an anemic patient.

    3. Stenosis is more than 50% in the left coronary artery.

    4. Stenosis is more than 50% in one of the epicardial arteries with well-developed collateral.

250. A 65-year-old man with a known history of diabetes mellitus was recently discharged from the coronary care unit after he had an inferior myocardial infarction (MI). Which of the following is the best measure for reducing secondary MI risk?

    1. Prescribe omega-3 fatty acid capsule.

    2. Take vitamin C 500 mg daily.

    3. Stop drinking alcohol.

    4. Exercise for 20 to 30 minutes daily.

251. A 55-year-old female patient was admitted to the hospital because of a femoral neck fracture. Five days later, she started to complain of weakness on the right side with change in her mental status. On physical exam, her blood pressure is 120/70 mmHg and her pulse is 90 beats/min. Neurological exam revealed muscle power in the right arm is 0/5 and in the right leg is 2/5 with dysarthria. Leg exam revealed right thigh swelling. Brain computed tomography (CT) showed evidence of infarction in the left middle cerebral artery zone. After treating this patient with appropriate management, which of the following tests will help to discover the cause of her illness?

    1. Echocardiography.

    2. Carotid Doppler.

    3. Abdominal CT angiography.

    4. Anticardiolipin antibody.

252. A 65-year-old woman who has no past medical history presented to the emergency department with retrosternal chest pain that radiates to her left arm and jaw and began 60 minutes ago. She complains of nausea and diaphoresis. On physical exam, her blood pressure is 170/70 mmHg and her pulse is 140 beats/min. Electrocardiogram showed ST elevation in leads II, III, and aVF. Which of the following arteries is responsible for this patient's symptoms?

    1. Right coronary artery.

    2. Left anterior descending artery.

    3. Circumflex branch of left coronary artery.

    4. Diagonal branch of the left coronary artery.

253. A 30-year-old female patient presented with shortness of breath that started a couple months ago; it is progressive and worsens during exercise. On physical exam, her blood pressure was 130/80 mmHg and her pulse was irregularly irregular. The cardiac survey revealed a mid-diastolic rumble. Which of the following findings will appear on her electrocardiogram?

    1. ST depression in V1.

    2. Inverted T wave in aVF.

    3. Peaked P-wave.

    4. PR depression in all leads.

254. A 30-year-old female patient presented with shortness of breath that started a couple of months ago; it is progressive and increases during exercise. On physical exam,

her blood pressure was 130/80 mmHg and her pulse was irregularly irregular. Her cardiac survey revealed a middiastolic rumble. Echocardiography showed mitral stenosis. What is the cause of her symptoms?

1. Calcified mitral stenosis.

2. Rheumatic fever.

3. Mitral valve prolapse.

4. Carcinoid syndrome.

255. A 60-year-old woman is diagnosed with hypertension by her nurse practitioner who prescribed enalapril to manage her blood pressure. Which of the following tests should be ordered before the patient starts taking enalapril?

    1. Liver enzymes.

    2. Electrolytes.

    3. Electrocardiogram.

    4. Cortisol level.

256. A 35-year-old healthy woman visits the outpatient clinic because of chest discomfort and lightheadedness that began a couple of days ago. She has no medical history, but she recently had a viral upper respiratory tract infection. On physical exam, she appears well, her blood pressure is 130/80 mmHg, and her pulse is regular and within the normal range. Cardiac auscultation reveals distant heart sounds. What does the nurse practitioner suspect the electrocardiogram will show?

    1. Diffuse ST elevation in pericardial leads.

    2. Large P-wave.

    3. Electrical alternans.

    4. PR depression.

257. A 30-year-old homeless man presented to the emergency department with fever, fatigue, and sudden shortness of breath that began yesterday. After undergoing an appropriate exam, he was diagnosed with infective endocarditis. Which of the following will raise the suspicion that this patient has an acute aortic regurgitation?

    1. Narrow pulse pressure.

    2. High blood pressure.

    3. Systolic ejection murmur.

    4. Peripheral vasoconstriction.

258. A 50-year-old man with uncontrolled hypertension on three different medications visited his nurse practitioner for routine follow-up. On physical exam, his blood pressure is 180/100 mmHg and his pulse is 120 beats/min. His lab results show sodium 150 mEq/L, potassium 2.9 mEq/L, and creatinine 0.9 mg/dL. Abdominal ultrasound was normal. Which of the following is the leading cause of the patient's condition?

    1. Polycystic kidney disease.

    2. Renal artery stenosis.

    3. Primary hyperaldosteronism.

    4. Pheochromocytoma.

259. A 58-year-old man complains of calf pain after walking three blocks. He has no history of coronary artery disease or transient ischemic attacks. He is allergic to aspirin. The physical exam reveals multiple leg ulcers. Computed tomography angiography shows peripheral artery disease. What is the best management option in this patient?

    1. Heparin.

    2. Warfarin.

    3. Clopidogrel.

    4. Dabigatran.

260. A 66-year-old woman presented with retrosternal chest pain that began 40 minutes ago. Electrocardiogram showed ST elevation in leads V1 to V4. She was managed by aspirin and clopidogrel. Minutes later, she developed ventricular fibrillation and resuscitation was done. Which of the following can improve long-term survival in this patient?

    1. Thrombolysis.

    2. Warfarin.

    3. Implanted cardiac device.

    4. Bisoprolol.

261. A 50-year-old woman with no past medical history presented to the emergency department with retrosternal chest pain that radiates to her left arm and jaw and nausea and diaphoresis. The pain began 40 minutes ago. On physical exam, her blood pressure is 170/70 mmHg and his pulse is 140 beats/min. Electrocardiogram showed ST depression in leads V1 to V3. Which artery is responsible for the patient's symptoms?

    1. Right coronary artery.

    2. Left anterior descending artery.

    3. Circumflex branch of left coronary artery.

    4. Diagonal branch of the left coronary artery.

262. A young female patient with a history of end-stage renal disease presented with sharp chest pain relieved by leaning forward. On physical exam, she appears pale and tired. Electrocardiogram showed T-wave inversion in V4 to V5. Her laboratory results show creatinine 4 mg/dL and urea 120 mg/dL. What is the appropriate next step in this patient's management?

    1. Nonsteroidal antiinflammatory drugs.

    2. Heparin.

    3. Steroid.

    4. Hemodialysis.

263. A 60-year-old gentleman is prepared for laparoscopic cholecystectomy. An abdominal ultrasound was done before surgery and showed an aortic aneurysm 4 cm below the level of the renal artery. Which of the following factors increase the risk of expansion and rupture?

    1. Smoking.

    2. Diabetes mellitus.

    3. Male.

    4. Hypertension.

264. A 35-year-old healthy female patient comes to the outpatient clinic because of chest discomfort and lightheadedness that began a couple of days ago. She has no past medical history, but she recently recovered from an upper respiratory tract infection. On physical exam, she appears well, her blood pressure is 130/80 mmHg, and her pulse is regular within the normal range. Cardiac auscultation reveals distant heart sounds, and the nurse practitioner suspects this patient has a pericardial effusion. Which of the following tests will establish the patient's diagnosis?

    1. Electrocardiogram (ECG).

    2. Chest computed tomography.

    3. Echocardiography.

    4. Exercise ECG.

265. A 60-year-old man who works as an accountant presented to his nurse practitioner with complaints of right calf pain. The pain begins after he has walked for three blocks and is relieved by rest. The right ankle-brachial index was 0.6. This patient has a high risk for which of the following in the next 5 years?

    1. Leg amputation.

    2. Myocardial infarction.

    3. Lung cancer.

    4. Aortic dissection.

266. A 60-year-old man was admitted to the coronary care unit because of an inferior wall myocardial infarction 5 days ago, and he was treated by thrombolysis. Today he started to complain of chest pain similar to the chest pain he previously experienced. His vital signs are within normal limits and cardiac exam revealed normal S1, S2 with no murmur. Which of the following tests will be useful in this situation?

    1. Lactic acid dehydrogenase.

    2. Troponin I.

    3. Creatine kinase myocardial band.

    4. Alkaline phosphatase.

267. A 30-year-old female patient visited her nurse practitioner with complaints of recurrent shortness of breath during exercise that has been getting progressively worse. On physical exam, her vital signs are within normal limits and her cardiac exam revealed systolic ejection murmur. Echocardiography discovered an ostium secundum atrial septal defect. Which of the following is correct?

    1. Ostium secundum is associated with left axis deviation on electrocardiogram.

    2. Surgical indication only when pulmonary pressure is less than 1.5 systematic pressure.

    3. Usually asymptomatic in childhood.

    4. Echocardiography will reveal left ventricular volume overload.

268. A 60-year-old female patient with a history of end-stage renal disease on hemodialysis was found dead in her bed by her husband. The postmortem report revealed the cause of death as myocardial infarction (MI). Which of the following is the likely cause of MI in this patient?

    1. Atherosclerosis.

    2. Coronary artery aneurysm.

    3. Arterial calcification.

    4. Aortic dissection.

269. A young man goes to his nurse practitioner for his annual physical exam. He is in good health, he does not smoke, and he has no past medical history. On physical exam, his blood pressure is 120/70 mmHg and his pulse is 80 beats/min. The cardiac exam revealed systolic click with late systolic murmur. All his laboratory results are within the normal range. Which test will aid in diagnosing this patient?

    1. Electrocardiogram (ECG).

    2. Echocardiography.

    3. Exercise ECG.

    4. Computed tomography angiography.

270. A 50-year-old man who is a heavy smoker and has a history of chronic kidney disease presented with sudden-onset chest pain that radiates to the back. On physical exam, his blood pressure in the left arm is 190/90 mmHg and in the right arm is 140/70 mmHg. The cardiac auscultation revealed regular S1, S2 with no murmur. Chest x-ray showed widened mediastinum, and his creatinine is 2.5 mg/dL. What is the best next step of management for this patient?

    1. Transesophageal echocardiography.

    2. Trans-sternum echocardiography.

    3. Coronary angiography.

    4. Computed tomography pulmonary angiography.

271. A young man visits his nurse practitioner for his annual physical exam. He has no past medical history and he does not smoke. On physical exam, his blood pressure is 120/70 mmHg and his pulse is 80 beats/min. The cardiac exam revealed systolic click with a late systolic murmur. The rest of the checkup was normal, and all his laboratory results are within the normal range. What is the most likely cause of murmur in this patient?

    1. Physiological variant.

    2. Atrial septal defect.

    3. Mitral valve prolapse.

    4. Ventricular septal defect.

272. A 70-year-old man was admitted to the coronary care unit for elective angiography after he complained of recurrent retrosternal chest pain that happens mainly after exercise and is relieved by rest. His electrocardiogram (ECG) was normal and exercise ECG was positive. Angiography did not find any significant stenosis in the coronary branches. Which of the following may help the physician to diagnose this patient?

    1. Computed tomography (CT) calcium score.

    2. Echocardiography.

    3. High-resolution CT scan.

    4. Cardiac enzymes.

273. A young man presented to the emergency department with increased shortness of breath during exercise. He feels anxious and fatigued. Cardiac auscultation revealed systolic click with a late systolic murmur. His electrocardiogram was normal. The nurse practitioner suspects he has mitral valve prolapse. Which of these diseases is not a complication of the patient's condition?

1. Atrial fibrillation.

2. Myocardial infarction.

3. Infective endocarditis.

4. Mitral regurgitation.

274. A 45-year-old female patient who has a history of systemic lupus and antiphospholipid syndrome presented to the emergency department with sudden-onset chest pain associated with shortness of breath and hemoptysis. She is hypotensive and her pulse is 150 beats/min. Oxygen saturation was 80% on room air and she has right thigh swelling. Computed tomography angiography confirmed pulmonary embolism. What is the next step in treating this patient?

1. Heparin.

2. Echocardiography.

3. Thrombolysis.

4. Warfarin.

275. A 70-year-old man presented to the emergency department with sudden pain in his left arm and paresthesia. He denies any history of trauma. The muscle power in his left arm is 0/5 but in his left leg it is 5/5. His left radial pulse is absent, but the pulse is palpable in the contralateral side. Electrocardiogram showed atrial fibrillation. Which of the following is the next step in treating this patient?

1. Warfarin.

2. Intravenous heparin.

3. Trans-sternum echocardiography.

4. Clopidogrel.

276. A 60-year-old male patient with a history of diabetes mellitus, hypertension, and dyslipidemia presented with right calf muscle pain after walking four blocks; it is relieved by rest. The right posterior tibial artery pulse is palpable but weak. Which of the following is the next step in treating this patient?

1. Computed tomography angiography.

2. Ankle-brachial index.

3. Ultrasound for lower limbs.

4. Exercise tolerance test.

Cardiovascular Answers & Rationales

2

1. Answer: 1

Rationale: This patient with a previous history of upper respiratory tract infection probably suffered from a developing cardiac tamponade. This resulted in a pericardial effusion that formed as a complication of the previous upper respiratory infection. The electrocardiogram findings described the typical electrical alternans that is seen in cardiac tamponade as a result of the heart swinging back and forth within the increased amount of fluid in the pericardial cavity.

2. Answer: 4

Rationale: Beck's triad alerts clinicians that cardiac tamponade is potentially present. The main components of cardiac tamponade are hypotension, muffled heart sounds, and jugular venous distension. This triad is often associated with prominent x-descent and absent y-descent and pulsus paradoxus. These features are caused by failure of ventricular filling and limited cardiac output. The Kussmaul sign is seen in restrictive cardiomyopathy and constrictive pericarditis. A friction rub can be seen in any condition associated with pericardial inflammation.

3. Answer: 3

Rationale: This patient most likely has a developing cardiac tamponade from a previously formed pericardial effusion. Melanoma is a known tumor to infiltrate the pericardium. Cardiac tamponade is characterized by increased jugular venous pressure, muffled heart sounds, hypotension, and pulsus paradoxus (greater than 10 mmHg drop in systolic blood pressure with inspiration). Answer 1 is not correct because the JVP increases. A pericardial knock is more likely to be noted in constrictive pericarditis.

4. Answer: 3

Rationale: This patient most likely has cardiac tamponade, which is characterized by altered and varied QRS complexes from beat to beat caused by the heart swinging in the accumulating fluid in the pericardial cavity.

5. Answer: 4

Rationale: Cardiac tamponade is associated with sinus tachycardia in almost all cases, but sinus bradycardia could be found in subacute cardiac tamponade associated with hypothyroidism. The Beck triad (hypotension, increased jugular venous pressure, muffled heart sounds), pulsus paradoxus, and peripheral edema also are present in patients with cardiac tamponade.

6. Answer: 3

Rationale: All the previous facts are true about cardiac tamponade except that the Beck triad, which consists of hypotension, elevated jugular venous pressure, and muffled heart sounds, is present in only a minority of patients.

7. Answer: 4

Rationale: Drug-induced cardiac tamponade is rare. Procainamide, isoniazid, and hydralazine (drug-induced lupus) are involved in cardiac tamponade formation. Others drugs found in drug-induced cardiac tamponade include dantrolene, anticoagulants, thrombolytics, phenytoin, penicillin, and doxorubicin.

8. Answer: 2

Rationale: This patient with suspected acute cardiac tamponade is hemodynamically unstable. Both catheter pericardiocentesis and surgical drainage of a pericardial effusion are highly effective at removal of pericardial fluid. Catheter pericardiocentesis is the treatment of choice because it is less invasive, less expensive, and does not need general anesthesia, which may worsen the hemodynamic compromise if needle drainage is not performed first to reduce the severity of the cardiac tamponade.

9. Answer: 4

Rationale: This patient with a previous history of diabetes mellitus, hypertension, and long history of heavy smoking with presentation of sudden stabbing back pain, severe hypotension, muffled heart sounds, and increased jugular venous pressure is most likely suffering from aortic dissection complicated by cardiac tamponade. Aortic dissection and myocardial rupture are contraindications for catheter pericardiocentesis because the relief of cardiac tamponade may lead to more severe bleeding. Such patients require immediate surgical intervention.

10. Answer: 2

Rationale: This patient with a history of acute pericarditis now presents with cardiac tamponade, which occurs in 15% of cases of acute pericarditis. He is unlikely to have Kussmaul sign (increase un jugular venous pressure with inspiration) because this is usually seen in constrictive pericarditis. The other choices are true, and all can be found in cardiac tamponade.

11. Answer: 1

Rationale: Pulsus paradoxus (drop in systolic blood pressure [SBP] more than 10 mmHg during inspiration) is the most sensitive sign in cardiac tamponade. A drop in SBP more than 20 mmHg while changing the position of the patient is characteristic for orthostatic hypotension. Distant heart sounds can be found in cardiac tamponade, but it is not the most sensitive sign.

12. Answer: 4

Rationale: This patient with cardiac tamponade is hemodynamically unstable and preload dependent. He should not be given diuretics, nitrates, or morphine because they could exacerbate his compromise. The patient should be supported with intravenous fluid while waiting for the pericardiocentesis to protect him from more deterioration.

13. Answer: 1

Rationale: This patient presents with cardiac tamponade. He is hypotensive, has muffled heart sounds, and increased jugular venous pressure, so the three components of the Beck triad are present. The accumulated fluid in the pericardial cavity will increase the intrapericardial pressure above the diastolic ventricular pressure. This restricts venous return to the heart and lowers right and left ventricular filling. The net result is decreased preload, stroke volume, and cardiac output. Cardiac tamponade is caused by fluid accumulation in the pericardial cavity that increases the intrapericardial pressure above the diastolic ventricular pressure. This restricts venous return to the heart and lowers right and left ventricular filling. Cardiac tamponade will decrease the compliance of the right ventricle, so during inspiration and because of increased intrathoracic pressure and increased venous return the right ventricle will shift the interventricular septum toward the left ventricle and reduce its filling.

14. Answer: 4

Rationale: This patient most likely has cardiac tamponade. She is hypotensive, her jugular veins are distended, and her heart sounds are muffled. Intraarterial catheter in the radial artery shows pulsus paradoxus (more than 10 mmHg drop in the systolic blood pressure during inspiration), which is common in patients with cardiac tamponade.

15. Answer: 4

Rationale: This patient with low blood pressure, tachycardia, and distended jugular veins after blunt thoracic trauma most likely has acute cardiac tamponade. Only 100 to 200 mL of fluid is sufficient to accumulate in the pericardial cavity to compress the four cardiac chambers and compromise both venous return and cardiac output. A chest x-ray could be normal because of the small amount of fluid present.

16. Answer: 1

Rationale: This patient most likely presents with dilated cardiomyopathy. Dilated left ventricle on echocardiography with a reduced ejection fraction of 24% (systolic dysfunction) with heavy alcohol intake and normal angiography all suggest the diagnosis. Dilated cardiomyopathy can lead to heart failure, which is demonstrated by his dyspnea, S3 sound, and systolic dysfunction. Alcohol-related dilated cardiomyopathy should not be diagnosed until the exclusion of other causes of cardiomyopathy such as coronary artery disease and valvular diseases. Abstinence from alcohol will improve left ventricular function over time.

17. Answer: 4

Rationale: This patient most likely presents with heart failure as a result of dilated cardiomyopathy, which results from viral myocarditis. Many viruses are involved in myocarditis, such as adenovirus, human immunodeficiency virus, influenza, parvovirus B19, coxsackievirus, and human herpesvirus 6. In most cases of viral myocarditis, there will be dilated cardiomyopathy and the patient will present to the clinic with a picture of heart failure (dyspnea, edema, S3 sound) caused by systolic dysfunction of the heart. Few patients with viral myocarditis will not develop dilated cardiomyopathy and will only suffer from chest pain that mimics myocardial infarction.

18. Answer: 3

Rationale: This patient most likely presents with heart failure (dyspnea, elevated jugular venous pressure, S3 sound, edema), which results from dilated cardiomyopathy and is a complication of viral myocarditis. Many viruses are involved in myocarditis such as adenovirus, human immunodeficiency virus, influenza, parvovirus B19, coxsackievirus, and human herpesvirus 6. In most cases of viral myocarditis, there will be dilated cardiomyopathy and the patient will present to emergency department with a picture of heart failure.

19. Answer: 2

20. Answer: 2

21. Answer: 4

22. Answer: 4

23. Answer: 4

Rationale: This patient presents with a sudden attack of syncope during exercise, S4 sound, systolic murmur on the left sternal border, and family history of sudden cardiac death at a young age. This all suggests the diagnosis of hypertrophic cardiomyopathy. This disease is inherited as an autosomal dominant caused by mutations in one of several sarcomere genes encoding the myocardial contractile proteins of the heart. This mutation will lead to asymmetrical hypertrophy of the interventricular septum causing obstruction for the ventricular output, which is responsible for the harsh systolic murmur best heard at the apex and left lower sternal border. The main abnormality of the mitral valve in this lesion is systolic anterior motion (SAM; or prolapse) of the mitral valve, so the anterior motion of the mitral valve leaflets will move toward the interventricular septum during systole causing obstruction and murmur. Patients with symptoms (heart failure, angina, syncope) should be treated with negative inotropic agents (beta-blockers, nondihydropyridine calcium channel blockers) as the initial medical therapy because they prolong diastole and decrease myocardial contractility. The best initial medical monotherapy is a beta-blocker (metoprolol). Any maneuver that increases the venous return to the heart will decrease left ventricular filling, increasing the intensity of the murmur. Valsalva maneuver and standing will increase the intensity of the hypertrophic cardiomyopathy murmur.

24. Answer: 3

Rationale: Amyloidosis, which is a systemic disease caused by fibril deposition in multiple organs, is the most likely diagnosis in this patient. Cardiac amyloidosis should be suspected in patients who have manifestations of congestive heart failure (dyspnea, lower extremity edema, jugular venous distention, ascites) with echocardiographic findings of concentric left ventricular hypertrophy and a nondilated left ventricular cavity (diastolic dysfunction). As the fibril deposition occurs, the left ventricular wall thickness increases, and cavity size decreases and restrictive physiology develops. Atrial enlargement is common and cardiac conduction abnormalities may occur. Restrictive cardiomyopathy is less common than dilated and hypertrophic cardiomyopathy, but it is such an important cause of heart failure with preserved ejection fraction. Other manifestations of amyloidosis are nephrotic syndrome, anemia, waxy skin, easy bruising with ecchymosis, hepatomegaly, gastrointestinal bleeding, early satiety, subcutaneous nodules, enlarged tongue, and peripheral or autonomic neuropathy.

25. Answer: 4

Rationale: This patient most likely has hypertrophic cardiomyopathy, which is the most common cause for sudden cardiac death in athletes. His positive family history also suggests the diagnosis. This disease causes a systolic murmur best heard at the apex and left sternal border, and its intensity is increased by decreased venous return to the heart. Valsalva maneuver and standing both increase the intensity of the murmur. In contrast to patients with aortic stenosis, these patients have strong carotid pulses.

26. Answer: 1

Rationale: Maneuvers that decrease venous return to the heart and so decrease left ventricular filling will enhance the intensity of hypertrophic cardiomyopathy murmur such as the Valsalva maneuver and changing from the squatting position to the standing position. Squatting, leaning forward while sitting, and handgrip will increase left ventricular filling thus decreasing the intensity of the murmur.

27. Answer: 4

Rationale: Familial cardiomyopathy is associated with many cytoskeletal abnormalities; cardiac biopsy is not generally indicated unless the patient is referred to specialist care centers. A chest x-ray can show enlargement of the heart. An electrocardiogram can show ST segment changes. Echocardiography can show ventricular dilation on either the left or right side. Cardiac magnetic resonance is useful in exploring the presence of thrombus in dilated cardiomyopathy.

28. Answer: 1

Rationale: This patient with atrial fibrillation most likely presents with tachycardia-induced cardiomyopathy. A variety of tachyarrhythmias with prolonged periods of rapid ventricular rates can lead to this condition. These tachyarrhythmias include atrial fibrillation, atrial flutter, and ventricular tachycardia. Chronic tachycardia causes structural changes in the heart including left ventricular dilation and myocardial dysfunction. Most patients will present with signs and symptoms of congestive heart failure. This condition is treated by aggressive rate control or restoration of normal sinus rhythm because of the potential reversibility of tachycardia-induced cardiomyopathy.

29. Answer: 2

Rationale: Selenium deficiency is one of the reversible causes of dilated cardiomyopathy.

30. Answer: 1

Rationale: The main feature of hypertrophic cardiomyopathy that leads to its signs and symptoms is asymmetrical septal hypertrophy along with systolic anterior motion of the mitral valve leaflets. Both cause obstruction and the appearance of consequent complications.

31. Answer: 4

Rationale: Hypertrophic cardiomyopathy (HCM) puts the patient at risk of sudden cardiac death caused by ventricular fibrillation/ventricular tachycardia (VT).

There are five poor prognostic factors that are predictive of sudden cardiac death:

1. Family history of HCM and sudden cardiac death.
2. Maximum left ventricular wall thickness greater than 3 cm.
3. Syncope.
4. Blood pressure drop during peak exercise on stress testing.
5. Documented runs of nonsustained VT on 24-hour tape.

Left ventricular (LV) outflow obstruction causes symptoms and can deteriorate LV function, but it does not predict sudden cardiac death.

32. Answer: 2

33. Answer: 2

Rationale: This patient most likely presents with myocarditis that often causes dilated cardiomyopathy and heart failure. Some patients do not develop dilated cardiomyopathy and will only complain of chest pain, palpitation, and fever with complete recovery. With myocarditis, troponin I is elevated. One of the most likely causes for myocarditis is coxsackie B virus.

34. Answer: 3

Rationale: This patient most likely has hereditary hemochromatosis, an autosomal recessive disease characterized by accumulation of iron in multiple organ system. It is also called bronze diabetes because it causes hyperpigmentation of the skin (bronze color) and diabetes mellitus. Hereditary hemochromatosis also causes reversible dilated cardiomyopathy and arthropathy. This young male patient who presents with a typical picture of hemochromatosis must be further investigated to rule out the disease, so we will request a ferritin level.

35. Answer: 3

Rationale: Hereditary hemochromatosis causes reversible dilated cardiomyopathy. The only reversible complications of hemochromatosis when treated probably are skin manifestations and dilated cardiomyopathy.

36. Answer: 2

Rationale: Trastuzumab is a monoclonal antibody used to treat breast cancer. It is specifically used for breast cancer that is HER2 receptor positive. Doxorubicin is an anthracycline drug used as chemotherapy. It activates the stress signal pathway within the heart, so it inhibits these receptors. Although HER2 activation is protective against the damage that stress signaling induces, its inhibition removes this protection leading to dilated cardiomyopathy.

37. Answer: 2

Rationale: This patient with alcoholic liver disease and cirrhotic liver most likely has cardiomyopathy of alcoholism that is in its dilated or congestive form.

38. Answer: 1

Rationale: Jerky pulse (in which the artery is suddenly and markedly distended) is typically associated with hypertrophic cardiomyopathy, but hypertrophic cardiomyopathy can present with a completely normal physical exam.

39. Answer: 3

Rationale: Resting electrocardiogram and transthoracic echocardiography are the most effective screening strategies for relatives of patients with hypertrophic cardiomyopathy. Genetic study is not used as a first-line screening tool because of varying rates of penetrance.

40. Answer: 4

Rationale: This patient with hypertrophic cardiomyopathy is at increased risk for sudden cardiac death caused by ventricular fibrillation or ventricular tachycardia. Implantable cardiac defibrillators (ICDs) are superior to amiodarone or beta-blockers for preventing this. Other indications for ICD implantation include the following:

1. Cardiac arrest after ventricular fibrillation/ventricular tachycardia (VT).
2. Sustained VT causing hemodynamic compromise.
3. Chronic heart failure or left ventricular ejection fraction of less than 40% and associated syncopal episodes caused by nonsustained VT post myocardial infarction, nonsustained VT with left ventricular ejection fraction less than 40%.
4. Arrhythmogenic right ventricular cardiomyopathy causing cardiac arrest.
5. Congenital long QT with family history of sudden cardiac death at young age.

41. Answer: 3

Rationale: The most common electrocardiogram abnormality in patients with pulmonary embolism is sinus tachycardia.

42. Answer: 4

Rationale: Second-degree heart block (Mobitz II) is not treated with atropine because it has no effect on this conduction disease. The first line of management for both third-degree heart block and Mobitz II is pacing.

43. Answer: 4

Rationale: The most common cause of third-degree heart block is simple fibrous degenerative changes. Third-degree heart block is characterized by complete dissociation between QRS complexes and P-waves. It also can be caused by other factors mentioned in the question's options, but simple fibrous degenerative change is the most common cause for it.

44. Answer: 4

Rationale: All of the described statements about multifocal atrial tachycardia (MAT) are true, except the last one. We prefer to use diltiazem, verapamil, or digoxin and avoid beta-blockers because of the lung disease that most often presents in patients with MAT.

45. Answer: 4

Rationale: Amiodarone is a class III antiarrhythmic drug that is often used for management of ventricular arrhythmias in patients with coronary artery disease and ischemic cardiomyopathy. It causes several potential adverse effects. Pulmonary toxicity is a serious side effect of long-term use of this drug. Chronic interstitial pneumonitis is the most common complication, but acute respiratory distress syndrome can occur. Long-term monitoring of several parameters (pulmonary function and thyroid tests) is recommended for early detection and recognition of potential side effects from its use.

46. Answer: 3

47. Answer: 3

Rationale: This hypertensive and diabetic patient suffers from atrial fibrillation as his electrocardiogram illustrates. Management of new-onset atrial fibrillation includes assessing for a rate versus rhythm control strategy and preventing embolization. A stable patient can receive medical therapy (e.g., beta-blockers, diltiazem, digoxin) to control ventricular rate. Emergent cardioversion is indicated for the hemodynamically unstable patient. Rhythm control should be considered in patients unable to achieve adequate heart rate control, those with recurrent symptomatic episodes (palpitations, lightheadedness, dyspnea, angina), and those with heart failure symptoms in the setting of underlying left ventricular systolic dysfunction.

48. Answer: 1

Rationale: This stable symptomatic patient with supraventricular tachycardia should be treated by carotid massage, which is a vagal maneuver that will increase vagal tone and so decrease heart rate. This is the best initial step. Carotid massage is followed by adenosine.

49. Answer: 2

Rationale: Adenosine is used only in supraventricular tachycardia and it is effective in more than 90% of cases.

50. Answer: 3

Rationale: According to the CHADS2 score, the third patient in the third answer choice of the question has a score of 3, thus she needs an oral anticoagulant. The patients in the first, second, and last choices all have a score of 1.

51. Answer: 2

Rationale: According to the CHADS2 score, age greater than 75 and the presence of stroke/transient ischemic attach/thromboembolism has the highest risk score for systemic embolization.

52. Answer: 4

Rationale: The only role for digoxin in patients with atrial fibrillation is comorbid congestive heart failure.

53. Answer: 4

Rationale: This stable athlete patient with nonsymptomatic bradycardia does not need any treatment. If symptoms are present then give atropine; if atropine does not resolve symptoms, then pacing is indicated.

54. Answer: 1

Rationale: This unstable patient with atrial fibrillation on the second postoperative day needs immediate direct current cardioversion. He is hemodynamically unstable with signs of cardiogenic shock and acute pulmonary edema. All patients with a pulse who have persistent tachyarrhythmia causing clinical or hemodynamic instability should be managed by immediate direct current cardioversion at which energy delivery is synchronized to the QRS complex to minimize the occurrence of shock during repolarization, which can precipitate ventricular fibrillation.

55. Answer: 1

Rationale: This patient with atrial fibrillation most likely has tachycardia-induced cardiomyopathy. His clinical picture of fatigue, dyspnea on exertion, and decreased exercise tolerance with low ejection fraction (systolic dysfunction) suggests dilated cardiomyopathy induced by atrial fibrillation. Chronic tachycardia causes structural changes to the heart including left ventricular dilatation and myocardial dysfunction. This patient can be treated by aggressive rate or rhythm control because of the potential reversibility of tachycardia-induced cardiomyopathy and normalization of left ventricular systolic function.

56. Answer: 1

57. Answer: 1

58. Answer: 2

59. Answer: 1

60. Answer: 3

Rationale: This patient with atrial fibrillation and a CHADS2 score of 4 most likely has tachycardia-induced cardiomyopathy, which is reversible if the normal rate or rhythm of the heart is restored. Atrial fibrillation is the criminal tachycardia in this case. According to his score, he needs warfarin to prevent systemic embolization, and according to his history, his age (80 years old) is the strongest risk factor for systemic embolization.

61. Answer: 4

Rationale: This patient has of what is called "lone atrial fibrillation." It is used for patients with paroxysmal, persistent, or permanent atrial fibrillation with no evidence of cardiopulmonary or structural heart disease. The risk of systemic embolization in this patient is extremely low and anticoagulant therapy is not indicated.

62. Answer: 2

Rationale: Atrial fibrillation (AF) can be caused by a variety of cardiac and or systemic disorders. Among the answer choices, hyperthyroidism is the most common and likely cause for new-onset AF. All such patients with new-onset AF should be evaluated for hyperthyroidism as the underlying cause.

63. Answer: 2

Rationale: Hyperthyroidism is the most common risk factor for atrial fibrillation. There are many associated conditions that lead to atrial fibrillation such as coronary artery disease, rheumatic heart disease, congestive heart failure, congenital heart disease like atrial septal defect, obstructive sleep apnea, pulmonary embolism, chronic obstructive pulmonary disease, obesity, diabetes mellitus, hyperthyroidism, and drugs like cocaine and theophylline.

64. Answer: 2

Rationale: It is obvious from the electrocardiogram that this patient has Mobitz II second-degree atrioventricular block. Pacing is highly recommended and is the definite treatment.

65. Answer: 2

Rationale: This patient's electrocardiogram shows third-degree heart block. All atrial beats in this conduction abnormality are blocked, and the ventricles are driven by escape focus distal to the site of block. The most common cause in adults is simple fibrous degenerative changes in the conductive system as a result of aging. The definitive treatment is pacing.

66. Answer: 2

Rationale: Amiodarone is a very effective antiarrhythmic drug and can be used in ventricular tachycardia, atrial fibrillation, and atrial flutter. It has a long half-life of more than 50 days, so drug interactions are possible for weeks after discontinuation. The most severe side effects of this drug are related to the lungs, and the patient presents with cough, fever, and painful breathing. Thyroid dysfunction is also common because the drug molecule is chemically related to thyroxin. Hypothyroidism seems to be more common, but hyperthyroidism also can occur.

67. Answer: 3

Rationale: Calcium channel blockers are a known cause for constipation and lower limb edema. They cause congestive heart failure and asystole. Each patient that receives this type of drug should be informed and educated about its possible side effects.

68. Answer: 1

Rationale: Procainamide is a known antiarrhythmic drug and a sodium channel blocker of cardiomyocytes. It is the best drug for Wolff-Parkinson-White syndrome. Procainamide also can cause gastrointestinal upset, rash, hypotension, and aggravation of arrhythmia and blood dyscrasias.

69. Answer: 2

Rationale: Phenytoin is an anticonvulsant and antiarrhythmic drug that should be injected carefully and slowly because it can cause heart block with rapid injection. It also can cause hypotension and central nervous system toxicity (ataxia, nystagmus, and drowsiness).

70. Answer: 2

Rationale: A beta-blocker is a commonly used type of medication, but it can cause multiple side effects that must be considered.

71. Answer: 2

Rationale: This patient most likely has atrial fibrillation (AF). The most frequent site for ectopic foci that cause AF are the pulmonary veins because this tissue site has different electrical properties than the surrounding atrial myocytes and is prone to ectopic foci and/or aberrant conduction. In these patients, the myocardial tissue that surrounds the pulmonary veins can be disrupted by catheter-based radiofrequency ablation, thus disconnecting the pulmonary veins from the left atrium.

72. Answer: 2

Rationale: Atrial premature beats or what are called premature atrial contractions represent benign arrhythmia that can occur both in healthy individuals and in patients with cardiovascular and systemic disease. They are usually asymptomatic; however, in some patients, they can cause symptoms of palpitations. Treatment is needed only when atrial premature beats cause distress or when there is supraventricular tachycardia. In asymptomatic patients, precipitating factors such as tobacco, alcohol, caffeine, and stress should be considered.

73. Answer: 3

Rationale: This patient with symptomatic bradycardia and low blood pressure must be treated with atropine. Most patients with bradycardia are asymptomatic, but some can develop fatigue, dizziness, lightheadedness, hypotension, syncope, angina, and congestive heart failure. If intravenous (IV) atropine fails to improve symptoms, further treatment options include IV epinephrine or dopamine or transcutaneous pacing.

74. Answer: 2

Rationale: This patient's rhythm definitely shows first-degree heart block, which is caused by delayed impulse transmission at a number of possible sites from the atria to the ventricles. Most cases are caused by conduction delay in the atrioventricular node and require no further evaluation unless there are no significant associated bradycardia symptoms. In general, it is a benign finding, but its presence has been associated with a higher risk of heart failure, atrial fibrillation, and overall mortality. In this patient, constant chest pain that is worse with movement and induced by palpation is more consistent with musculoskeletal rather than cardiac cause and can be observed.

75. Answer: 1

Rationale: This patient with regular narrow complex tachycardia most likely suffers from supraventricular tachycardia. Because of his unstable hemodynamic status, he needs immediate synchronized cardioversion for which low-energy electrical shock is delivered synchronized to the QRS complex.

76. Answer: 2

Rationale: This hemodynamically unstable patient with ventricular fibrillation needs immediate unsynchronized cardioversion. No synchronicity is needed between the electrical shock and the QRS complex. Unsynchronized cardioversion is indicated only in pulseless ventricular tachycardia and ventricular fibrillation.

77. Answer: 3

Rationale: Intravenous magnesium is effective for the treatment of torsade de pointes, even with a normal magnesium level.

78. Answer: 3

Rationale: Atrial fibrillation (AF) is present in 10% to 30% of patients with Wolff-Parkinson-White syndrome (WPWS) and is potentially a life-threatening condition. Persistent AF with rapid ventricular response in patients with WPWS can ultimately deteriorate into ventricular fibrillation. Acute treatment of AF in stable patients with WPWS is procainamide.

79. Answer: 1

Rationale: Acute treatment of atrial fibrillation in unstable patients with Wolff-Parkinson-White syndrome is synchronized cardioversion.

80. Answer: 1

Rationale: The main pathophysiology of WPWS is the presence of accessory pathways between both atria and ventricles, which leads to preexcitation of ventricles via an abnormal bypass tract.

81. Answer: 3

Rationale: Nitroglycerin increases the capacity of the veins, so preload decreases and heart size decreases, and oxygen demand falls. Nitroglycerin causes atrial dilation and this leads to decrease afterload, but this drug has no approved effect on the coronary arteries.

82. Answer: 2

Rationale: The patient has a history of myocardial infarction (MI). One of the complications of MI is ventricular remodeling; this can happen months after an MI, and can cause heart failure. Therefore you must exclude heart failure before treating the patient.

83. Answer: 1

Rationale: This is a 50-year-old male patient with body mass index greater than 30 and high alcohol intake. His hypertension is most likely caused by obesity; therefore lifestyle modifications such as weight reduction and decrease of alcohol intake can control his blood pressure.

84. Answer: 3

Rationale: This patient suffered from acute myocardial infarct. Initial stabilization of this patient includes oxygen, aspirin, statin, clopidogrel, and sublingual nitrate.

85. Answer: 4

Rationale: Any patient newly diagnosed with hypertension (HTN) should undergo investigations including chemistry, lipid panel, baseline electrocardiogram, and urinalysis to exclude secondary causes of HTN or target organ damage.

86. Answer: 2

Rationale: This patient has an inferior myocardial infarction (MI) associated with hypotension, so we suspect acute decompensated heart failure. Beta-blockers are contraindicated in such cases, but furosemide is the drug of choice in acute heart failure. A calcium channel blocker is not indicated in this case.

87. Answer: 2

Rationale: The first choice for this African American patient who is less than 55 years old is a calcium channel blocker. Diuretics such as furosemide and spironolactone are not used to treat hypertension. A beta-blocker is not the first choice of treatment for hypertension.

88. Answer: 3

Rationale: This patient suffered from acute pericardial effusion symptoms (cardiac tamponade). He has the classic symptomatology triad of hypotension, distended jugular vein, and muffled heart sounds. Cardiac tamponade can be diagnosed by echocardiography, so there is no need for the rest of the mentioned investigations.

89. Answer: 3

Rationale: The patient suffered from inferior myocardial infarction, and there is evidence of right ventricular failure. The management here is different from management in left ventricular failure. Intravenous fluid is indicated to raise systolic blood pressure. In such a case, a beta-blocker is contraindicated. In addition, there is no sign of heart failure so furosemide is not indicated.

90. Answer: 1

Rationale: Heparin is the drug of choice in a non–ST-elevated myocardial infarction (NSTEMI), which can reduce mortality and morbidity. There is no role for thrombolysis in NSTEMI. Furosemide also has no role in this case because there is no sign of heart failure.

91. Answer: 2

Rationale: According to the Joint National Committee on prevention, detection, evaluation, and treatment of hypertension, all of these modifications can cause a reduction in blood pressure, but the most significant one is weight loss in overweight patients.

92. Answer: 4

Rationale: This patient is suffering from giant cell arteritis, which can affect medium and large arteries. One of these arteries is the aorta, which can cause aortic aneurysms.

93. Answer: 3

Rationale: This patient has symptoms of ischemic heart disease. Hypertension is a risk factor for angina, which happens during exercise only. His electrocardiogram is normal because of the absence of effort, so we induce the pain by exercise without any imaging.

94. Answer: 2

Rationale: Three weeks ago this patient started enalapril, which is an angiotensin-converting enzyme inhibitor (ACEi). One of the most common side effects of an ACEi is a dry cough. The cough will subside after switching to angiotensin receptor blockers.

95. Answer: 4

Rationale: Heart failure is one of the complications of myocardial infarction, and nitroglycerin will be a very useful medication in those patients, especially those with normal blood pressure.

96. Answer: 1

Rationale: Low high-density lipoprotein (HDL) and high total cholesterol can increase the risk of coronary artery disease. HDL is protective for cardiac ischemia, so when it decreases, the risk of MI increases.

97. Answer: 4

Rationale: Hypertension, headache, and weak femoral pulse are all symptoms of coarctation of the aorta, which is a congenital disease. Echocardiogram is used to diagnose this disease.

98. Answer: 1

Rationale: Hypertension, headache, and weak femoral pulse are symptoms of coarctation of the aorta, which is a congenital disease. Primary hypertension is diagnosed after exclusion of all other differential diagnoses. Hyperaldosteronism and Cushing cannot cause weak femoral pulse or murmur.

99. Answer: 3

Rationale: Patients with a prolonged history of hypertension can develop left ventricular hypertrophy, which appears on chest x-ray as cardiomegaly and on electrocardiogram as left axis deviation with high QRS voltage in leads V5 and V6.

100. Answer: 1

Rationale: One complication of prolonged hypertension is left ventricular hypertrophy, which appears on chest x-ray as cardiomegaly and on electrocardiogram as left axis deviation.

101. Answer: 3

Rationale: Patients with uncontrolled hypertension can present with many complications, one of which is a hypertensive crisis associated with end-organ damage, so cotton wool spots can be seen in the retina.

102. Answer: 2

Rationale: The patient presented with symptoms of myocardial infarction (MI), and the first step to diagnosing MI is by electrocardiogram.

103. Answer: 2

Rationale: Myocardial infarction (MI) can present in diabetic patients and elderly people in atypical presentations. Also, the Q change in the electrocardiogram is very specific to MI.

104. Answer: 3

Rationale: The most common cause of myocardial infarction (MI) is atherosclerotic plaque rupture, leading to the closure of the coronary artery, which decreases blood perfusion to the heart muscle.

105. Answer: 1

Rationale: Subarachnoid hemorrhage and intracerebral hemorrhage are complications of hypertensive crisis, which can happen when blood pressure is greater than 220/110 mmHg. This is an emergency that needs immediate intervention.

106. Answer: 2

Rationale: Myocardial infarction can present in the patient with diabetes mellitus as atypical pain. One of these scenarios is epigastric pain, so the first step in an elderly patient who comes in with epigastric pain not relieved by antacid is performing an electrocardiogram.

107. Answer: 4

Rationale: Primary or essential hypertension is the most common cause of hypertension but cannot be diagnosed until exclusion of all other differential diagnoses especially in the young patients.

108. Answer: 2

Rationale: The patient's clinical presentation suggests interventricular septum rupture, which can happen within 5 days of a myocardial infarction. There are no distant heart sounds or changes on the electrocardiogram, so pericarditis and free wall rupture are not expected.

109. Answer: 3

Rationale: This patient suffered from free wall rupture and pericardial effusion, which mainly happens after left anterior descending occlusion. Right coronary artery occlusion can cause right heart failure.

110. Answer: 3

Rationale: One of the complications of myocardial infarction (MI) is pericarditis, which can happen within a week after MI. This presents as chest pain relieved by leaning forward and is diagnosed by diffuse ST elevation in all leads.

111. Answer: 3

Rationale: The patient who underwent percutaneous coronary intervention (PCI) because of angina symptoms can drive a car 1 week after PCI according to the latest guideline, but if he underwent PCI because of myocardial infarction he needs at least 3 weeks to recover before driving a car.

112. Answer: 4

Rationale: Clopidogrel works as antagonist to the adenosine diphosphate receptor, whereas aspirin inhibits platelet aggregation through inhibition of the cyclooxygenase pathway.

113. Answer: 2

Rationale: The right coronary artery (RCA) supplies the atrioventricular (AV) node, so when the RCA is occluded both the right ventricle and AV node will be affected, which can lead to heart block.

114. Answer: 4

Rationale: One of the complications of myocardial infarction is rupture of the papillary muscle, which can lead to mitral valve regurgitation and pulmonary edema.

115. Answer: 1

Rationale: This patient has signs of left ventricular heart failure, which is a complication from hypertension (HTN). HTN leads to left ventricular hypertrophy, leading to increased afterload, so the lung will be congested.

116. Answer: 2

Rationale: This gentleman has isolated hypertension, which has high risk in elderly people. The drug of choice for this patient is either a calcium channel blocker or a diuretic.

117. Answer: 2

Rationale: The most specific change related to myocardial infarction is change of the Q wave. ST elevation can happen with multiple diseases. Also, cardiac enzymes can increase in several diseases.

118. Answer: 4

Rationale: The patient suffered from myocardial infarction, which is confirmed by electrocardiogram changes. The next step in such cases according to guidelines is either percutaneous coronary intervention PCI or thrombolysis.

119. Answer: 3

Rationale: According to National Cholesterol Education Program Adult Treatment Panel III, the most effective method to reduce risk of myocardial infarction in patients with high cholesterol level is to use a statin.

120. Answer: 3

Rationale: Mitral valve regurgitation is one of the complications of myocardial infarction. This condition appears on exam as holosystolic murmur and pulmonary edema. Leg swelling occurs in heart failure. Jugular venous distention and muffled heart sounds occur in cardiac tamponade but not in mitral valve regurgitation.

121. Answer: 1

Rationale: Aortic aneurysm dissection is one of the complications of uncontrolled hypertension. It can present with chest pain and can be associated with myocardial infarction, especially if dissection happens in the root of the aorta. The first step of management is surgery to repair the aneurysm.

122. Answer: 2

Rationale: One of the side effects of statins is muscle aches, which can disappear by decreasing the dose or changing the drug. Rosuvastatin can give the appropriate effect with low doses such as 5 mg or 10 mg.

123. Answer: 1

Rationale: There are several contraindications for thrombolytic therapy. These are ischemic stroke within 3 months, uncontrolled hypertension, non–ST-elevated myocardial infarction, brain trauma within 3 weeks, or brain surgery within 6 months.

124. Answer: 2

Rationale: Performing a bimanual palpation of the supraumbilical area suggests that the nurse practitioner suspects an aortic aneurysm.

125. Answer: 1

Rationale: Research confirms that the effect of thrombolysis in ST-elevated myocardial infarctions (STEMIs) improved reperfusion, but there is no role for thrombolysis in non-STEMIs, and heparin should be used.

126. Answer: 4

Rationale: There are two types of myocardial infarction: ST-elevated and non–ST-elevated. The management of these two types is different. There is no role for percutaneous coronary intervention or thrombolysis in non–ST-elevated myocardial infarction, and the drug we can use is heparin.

127. Answer: 2

Rationale: For prevention of future cardiovascular events, any patient who underwent coronary revascularization should take a moderate-intensity or high-intensity statin for life.

128. Answer: 3

Rationale: This clinical presentation is consistent with aortic dissection affecting the ascending aorta. There are many risk factors for this condition including hypertension, Marfan syndrome, and cocaine use. Systemic hypertension is the most important risk factor associated with the risk of developing aortic dissection because a sudden, dramatic, and transient increase in blood pressure is frequently noticed in patients who present with acute aortic dissection.

129. Answer: 3

Rationale: Weight loss of 10% of his current weight is an established way to control blood pressure (BP). Reduction in alcohol use and sodium intake also are ways to control BP.

130. Answer: 1

Rationale: In addition to a detailed history and physical exam, patients who are newly diagnosed with hypertension should have the following:

- Urinalysis and urine protein/creatinine ratio
- Chemistry panel
- Lipid profile (to assess the risk for coronary artery disease)
- Electrocardiogram (to check for coronary artery disease and left ventricular hypertrophy)

These tests are done to assess possible secondary causes for hypertension, duration of hypertension, and the extent of organ damage.

131. Answer: 2

132. Answer: 1

133. Answer: 2

Rationale: Ventricular septal defect (VSD) is the most likely congenital abnormality in this patient, and it is the most common cause of congenital heart disease (25%). There are many types of VSD: muscular, membranous (the most common type), perimembranous, inlet, and outlet. All patients with suspected VSD need echocardiography to determine both type and size of the defect. VSD is characterized by a holosystolic murmur at the left lower sternal border.

134. Answer: 2

135. Answer: 2

136. Answer: 4

Rationale: This patient presentation is consistent with tetralogy of Fallot, which is the most common cyanotic congenital cardiac disease. It is characterized by the following four abnormalities:

1. Right ventricular outflow obstruction (pulmonary stenosis or atresia)
2. Right ventricular hypertrophy
3. Ventricular septal defect
4. Overriding aorta

The varying degree of pulmonary blood flow results in a range of clinical manifestations. During exertion or agitation, the right ventricular outflow can be completely obstructed, so the diversion of blood from the right ventricle to the aorta instead of pulmonary artery results in sudden hypoxemia and cyanosis.

137. Answer: 1

Rationale: This infant most likely has an atrial septal defect, which is characterized by the presence of a defect between both atria. It leads to a left-to-right shunt and increased outflow of the blood through the pulmonary valve, so a systolic ejection murmur at the left upper sternal border will be heard. Wide fixed splitting of S2 is characteristic of an atrial septal defect.

138. Answer: 2

Rationale: The most common type of atrial septal defect is ostium secundum, which is caused by failure of the septum secundum to close the foramen secundum.

139. Answer: 4

Rationale: Cyanotic congenital heart diseases are most commonly characterized by a right-to-left shunt, which leads to an increased level of deoxygenated blood and cyanosis. Cyanotic congenital heart diseases include tetralogy of Fallot, truncus arteriosus, transposition of great vessels, tricuspid atresia, and Ebstein anomaly.

140. Answer: 1

Rationale: The most common congenital cardiac abnormality in Down syndrome patients is endocardial Cushing defect. Ventricular septal defect, atrial septal defect, and patent ductus arteriosus also can occur.

141. Answer: 1

Rationale: Conditions associated with high risk for infective endocarditis include prosthetic valves, aortic valve disease, mitral regurgitation, patent ductus arteriosus, arteriovenous fistula, coarctation of the aorta, previous infective endocarditis, and Marfan syndrome. Atrial septal defect is associated with low risk for infective endocarditis.

142. Answer: 1

Rationale: The most common cause for acute endocarditis is *Staphylococcus aureus.*

143. Answer: 2

Rationale: The most common cause for death in patients with infective endocarditis is congestive heart failure.

144. Answer: 3

Rationale: The two major criteria for infective endocarditis are abnormal echocardiography and positive blood cultures for typical microorganisms (*Staphylococcus aureus*, streptococcus, enterococcus). To diagnose infective endocarditis, these two major criteria are required. If one major criterion is present, then three minor criteria are required. Minor criteria for the diagnosis of infective endocarditis are

1. Fever
2. Intravenous drug use
3. Vascular phenomena (arterial embolic, septic pulmonary infarcts, Janeway lesions)
4. Immunological phenomena (Osler nodes, Roth spots, glomerulonephritis, or a positive rheumatoid factor)
5. Microbiological evidence (positive blood cultures not meeting major criteria or evidence of active infection with an organism consistent with infective endocarditis)
6. Predisposing cardiac lesions

145. Answer: 4

146. Answer: 3

147. Answer: 2

148. Answer: 3

149. Answer: 3

Rationale: This young female patient with a history of cellulitis 6 months ago and track marks on her right arm is most likely an intravenous (IV) drug abuser. Her generalized weakness, fever, and tricuspid regurgitation are consistent with IV drug abuse and infective endocarditis. IV drug abuse is a significant risk factor for infective endocarditis. The most common causative organism for infective endocarditis in an IV drug abuser is *Staphylococcus aureus*. And the most commonly involved valve in IV drug abusers with infective endocarditis is the tricuspid valve. The murmur described in the question is the murmur of tricuspid regurgitation (holosystolic murmur at the left lower sternal area that increases with inspiration). Human immunodeficiency virus infection increases the risk of infective endocarditis in patients with IV drug abuse. Septic pulmonary emboli are common in this situation. Peripheral infective endocarditis manifestations (like Janeway lesions) are less likely present in the case of IV drug abuse. Heart failure is more common with aortic valve involvement rather than tricuspid valve involvement. Vancomycin is the most appropriate antibiotic for empiric therapy in patients with native valve (not prosthetic valve) involvement. The empiric therapy in the native valve should cover methicillin-susceptible and methicillin-resistant staphylococci, streptococci, and enterococci. Once the organism is identified in blood cultures, antibiotics can be changed to cover the appropriate organism.

150. Answer: 3

Rationale: The most frequent clinical finding in patients with infective endocarditis is fever, and it is present in more than 90% of cases. Then heart murmurs, petechiae, and subungual splinter hemorrhages follow fever in their frequency, respectively.

151. Answer: 2

Rationale: Roth spots are the least common clinical finding in patients with infective endocarditis because it is present in only less than 5% of cases.

152. Answer: 4

153. Answer: 4

154. Answer: 4

155. Answer: 1

Rationale: Low-grade fever, anorexia, generalized weakness, aortic regurgitation, hematuria, and a history of invasive dental procedure are suggestive of infective endocarditis. Early diastolic murmur indicates aortic regurgitation. *Streptococcus viridians* is the most likely causative organism for infective endocarditis after gingival manipulation (dental procedure). The diagnosis of infective endocarditis is based on the patient's clinical presentation and cardiac imaging and laboratory studies. The most appropriate next step is to obtain serial blood cultures over a specified period before initiation antibiotic therapy. An early diastolic murmur indicates aortic or pulmonary regurgitation.

156. Answer: 1

Rationale: Mitral valve disease, usually coexisting mitral regurgitation, is the most common valvular abnormality detected in patients with infective endocarditis.

157. Answer: 3

Rationale: The most common cause for infective endocarditis in patients with nosocomial urinary tract infection is enterococci, especially *Enterococcus faecalis.*

158. Answer: 3

Rationale: This patient most likely has infective endocarditis of the mitral valve caused by infection with *Streptococcus bovis* biotype 1. Meta-analysis showed a significantly increased risk of colorectal cancer and endocarditis in patients with infection caused by *S. bovis* biotype 1 compared with patients with *S. bovis* biotype 2 infection. Thus the patient should have a colonoscopy to look for an underlying occult malignancy.

159. Answer: 2

160. Answer: 2

161. Answer: 1

Rationale: This patient with a presentation of acute renal failure secondary to post-streptococcal glomerulonephritis and a urea level of greater than 60 mg/dL (62 mg/dL) most likely suffers from uremic pericarditis. Retrosternal nonradiating chest pain relieved by leaning forward, a pericardial friction rub, and a urea level of greater than 60 mg/dL typically confirm the diagnosis. Pericarditis in patients with acute renal failure is an indication for hemodialysis. Indications for hemodialysis in patients with acute renal failure can be memorized from AEIOU (vowel letters mnemonic):

A: Acidosis (pH less than 7.1 that is refractory to treatment)

E: Electrolytes imbalance (symptomatic hyperkalemia, potassium level of greater than 6.5)
I: Ingestion (toxic alcohol, carbamazepine, salicylate, lithium, sodium valproate)
O: Volume overload refractory to medical treatment
U: Symptomatic uremia (uremic encephalopathy, uremic pericarditis, uremic bleeding)

The typical electrocardiogram finding in patients with pericarditis is diffuse ST elevation with typical depressed PR depression.

162. Answer: 2

163. Answer: 3

164. Answer: 2

165. Answer: 4

166. Answer: 2

167. Answer: 1

Rationale: This male patient, who recently emigrated from China to the United States, most likely has constrictive pericarditis secondary to tuberculosis (TB) infection. His shortness of breath, fatigue, abdominal ascites, pericardial knob heard during cardiac auscultation, and ring of calcification around the heart on chest x-ray all confirm the diagnosis. China is one of the countries most highly burdened with tuberculosis. Although in the United States the most common cause for constrictive pericarditis is idiopathic or viral pericarditis, then radiation therapy, then cardiac surgery, and then connective tissue disease. Elevated jugular venous pressure (JVP) on inspiration typically describes the Kussmaul sign, which is present on the physical exam of patients with constrictive pericarditis. JVP tracing typically shows prominent descent of the x and y waves. Pulsus paradoxus (decreased systolic blood pressure of greater than 10 mmHg during inspiration) can be found on the physical exam of patients with constrictive pericarditis.

168. Answer: 4

169. Answer: 1

170. Answer: 4

171. Answer: 4

Rationale: This patient with a history of upper respiratory tract infection most likely is suffering from viral myocarditis. Coxsackievirus B and adenovirus are the most causative organisms.

The pathogenesis is proposed to be direct viral injury and autoimmune inflammation, which leads to myocyte necrosis with impaired systolic and diastolic function. A viral prodrome (e.g., upper respiratory tract infection) typically precedes worsening respiratory distress from acute left heart failure and pulmonary edema. A holosystolic murmur may be identified secondary to dilated cardiomyopathy and the resulting functional mitral regurgitation. Hepatomegaly can be seen on physical exam, and pulmonary edema can be seen on chest x-ray. The gold standard for the diagnosis is myocardial biopsy, but treatment should be initiated based on clinical suspicion of the diagnosis. Management includes supportive measures such as inotropes and diuretics.

172. Answer: 3

173. Answer: 3

174. Answer: 3

Rationale: This patient's clinical features with shortness of breath, orthopnea, lower edema, bilateral lung crackles, and past history of myocardial infarction are consistent with decompensated heart failure caused by left ventricular dysfunction. In patients with congestive heart failure (CHF), hyponatremia usually parallels the severity of heart failure and is an independent predictor of adverse clinical outcomes. In CHF, decreased cardiac output with renal hypoperfusion will lead to the activation of the renin-angiotensin-aldosterone system, which will increase the level of epinephrine and norepinephrine. These actions will increase water absorption and lead to dilutional hyponatremia. The third heart sound (S3) is a low-frequency diastolic sound produced by passive ventricular filling during early diastole. This sound is best heard over the cardiac apex. An abnormal S3 (louder and higher pitch, S3 gallop) is commonly heard in patients with CHF because of left ventricular dysfunction.

175. Answer: 4

Rationale: Patients with congestive heart failure will have decreased cardiac output and renal hypoperfusion. This will lead to activation of the renin-angiotensin-aldosterone system. Angiotensin II will lead to constriction of both efferent and afferent arterioles of the kidney leading to increased renal vascular resistance and net decrease in renal blood flow.

176. Answer: 2

Rationale: Acute decompensated heart failure is most commonly caused by left ventricular systolic or diastolic dysfunction with or without additional cardiac disease. Pulmonary edema can also occur in the setting of normal left ventricular function in conditions such as severe hypertension, renal artery stenosis, or severe renal disease with fluid overload. Uncontrolled hypertension is the underlying cause for decompensated heart failure in this patient. Acute management of acute decompensated heart failure includes supplemental oxygen and intravenous loop diuretics (e.g., furosemide). This patient also requires further evaluation (serial cardiac markers, echocardiography) to identify any additional factors contributing to heart failure.

177. Answer: 2

Rationale: Beta-blockers significantly reduce morbidity and mortality in heart failure. Spironolactone, angiotensin-converting enzyme inhibitors, and angiotensin receptor blockers all reduce mortality and morbidity in patients with heart failure.

178. Answer: 4

Rationale: There are many factors that suggest poor prognosis in patients with heart failure such as elevated pro-brain natriuretic peptide levels, hyponatremia, anemia, and elevated uric acid. Serum potassium is not useful in the prognosis of heart failure.

179. Answer: 4

Rationale: Pioglitazone can result in retention of fluid, and the mechanism for that is unknown. This will cause mild dilutional anemia and ankle edema. It is contraindicated in congestive heart failure patients.

180. Answer: 1

Rationale: There are many drugs that are known to cause gynecomastia including spironolactone, cimetidine, cyclosporine, omeprazole, and digoxin. The other drugs are less likely to cause gynecomastia.

181. Answer: 4

Rationale: This patient most likely has cardiogenic shock caused by acute right ventricular myocardial infarction, which is seen in 30% to 50% of patients with acute ST-elevation of the inferior wall and is caused by occlusion of the right coronary artery proximal to the origin of right ventricular branches. We suspect right ventricular myocardial infarction if the patient has symptoms of myocardial injury (chest pain, diaphoresis, dyspnea), hypotension, and distended jugular veins with clear lung fields caused by right ventricular dysfunction. These patients are treated similarly to others with acute myocardial infarct with dual antiplatelets, statins, anticoagulation, and urgent revascularization; yet these patients require a high preload to maintain adequate right heart output. Therefore patients with hypotension should be given high-flow intravenous fluids to increase right ventricular preload. Drugs that decrease preload, such as nitrates, opioids, and diuretics, can cause profound hypotension and should not be given.

182. Answer: 3

Rationale: This patient with suspected inferior myocardial infarction (MI) possibly has right ventricular wall infarction, so his preload needs to be supported not reduced. If this patient receives nitroglycerin, he will be at risk for cardiogenic shock if he really has right ventricular wall infarction. Do not give nitroglycerin to patients with inferior wall MI unless and until you exclude right ventricular wall infarction.

183. Answer: 3

Rationale: Thirty to 50% of patients with inferior myocardial infarction have right ventricular wall infarction. This should be strongly considered because it plays a critical role in the management of the patient. Right-sided chest electrocardiography should be done to exclude right ventricular infarction.

184. Answer: 4

Rationale: Patients with cardiogenic shock will have decreased cardiac index and elevated pulmonary capillary wedge pressure caused by pump failure. In this case, the heart is not pumping efficiently. Systemic vascular resistance is typically increased to maintain adequate tissue perfusion. Cardiac preload is typically increased in patients with cardiogenic shock.

185. Answer: 1

Rationale: High-output heart failure is a heart condition that occurs when the cardiac output is higher than normal. This increase in cardiac output is caused by increased peripheral demand. It is also characterized by low systemic vascular resistance and low arteriovenous oxygen content difference. There are many causes for high-output heart failure, for example, morbid obesity, arteriovenous fistula, cirrhosis, erythroderma, carcinoid syndrome, myeloproliferative disorders, hyperthyroidism, sepsis, beriberi, acromegaly, anemia, pregnancy, and chronic pulmonary disease. Dilated cardiomyopathy is not a cause for high-output heart failure.

186. Answer: 4

Rationale: Acute respiratory distress syndrome (ARDS) is a pulmonary syndrome characterized by noncardiogenic and high-protein pulmonary edema. It can be caused by sepsis, acute pancreatitis, blood transfusion, and massive trauma. Systemic inflammation is the most common insult for ARDS. It is caused by injury to the alveolar–capillary interface, with increase in the capillary permeability and exudation of protein-rich fluid into the interstitium and alveoli. In addition, there is a deficiency in surfactant, which reduces lung compliance and predisposes to collapse. Bilateral infiltration is seen on chest radiography. The PaO_2/FiO_2 ratio is less than 200, and pulmonary capillary wedge pressure is less than 18 mmHg.

187. Answer: 3

Rationale: There are many causes for acute respiratory distress syndrome (ARDS). Direct causes include infections, near drowning, toxic gas inhalation, pulmonary trauma, aspiration, and oxygen toxicity. Indirect causes are uremia, anaphylaxis, sepsis, bowel infarction, nonthoracic trauma, and burns. ARDS mortality rate is generally high (40%). When associated with aspiration pneumonia the mortality rate is 80%.

188. Answer: 4

Rationale: This patient most probably has aspiration pneumonia and developed acute respiratory distress syndrome (ARDS). The mortality rate for ARDS with aspiration pneumonia increases up to 80%. Damage to the alveolar–capillary interface is the main pathophysiological feature for this syndrome, which will lead to release of proteins, cytokines, and neutrophils into the alveolar space. This leads to leakage of bloody and proteinaceous fluid into the alveoli and alveolar collapse (decreased lung compliance) caused by loss of surfactant and diffuse alveolar damage. Pulmonary arterial pressure is increased (pulmonary hypertension) because of hypoxic vasoconstriction, destruction of lung parenchyma, and compression of vascular structure from positive airway pressure in mechanically ventilated patients.

189. Answer: 4

Rationale: Mechanical ventilation is an important cornerstone in the management of acute respiratory distress syndrome. The correct parameters that will help to improve the patient's condition are low tidal volume, permissive hypercapnia, and high positive-end expiratory pressure.

190. Answer: 2

Rationale: One of the complications of myocardial infarct is vagal attack, which presents with hypotension and bradycardia. The first choice of treatment in this case is an anticholinergic drug like atropine. If symptoms persist after atropine, then we use a temporary pacemaker. Fluid can be used after correction of the bradycardia. There is no role for digoxin.

191. Answer: 1

Rationale: Enalapril is an angiotensin-converting enzyme inhibitor that is used as first-line treatment in hypertension management. It is the drug of choice in the patient with microalbuminuria. This drug has side effects such as cough and angioedema. One of the contraindications of this drug is bilateral renal artery stenosis because renal hypoperfusion can occur with a decrease in systemic pressure caused by enalapril.

192. Answer: 2

Rationale: Diastolic heart failure is one of the complications of prolonged hypertension caused by left ventricular hypertrophy, so it leads to decreased elasticity of the left ventricle during diastole. The first line of management is a beta-blocker or calcium channel blocker. Other drugs such as angiotensin-converting enzyme inhibitors and thiazides can be used if there is a contraindication for a beta-blocker or a calcium channel blocker (A and C).

193. Answer: 2

Rationale: Percutaneous transluminal coronary angioplasty (PTCA) is used to treat angina that is unresponsive to medical therapy. The success rate of PTCA is more than 90%. Ischemic symptoms that happen within 6 months after the procedure are mainly caused by restenosis, which happens in the dilated part before the stent region, whereas the ischemic symptoms that happen after 6 months are mainly caused by stenosis in another site.

194. Answer: 1

Rationale: Diastolic heart failure can happen because of left ventricular hypertension, which is caused by long-term uncontrolled hypertension. Left ventricular hypertension can lead to decreased expansion of the left ventricle during diastole, so preload decreases, which explains this patient's symptoms.

195. Answer: 3

Rationale: Right ventricular infarction can present by the triad of hypotension, elevated jugular venous pressure, and clear lungs. On the electrocardiogram, right ventricular infarction appears as elevation of ST in lead V4 and can present with a heart block.

196. Answer: 4

Rationale: Left ventricular hypertrophy is one of the complications of long-standing hypertension, which can cause diastolic heart failure with a normal ejection fraction. Left ventricular hypertrophy causes decreased elasticity of the left ventricle, which causes decreased of preload. There is no sign of aortic valve stenosis like syncope or angina symptoms (B). Foramen ovale usually does not present with shortness of breath; it is associated with ejection murmur and does not cause ventricular hypertrophy.

197. Answer: 2

Rationale: The most common cause of congenital heart disease in adults is foramen ovale, which is usually asymptomatic but can present with systolic murmur. Secondary foramen ovale presents on electrocardiogram as right axis deviation.

Left bundle branch block happens with myocardial infarction, whereas ST elevation in all leads occurs in pericarditis.

198. Answer: 2

Rationale: Hypertensive emergency is one of the acute complications of hypertension, defined as elevated blood pressure greater than 220/110 mmHg with end-organ damage. End-organ damage may include intracerebral hemorrhage, encephalopathy, myocardial infarction, acute renal failure, and aortic dissection. The main treatment in such a case is lowering blood pressure by 25% over a number of hours. The drug of choice is nitroprusside, but this drug needs blood pressure monitoring to avoid hypotension.

199. Answer: 2

Rationale: The main cause of aortic aneurysm is atherosclerosis with most of them located below the renal arteries. Indications for repair include the aneurysm is greater than 6 cm or it is expanding more than 0.5 cm per year. There are several contraindications for surgical repair such as chronic kidney failure, severe chronic obstructive pulmonary disease, life expectancy less than 2 years like in this case, and history of myocardial infarction within 6 months.

200. Answer: 2

Rationale: The main cause of aortic aneurysm is atherosclerosis. More than two-thirds of cases are located just distal to the renal artery. The indication for elective repair is either the size of the aneurysm is greater than 6 cm or the expansion rate is greater than 0.5 cm per year. The mortality rate in this case is more than 50%. Aneurysms less than 6 cm only need serial ultrasound follow-up.

201. Answer: 2

Rationale: According to the last update in the treatment of hypertension in patients with chronic obstructive pulmonary disease, thiazide diuretics are the first line of management. You can use an angiotensin-converting enzyme inhibitor (ACEi) instead, but the side effects of an ACEi, such as cough, may decrease the patient's quality of life. Beta-blockers can exacerbate the patient's disease, so this class should not be used. Alpha-blocker drugs can be used as a second-line or third-line management if there is any contraindication for thiazides.

202. Answer: 3

Rationale: This man complains of symptoms of gout, which can be associated with thiazide drugs. Thiazides increase reabsorption of uric acid from the urinary system, so they can cause hyperuricemia. The complications of angiotensin-converting enzyme inhibitors mainly include cough and angioedema in rare cases.

203. Answer: 4

Rationale: This patient has Marfan syndrome, which is a genetic disease A patient with Marfan syndrome looks tall with disproportionately long arms and legs. They often have mitral regurgitation because of tissue involvement.

204. Answer: 1

Rationale: The patient is suspected to have atrial fibrillation, which is associated with embolic events, dilated left atrium, and demarcated left heart border. The main cause of atrial fibrillation is mitral stenosis.

205. Answer: 2

Rationale: Atrial fibrillation is mainly happens caused by mitral valve stenosis, which leads to atrium dilation. In this patient, the main cause of atrial fibrillation is rheumatic fever. Neither atrial septal defect nor aortic aneurysm can cause atrial fibrillation. Senile aortic stenosis mainly happens in patients over 60 and does not cause atrial fibrillation.

206. Answer: 2

Rationale: This man complains of symptoms of gout, which can be associated with thiazide drugs. Thiazides increase reabsorption of uric acid from the urinary system, so they can cause hyperuricemia. Thiazides have no effect on kidney or liver function.

207. Answer: 3

Rationale: Patients with long-standing uncontrolled diabetes mellitus mainly have a neuropathic disease, so she will not feel the symptoms of myocardial infarction. There is no risk factor for pulmonary embolism in this woman such as embolization or cancer. Neither stroke nor septic shock can cause sudden death.

208. Answer: 3

Rationale: An angiotensin-converting enzyme inhibitor (ACEi) is the first choice in diabetic patients with microalbuminuria according to the last update of the last update of the Eighth Joint National Committee (JNC8) guidelines. Thiazides and alpha-blocker drugs are not superior to ACEis.

209. Answer: 2

Rationale: Myocardial infarction has several complications such as rupture of the free ventricular wall, mitral regurgitation, rupture of interventricular septum, and dysrhythmia. The main cause of death in this patient is arrhythmia, most likely ventricular fibrillation.

210. Answer: 2

Rationale: The pharmacological treatment of dyslipidemia includes a wide range of choices, all of which can lead to a decrease in cardiovascular mortality rate. According to the Eighth Joint National Committee (JNC8) guidelines, pharmacological treatment should begin in any patient with coronary artery disease and a low-density lipoprotein level (LDL) greater than 130 or in diabetic patients with LDL levels greater than 100; the target level should be less than 100 mg/dL.

211. Answer: 1

Rationale: This patient has dilated cardiomegaly, which presented with progressive dyspnea, orthopnea, and cardiomegaly. The most common cause of dilated cardiomyopathy in the patient with risk factors for atherosclerosis is coronary artery disease. The most accurate test for coronary artery disease is coronary angiography.

212. Answer: 3

Rationale: Prasugrel works by irreversibly blocking adenosine diphosphate receptors so it can prevent platelet activation and aggregation. It can be used in unstable angina, non–ST-elevated myocardial infarction, and ST-elevated myocardial infarction treated by percutaneous coronary intervention. The contraindication for this drug is bleeding diathesis or history of a previous stroke.

213. Answer: 3

Rationale: Treatment for multivessel disease with a decreased ejection fraction is coronary artery bypass graft (CABG). Medical therapy in such cases is associated with a bad outcome. There is no role for antithrombolytic therapy in this case. Percutaneous coronary intervention can be used, but the outcome of this procedure is not as satisfactory as CABG.

214. Answer: 2

Rationale: According to the latest Eighth Joint National Committee (JNC8) guidelines for the treatment of hypertension, the main choice in the patient older than 55 is a calcium channel blocker or thiazide, but if one of these drugs does not control blood pressure, the second choice will be an angiotensin-converting enzyme inhibitor. A beta-blocker is the second choice; it can be used in fourth-line management.

215. Answer: 3

Rationale: Angiotensin-converting enzyme inhibitors can prevent remodeling, which happens after myocardial infarction (MI). Recent studies show it can lead to the reduction of mortality in patients with hypertension, and it is a first-line treatment for diabetic nephropathy. Beta-blockers can be used in the patient with MI, but it is not the first-line management. There is no role for diuretics in such cases.

216. Answer: 2

Rationale: Aspirin works by irreversible inhibition of the cyclooxygenase pathway, so it can prevent platelet aggregation. The only contraindication to aspirin is allergy. History of peptic ulcer or upper gastrointestinal bleeding is not a contraindication to aspirin.

217. Answer: 3

Rationale: ST elevation 6 months after a myocardial infarction (MI) with no other major symptoms for a new MI could be caused by a left ventricular aneurysm (especially an anterolateral one), which is one of the complications of MI. Left ventricular aneurysm will appear on electrocardiogram as a sustained elevation of the ST segment in leads V1 to V4. It is diagnosed by echocardiogram.

218. Answer: 4

Rationale: Left ventricular aneurysm is one of the complications of anterolateral myocardial infarction (MI) that results from weakness of the left ventricular muscle after left anterior descending (LAD) occlusion. It appears as a sustained elevation of the ST segment in the same leads as the previous MI with an absence of major symptoms. It is more common with an LAD occlusion.

219. Answer: 2

Rationale: The main cause for an aortic aneurysm in elderly people is atheroma. Several risk factors include smoking, hyperlipidemia, hypertension, and aging. The patient has no headache or any symptoms of giant cell arteritis, and thromboangiitis obliterans happens mainly in the peripheral arteries.

220. Answer: 3

Rationale: The majority of aortic aneurysms are degenerative and associated with the risk factors for atherosclerosis such as hypertension, smoking, hypercholesterolemia, and aging. Although diabetes mellitus is associated with atherosclerosis, it is negatively correlated with aortic aneurysm.

221. Answer: 2

Rationale: Decubitus angina is a variant type of angina that occurs in the night when the patient in a recumbent position. It happens mainly in the patient with severe heart failure as a result of an increasing demand for oxygen caused by increased venous return to the heart in the recumbent position.

222. Answer: 2

Rationale: Aortic dissection is an emergent condition because it has a high mortality rate. It can present with sudden-onset chest pain that radiates to the interscapular region. Management can be medical or surgical according to the type of dissection. In a stable dissection, blood pressure should be reduced and the drug of choice is a beta-blocker. In an unstable patient, surgical treatment is preferred, but blood pressure should be reduced using beta-blockers. Angiotensin-converting enzyme inhibitors are the drug of choice in a patient with chronic renal disease or in a diabetic patient. Calcium channel blockers or thiazides can be used as the first choice in a Caucasian man greater than 55 years of age, but is not the first line of treatment for aortic dissection.

223. Answer: 1

Rationale: A patient with a history of rheumatic heart disease has a risk for embolus because of atrial fibrillation. The patient has dyspnea, which is a symptom of atrial fibrillation. The treatment plan for this patient includes embolectomy or antithrombotic therapy. Atherosclerosis cannot cause this sudden pain and deep vein thrombosis does not cause the pulse to be absent.

224. Answer: 1

Rationale: Patients with atrial fibrillation caused by rheumatic heart disease are at risk of developing thrombi, which can transfer to any site, causing sudden ischemia. The main treatment of embolus is embolectomy. Atrial septal defect and aortic aneurysm do not cause irregularity of the pulse.

225. Answer: 1

Rationale: Acute limb ischemia is a medical emergency, so an immediate intervention is necessary to prevent leg death. There are several ways to treat this including anticoagulant heparin, direct embolectomy, and catheter-directed thrombolysis. In contrast to chronic limb ischemia, aspirin is not used in the treatment of acute limb ischemia.

226. Answer: 4

Rationale: Myocardial infarction is one of the coronary artery diseases that results when one of the coronary artery branches become totally occluded. It is can appear on electrocardiogram in different ways such as elevation or depression of the ST, pathological Q wave, and new left bundle branch block. The right bundle branch block is a normal variant related to age.

227. Answer: 3

Rationale: Thiazide diuretics are one of the options used in the treatment of hypertension. They work by inhibition of sodium absorption in the distal convoluted tubule. The adverse effects of this drug include hypokalemia, postural hypotension, gout, and impaired glucose tolerance.

228. Answer: 3

Rationale: Pericarditis or Dressler syndrome is one of the complications of a myocardial infarction (MI), which happens mainly 2 weeks after the MI. Electrocardiogram shows elevation of the ST segment in all leads and can be treated by aspirin or nonsteroidal antiinflammatory drugs. Echocardiogram is used in pericarditis to exclude pericardial effusion but does not diagnose it. Cardiac markers and chest x-ray are not diagnostic in these cases.

229. Answer: 1

Rationale: Pericarditis or Dressler syndrome is one of the complications of myocardial infarction (MI), which happens mainly 2 weeks after the MI. Electrocardiogram shows an elevation of the ST segment in all leads. The treatment options for pericarditis include aspirin or nonsteroidal antiinflammatory drugs; steroids can be used in refractory cases.

230. Answer: 2

Rationale: A calcium channel blocker is first-line treatment for hypertension. It works by relaxing the smooth muscle in the vessel wall. Side effects for calcium channel blockers include ankle swelling, bradycardia, constipation, and gastroesophageal reflux disease. This patient has no dyspnea or orthopnea, so we can exclude heart failure. Deep vein thrombosis is rarely bilateral.

231. Answer: 2

Rationale: Calcium channel blockers work by relaxing the smooth muscle in the vessel wall. Side effects for calcium channel blockers include ankle swelling, bradycardia, constipation, and gastroesophageal reflux disease. Thiazides do not cause ankle swelling, but they cause hypokalemia and orthostatic hypotension, whereas angiotensin-converting enzyme inhibitors can cause cough and angioedema, but not ankle edema.

232. Answer: 3

Rationale: There are four initial drug classes used to control blood pressure including angiotensin-converting enzyme inhibitors, beta-blockers, calcium channel blockers, and thiazide diuretics. In the beginning, a single drug is used for 3 months; if the blood pressure remains uncontrolled, another drug from a different group is added. If the patient receives four drugs from different groups and blood pressure is still uncontrolled, then he is referred to a hypertension specialist.

233. Answer: 2

Rationale: Cardiac tamponade can be diagnosed by using the Beck triad, which includes hypotension, distention of the jugular vein, and muffled heart sounds. On chest x-ray the heart appears as a globular shape. Kerley B lines are found in pulmonary edema and pulmonary congestion, whereas widening of the mediastinum can happen in a patient with aortic dissection or mediastinal mass.

234. Answer: 4

Rationale: Angiotensin-converting enzyme inhibitors are the first-line management of hypertension in a patient with chronic kidney failure, chronic heart failure, and diabetes. Side effects include cough, hyperkalemia, and hypotension, and angioedema in rare cases. Bisoprolol can exacerbate asthma symptoms but does not cause hyperkalemia. In contrast, thiazides cause hypokalemia but not hyperkalemia.

235. Answer: 1

Rationale: Polycystic kidney disease is an autosomal dominant disease characterized by the development of multiple cysts on the kidney and different organs. It can present with flank pain, hypertension, and an increased creatinine. The most useful tool for diagnosis is abdominal ultrasound. Echocardiograph and arterial angiography will not help to diagnose polycystic kidneys. A 24-hour urine collection is used to diagnose nephrotic syndrome.

236. Answer: 1

Rationale: Polycystic kidney disease is an autosomal dominant disease characterized by the development of multiple cysts in the kidney and different organs. It can present with flank pain, hypertension, and an increased level of creatinine. The drug of choice for polycystic kidney and chronic kidney disease is an angiotensin-converting enzyme inhibitor or angiotensin receptor blocker.

237. Answer: 3

Rationale: Aortic dissection is an emergency condition with a high mortality rate and needs high suspicion. It can present with sudden chest pain radiated to the interscapular region. The definitive diagnosis in most patients is seen on computed tomography with contrast, whereas the most sensitive is a magnetic resonance imaging scan. An echocardiograph can be used but will not be accurate, especially a transthoracic echo.

238. Answer: 3

Rationale: The patient has symptoms of decubitus angina, which happens mainly in a patient with moderate to severe heart failure; it is caused by the increase in oxygen demand due to the increase of venous return to the heart muscle while lying down. Decubitus angina is associated with severe coronary artery stenosis, so we should do a coronary angiography to discover which artery is affected and treat it.

239. Answer: 1

Rationale: The patient with uncontrolled diabetes mellitus is at high risk for worsening elevated triglycerides and a low high-density lipoprotein; another cause of this problem is hypothyroidism. Hemoglobin A1c can help the physician discover if his patient is compliant with the treatment. Liver function tests can be used to diagnose if the patient has liver disease, but this will not help us in this case. Antinuclear antibodies and erythrocyte sedimentation rate tests show if the patient has a rheumatological condition or any inflammatory reaction.

240. Answer: 3

Rationale: Patients with diabetes mellitus mainly have low high-density lipoprotein and high triglyceride levels, which can improve in some patients with greater control of their glucose level.

241. Answer: 2

Rationale: Aortic stenosis can happen for different reasons, such as senile aortic stenosis or rheumatic heart disease. Indications of surgery for these patients include a gradient of more than 50 mmHg or if the patient has a symptom of aortic stenosis, such as syncope, breathlessness, or pulmonary edema.

242. Answer: 3

Rationale: Statin drugs work through inhibition of β-hydroxy β-methylglutaryl-CoA (HMG-CoA) reductase, which is the main enzyme in the HMG-CoA reductase pathway; this pathway is responsible for internal cholesterol production. Sequestration of bile acid is the mechanism of action of cholestyramine, not a statin, whereas ezetimibe works by decreasing absorption of cholesterol.

243. Answer: 4

Rationale: Aliskiren is a direct renin inhibitor. It blocks the renin-angiotensin-aldosterone system when aliskiren binds to renin and inhibits renin from converting angiotensin I to angiotensin II. Inhibition of the angiotensin-converting enzyme (ACE) is the mechanism of action of the ACE inhibitor drug, whereas diuretics are responsible for decreasing the absorption of sodium from the convoluted tubule.

244. Answer: 2

Rationale: A transient ischemic attack (TIA) is mainly present because of a small embolus. According to National Institute for Health and Care Excellence recommendations, any patient who presents with TIA is highly suspected of having a stroke

and treatment options depend on the patient's ABCD score. Because of this, in a symptomatic patient carotid endarterectomy is more useful than the other options. Brain magnetic resonance imaging will not help us to discover the severity of carotid stenosis because it is used to diagnose brain ischemia. Neither electrocardiogram nor echocardiograph has any role in management.

245. Answer: 2

Rationale: According to National Institute for Health and Care Excellence recommendations, carotid endarterectomy is the best option in symptomatic patients with a stenosis greater than 70%.

246. Answer: 3

Rationale: In any patient with a history of cancer and major surgery in the last few months, thrombolysis is a contraindication. Recent studies suggest the superiority of angioplasty in the treatment of myocardial infarction, especially in the first 120 minutes of patient presentation.

247. Answer: 1

Rationale: The target blood pressure in a pregnant woman with chronic hypertension is 110 to 129/65 to 79 mmHg.

248. Answer: 1

Rationale: Health care providers need to weigh the benefits and risks of side effects of hypertensive drugs in this older patients. In this patient, the diagnosis is confirmed by regular blood pressure checks during admission. He has a few lifestyle factors that need to be modified, so antihypertensive drugs should be started.

249. Answer: 3

Rationale: Significant coronary artery disease is defined according to the American Heart Association as stenosis greater than 70% in diameter of one major epicardial artery or 50% of width in the left coronary artery. If the patient suffered from anemia or coronary spasm, the percentage is reduced to 50% in the epicardial artery.

250. Answer: 4

Rationale: According to the guidelines of the American Heart Association and the American College of Cardiology for the secondary prevention of myocardial infarction (MI), the most effective measures are to be active for more than 20 minutes per day. Quitting alcohol has no effect on prevention, but decreasing the amount of alcohol can be useful. A recent study suggests that omega-3 and vitamin C have no role in the prevention of MI.

251. Answer: 1

Rationale: Patients with prolonged immobilization have a high risk of getting a deep vein thrombosis (DVT), which is what happened to this patient. If the DVT is not discovered and treated adequately, then the patient can develop an embolus, which can then lead to a pulmonary embolism. In some patients with right-to-left shunts, due to structural heart defects such as atrial septal defect, ventricular septal defect, and atrioventricular septal defect, the embolism can reach the brain and cause a brain infarction. Carotid Doppler is used when we suspect the presence of carotid stenosis like in the patient with transient ischemic attack.

252. Answer: 1

Rationale: This patient has an inferior myocardial infarction that involves the right ventricle. The right coronary artery supplies the right ventricle and interventricular septum. The left coronary artery supplies the anterior side of the heart and the left circumflex artery supplies left atrium and the posterolateral surface of the left ventricle.

253. Answer: 3

Rationale: Mitral stenosis has many causes, but the most common is rheumatic fever. Mitral stenosis can lead to atrial dilation and this may lead to atrial fibrillation. If the patient has a past medical history of mitral stenosis that lead to atrial enlargement, a peaked P-wave will appear, especially in lead V1.

254. Answer: 2

Rationale: The most common reason for mitral stenosis in this age group is rheumatic fever; it may take years before symptoms begin to appear. In older people, the most common reason for stenosis is aging. A long history of mitral stenosis can lead to atrial dilation, which may lead to atrial fibrillation.

255. Answer: 2

Rationale: Angiotensin-converting enzyme inhibitors inhibit the conversion of angiotensin I to angiotensin II. They have many side effects including chronic cough, hypokalemia, and angioedema, and can raise the creatinine level. Thus this medication can make the kidney function worse in some patients. This drug does not affect the liver, so there is no need to monitor liver enzymes and no need for a baseline electrocardiogram in this case.

256. Answer: 3

Rationale: Pericardial effusion is a collection of fluid in pericardial space. This can happen for different reasons including cardiological causes such as pericarditis and systemic causes such as a viral infection or metastatic cancer. Pericardial effusion can be suspected by history and physical exam and. On electrocardiogram it will appear as electrical alternans.

257. Answer: 4

Rationale: Acute aortic regurgitation is one of the fatal complications of infective endocarditis, which can be associated with large pulse volume, increase in pulse pressure, decrescendo murmur, and low blood pressure. It has a high mortality rate and needs immediate intervention to save patient's lives and prevent heart failure.

258. Answer: 3

Rationale: Primary hyperaldosteronism presents typically with uncontrolled hypertension, hypokalemic alkalosis, and hypernatremia, which are present in this this patient. Patients with polycystic kidney will have impaired renal function and cysts will appear on ultrasound. Pheochromocytoma will cause paroxysmal hypertension with recurrent headache. Patients with renal artery stenosis will be normal in the early stage with normal renal function tests, but will worsen when an angiotensin-converting enzyme inhibitor is added.

259. Answer: 3

Rationale: According to recommendations of the European Society of Cardiology (ESC), clopidogrel is the first line of management in a patient with peripheral artery disease (PAD) who cannot tolerate aspirin. Heparin has no role in PAD, and there is no indication for warfarin in a patient with sinus rhythm. Dabigatran is only indicated to treat patients with a thromboembolic event postsurgery or in the patient who has a history of atrial fibrillation.

260. Answer: 3

Rationale: The most common cause of death in myocardial infarction (MI) is arrhythmia. A patient who has at least one episode of ventricular tachycardia or ventricular fibrillation will be at high risk for developing arrhythmia. The best treatment option for those patients is an implanted cardiac device. Thrombolysis or warfarin cannot reduce the risk of arrhythmia. Bisoprolol is essential after MI to decrease oxygen consumption of the heart muscle, and not for arrhythmia.

261. Answer: 3

Rationale: This patient has a posterior wall myocardial infarction, which involves the posterolateral surface of the left ventricle and the right ventricle. The left circumflex artery supplies the left atrium with the posterolateral surface of the left ventricle and right ventricle. The right coronary artery supplies the right ventricle and interventricular septum, whereas the left coronary artery supplies the anterior side of the heart.

262. Answer: 4

Rationale: Uremic pericarditis is one of the complications of chronic kidney disease; it typically occurs in end-stage renal disease. Pericarditis can present with chest pain that increases by leaning forward. Uremic pericarditis appears as T-wave changes with ST elevation on electrocardiogram, which may disappear in some patients. The treatment of this condition includes urgent dialysis and follow-up blood, urea, nitrogen level.

263. Answer: 1

Rationale: Multiple factors can increase the risk of aortic aneurysm expansion and rupture, and the most important factor is smoking and the diameter of the aortic aneurysm. An aortic aneurysm that expands greater than 5 mm per year has a high risk for rupture. Other factors include a history of cardiac or renal transplant, female gender, and elevated aortic wall stress.

264. Answer: 3

Rationale: Pericardial effusion is a collection of fluid in the pericardial space, which can happen for different reasons including cardiological causes such as pericarditis and systemic causes such as a viral infection or metastatic cancer. Pericardial effusion can be suspected by history, physical exam, and electrocardiogram, but the diagnosis can be established only by echocardiography.

265. Answer: 2

Rationale: Recent studies showed that patients who have intermittent claudication and peripheral artery disease (PAD) are at risk for developing cardiovascular events in the future. Thus cardiovascular disease is the primary cause of morbidity and mortality in patients with PAD, so aggressive risk factor modification should be initiated as soon as possible.

266. Answer: 3

Rationale: The patient has a symptom of myocardial infarction (MI), which can happen because of reocclusion in the same artery due to failure of thrombolysis therapy. The most sensitive and specific test for MI is a troponin level, but it takes time to return to normal range. Creatine kinase myocardial band returns to normal range within 2 days, so it can aid in the diagnosis when we suspect new ischemia.

267. Answer: 3

Rationale: Ostium secundum atrial septal defect is a large opening in the atrial septum; it is the second most common congenital heart defect. It is asymptomatic in childhood and symptoms appear when pulmonary pressure exceeds the systemic pressure, which happens mainly in adults if the opening is large. The only indication for surgery is when pulmonary pressure is greater than 1.5 systemic pressure. It is associated with right axis deviation seen on electrocardiogram with right ventricular volume overload in echocardiography.

268. Answer: 3

Rationale: The cardiovascular mortality in the patient who is on hemodialysis is higher than the general population. Hemodialysis causes arterial calcification, which decreases the artery recoil, so the blood flow that reaches the cardiac muscle decreases. Atherosclerosis is the leading cause of myocardial infarction in the general population but not in hemodialysis patients. This patient has no risk factor for aortic dissection.

269. Answer: 2

Rationale: Mitral valve prolapse is the most common valvular abnormality; it affects 1% of the population. Usually it has a benign course and is asymptomatic in most patients, but some patients have severe complications such as infective endocarditis and aortic regurgitation. It can be diagnosed by echocardiography and appears on physical exam as a late systolic murmur associated with systolic click.

270. Answer: 1

Rationale: Aortic dissection is an emergency condition that has a high mortality rate and should be met with high clinical suspicion. It can present with sudden chest pain radiating to the interscapular region. Aortic dissection can be diagnosed in stable patients by computed tomography (CT) angiography, but if the patient has any contraindications for CT angiography, transesophageal echocardiography is the second option and it has the same validity as CT angiography. Management can be medical or surgical according to the type of dissection.

271. Answer: 3

Rationale: Mitral valve prolapse is the most common valvular abnormality, and it affects 1% of the population. Usually it has a benign course and can be asymptomatic in most patients, but some patients have serious complications such as infective endocarditis and aortic regurgitation. It can be diagnosed by echocardiography. Mitral valve prolapse appears on physical exam as a late systolic murmur associated with systolic click.

272. Answer: 2

Rationale: Angina symptoms can be caused by coronary artery disease or aortic stenosis. Aortic stenosis can present with angina, syncopal attack, or heart failure. If the arteriography does not show any stenosis, then the second option would be aortic stenosis, which also can be diagnosed by echocardiography. The calcium score is used to assess the calcification of the coronary arteries, but this test is out of date. High-resolution computed tomography scan is used to evaluate the lung, but there is no need for our patient to have this test.

273. Answer: 2

Rationale: Mitral valve prolapse is the most common valvular abnormality; it affects 1% of the population. Usually it has a benign course and can be asymptomatic in most patients, but some patients have serious complications such as infective endocarditis and aortic regurgitation. It can be diagnosed by echocardiography. Mitral valve prolapse appears on physical exam as a late systolic murmur associated with systolic click. Its complications include severe mitral regurgitation, atrial fibrillation, infective endocarditis, and sudden cardiac death.

274. Answer: 2

Rationale: Pulmonary embolism mainly originates from deep vein thrombus (DVT), which can cause pulmonary infarction. It presents with sudden chest pain, hemoptysis, and dyspnea. Pulmonary embolism is usually treated as a DVT with heparin and warfarin or other anticoagulants. In some cases, such as significant pulmonary embolism or hemodynamic instability, thrombolysis is the best treatment option.

275. Answer: 2

Rationale: This patient has an acute occlusion of the radial artery. The cause of occlusion in this patient is arterial embolism, which can originate from cardiogenic or noncardiogenic sources. In this patient, the cause is atrial fibrillation, which appears on his electrocardiogram. Pain in embolic occlusion happens suddenly and the pulse disappears on the same side. The treatment of extremity embolism includes a systemic anticoagulant such as heparin, which should be started as soon as possible. Some patients may need embolectomy plus a systemic anticoagulant. Warfarin and clopidogrel are not used to treat acute arterial embolism. Warfarin is mainly used to treat atrial fibrillation, and clopidogrel is used to treat peripheral artery disease.

276. Answer: 2

Rationale: This patient has many risk factors for atherosclerosis such as diabetes mellitus, hypertension, and dyslipidemia. He also has symptoms of peripheral artery disease (PAD), which are caused by claudication. PAD can be confirmed by the ankle-brachial index, which is defined as the ratio of systolic pressure at the ankle to systolic pressure at the brachial artery. This test is very sensitive and specific to PAD in the symptomatic patient.

3

Pulmonary

1. A 56-year-old white female patient presents to the intensive care unit with some respiratory distress following an elective total hysterectomy. Before the procedure she was in good overall health. The patient received cefotetan 1 g intravenous × 1 dose before her surgery. She had issues during surgery with her respiratory status and required mechanical ventilation at that time. The patient has been on a ventilator for 3 days and the staff now notices increased sputum production, decreased pulmonary function, elevated temperature, and elevated white blood cell count. A chest radiograph was ordered and shows significant left lower lobe infiltrates. She has been diagnosed with health care–associated pneumonia to be treated in the intensive care unit. Which of the following drug regimens would be appropriate for empiric therapy if you determine that she is at risk for multidrug-resistant pathogens?

   1. Cefepime (Maxipime) + levofloxacin (Levaquin) + vancomycin.

   2. Ertapenem (Invanz) + gentamicin.

   3. Cefepime (Maxipime) + tobramycin + daptomycin.

   4. Levofloxacin (Levaquin) alone.

2. A patient was properly cultured and was found to be growing methicillin-resistant *Staphylococcus aureus* (MRSA) in the sputum. Which of the following medications would best treat this organism?

   1. Amikacin.

   2. Gentamicin (Garamycin).

   3. Linezolid (Zyvox).

   4. Levofloxacin (Levaquin).

3. Which of the following regimens would be appropriate empiric therapy for a patient with community-acquired pneumonia (CAP) that requires admission to the intensive care unit?

   1. Azithromycin (Zithromax) intravenously (IV).

   2. Azithromycin IV + ceftriaxone (Rocephin) IV.

   3. Azithromycin oral + amoxicillin/clavulanate (Augmentin) oral.

   4. Levofloxacin (Levaquin) oral.

4. You are working in the walk-in clinic today and your first patient is a 62-year-old male patient with chronic diabetes mellitus, hypertension, and hyperlipidemia. He was recently on some antibiotics for a tooth infection this last month. He presents with a mild case of community-acquired pneumonia, and you determine that he is a good candidate for outpatient therapy. Which antibiotics choice would be the most appropriate on which to send him home?

   1. A macrolide alone.

   2. Doxycycline alone.

   3. Fluoroquinolone alone.

   4. β-lactam plus a fluoroquinolone.

5. KS had a complicated intensive care unit (ICU) stay. He developed heparin-induced thrombocytopenia, resulting in a pulmonary embolus. He was unable to be extubated. He remains on the ventilator. It is day 8 of his ICU stay. Today you note that he has developed fever and decreasing oxygen saturation. Chest x-ray reveals a right lower lobe infiltrate with a small effusion. What would be the empiric treatment?

   1. Cefepime 2 g intravenously (IV) every 12 hours, doxycycline 100 mg twice a day, Zyvox 600 mg twice a day.

   2. Azactam 2 g IV every 8 hours and tobramycin 7 mg/kg every 24 hours, vancomycin 1 g every 12 hours.

   3. Rocephin 2 g IV every 24 hours, Zithromax 500 mg IV every 24 hours.

   4. Tobramycin 7 mg/kg every 24 hours, daptomycin 6 mg/kg every 24 hours.

6. You also sent a sputum culture for this patient. Your results are *Acinetobacter baumannii*, which is resistant to Primaxin and Zosyn, and intermediate to tobramycin and minocycline. What would be an appropriate antibiotic regimen for this, including the appropriate length of treatment?

    1. Continue Azactam and tobramycin for 14 days.

    2. Change vancomycin to linezolid.

    3. Change tobramycin to amikacin for 14 days.

    4. Minocycline with Colistin for 14 days.

7. A 52-year-old white male patient presenting to the emergency department with shortness of breath. He claims that he has felt a little short of breath over the last few days, but today it became extremely difficult to breathe and he generally feels bloated and uncomfortable. He has had difficulty trying to button his pants, tie his shoes, and noted a 15-lb weight gain over the last week or so. His blood pressure is 138/92 with a heart rate of 98 beats/min. His past medical history includes idiopathic heart failure. His current medications are enalapril, furosemide, digoxin, and carvedilol. Which of the following should be added to his regimen?

    1. Bumetanide.

    2. Metoprolol XL.

    3. Sotalol.

    4. Spironolactone.

8. A 71-year-old male patient comes to the clinic 2 months ahead of his scheduled appointment with concerns of increasing shortness of breath, which first started a month ago. The shortness of breath appears to have coincided with daily walks with his granddaughter. He has noticed a nonproductive cough but no other associated symptoms. His past medical history includes chronic obstructive pulmonary disease, benign prostatic hypertrophy, and hypertension. He has a 50 pack-year smoking history and continues to smoke his pipe daily. He also admits to two to three beers daily. His current medications are Flomax 0.4 mg daily; Spirival 8 mcg, one inhalation daily; and Norvasc 5 mg daily. The patient should have been counseled on which of the following when started on Spiriva?

    1. Not to swallow the capsule.

    2. A side effect can be a brown coating on the tongue.

    3. To call the office if he develops symptoms of depression.

    4. Do not eat or drink anything for 2 hours after inhalation.

9. A 71-year-old male comes to the clinic with complaints of worsening shortness of breath after adding Spiriva to his medication regimen. He has noticed a nonproductive cough but no other associated symptoms. His past medical history includes chronic obstructive pulmonary disease, benign prostatic hypertrophy, and hypertension. He has a 50 pack-year smoking history and continues to smoke his pipe daily. He also admits to two to three beers daily. His current medications are Flomax 0.4 mg daily; Spirival 8 mcg, one inhalation daily; and Norvasc 5 mg daily. What medication change should the nurse practitioner make to the patient's therapy?

    1. Increase Spiriva dose to 36 mcg daily.

    2. Increase Flomax to 2 tablets daily.

    3. Add Combivent 2 puffs 4 times a day.

    4. Add an albuterol inhaler.

10. A patient picks up several over-the-counter products when he picks up his prescriptions. Which one of these is cause for concern for patients with chronic obstructive pulmonary disease?

    1. Acetaminophen.

    2. Multivitamin with iron and zinc.

    3. Robitussin DM.

    4. Tums.

11. A patient who weighs 70 kg is intubated after a motor vehicle accident. He has the following arterial blood gas: pH 7.20, Paco2 60 mmHg, Pao2 89 mmHg, and HCO_3 22 mEq/L. The ventilator settings are tidal volume 650 ml, synchronized intermittent mandatory ventilation (SIMV) rate 12, and fraction of inspired oxygen of 0.50. What adjustment needs to be made to the ventilator settings?

    1. Administer 1 ampule of $NaHCO_3$ intravenously.

    2. Increase the tidal volume.

    3. Increase the SIMV rate.

    4. Increase the Fio_2.

12. Which of the following conditions can cause acute hypoxic respiratory failure?

    1. Pneumonia.

    2. Chronic obstructive pulmonary disease.

    3. Congestive heart failure.

    4. Obstructive sleep apnea.

13. Alveolar edema can be classified as high-pressure pulmonary edema, low-pressure pulmonary edema, and:

    1. Psychogenic pulmonary edema.

    2. Neurological pulmonary edema.

    3. Adnexa pulmonary edema.

    4. High-altitude pulmonary edema.

14. High-pressure pulmonary edema can be seen in which diagnosis?

    1. Acute respiratory distress syndrome.

    2. Inhaling toxic chemicals such as terbutaline.

    3. Congestive heart failure.

    4. Acute lung injury.

15. Interpret the following arterial blood gas: $Po_2 = 45$ mmHg, $Pco_2 = 30$ mmHg, $HCO_3 = 24$ mEq/L, and pH is 7.47.

    1. Acute respiratory alkalosis.

    2. Acute respiratory acidosis.

    3. Acute metabolic acidosis.

    4. Acute metabolic alkalosis.

16. The classic triad of asthma includes wheezing, dyspnea, and what?

    1. Pallor.

    2. Cough.

    3. Airway hyporesponsiveness.

    4. Rash.

17. How could total lung capacity be described?

    1. Forced expiratory volume.

    2. Forced vital capacity.

    3. Volume of air in the lungs at end of inspiration.

    4. Volume of air in the lungs at end of exhalation.

18. How can the work of breathing be described?

    1. Amount of effort needed to inhale and exhale.

    2. Tendency of the lungs to return to their original shape.

    3. How easy the lungs can inhale and exhale.

    4. Stimulation of the chemoreceptors in the brain stem.

19. In respiratory acidosis, what is the goal?

    1. Increase the Pco_2.

    2. Decrease the Pco_2.

    3. Increase the Po_2.

    4. Decrease the Po_2.

20. In a ventilated patient, peak inspiratory pressures may be seen in what circumstance?

    1. Decreased airway resistance.

    2. Increased Po_2.

    3. Metabolic acidosis.

    4. Worsening airspace disease.

21. What allows oxygen to be transported in the blood?

    1. Hematocrit.

    2. Lymphocytes.

    3. Hemoglobin.

    4. White blood cells.

22. What is an example of an airway disease that is restrictive in the extraparenchymal tissue?

    1. Cystic fibrosis.

    2. Myasthenia gravis.

    3. Sarcoidosis.

    4. Asthma.

23. Pulmonary vasculature requires measuring the pulmonary vascular resistance (PVR). The PVR will rise because of what condition?

    1. Metabolic alkalosis.

    2. Sarcoidosis.

    3. Running a 5K.

    4. Intraluminal thrombi.

24. What can pulmonary hypertension be caused by?

    1. Ankylosing spondylitis.

    2. Pneumonia.

    3. Interstitial lung disease.

    4. 25 pack-year history of smoking.

25. What does the alveolar to arterial gradient measure?

    1. The difference between the pH in the alveoli and the pH in the arteries.

    2. The difference between the tidal volume in the alveoli and the tidal volume in the arteries.

    3. The difference between the partial pressure of carbon dioxide in the alveoli and the arterial partial pressure of carbon dioxide.

    4. The difference between the partial pressure of oxygen in the alveoli and the arterial partial pressure of oxygen.

26. What does the diffusion capacity of the lungs for carbon monoxide measure?

    1. How much oxygen travels from the blood stream to the alveoli.

    2. How much oxygen travels from the alveoli to the blood stream.

    3. How much carbon monoxide travels from the blood stream to the alveoli.

    4. How much carbon monoxide travels from the alveoli to the blood stream.

27. What is the gold standard used to measure obstructive airway disease?

    1. Forced expiratory volume in 1 second.

    2. Forced vital capacity.

    3. Total lung capacity.

    4. Forced expiratory capacity.

28. Short-acting β_2 agonists are often used in asthma treatment because they focus on which of the following?

    1. Increasing forced vital capacity.

    2. Increasing total lung capacity.

    3. Prohibiting airway inflammation.

    4. Relaxing airway smooth muscles.

29. What is a common side effect of β_2 agonists?

    1. Muscle tremors.

    2. Dry mouth.

    3. Headache.

    4. Somnolence.

30. Kaden, a 23-year-old male patient, is having an asthma exacerbation. The nurse practitioner would prescribe which of the following medications?

    1. Long-acting β_2 agonist, metered-dose inhaler, 1 puff twice a day.

    2. Short-acting β_2 agonist, metered-dose inhaler, 4 to 8 puffs every 20 minutes up to 4 hours.

    3. Tapering dose of oral prednisone starting with 10 mg a day and tapering over 1 week.

    4. Leukotriene modifier, 1 tablet by mouth daily.

31. Jennifer, a 35-year-old female patient, has moderate persistent asthma. The mainstays of treatment require the nurse practitioner to prescribe which of the following?

    1. Long-acting β_2 agonists (LABAs) and high-dose inhaled corticosteroid and an oral corticosteroid.

    2. LABAs and high-dose inhaled corticosteroid.

    3. LABAs and low-dose inhaled corticosteroid.

    4. Low-dose corticosteroid.

32. What is the most common cause of community-acquired pneumonia in adults?

    1. *Chlamydia pneumoniae.*

    2. Respiratory syncytial virus.

    3. *Streptococcus pneumoniae.*

    4. Aspiration pneumonia.

33. The nurse practitioner is evaluating a patient who complains of a cough for the last several months. He denies fever or shortness of breath. He has worked as an interior house painter for the last 20 years. What test would be ordered first to aid in diagnosis?

    1. Arterial blood gas.

    2. Chest x-ray.

    3. Pulmonary function test.

    4. Pulse oximetry.

34. The nurse practitioner has diagnosed John with asbestosis. What would the patient education include?

    1. Moving to a dry environment.

    2. Using supplemental oxygen.

    3. Weight loss.

    4. Smoking cessation.

35. Which of the following is *not* a risk factor for a pulmonary embolism?

    1. Recent surgery.

    2. Trauma.

    3. Coronary artery disease.

    4. Immobilization.

36. Which of the following is *not* part of the Virchow triad?

    1. Factor V Leiden.

    2. Venous stasis.

    3. Endothelial injury.

    4. Hypercoagulable state.

37. Most emboli that cause a pulmonary embolus are thought to arise from what vein?

    1. Pulmonary.

    2. Popliteal.

    3. Brachial.

    4. Iliac.

38. What causes the impaired gas exchange that results from a pulmonary embolus?

    1. Altered alveolar to arterial gradient.

    2. Altered pulmonary recoil.

    3. Altered ventilation to perfusion ratio.

    4. Altered pulmonary elasticity.

39. What causes hypotension due to a pulmonary embolus?

    1. Increased right ventricular outflow.

    2. High venous outflow from the inferior vena cava.

    3. Decreased pulmonary vascular resistance.

    4. Increased pulmonary vascular resistance.

40. The nurse practitioner is seeing a 40-year-old hemodynamically stable patient in the emergency department with a suspected pulmonary embolus (PE). What does treatment of a PE include?

    1. Low-molecular-weight heparin.

    2. Oxygen.

    3. Inferior vena cava filter.

    4. Admission to the hospital.

41. According to the Global Initiative for Obstructive Lung Disease (GOLD) criteria, how would a patient with an forced expiratory volume in 1 second (FEV_1)/forced vital capacity less than 0.7 and FEV_1 less than 30% predicted, be classified?

    1. GOLD stage I.

    2. GOLD stage II.

    3. GOLD stage III.

    4. GOLD stage IV.

42. Which of the following criteria suggests a diagnosis of chronic bronchitis?

    1. Chronic productive cough for 3 months per year for the last 2 years.

    2. Dyspnea that has gotten progressively worse over the last 3 months.

    3. Being diagnosed with acute bronchitis more than twice in a 12-month period.

    4. Having pneumonia that required hospitalization.

43. The nurse practitioner is reviewing the chest x-ray of a patient with chronic obstructive pulmonary disease. Which of the findings would *not* be expected?

    1. Hyperinflation of lungs.

    2. Pulmonary hypertension.

    3. Consolidation in one lung lobe.

    4. Flattened diaphragm.

44. Which of the following pulmonary function test findings is not expected in a patient with emphysema?

    1. Increased total lung capacity.

    2. Increased residual volume.

    3. Decreased total lung capacity.

    4. Decreased residual volume.

45. The nurse practitioner (NP) is examining Mrs. Jones, a 69-year-old female patient in the intensive care unit for exacerbation of her emphysema. Mrs. Jones is usually very pleasant and talkative. However, today she tells the NP to "get away from her" and then she starts yelling for the police because the NP is "trying to kill me!" The NP notes the change in mental status of Mrs. Jones. What is the next most likely order?

    1. Restraints.

    2. Arterial blood gas.

    3. Pulse oximetry.

    4. Intravenous fluids.

46. Which of the following is *not* part of the criteria for diagnosing acute respiratory distress syndrome?

    1. Respiratory symptoms must have begun within 1 week of a known clinical insult.

    2. Bilateral opacities must be present on a chest radiograph or computed tomography scan.

    3. The patient must be on mechanical ventilation with an Fio_2 of at least 0.6 or greater.

    4. The patient's respiratory failure must not be fully explained by cardiac failure or fluid overload.

47. The nurse practitioner suspects a patient has acute respiratory distress syndrome. Which diagnostic test should the NP order to confirm or deny this diagnosis?

    1. Computed tomography scan of the chest.

    2. Chest nuclear medicine study.

    3. Pulmonary function test.

    4. Chest x-ray.

48. Which complication is a cause of morbidity and mortality in a patient with acute respiratory distress syndrome?

    1. Nosocomial infections.

    2. Delirium.

    3. Poor nutrition.

    4. Myopathies.

49. The release of which cytokines causes acute respiratory distress syndrome?

    1. Cardiotrophin.

    2. Tumor necrosis factor.

    3. Adiponectin.

    4. Apolipoprotein.

50. What are the three pathological stages that acute respiratory distress syndrome goes through?

    1. Reactive stage, proliferative stage, and exudative stage.

    2. Injury stage, proliferative stage, and reactive stage.

    3. Proliferative stage, the fibrotic stage, and the injury stage.

    4. Exudative stage, proliferative stage, and fibrotic stage.

51. What predisposing diagnosis is the most common cause of acute respiratory distress syndrome?

    1. Chronic obstructive pulmonary disease.

    2. Sepsis.

    3. Pneumonia.

    4. Transfusion-related acute lung injury.

52. Which patient type is at an increased risk of death from acute respiratory distress syndrome?

    1. A 20-year-old male patient who was in a motor vehicle accident.

    2. A 39-year-old female patient who is pregnant and had an emergency cesarian section.

    3. A 60-year-old male patient who has worked in a factory producing weed killer for the last 20 years.

    4. An 80-year-old female patient who smoked in her early 20s but has not smoked since.

53. The nurse practitioner is seeing JR, a 50-year-old male patient, today in the clinic. He was released from the hospital a month ago after being intubated for 6 days for acute respiratory distress syndrome. He asks, "When will my lungs be completely healed from this?" What is the correct answer?

    1. Lung function can be compromised for as long as 5 years.

    2. Lung function can be compromised for as long as 3 years.

    3. Lung function can be compromised for as long as 12 months.

    4. Lung function can be compromised for as long as 6 months.

54. Why are sedatives and analgesic medications used in patients with acute respiratory distress syndrome?

    1. Decrease the need for restraints.

    2. Maximize oxygen consumption.

    3. Increase energy expenditure.

    4. Decrease the incidence of intensive care unit psychosis.

55. What should the initial ventilator settings for a patient with acute respiratory distress syndrome begin with?

    1. Low tidal volume ventilation.

    2. Synchronous intermittent mandatory ventilation.

    3. Pressure controlled ventilation.

    4. Pressure support ventilation.

56. Which of the following is a risk factor for transfusion-related acute lung injury (TRALI)?

    1. History of diabetes.

    2. History of obesity.

    3. History of hypertension.

    4. There are no risk factors for TRALI.

57. Which component is involved in the pathogenesis of transfusion-related acute lung injury?

    1. Eosinophils.

    2. Neutrophils.

    3. Lymphocytes.

    4. Monocytes.

58. Transfusion-related acute lung injury presents with a sudden onset of hypoxemia during or shortly after receiving a blood product. Which of the following symptoms will most likely *not* be present?

    1. Fever.

    2. Mental status change.

    3. Hypotension.

    4. Cyanosis.

59. The nurse practitioner (NP) suspects his patient has transfusion-related acute lung injury. The patient is hypoxic with a room air O_2 saturation of 85%. The patient received a unit of whole blood 30 minutes ago. What diagnostic test should the NP order first?

    1. Arterial blood gas.

    2. Beside pulmonary function test.

    3. Chest x-ray.

    4. Chest computed tomography scan.

60. The nurse practitioner (NP) is called into the intensive care unit for a patient who complains of being short of breath. The patient is a 53-year-old female with triple-negative breast cancer. When the NP arrives, the vital signs are temperature 99.8°F, heart rate 112 beats/min, respiratory rate 14 breaths/min, blood pressure 88/60 mmHg, and oxygen saturation is 89% on room air. The patient is receiving 0.9% normal saline at 25 mL/hr and a unit of packed red blood cells at 75 mL/hr. What should the NP order first?

    1. Place the patient on oxygen at 2 L via nasal cannula.

    2. Arterial blood gas.

    3. Increase the 0.9% normal saline to 100 mL/hr.

    4. Stop the blood transfusion.

61. Which of the following is a risk factor for chronic obstructive pulmonary disease?

    1. Obesity.

    2. Hypertension.

    3. Gastroesophageal reflux.

    4. Lung cancer.

62. Which diagnosis is *not* considered to be a type of chronic obstructive pulmonary disease?

    1. Asthma.

    2. Chronic bronchitis.

    3. Cystic fibrosis.

    4. Emphysema.

63. Where do the pathological changes of chronic obstructive pulmonary disease occur?

    1. Goblet cells.

    2. Mast cells.

    3. Endothelial cells.

    4. Cytoplasmic cells.

64. Chronic inflammation associated with chronic bronchitis is characterized by which of the following?

    1. CD4+ cells.

    2. CD8+ cells.

    3. CD14+ cells.

    4. CD3+ cells.

65. Bronchial inflammation associated with asthma is characterized by which of the following?

    1. CD4+ cells.

    2. CD8+ cells.

    3. CD14+ cells.

    4. CD3+ cells.

66. Proximal acinar or centrilobular emphysema is commonly associated with which of the following?

    1. Pulmonary hypertension.

    2. Working around birds.

    3. Cigarette smoking.

    4. Traveling to a foreign country.

67. Panacinar emphysema is most commonly seen in people with which of the following?

    1. Sarcoidosis.

    2. Bronchopulmonary dysplasia.

    3. Henoch-Schönlein purpura.

    4. α_1-antitrypsin deficiency.

68. Which part of the airway is affected in distal acinar, or paraseptal, emphysema?

    1. Bronchioles.

    2. Pleura.

    3. Bronchi.

    4. Alveoli.

69. What is *not* a risk factor for developing chronic obstructive pulmonary disease?

    1. Exposure to cigarette smoke.

    2. Exposure to animals with heavily shed coats.

    3. Exposure to fumes.

    4. Exposure to organic dusts.

70. What are the three cardinal symptoms of chronic obstructive pulmonary disease?

    1. Dyspnea, chronic cough, and sputum production.

    2. Dyspnea, chronic cough, and snoring.

    3. Dyspnea, chronic cough, and accessory muscle use when breathing.

    4. Dyspnea, chronic cough, and wheezing.

71. Which of the following is an associated symptom of chronic obstructive pulmonary disease?

    1. Clubbing of fingers.

    2. Weight loss.

    3. Depression.

    4. Irritability.

72. The Global Initiative for Chronic Obstructive Lung Disease classification for chronic obstructive pulmonary disease is based on which of the following?

    1. Pack-year smoking history.

    2. Risk of exacerbation.

    3. Sputum production in 24 hours.

    4. Number of inhalers the patient is prescribed.

73. The nurse practitioner is seeing a new patient who presents with cough, dyspnea, and sputum production. The patient has a 70 pack-year history of smoking and continues to smoke two packs a day. The patient only gets short of breath with strenuous exercise or when walking uphill. According to the Global Initiative for Chronic Obstructive Lung Disease classification, which class would this patient be in?

    1. Class D.

    2. Class C.

    3. Class B.

    4. Class A.

74. The nurse practitioner (NP) is seeing a new patient who presents with cough, dyspnea, and sputum production. The patient has a 70 pack-year history of smoking and continues to smoke two packs a day. The patient only gets short of breath with strenuous exercise or when walking uphill. What should the NP prescribe for the patient?

    1. Short-acting bronchodilator.

    2. Long-acting bronchodilator.

    3. Oral steroids.

    4. Inhaled corticosteroids.

75. The nurse practitioner (NP) is seeing a patient who presents with cough, dyspnea, and sputum production. The patient has a 70 pack-year history of smoking and continues to smoke two packs a day. The patient was started on a short-acting bronchodilator 2 months ago. The patient reports that the dyspnea is worse, and he must stop to "catch his breath" frequently. What should the NP prescribe for the patient?

    1. Short-acting bronchodilator.

    2. Long-acting bronchodilator.

    3. Oral steroids.

    4. Inhaled corticosteroids.

76. What is a radiographic finding suggestive of chronic obstructive pulmonary disease?

    1. Cloudiness in lung fields.

    2. Flattened diaphragm.

    3. Segmented opacities in lower lobes.

    4. Lobar consolidation.

77. Which diagnostic test has the best sensitivity and specificity for chronic obstructive pulmonary disease (COPD)?

    1. Computed tomography scan.

    2. Arterial blood gas.

    3. Chest x-ray.

    4. Pulmonary function test.

78. The nurse practitioner (NP) is seeing a patient in the emergency department (ED) for exacerbation of chronic obstructive pulmonary disease (COPD). This patient was in the ED 6 weeks ago for the same diagnosis. The patient continues to smoke two to three packs a day and works in a popcorn factory. Her vital signs are temperature 99.9°F, heart rate 101 beats/min, respiratory rate 20 breaths/min, blood pressure 102/86 mmHg, and oxygen saturation of 90% on room air. The patient appears comfortable. The patient asks the NP "for an antibiotic this time so I won't end up here 6 weeks from now." The NP knows that prescribing antibiotics for COPD exacerbation is which of the following?

    1. The standard of care for a patient with worsening COPD and fever.

    2. Based on the results of a sputum culture.

    3. Based on the clinical severity of the disease.

    4. Not indicated at this time because the patient is stable.

79. The nurse practitioner (NP) is seeing a patient in the emergency department (ED) for exacerbation of chronic obstructive pulmonary disease (COPD). This patient was in the ED 6 weeks ago for the same diagnosis. The patient continues to smoke two to three packs a day and works in a popcorn factory. Her vital signs are temperature 99.9°F, heart rate 101 beats/min, respiratory rate 20 breaths/min, blood pressure 102/86 mmHg, and oxygen saturation of 90% on room air. The patient appears comfortable. The patient asks the NP, "for some prednisone to help me breathe, like the other doctors always give me." The NP knows which of the following is *not* true when prescribing prednisone for COPD exacerbation?

    1. 7 to 10 days of corticosteroid therapy is associated with fewer treatment failures.

    2. 7 to 10 days of corticosteroid therapy is the standard of care for hemodynamically stable patients with a COPD exacerbation.

    3. The dose range for corticosteroid therapy is lower than that for treating asthma.

    4. Intravenous steroids offer no benefit over oral steroids.

80. The nurse practitioner is seeing a patient who was just admitted to the intensive care unit for exacerbation of chronic obstructive pulmonary disease. What would the recommended ventilator settings include?

    1. Pressure support mode.

    2. High tidal volumes.

    3. Low tidal volumes.

    4. High positive end-expiratory pressures.

81. The nurse practitioner (NP) is seeing a patient who was just admitted to the intensive care unit for exacerbation of chronic obstructive pulmonary disease. The patient's arterial blood gas shows pH 7.34, Pao_2 85, $Paco_2$ 58, and HCO_3 28. The NP is considering noninvasive ventilation support for this patient. The NP knows that noninvasive ventilatory support is

    1. Not indicated in this patient.

    2. Only used in patients who have exacerbation of asthma.

    3. Can only be used on patients for 48 hours.

    4. Indicated in patients with progressing hypercapnia.

82. Which of the following is an indication for a pneumonectomy?

    1. Lung cancer.

    2. Well-controlled chronic obstructive pulmonary disease.

    3. Asthma.

    4. Chronic bronchitis.

83. The nurse practitioner (NP) is performing a preoperative assessment for Joe, a 70-year-old patient with lung cancer, who is scheduled to undergo a right middle lobe lobectomy. The NP is reviewing Joe's pulmonary function test. The predicted postoperative value for the diffusing capacity of the lung for carbon monoxide is 38%. What does this value mean to the NP?

    1. Joe needs to repeat the test because this is an incorrect value.

    2. Joe is at a low to medium risk for postoperative morbidity.

    3. Joe is at no increased risk for postoperative morbidity.

    4. Joe is at a moderate-to-high risk for postoperative morbidity.

84. The nurse practitioner is performing a preoperative assessment for Joe, a 70-year-old patient with lung cancer, who is scheduled to undergo a right middle lobe lobectomy. Which diagnostic test is *not* part of the preoperative assessment?

    1. Pulmonary function test.
    2. Evaluation of tuberculosis status.
    3. Chest x-ray.
    4. Cardiac risk assessment.

85. Pulmonary function testing (PFT) is an important part of the preoperative assessment for a patient undergoing lung surgery. The diffusing capacity of the lung for carbon monoxide and what other measurement from the PFT provide the best estimate of postoperative morbidity and mortality?

    1. Tidal volume.
    2. Functional residual capacity.
    3. Forced expiratory volume in 1 second.
    4. Total lung capacity.

86. The nurse practitioner is performing a preoperative assessment for Joe, a 70-year-old patient with lung cancer, who is scheduled to undergo a right pneumonectomy. The nurse practitioner knows that Joe has a 10% to 20% chance of going into which cardiac arrhythmia?

    1. Sinus tachycardia.
    2. Sick sinus syndrome.
    3. Bradycardia.
    4. Atrial fibrillation.

87. The nurse practitioner is performing a preoperative assessment for Joe, a 70-year-old patient with lung cancer, who is scheduled to undergo a right pneumonectomy. The nurse practitioner knows that cardiac arrhythmias can occur in 10% to 20% of patients and if they do occur, they usually happen during which postoperative time frame?

    1. 1 to 2 days postoperatively.
    2. 2 to 4 days postoperatively.
    3. 4 to 6 days postoperatively.
    4. 6 to 8 days postoperatively.

88. The nurse practitioner (NP) has just admitted Joe, a 70-year-old patient with lung cancer, who just underwent a right pneumonectomy. The NP knows that cardiac arrhythmias can occur postoperatively, so which serum electrolyte is ordered to be checked every morning?

    1. Magnesium.
    2. Potassium.
    3. Sodium.
    4. Chloride.

89. Which of the following is *not* a potential complication after a pneumonectomy?

    1. Chronic obstructive pulmonary disease.
    2. Pulmonary edema.
    3. Postpneumonectomy syndrome.
    4. Intraoperative spillage.

90. Which of the following is *not* a potential complication of the pleural space after a pneumonectomy?

    1. Empyema.
    2. Chylothorax.
    3. Cardiopleural fistula.
    4. Bronchopleural fistula.

91. Which of the following is an indication for one-lung ventilation?

    1. Pulmonary resection.
    2. *Staphylococcus* aureus pneumonia infection.
    3. Open heart surgery.
    4. Acute respiratory distress syndrome.

92. Which three factors are taken into consideration when determining treatment for lung cancer?

    1. Tumor histology, extent of disease, and gender of patient.
    2. Tumor histology, comorbidity, and which lung lobe is involved.
    3. Tumor histology, extent of disease, and comorbidity.
    4. Tumor histology, smoking history, and comorbidity.

93. The nurse practitioner (NP) is reviewing a chest x-ray of a patient in status asthmaticus. What finding would the NP expect to see?

    1. Expanded diaphragm.
    2. Pulmonary nodules.
    3. Consolidation.
    4. Hyperinflation.

94. Ipratropium bromide (Atrovent) is used in the treatment of asthma and has shown to increase the forced expiratory volume in 1 second. What other statement is true about Atrovent?

    1. It is only available as a metered-dose inhaler.

    2. It is a short-acting muscarinic agent used in the treatment of chronic asthma.

    3. There are no side effects.

    4. Patients must be educated about storing the medication in an area that is less than 40°F.

95. What is tuberculosis of the lung caused by?

    1. Gram-negative, rod-shaped aerobic bacteria.

    2. Gram-negative, spherical-shaped anaerobic bacteria.

    3. Gram-positive, spherical-shaped anaerobic bacteria.

    4. Gram-positive, rod-shaped aerobic bacteria.

96. Tuberculosis of the lung is caused by what bacteria?

    1. *Streptococcus.*

    2. *Acinetobacter.*

    3. *Mycobacterium.*

    4. *Bifidobacterium.*

97. Sally has just been diagnosed with *Mycobacterium* tuberculosis. The nurse practitioner (NP) is educating Sally on how *M. tuberculosis* is spread. The NP knows that Sally has understood the education when Sally says which of the following?

    1. "Tuberculosis can be spread when I cough or sneeze and don't cover my mouth."

    2. "Tuberculosis can be spread when someone hugs me or shakes my hand."

    3. "Tuberculosis can be spread when I have sex with my boyfriend."

    4. "Tuberculosis can be spread if someone drinks from the same cup as me."

98. The nurse practitioner (NP) is performing a preoperative assessment for Joe, a 70-year-old patient with small cell lung cancer, who is scheduled to start chemotherapy. Joe asks the NP if chemotherapy is the best treatment for this disease. What does the NP explains to Joe about the disease?

    1. "There is no 'best' treatment. All treatments have the same probably outcome."

    2. "Chemotherapy has been shown to increase survival compared with best supportive care."

    3. "Your insurance will only pay for chemotherapy so that is why you're going to get chemotherapy."

    4. "Chemotherapy is only going to shrink the cancer. You'll need radiation too."

99. The nurse practitioner is seeing a new patient, Fred, in the pulmonary clinic. The NP sees the diagnosis of "latent tuberculosis (TB)" in the past medical history section of the patient's chart. What does latent TB mean?

    1. The person had a history of TB, but he is now cured.

    2. The patient shared a home with someone with a history of TB.

    3. The patient has TB that is silent but can be reactivated to active disease.

    4. The patient has active TB and is contagious.

100. The nurse practitioner (NP) is seeing Celia, a 39-year-old patient with a history of low-grade fever that has been present for the last 2 weeks. A chest x-ray is ordered. Celia suspects tuberculosis. If this suspicion is correct, what will the NP see on the chest x-ray?

    1. Hyperinflation.

    2. Hilar adenopathy.

    3. Pleural effusions.

    4. Pulmonary infiltrates.

101. What type of physiological changes are seen as a result of poorly controlled asthma?

    1. Increase in lung function.

    2. Chronic bronchitis.

    3. Airway remodeling.

    4. Barrel chest.

102. Which patient should be screened for latent tuberculosis?

    1. An 80-year-old male patient who has a history of chronic obstructive pulmonary disease.

    2. A 35-year-old female patient who was just released from prison.

    3. A 55-year-old male patient who works as a corporate lawyer who has a chronic, nighttime cough.

    4. A 41-year-old female patient who works for the postal service with a sudden 25-pound weight loss.

103. Pulmonary hypertension (PH) is classified into five groups. Persons in group 1 are considered to have which of the following?

    1. PH caused by left heart disease.

    2. PH caused by idiopathic causes.

    3. PH caused by lung disease.

    4. PH caused by pulmonary artery obstruction.

104. Pulmonary hypertension (PH) can be classified as precapillary or postcapillary. Although patients can have a mixture of both, what causes precapillary PH?

    1. An elevation of pressure in the pulmonary venous system.

    2. A primary elevation of pressure in the pulmonary arterial system.

    3. An elevation of pressure in the pulmonary capillary system.

    4. An elevation of pressure in the superior vena cava.

105. What are the most common initial symptoms of pulmonary hypertension?

    1. Exertional dyspnea, fatigue, weight loss.

    2. Exertional dyspnea, fatigue, excess sweating.

    3. Exertional dyspnea, fatigue, weight gain.

    4. Exertional dyspnea, fatigue, lethargy.

106. Exertional dyspnea and fatigue are common symptoms in a patient with pulmonary hypertension. What is the cause of these symptoms?

    1. Inadequate increase in cardiac output during exercise.
    2. Decrease in total lung volume.
    3. Right atrial bundle branch block.
    4. Respiratory muscle fatigue.

107. A patient with pulmonary hypertension may also develop right heart failure. What is the pathophysiology of right heart failure caused by pulmonary hypertension?

    1. Impaired cardiac filling and decrease left ventricular output lead to weakened right ventricle muscle.

    2. Subendocardial hypoperfusion caused by increased right ventricular wall stress and myocardial oxygen demand.

    3. Chronic hypertension causes increased afterload and therefore increased cardiac workload.

    4. Chronic hyperperfusion from the right ventricle leads to overstressed right ventricular contractility.

108. The initial physical symptoms of pulmonary hypertension are symptoms related to which of the following?

    1. Right ventricular failure.

    2. Right atrial failure.

    3. Left ventricular failure.

    4. Left atrial failure.

109. The nurse practitioner is reviewing the chest x-ray of a patient with pulmonary hypertension. What would the nurse practitioner expect to see on the x-ray?

    1. Enlargement of the heart muscle.

    2. Accentuated left atrial border.

    3. Enlargement of the central pulmonary arteries.

    4. Attenuation of aortic notch.

110. Which abnormal lab value is seen in patients with pulmonary hypertension?

    1. Elevated brain natriuretic peptide.

    2. Elevated serum creatinine.

    3. Decreased serum sodium.

    4. There is no specific lab abnormality in a patient with pulmonary hypertension.

111. The nurse practitioner (NP) is evaluating James, a 59-year-old with a history of dyspnea, lethargy, and fatigue along with signs of heart failure. The NP suspects James has pulmonary hypertension. What is the initial test of choice?

    1. Chest computed tomography scan.

    2. Magnetic resonance imaging.

    3. Transthoracic echocardiography.

    4. Electrocardiogram.

112. What is a general recommendation for someone with pulmonary hypertension?

    1. Regular exercise.

    2. Low-fat diet.

    3. Avoid air travel.

    4. No scuba diving.

113. Patients with pulmonary hypertension may experience edema in their extremities. Which diuretic would be recommended?

    1. Spironolactone (Aldactone).

    2. Furosemide (Lasix).

    3. Hydrochlorothiazide (HCTZ or Microzide).

    4. Triamterene (Dyrenium).

114. The nurse practitioner (NP) is treating Tracy, a 28-year-old female patient with pulmonary arterial hypertension (PAH). The NP knows that Tracy understands the education when Tracy says

    1. "I can keep smoking a pack a day."

    2. "It's important for me to not stress myself too much."

    3. "I'll have to apply for disability."

    4. "I need to use birth control because pregnancy can worsen my PAH."

115. A 75-year-old male living in an extended care facility develops a fever of 100.9°F. He is also coughing up copious amounts of yellow sputum. His past medical history is significant for dementia. A portable chest x-ray shows an infiltrate in the left lower lobe. What is the most likely cause for this?

    1. *Legionella pneumophilia*

    2. *Streptococcus pneumoniae*

    3. *Mycobacterium tuberculosis*

    4. *Pneumocystis jirovecii*

116. Which of the following patients with pulmonary hypertension has the worst prognosis?

    1. A 31-year-old female patient.

    2. A 25-year-old pregnant female patient.

    3. A 53-year-old male patient.

    4. A 25-year-old male marathoner.

117. Obstructive sleep apnea is defined broadly as an Apnea–Hypopnea Index greater than how many events per hour of sleep?

    1. Three.

    2. Four.

    3. Five.

    4. Six.

118. Which of the following are risk factors for obstructive sleep apnea?

    1. Obesity, female, smoking.

    2. Obesity, perimenopause, older age.

    3. Obesity, male, older age.

    4. Obesity, history of snoring as a child, ankyloglossia.

119. The prevalence of obstructive sleep apnea is higher in patients who also have

    1. Hypertension.

    2. Diabetes type 2.

    3. Hyperthyroidism.

    4. Stage 3 chronic kidney disease.

120. Which of the following is *not* a sign of obstructive sleep apnea?

    1. Daytime sleepiness.

    2. Loud snoring.

    3. Lack of concentration.

    4. Evening headaches.

121. The nurse practitioner (NP) is getting ready to examine a patient who complains of being tired all day and his wife says that he often wakes up in the middle of the night feeling like he is choking or gasping. The NP suspects obstructive sleep apnea. Which physical exam finding is the NP likely to see?

    1. Crowded airway.

    2. Neck size less than 15 inches.

    3. Yawning during exam.

    4. Tonsils and adenoids.

122. Obstructive sleep apnea (OSA) is not a clinical diagnosis, and diagnostic testing must be performed. Diagnostic testing for OSA should be performed on patients with which of the following?

    1. Excessive daytime sleepiness, difficulty concentrating, and moodiness.

    2. Excessive daytime sleepiness, chronic obstructive pulmonary disease, and moodiness.

    3. Excessive daytime sleepiness, hypertension, and difficulty concentrating.

    4. Excessive daytime sleepiness, habitual loud snoring, and hypertension.

123. The nurse practitioner (NP) is examining a patient that she suspects has obstructive sleep apnea. Which tool can the NP use to diagnose the patient?

    1. STOP-BANG questionnaire.

    2. Epworth Sleepiness Scale.

    3. Berlin score.

    4. None of the above.

124. What is the gold standard for diagnosing obstructive sleep apnea?

    1. STOP-BANG questionnaire.

    2. Epworth Sleepiness Scale.

    3. In-laboratory polysomnography.

    4. None of the above.

125. The nurse practitioner (NP) thinks his patient has obstructive sleep apnea and would like to perform a polysomnogram on the patient. Which factor will influence the NP's decision to order the polysomnogram to be performed in the lab instead of at home?

    1. The patient has anxiety.

    2. The patient is an airline pilot.

    3. The patient works night shift in a factory.

    4. The patient is breast-feeding a newborn.

126. Which of the following is a nonobstructive sleep apnea conditions that is *not* associated with sleep-disordered breathing?

    1. Intracardiac shunts.

    2. Muscular dystrophy.

    3. Myasthenia gravis.

    4. Myocardial infarction.

127. What is the treatment for chronic obstructive pulmonary disease based on?

    1. CAT score.

    2. STOP-BANG score.

    3. Berlin score.

    4. Breathlessness rating.

128. Bronchial breath sounds:

    1. Are soft and high-pitched and are heard over the manubrium.

    2. Are hollow sounds heard when auscultating over the large airways.

    3. Have an inspiratory phase that is longer than the expiratory phase.

    4. Are low-pitched sounds that can be heard over both lung fields.

129. The nurse practitioner (NP) is viewing the chest x-ray of a patient she suspects has pneumonia. What would the NP expect to see on the chest x-ray?

    1. Consolidations or infiltrates.

    2. Patchy air space disease.

    3. Diffuse bilateral coalescent opacities.

    4. Hyperlucent lungs.

130. Which medication is used as a treatment for tuberculosis?

    1. Linezolid.

    2. Lenvatinib.

    3. Ethambutol.

    4. Eumovate.

131. Which medication is used as a treatment for multi-drug-resistant tuberculosis?

    1. Clofazimine.

    2. Isoniazid.

    3. Eumovate.

    4. Rifampin.

132. Which of the following is a risk factor for transmission of tuberculosis via droplet nuclei?

    1. Presence of cavitary disease.

    2. Decreased forced expiratory volumes.

    3. History of chronic obstructive pulmonary disease.

    4. History of chain-smoking.

133. Tuberculosis is spread person to person via which modality?

    1. Sexual intercourse.

    2. Droplet nuclei.

    3. Contaminated food and/or water.

    4. Contact with another person.

134. The World Health Organization recommends how many drugs for treating multidrug-resistant tuberculosis?

    1. Three.

    2. Four.

    3. Five.

    4. Six.

135. The World Health Organization recommends how many months of intensive-phase treatment for multidrug-resistant tuberculosis?

    1. Three.

    2. Four.

    3. Five.

    4. Six.

136. Treatment of drug-sensitive pulmonary tuberculosis includes four medications often referred to as what kind of therapy?

    1. LIPS.

    2. RIPE.

    3. PAIL.

    4. RICE.

137. How many months does the intensive-phase treatment of drug-sensitive pulmonary tuberculosis last?

    1. One.

    2. Two.

    3. Three.

    4. Four.

138. How many drugs are used to treat drug-sensitive pulmonary tuberculosis in the continuation phase?

    1. One.

    2. Two.

    3. Three.

    4. Four.

139. Which of the following drugs are part of the treatment of drug-sensitive pulmonary tuberculosis in the continuation phase?

    1. Isoniazid and rifampin.

    2. Isoniazid and ethambutol.

    3. Pyrazinamide and rifampin.

    4. Ethambutol and pyrazinamide.

140. A 40-year-old male patient with persistent asthma will be discharged soon from the hospital after admission because of asthma exacerbation. He has been taking a low-dose beclomethasone inhaler daily and inhaled albuterol as needed for the last 2 years. He is completely stable now. Before discharge, he asks about the complications of prolonged beclomethasone use because he has some concerns about it. Which of the following is the most common complication of this drug?

    1. Osteoporosis.

    2. Purpura.

    3. Thrush.

    4. Cushing syndrome.

141. Which of the following is *not* a risk factor for a spontaneous pneumothorax?

    1. Genetics.

    2. Smoking.

    3. Subpleural blebs.

    4. Older age.

142. Secondary spontaneous pneumothorax is caused by an underlying disease. Which of the following is an example of an underlying disease that may cause a secondary spontaneous pneumothorax?

    1. Respiratory syncytial virus.

    2. Lymphocytic lymphoma.

    3. Langerhans cell granulomatosis.

    4. Pulmonary embolus.

143. What are the two diseases most commonly seen with secondary spontaneous pneumothorax?

    1. Pulmonary embolus and tuberculosis.

    2. Tuberculosis and chronic obstructive pulmonary disease.

    3. Marfan syndrome and pulmonary Langerhans cell granulomatosis.

    4. Respiratory syncytial virus and lymphocytic lymphoma.

144. Pathologically, what is the most common cause of a secondary spontaneous pneumothorax?

    1. Dysfunction of the alveoli sacs.

    2. Rupture of apical blebs or bullae.

    3. Thinning of the bronchial tissue.

    4. Fibrosis of the thoracic cavity.

145. Cystic fibrosis (CF) patients 18 years and older have an increased incidence of having secondary spontaneous pneumothorax. Other than CF, what else increases a CF patient's risk of having a secondary spontaneous pneumothorax?

    1. *Acinetobacter moori.*

    2. *Pseudomonas aeruginosa.*

    3. *Streptococcus pneumoniae.*

    4. *Bifidobacterium bifidum.*

146. A pneumothorax should be suspected in which patient?

    1. A 37-year-old female patient who complains of a productive cough with white sputum.

    2. A 43-year-old male patient with complaints of pleuritic chest pain and cough.

    3. A 48-year-old female patient with complaints of sudden-onset chest pain and shortness of breath.

    4. A 50-year-old male patient with complaints of a productive cough and fever.

147. The nurse practitioner (NP), suspects that his patient has a spontaneous pneumothorax. What would the NP expect to find on physical exam?

    1. Decreased chest excursion on the affected side.

    2. Circumoral cyanosis and cyanotic nail beds.

    3. Clubbing of fingers.

    4. Barrel chest.

148. Which diagnostic test would the nurse practitioner order on a hemodynamically stable patient to diagnose a spontaneous pneumothorax?

    1. Arterial blood gas.

    2. Chest x-ray.

    3. Electrocardiography.

    4. D-dimer and troponin.

149. What is a tension pneumothorax?

    1. One without mediastinal shift to the contralateral side.

    2. One with both fluid and air in the pleural space.

    3. One formed when air in the pleural space builds up enough to rupture part of the lung.

    4. One seen following pleural fluid removal of the lung cavity.

150. The nurse practitioner (NP) is seeing a patient with a complaint of a dry cough for the last 4 weeks. The patient has a history of diabetes and hypertension. The patient complains of no other symptoms. The NP reports a negative physical exam and suspects which of the following as the cause of the cough?

    1. Bronchitis.

    2. Metformin.

    3. Angiotensin-converting inhibitor.

    4. Allergies.

151. Which of the following is a predisposing factor for aspiration pneumonia?

    1. Protracted vomiting.

    2. Cystic fibrosis.

    3. Chronic obstructive pulmonary disease.

    4. Toxoplasmosis.

152. Which of the following is *not* an appropriate intervention to prevent aspiration pneumonia?

    1. Dietary changes.

    2. Improved oral hygiene.

    3. Sitting upright while eating.

    4. Chewing food 20 times before swallowing.

153. The term "chemical pneumonitis" refers to which of the following?

    1. The aspiration of substances that are toxic to the lower airways, independent of bacterial infection.

    2. A disease commonly associated with people who work in chemical factories.

    3. The inhalation of electronic cigarettes.

    4. A hypersensitive reaction to airborne pollutants.

154. Which of the following is *not* a symptom of chemical pneumonitis?

    1. Sudden-onset of dyspnea.

    2. Purulent sputum production.

    3. Low-grade fever.

    4. Diffuse crackles in lung fields.

155. What is the mainstay of treatment in chemical pneumonitis?

    1. Supplemental oxygen.

    2. Support of pulmonary function.

    3. Antibiotics.

    4. Mechanical ventilation.

156. Which of the following is a common microbe responsible for aspiration pneumonia?

    1. *Peptostreptococcus.*

    2. *Fusobacterium nucleatum.*

    3. *Bacteroides melaninogenicus.*

    4. *Staphylococcus aureus.*

Pulmonary Answers & Rationales

3

1. Answer: 1

Rationale: When empiric treatment that includes coverage for methicillin-sensitive *Staphylococcus aureus* (and not methicillin-resistant *S. aureus* [MRSA]) is indicated, the guidelines suggest a regimen, including piperacillin-tazobactam, cefepime, levofloxacin, imipenem, or meropenem. If empiric coverage for MRSA is indicated, either vancomycin or linezolid is recommended.

2. Answer: 3

Rationale: In an effort to minimize patient harm and exposure to unnecessary antibiotics and reduce the development of antibiotic resistance, the Infectious Diseases Society of America (IDSA) and the American Thoracic Society (ATS) guidelines recommend that the antibiogram data be used to decrease the unnecessary use of dual gram-negative and empiric methicillin-resistant *Staphylococcus aureus* (MRSA) antibiotic treatment. If empiric coverage for MRSA is indicated, either vancomycin or linezolid is recommended.

3. Answer: 2

Rationale: Typical bacterial pathogens causing community-acquired pneumonia (CAP) include streptococcal pneumonia (penicillin-sensitive/resistant strains), *Haemophilus influenza* (ampicillin-sensitive/resistant strains), and *Moraxella catarrhalis* (all strains penicillin-resistant) and account for about 85% of CAP cases. Aspiration pneumonia is the only form of CAP caused by multiple pathogens (e.g., aerobic/anaerobic oral organisms). *Klebsiella pneumoniae* CAP occurs primarily in individuals with chronic alcoholism, and *Staphylococcus aureus* may cause CAP in influenza patients. *Pseudomonas aeruginosa* is a cause of CAP in patients with bronchiectasis or cystic fibrosis. Empiric therapy for a hospitalized intensive care patient is azithromycin intravenously (IV) + ceftriaxone (Rocephin) IV.

4. Answer: 3

Rationale: If there are comorbidities present (e.g., alcoholism, bronchiectasis/cystic fibrosis, chronic obstructive pulmonary disease, intravenous (IV) drug user, post influenza, asplenia, diabetes mellitus, lung/liver/renal diseases) then use levofloxacin 750 mg by mouth (PO) every 24 hours or moxifloxacin 400 mg PO every 24 hours or a combination of a β-lactam (amoxicillin 1 g PO every 8 hours or amoxicillin-clavulanate 2 g PO every 12 hours or ceftriaxone 1 g IV/intramuscularly every 24 hours or cefuroxime 500 mg PO twice daily) plus a macrolide (azithromycin or clarithromycin).

5. Answer: 2

Rationale: This patient has ventilator-associated pneumonia and the patient has been in the hospital for several days, so an infection with multidrug-resistant organisms is a possibility. For that reason, Azactam 2 g intravenously every 8 hours and tobramycin 7 mg/kg every 24 hours, and vancomycin 1 g every 12 hours is the best answer.

6. Answer: 4

Rationale: Extensively drug-resistant *Acinetobacter baumannii* should be treated with minocycline with Colistin for 14 days based on antibiograms.

7. Answer: 4

Rationale: Aldactone can be used for congestive heart failure for the management of edema and sodium retention when the patient is only partially responsive to, or is intolerant of, other therapeutic measures. Aldactone is also indicated for patients with congestive heart failure taking digitalis when other therapies are considered inappropriate.

8. Answer: 1

Rationale: Do not swallow Spiriva capsules. Spiriva capsules should only be used with the Spiriva Handihaler device and inhaled through your mouth (oral inhalation).

9. Answer: 4

Rationale: Inhaled short-acting β_2 agonists are effective in treating a person whose symptoms are rapidly getting worse (chronic obstructive pulmonary disease [COPD] exacerbation) and improving lung function and shortness of breath in stable COPD.

10. Answer: 3

Rationale: Robitussin DM is used as an expectorant and will not help these symptoms.

11. Answer: 1

Rationale: The patient is acidotic, so a buffering agent needs to be administered, such as 1 ampule of $NaHCO_3$ intravenously.

12. Answer: 1

Rationale: Acute respiratory distress syndrome, characterized by hypoxemic respiratory failure, is associated with a mortality of 30% to 50% and is precipitated by both direct and indirect pulmonary insults. Treatment is largely supportive, consisting of lung protective ventilation, necessitating intensive care unit admission. The most common precipitant is community-acquired bacterial pneumonia.

13. Answer: 4

Rationale: High-altitude pulmonary edema, which can be seen with quick assent or descent from high altitudes.

14. Answer: 3

Rationale: Congestive heart failure is considered high-pressure pulmonary edema caused by fluid backup.

15. Answer: 2

Rationale: The slight elevation in Po_2 indicates a shunt and the most likely cause is hypoxemia, so this exhibits acute respiratory alkalosis.

16. Answer: 2

Rationale: The classic asthma triad is cough, wheezing, and dyspnea.

17. Answer: 3

Rationale: Total lung capacity is the volume of air in the lungs at the end of inspiration.

18. Answer: 1

Rationale: The work of breathing is the amount of effort needed to inhale and exhale.

19. Answer: 2

Rationale: The goal of respirator acidosis is to improve alveolar ventilation and increase minute ventilation. This can be done by decreasing the Pco_2.

20. Answer: 4

Rationale: It is a worsening airspace disease, such as acute respiratory distress syndrome or pneumonia.

21. Answer: 3

Rationale: Hemoglobin allows for blood transport of oxygen.

22. Answer: 2

Rationale: Myasthenia gravis impacts the extraparenchymal tissue.

23. Answer: 4

Rationale: Intraluminal thrombi are caused by diminished cross-sectional area from obstruction.

24. Answer: 3

Rationale: Interstitial lung disease is caused by chronic prolonged hypoxemia.

25. Answer: 4

Rationale: The alveolar to arterial gradient measures the difference between the partial pressure of oxygen in the alveoli and the arterial partial pressure of oxygen.

26. Answer: 2

Rationale: Diffusing capacity of the lungs for carbon monoxide is a medical test that determines how much oxygen travels from the alveoli of the lungs to the blood stream.

27. Answer: 1

Rationale: Forced expiratory volume in 1 second is the gold standard for measuring obstructive airway disease.

28. Answer: 4

Rationale: short-acting β_2 agonists work by relaxing airway smooth muscles.

29. Answer: 1

Rationale: Muscle tremors and palpitations are a common side effect of β_2 agonists.

30. Answer: 2

Rationale: The Global Initiative for Asthma recommends a short-acting β_2 agonist, metered-dose inhaler, 4 to 8 puffs every 20 minutes up to 4 hours for mild asthma.

31. Answer: 3

Rationale: Using a stepwise approach, the nurse practitioner would prescribe a long-acting β_2 agonist and low-dose inhaled corticosteroid.

32. Answer: 3

Rationale: Community-acquired pneumonia (CAP) is one of the most common acute infections requiring admission to the hospital. The main causative pathogens of CAP are *Streptococcus pneumoniae*, influenza A, *Mycoplasma pneumoniae*, and *Chlamydophila pneumoniae*, and the dominant risk factors are age, smoking, and comorbidities.

33. Answer: 2

Rationale: House painters are at risk for asbestosis, silicosis, and alveolitis. A chest x-ray would be the first test to order for this patient because of its specificity.

34. Answer: 4

Rationale: In the Prospective Investigation of Pulmonary Embolism Diagnosis (PIOPED II) study, 94% of patients with pulmonary embolism had one or more of the following risk factors: immobilization, trauma, or surgery. There is no specific treatment for asbestosis, but smoking cessation will prevent further lung damage.

35. Answer: 3

Rationale: While there are many risk factors for a pulmonary embolism, coronary artery disease is not a risk factor.

36. Answer: 1

Rationale: Factor V Leiden is not part of the Virchow triad, which consists of three factors that may predispose a person to the development of venous thrombosis. These factors include hypercoagulability, stasis, and endothelial injury.

37. Answer: 2

Rationale: Most emboli that cause a pulmonary embolus (PE) arise from veins in the lower extremities. A PE is present in 60% to 80% of patients with deep vein thrombosis, even though more than half of these patients are asymptomatic.

38. Answer: 3

Rationale: In an altered ventilation to perfusion ratio, a low pressure of oxygen in venous blood also may contribute to arterial hypoxemia when PE causes right ventricular failure. Low cardiac output leads to increased extraction of oxygen in the tissues, decreasing the partial pressure of oxygen in venous blood below normal levels. Venous blood with an abnormally low Po_2 amplifies the effect of a low ventilation to perfusion ratio when it passes through diseased lung gas-exchange units to the systemic circulation.

39. Answer: 4

Rationale: Increased pulmonary vascular resistance decreases right ventricular outflow and causes right ventricular dilation and flattening or bowing of the intraventricular septum. Both diminished flow from the right ventricle and right ventricular dilation reduce left ventricular preload, compromising cardiac output.

40. Answer: 1

Rationale: Treatment options for the initial-phase management of a pulmonary embolism include thrombolytics, parenteral anticoagulants, oral anticoagulants, and nonpharmacological interventions. Because this patient is hemodynamically stable, low-molecular-weight heparin is the best option.

41. Answer: 3

Rationale: In pulmonary function testing, a postbronchodilator forced expiratory volume in 1 second (FEV_1)/forced vital capacity (FVC) ratio of less than 0.70 is commonly considered diagnostic for chronic obstructive pulmonary disease. The Global Initiative for Chronic Obstructive Lung Disease (GOLD) system categorizes airflow limitation into stages. In patients with an FEV_1/FVC ratio of less than 0.70, GOLD 3 or severe, FEV_1 is less than or equal to 30% of normal value and less than 50% of predicted value.

42. Answer: 1

Rationale: Chronic bronchitis is a clinical diagnosis characterized by a cough productive of sputum for over 3 months' duration during 2 consecutive years and the presence of airflow obstruction. Pulmonary function testing aids in the diagnosis of chronic bronchitis by documenting the extent of reversibility of airflow obstruction.

43. Answer: 3

Rationale: Although a chest x-ray may not show chronic obstructive pulmonary disease (COPD) until it is severe, the images may show enlarged lungs, air pockets (bullae), or a flattened diaphragm. A chest x-ray also may be used to determine whether another condition may be causing symptoms similar to COPD. Consolidation in one lung lobe suggests an infectious process.

44. Answer: 2

Rationale: Patients with emphysema have hyperinflated lungs, which can cause increased total lung capacity, but because of decreased recoil the lung can have a decreased capacity. The air gets trapped; thus an increased residual volume would not be expected on pulmonary function testing.

45. Answer: 2

Rationale: This patient probably has an acid-base disorder causing her mental status change, and this needs to be evaluated.

46. Answer: 3

Rationale: The patient must be on mechanical ventilation with an Fio_2 of at least 0.6 or greater. There is no Fio_2 requirement for acute respiratory distress syndrome.

47. Answer: 4

Rationale: Chest radiograph findings of acute respiratory distress syndrome vary widely depending on the stage of the disease. The most common chest radiograph findings are bilateral, predominantly peripheral, somewhat asymmetrical consolidation with air bronchograms.

48. Answer: 1

Rationale: Nosocomial infections, such as ventilator-associated pneumonia, catheter-related infections, or *Clostridium difficile*, can cause morbidity and mortality in a patient with acute respiratory distress syndrome.

49. Answer: 2

Rationale: The release of tumor necrosis factor, which goes on to recruit neutrophils to the lungs, which release toxins, causes acute respiratory distress syndrome.

50. Answer: 4

Rationale: Histopathologically, three phases are recognized during the evolution of acute respiratory distress syndrome: (1) an exudative early phase, which results from diffuse alveolar damage and endothelial injury; (2) a proliferative phase, which ensues about 7 to 14 days after the injury, incorporating repair of the damaged alveolar structure and reestablishment of the barrier function, together with proliferation of fibroblasts; and (3) a fibrotic phase with chronic inflammation and fibrosis of the alveoli, which follows in some patients.

51. Answer: 2

Rationale: Sepsis-induced acute respiratory distress syndrome (ARDS) is often caused by indirect injury to the lung. However, pneumonia can directly injure the lung leading to ARDS and can cause sepsis. Pathway sepsis is more likely to work indirectly because this pathway of injury has been shown to be caused by inflammatory mediators. These mediators cause systemic endothelial damage, causing the lung damage that precedes ARDS.

52. Answer: 4

Rationale: An 80-year-old female patient who smoked in her early 20s but has not smoked since is at an increased risk of death from acute respiratory distress syndrome. Older patients have a 41% higher mortality rate.

53. Answer: 1

Rationale: Patients who survived acute respiratory distress syndrome had persistent exercise limitations and a reduced physical quality of life 5 years after their critical illness.

54. Answer: 2

Rationale: Maximize oxygen consumption by improving tolerance of mechanical ventilation.

55. Answer: 1

Rationale: The initial ventilator settings for a patient with acute respiratory distress syndrome begin with low tidal volume ventilation, which is also known as lung protective ventilation, 4 to 8 mL/kg predicted body weight.

56. Answer: 4

Rationale: There are no risk factors for transfusion-related acute lung injury. Risk factors are associated with pretransfusion issues such as sepsis, cancer, or patients who had received multiple transfusions.

57. Answer: 2

Rationale: Polymorphonuclear leukocytes (PMNs) are generally considered to be key effector cells in transfusion-related acute lung injury (TRALI). Pulmonary PMN infiltration has been described to occur in multiple animal models of TRALI. Additionally, the abundance of PMNs has been observed in the pulmonary tissue of TRALI patients on autopsy. PMNs are major producers of reactive oxygen species (ROS), and ROS production has been suggested to damage the endothelium in murine antibody-mediated TRALI models and in human pulmonary microvascular endothelial cells in vitro.

58. Answer: 2

Rationale: The diagnostic features of transfusion-related acute lung injury (TRALI), as follows: onset within 1 to 6 hours of transfusion, are acute respiratory distress, acute bilateral pulmonary edema (noncardiogenic), severe hypoxemia, hypotension (rarely hypertension), and fever. Mental status change is not associated with TRALI.

59. Answer: 3

Rationale: The National Heart Lung and Blood Institute Working Group on transfusion-related acute lung injury (TRALI) developed a definition. In patients with no ALI immediately before transfusion, and no other ALI risk factor is present, a diagnosis of TRALI is made by chest x-ray.

60. Answer: 4

Rationale: Stop the blood transfusion. The patient is most likely suffering from a transfusion-related acute lung injury.

61. Answer: 3

Rationale: Obesity, lung cancer, and hypertension do not increase a patient's risk of chronic obstructive pulmonary disease. However, gastroesophageal reflux does, but the exact etiology is unclear.

62. Answer: 3

Rationale: Cystic fibrosis is not considered a type of chronic obstructive disease (COPD). Although cystic fibrosis impacts the lungs, it also impacts other body systems so it cannot fall under the classification of COPD.

63. Answer: 1

Rationale: The pathological changes occur in goblet cells. Goblet cells in the airways are increased in someone with chronic obstructive pulmonary disease (COPD). Chronic bronchitis involves an increase in goblet cell number, enlarged submucosal glands, mucus hypersecretion and plugging of the airways, and chronic cough. Even COPD patients without chronic bronchitis have mucus obstruction of the small airways.

64. Answer: 2

Rationale: CD8+ (also known as T lymphocytes) lymphocytes may be the predominant cellular element for direct mediation of tissue injuries, but the importance of CD4+ lymphocytes in orchestrating the inflammatory response and facilitating autoimmune humoral responses also appears to be considerable.

65. Answer: 1

Rationale: In asthma, eosinophils, mast cells, and CD4 T lymphocytes represent the predominant cell types in the inflammatory process. In contrast, chronic obstructive pulmonary disease and bronchiectasis demonstrate a greater number of neutrophils, macrophages, and CD8 T lymphocytes.

66. Answer: 3

Rationale: Proximal acinar or centrilobular emphysema are common associated with cigarette smoking. This type of emphysema refers to abnormal dilation or destruction of the respiratory bronchiole, the central portion of the acinus. Centrilobular (proximal acinar) emphysema is the most common type and is commonly associated with smoking. It also can be seen in coal workers pneumoconiosis.

67. Answer: 4

Rationale: Panacinar emphysema is most commonly seen in people with α_1-antitrypsin deficiency, but it also can been seen in a small percentage of smokers. An α_1-antitrypsin deficiency is most common in white people, and it most frequently affects the lungs and liver. In the lungs, the most common manifestation is early-onset (patients in their 30s and 40s) panacinar emphysema most pronounced in the lung bases.

68. Answer: 4

Rationale: In paraseptal emphysema, the distal respiratory acinus, including alveolar duct and alveoli, is expanded. It occurs primarily adjacent to the pleura and connective tissue septa, especially in the upper lobes. Extensive involvement of the lung is rare. Some cases of spontaneous pneumothorax may be caused by this type of emphysema.

69. Answer: 2

Rationale: Exposure to animals with heavily shed coats or animals with hair has not been shown to be a risk factor for chronic obstructive pulmonary disease.

70. Answer: 1

Rationale: The three cardinal symptoms of chronic obstructive pulmonary disease are dyspnea, chronic cough, and sputum production, and the most common early symptom is exertional dyspnea. Less common symptoms include wheezing and chest tightness.

71. Answer: 2

Rationale: Weight loss is common due to dyspnea. Clubbing of the digits is not typical in chronic obstructive pulmonary disease (even with associated hypoxemia) and suggests comorbidities such as lung cancer, interstitial lung disease, or bronchiectasis.

72. Answer: 2

Rationale: The assessment of chronic obstructive pulmonary disease proposed by the Global Initiative for Chronic Obstructive Lung Disease has been based on the patient's level of symptoms, future risk of exacerbations, the extent of airflow limitation, the spirometric abnormality, and the identification of comorbidities.

73. Answer: 4

Rationale: The patient's symptoms are mild or infrequent so this would be considered class A.

74. Answer: 1

Rationale: The patient should be prescribed a short-acting bronchodilator and is categorized as "A" or low risk.

75. Answer: 2

Rationale: The patient should be prescribed a long-acting bronchodilator because the patient's chronic obstructive pulmonary disease is getting worse.

76. Answer: 2

Rationale: Flattened diaphragm caused by hyperinflation is the most likely radiographic finding.

77. Answer: 1

Rationale: The computed tomography scan has greater sensitivity and specificity than standard chest radiography for the detection of emphysema.

78. Answer: 3

Rationale: Using clinical indicators (dyspnea, sputum purulence, sputum volume) and severity of illness (advanced airflow limitation, presence of comorbidities, need for mechanical ventilation) can help identify patients who may benefit most from antibiotics; laboratory data (sputum culture, C-reactive protein, procalcitonin) alone should not be used to guide initiation of antibiotics.

79. Answer: 2

Rationale: 7 to 10 days of corticosteroid therapy is the standard of care for hemodynamically stable patients. Systemic corticosteroids are efficacious in the treatment of acute exacerbations of chronic obstructive pulmonary disease (AECOPD) and considered a standard of care for patients experiencing an AECOPD. Therefore systemic corticosteroids should be administered to all patients experiencing AECOPD severe enough to seek emergent medical care.

The lowest effective dose and shortest duration of therapy is the standard.

80. Answer: 3

Rationale: Low tidal volumes will help to prevent dynamic hyperinflation of the lungs.

81. Answer: 4

Rationale: Noninvasive ventilation is considered the standard of care in the management of acute hypercapnic respiratory failure secondary to chronic obstructive pulmonary disease. It can be delivered safely in any dedicated setting.

82. Answer: 1

Rationale: Lung cancer in an indication for pneumonectomy. Traditional/standard pneumonectomy is removal of the entire lung. Extrapleural pneumonectomy is removal of the entire lung, as well as a part of the membrane that covers the heart (pericardium), part of the diaphragm, and the membrane, which lines the inside of the chest (pleura).

83. Answer: 4

Rationale: The patient is at a moderate-to-high risk for postoperative morbidity. Diffusing capacity is an independent predictor of morbidity after major lung resection. Diffusing capacity is an important predictor of postoperative morbidity after lung resection, even in patients with normal spirometry.

84. Answer: 2

Rationale: Evaluation of tuberculosis status is not part of preoperative assessment.

85. Answer: 3

Rationale: Forced expiratory volume in 1 second and the diffusion capacity of the lungs for carbon monoxide are the best predictors of morbidity and mortality.

86. Answer: 4

Rationale: Cardiac complications are the second most common cause of morbidity and mortality in patients subjected to thoracic surgery after respiratory complications. Postoperative arrhythmia is one of the most common cardiac complications in these patients. Atrial fibrillation is the most common arrhythmia seen after pneumonectomy. The pathophysiology involved in the development of postoperative atrial fibrillation is multifactorial, and it involves a complex interaction between "triggering" stimuli and "sustaining" processes acting on a myocardial substrate that may be predisposed to developing tachyarrhythmia.

87. Answer: 2

Rationale: Arrhythmias most often occur 2 to 4 days post-operatively. Postoperative atrial fibrillation (POAF) is a common and potentially morbid complication following cardiac surgery. POAF occurs in around 35% of cardiac surgery cases and has a peak incidence on between postoperative days 2 and 4.

88. Answer: 1

Rationale: Keeping serum magnesium levels normal can decrease the likelihood of a postoperative arrhythmia. Magnesium plays an essential role in many fundamental biological reactions because it is involved in more than 300 metabolic reactions. Deficiency of magnesium may result in many disorders, including cardiac arrhythmias.

89. Answer: 1

Rationale: Chronic obstructive pulmonary disease is not a potential postoperative complication of a pneumonectomy.

90. Answer: 3

Rationale: Cardiopleural fistula is not a complication of the pleural space after a pneumonectomy. A true fistula of the circulatory system is characterized by a clearly ectatic vascular segment that exhibits fistulous flow and connects two vascular territories governed by widely variant hemodynamic environments.

91. Answer: 1

Rationale: Pulmonary resection, including pneumonectomy, lobectomy, and wedge resection are indications for one-lung ventilation.

92. Answer: 3

Rationale: Tumor histology, extent of disease, and comorbidity are considered when determining treatment for lung cancer. These 3 factors have the most impact on treatment.

93. Answer: 4

Rationale: Plain chest radiographs can be normal in up to 75% of patients with asthma. Reported features with asthma include pulmonary hyperinflation bronchial wall thickening, peribronchial cuffing (nonspecific finding but may be present in ~48% of cases with asthma), pulmonary edema (rare), and/or pulmonary edema caused asthma (usually occurs with acute asthma).

94. Answer: 2

Rationale: It is a short-acting muscarinic agent used in the treatment of chronic asthma.

95. Answer: 4

Rationale: *Mycobacterium tuberculosis* is a gram-positive, rod-shaped aerobic bacteria.

96. Answer: 3

Rationale: *Mycobacterium* is the cause of pulmonary tuberculosis.

97. Answer: 1

Rationale: "Tuberculosis can be spread when I cough or sneeze and don't cover my mouth." Tuberculosis is spread by airborne droplets and can be spread when someone speaks or sings.

98. Answer: 2

Rationale: Chemotherapy is the primary treatment for small-cell lung cancer because it spreads quickly. The most used chemotherapy regimen is etoposide (available as a generic drug) or irinotecan (Camptosar) plus a platinum-based drug such as cisplatin (available as a generic drug) or carboplatin (available as a generic drug).

99. Answer: 3

Rationale: Persons with latent tuberculosis (TB) infection do not feel sick and do not have any symptoms. They are infected with *Mycobacterium tuberculosis* but do not have TB disease. The only sign of TB infection is a positive reaction to the tuberculin skin test or a TB blood test.

100. Answer: 2

Rationale: Hilar adenopathy is the most common finding; changes were visible as early as 1 week after skin test conversion, and within 2 months in all cases.

101. Answer: 3

Rationale: Airway remodeling can result from poorly controlled asthma.

102. Answer: 2

Rationale: A 35-year-old female patient who was just released from prison should be screened for latent tuberculosis because this is an individual at risk of infection due to the close living quarters.

103. Answer: 2

Rationale: Pulmonary hypertension (PH) is due to idiopathic causes such as being drug and toxin induced, connective tissue disorder, portal hypertension, and so forth. Patients with this type of PH are in group 1.

104. Answer: 2

Rationale: Precapillary pulmonary hypertension includes the clinical groups 1 (pulmonary arterial hypertension), 3 (pulmonary hypertension caused by lung diseases and/or hypoxia), 4 (chronic thromboembolic pulmonary hypertension), and 5 (pulmonary hypertension with unclear and/or multifactorial mechanisms). Postcapillary pulmonary hypertension corresponds to clinical group 2 (pulmonary hypertension caused by left heart diseases).

105. Answer: 4

Rationale: Initial symptoms of pulmonary hypertension include exertional dyspnea, lethargy, and fatigue, but they also can include dizziness, chest pressure, or pain and ankle edema.

106. Answer: 1

Rationale: Impaired cardiac output on exercise and abnormal gas exchange both contribute to increased ventilatory drive, and this leads to an inadequate increase in cardiac output during exercise.

107. Answer: 2

Rationale: Subendocardial hypoperfusion caused by increased right ventricular wall stress and myocardial oxygen demand. The increase in pulmonary vascular resistance and pulmonary artery pressure imposes a sustained pressure load on the right ventricle (RV) resulting in its hypertrophy. Normally, perfusion to RV myocardium is maintained throughout systole and diastole because of the lower intraventricular pressures. However, in the presence of severe pulmonary artery hypertension its perfusion becomes like that of the left ventricle and depends on diastolic arterial pressure and diastolic duration.

108. Answer: 1

Rationale: Pulmonary arterial hypertension (PAH) is a right heart failure syndrome. In early-stage PAH, the right ventricle tends to remain adapted to afterload with increased contractility and little or no increase in right heart chamber dimensions.

109. Answer: 3

Rationale: Findings in patients with pulmonary artery hypertension include central pulmonary arterial dilatation, which contrasts with "pruning" (loss) of the peripheral blood vessels.

110. Answer: 4

Rationale: There is no specific lab abnormality in patients with pulmonary hypertension.

111. Answer: 3

Rationale: The transthoracic echocardiogram remains the most important noninvasive screening tool, and right heart catheterization remains mandatory to establish the diagnosis.

112. Answer: 1

Rationale: Many pulmonary hypertension (PH) patients become short of breath under mild-to-moderate exertion but feel fine at rest. Those who experience shortness of breath at rest or very mild exertion must be very closely monitored because exercise can induce fainting, excess stress to the right side of the heart, and other problems.

Because of the varying severity of PH from patient to patient (and other health-related factors), recommendations on exercise for PH patients are different for each individual and may change over time depending on symptoms and response to treatment.

113. Answer: 2

Rationale: Diuretic treatment is normally initiated alongside pulmonary artery hypertension–specific therapy. Loop diuretics (e.g., furosemide, torsemide, bumetanide), which inhibit reabsorption of sodium in the loops of Henle, are used when patients with pulmonary artery hypertension experience edema in their extremities.

114. Answer: 4

Rationale: "I need to use birth control because pregnancy can worsen my pulmonary hypertension (PH)." PH is associated with increased maternal and fetal risks, including high risk of maternal death.

115. Answer: 2

Rationale: The patient has lobar pneumonia in an extended care facility, which is considered a community setting. The most common bacteria for this type of pneumonia is *Streptococcus pneumoniae*.

116. Answer: 3

Rationale: A 53-year-old male patient has the worst prognosis. Increased age and male gender are frequently cited as factors associated with worse survival.

117. Answer: 3

Rationale: Obstructive sleep apnea is defined broadly as an Apnea–Hypopnea Index greater than 5 events per hour of sleep.

118. Answer: 3

Rationale: Factors that increase the risk of this form of sleep apnea include excess weight. Obesity greatly increases the risk of sleep apnea. Fat deposits around your upper airway can obstruct your breathing. Regarding neck circumference, people with thicker necks might have narrower airways. Men are 2 to 3 times more likely to have sleep apnea than are women.

119. Answer: 1

Rationale: The obstructive sleep apnea airway collapse leads to the blood pressure being driven up, and without treatment, the patient continues in a self-perpetuating pathophysiological cycle that leads to an increase in their cardiovascular and cerebrovascular risk.

120. Answer: 4

Rationale: The signs of obstructive sleep apnea include snoring, daytime sleepiness, pauses in breathing, difficulties with memory and concentration, unusual moodiness or irritability, frequently waking up to urinate at night, morning headaches, and dry mouth.

121. Answer: 1

Rationale: Crowded airway is the most like physical exam finding. Numerous craniofacial conditions can narrow the upper airway and contribute to the development of obstructive sleep apnea.

122. Answer: 4

Rationale: Excessive daytime sleepiness, habitual loud snoring, and hypertension are all signs of obstructive sleep apnea, and testing is warranted.

123. Answer: 4

Rationale: None of the tools can be used to diagnose the patient. Obstructive sleep apnea (OSA) is not a clinical diagnosis and diagnostic testing must be performed. Diagnostic testing for OSA should be performed.

124. Answer: 3

Rationale: In-laboratory polysomnography should be used for diagnosing obstructive sleep apnea. Either full-night ([i.e., diagnostic only] or split-night [i.e., diagnostic and therapeutic with positive airway pressure]) testing is the gold standard.

125. Answer: 2

Rationale: The patient is an airline pilot, so the nurse practitioner is more likely to perform a polysomnogram. Patients who are considered "mission critical workers," such as airline pilots, should have a polysomnography done in the lab. The rationale for this approach is that the risk to the patient and to others of missing a diagnosis of obstructive sleep apnea is sufficiently high to justify laboratory testing.

126. Answer: 4

Rationale: Myocardial infarction is *not* a condition associated with sleep-disordered breathing.

127. Answer: 1

Rationale: The COPD Assessment Test (CAT) is a questionnaire for people with chronic obstructive pulmonary disease (COPD). It is designed to measure the impact of COPD on a person's life and how this changes over time. The CAT is simple to administer, and aims to help clinicians, with their patients, better manage COPD.

128. Answer: 2

Rationale: Bronchial breath sounds are tubular, hollow sounds heard when auscultating over the large airways (e.g., second and third intercostal spaces). They will be louder and higher pitched than vesicular breath sounds.

129. Answer: 1

Rationale: The x-ray findings of pneumonia are airspace opacity, lobar consolidation, or interstitial opacities.

130. Answer: 3

Rationale: Ethambutol is one drug of the four-drug treatment for tuberculosis. The other medications are isoniazid, rifampin, and pyrazinamide.

131. Answer: 1

Rationale: Clofazimine and cycloserine/terizidone are just part of the choice of drugs needed to treat multidrug-resistant tuberculosis.

132. Answer: 1

Rationale: Presence of cavitary disease is associated with risk for tuberculosis transmission via droplet nuclei.

133. Answer: 2

Rationale: Droplet nuclei can be spread when speaking, singing, coughing, or sneezing.

134. Answer: 2

Rationale: In patients with confirmed rifampicin-susceptible and isoniazid-resistant tuberculosis, treatment with rifampicin, ethambutol, pyrazinamide, and levofloxacin is recommended for a duration of 6 months.

135. Answer: 4

Rationale: In patients with confirmed rifampicin-susceptible and isoniazid-resistant tuberculosis, treatment with rifampicin, ethambutol, pyrazinamide, and levofloxacin is recommended for a duration of 6 months.

136. Answer: 2

Rationale: The four-medication treatment is rifampin, isoniazid, pyrazinamide, and ethambutol (RIPE) therapy.

137. Answer: 2

Rationale: After 2 months of intensive-phase treatment (for a fully susceptible isolate), pyrazinamide can be stopped.

138. Answer: 2

Rationale: Isoniazid plus rifampin are continued as daily or intermittent therapy for 4 more months.

139. Answer: 1

Rationale: Isoniazid and rifampin are continued as daily or intermittent therapy for 4 more months.

140. Answer: 3

Rationale: The most common side effect associated with the use of inhaled corticosteroids is oropharyngeal candidiasis. Thrush occurs when the corticosteroid inhalers that depress the immune system in the lungs have the same effect on the surface of the throat.

141. Answer: 4

Rationale: Older age is not a risk factor for a spontaneous pneumothorax.

142. Answer: 3

Rationale: Underlying diseases that cause secondary spontaneous pneumothoraxes are emphysema, infections, pneumonitis, and granulomatosis.

143. Answer: 2

Rationale: Tuberculosis and chronic obstructive pulmonary disease are associated with secondary spontaneous pneumothorax.

144. Answer: 2

Rationale: Rupture of apical blebs or bullae are the most common pathological cause of secondary spontaneous pneumothoraxes.

145. Answer: 2

Rationale: *Pseudomonas aeruginosa* is a risk factor for secondary spontaneous pneumothorax.

146. Answer: 2

Rationale: A pneumothorax should be suspected in a 43-year-old male patient with complaints of pleuritic chest pain and cough. Sharp, sudden-onset chest pain; cough; shortness of breath; and tachycardia are just some of the signs of a pneumothorax.

147. Answer: 1

Rationale: Decreased chest excursion on the affected side would indicate a pneumothorax because there would not be any lung expansion on the affected side.

148. Answer: 2

Rationale: Chest x-ray is enough to diagnose a pneumothorax in this patient.

149. Answer: 3

Rationale: A tension pneumothorax develops when a lung or chest wall injury is such that it allows air into the pleural space but not out of it. As a result, air accumulates and compresses the lung, eventually shifting the mediastinum, compressing the contralateral lung, and increasing intrathoracic pressure enough to decrease venous return to the heart, causing shock. These effects can develop rapidly, particularly in patients undergoing positive pressure ventilation.

150. Answer: 3

Rationale: Angiotensin-converting enzyme (ACE) inhibitors are associated with a dry, persistent cough in 5% to 35% of patients who take them. The mechanism of cough is likely multifactorial. ACE inhibitors prevent the breakdown of bradykinin and substance P, resulting in an accumulation of protussive mediators in the respiratory tract.

151. Answer: 1

Rationale: Protracted vomiting is a predisposing factor because it interferes with closure of the glottis.

152. Answer: 4

Rationale: Chewing food 20 times before swallowing does not help prevent aspiration pneumonia.

153. Answer: 1

Rationale: Chemical pneumonitis refers to the aspiration of substances that are toxic to the lower airways, independent of bacterial infection.

154. Answer: 2

Rationale: Patients with chemical pneumonitis may present with an acute onset or abrupt development of symptoms within a few minutes to 2 hours of the aspiration event, as well as respiratory distress and rapid breathing, audible wheezing, and cough with pink or frothy sputum.

155. Answer: 2

Rationale: The patient with chemical pneumonitis will have compromised air exchange leading to a compromised respiratory system. Support of pulmonary function is the mainstay of pulmonary function.

156. Answer: 4

Rationale: The pathogens that commonly produce pneumonia, such as *Streptococcus pneumoniae*, *Haemophilus influenzae*, gram-negative bacilli, and *Staphylococcus aureus*, are relatively virulent bacteria so that only a small inoculum is required, and the aspiration is usually subtle.

4

Endocrine

1. A 25-year-old male patient is admitted to the intensive care unit after a motor vehicle collision resulting in an isolated severe traumatic brain injury causing elevated intracranial pressure. He is on a ventilator and minimally responsive. On the second day of hospitalization, he has increasing vasopressor requirements and hourly urine output of 400 mL. To address this problem, the nurse practitioner would:

   1. Order a fluid restriction.

   2. Order serum sodium, urine-specific gravity.

   3. Order 24-hour urine protein and creatinine.

   4. Order a stat noncontrast computed tomography of the head.

2. A 25-year-old male patient is admitted to the intensive care unit after a motor vehicle collision resulting in an isolated severe traumatic brain injury causing elevated intracranial pressure. He is on a ventilator and minimally responsive. On the second day of hospitalization, he has increasing vasopressor requirements and hourly urine output of 400 mL. His serum sodium increased from 146 to 155 in the last 6 hours and urine specific gravity (SG) is 1.001. To address this problem, the nurse practitioner would:

   1. Order 2 mcg desmopressin (DDAVP) intravenously (IV) and 1 L 0.9% saline.

   2. Increase maintenance fluids from 75 to 150 mL/hr and repeat sodium and SG in 6 hours.

   3. Order 2 mcg DDAVP IV and fluid restriction.

   4. Calculate the free water deficit and order free water via nasogastric tube.

3. A 68-year-old 70-kg male patient with a history of tobacco abuse was admitted with dyspnea. A chest x-ray revealed a pulmonary mass, flattened bilateral diaphragm, and no pulmonary edema. He is alert and breathing comfortably after being started on 4 L of oxygen via nasal cannula. His initial sodium is 128 mEq/L. Based on the nurse practitioner's knowledge of the probable diagnosis, how would the nurse practitioner correct his sodium?

   1. Start 3% saline at 75 mL/hr.

   2. Start 0.9% saline at 1000 mL/hr.

   3. Institute a fluid restriction.

   4. Order 40 mg furosemide and repeat sodium in 8 hours.

4. A 55-year-old female patient with a history of type 2 diabetes and diverticulitis is admitted to the intensive care unit following laparotomy for colectomy. She remains intubated and requires norepinephrine at 0.06 mcg/kg/min to maintain a mean arterial pressure greater than 65 mmHg despite adequate intraoperative fluid resuscitation. Her blood glucose is 220 mg/dL. The nurse practitioner's initial glucose management strategy will entail starting:

   1. Insulin(R) infusion with target glucose less than 120 mg/dL.

   2. Insulin(R) subcutaneous (SQ) sliding scale with target glucose 140 to 180 mg/dL.

   3. Insulin(R) SQ sliding scale with target glucose less than 120 mg/dL.

   4. Insulin(R) infusion with target glucose 140 to 180 mg/dL.

5. A 55-year-old female patient with a history of type 2 diabetes and diverticulitis was admitted to the intensive care unit after laparotomy for colectomy. She was briefly intubated and on vasopressors. She is now weaned off norepinephrine and transferred to a med/surg floor. She is tolerating oral nutrition with a carbohydrate-controlled diet and is still on insulin infusion at 0.5 units/hr with a 24-hour glucose range of 150 to 180 mg/dL. Her home regimen involves metformin 1000 mg twice a day (BID) by mouth and a carbohydrate-controlled diet. Hemoglobin A1c is 7.8%. The most appropriate next step in the management of this patient's diabetes is:

   1. Restart home metformin and monitor blood glucose Q achs.

   2. Continue the insulin infusion for 24 more hours.

   3. Restart and increase metformin to 2000 mg BID.

   4. Start insulin glargine 12 units daily and a subcutaneous sliding scale.

6. An 85-year-old female patient is admitted to a med/surg floor with a urinary tract infection and confusion. She is tolerating a regular diet and has no history of diabetes. The glucose on her initial chemistry panel is 230 mg/dL and hemoglobin A1c is 10%. The most appropriate management of this patient's glucose is:

   1. Start insulin infusion and follow glucose once every hour.

   2. Initiate a subcutaneous basal, prandial, correction regimen.

   3. Start metformin 1500 mg twice a day.

   4. Instruct patient to follow up with her primary care provider 2 weeks after discharge.

7. An 85-year-old female patient is admitted to a med/surg floor with urinary tract infection and confusion. She is tolerating a regular diet and has no history of diabetes. The glucose on her initial chemistry panel is 230 mg/dL and hemoglobin A1c is 10%. Her glucose was 140 mg/dL with glargine and lispro. When planning the discharge for this patient, you learn that she plans to return home but is confused during insulin teaching. What is the best way to manage this patient's hyperglycemia at home?

   1. Transition to an oral agent and confirm follow-up with primary care is available.

   2. Discharge with prescriptions for glargine, lispro, and syringes.

   3. Discharge with prescriptions for glargine and lispro pens.

   4. Refer the patient to her home county's adult protective services.

8. In a patient with fatigue and weight loss, what would confirm a tentative diagnosis of primary adrenal insufficiency?

   1. 2 p.m. serum cortisol 180 nmol/L.

   2. 8 a.m. serum cortisol 150 nmol/L.

   3. 24-hour urinary free cortisol 8 mcg/24 hr.

   4. Corticotropin test with peak cortisol less than 550 nmol/L.

9. A patient with recent chronic obstructive pulmonary disease exacerbation presents to the emergency department because of lethargy. She recently completed a month-long course of prednisone 50 mg daily. Blood pressure is 85/40 mmHg. Her most likely diagnosis is:

   1. Septic shock.

   2. Myxedema crisis.

   3. Thyroid storm.

   4. Adrenal insufficiency.

10. A 45-year-old male patient is admitted to the intensive care unit after resection of a pituitary adenoma. He develops vomiting, abdominal pain, myalgia, joint pains, and severe hypotension. This patient may have developed:

    1. Adrenal insufficiency.

    2. Diabetes insipidus.

    3. Abdominal compartment syndrome.

    4. Colonic ileus.

11. A 20-year-old college student with no past medical history is brought into the emergency department by friends after his mental status became altered. He has Kussmaul respirations, is confused, drowsy, and recently vomited. Which tests are required to confirm the most likely diagnosis?

    1. Serum glucose, bicarbonate, pH, and ketones.

    2. Serum sodium, chloride, and urinalysis.

    3. Arterial blood gas.

    4. Cerebrospinal fluid protein, glucose, and cell count.

12. A 20-year-old college student with no past medical history is brought into the emergency department by friends after his mental status became altered. He has Kussmaul respirations, is confused, drowsy, and recently vomited. His glucose is 380 mg/dL, bicarbonate 14 mEq/L, pH 7.27, and has ketonuria. Other than tachypnea, vital signs are normal. In a healthy young adult, what additional test should be obtained to avoid the commonly fatal complication of this disease process?

    1. Lactate.

    2. Potassium.

    3. Arterial pCO_2.

    4. Platelet count.

13. A 20-year-old college student with no past medical history is brought into the emergency department by friends after his mental status became altered. He has Kussmaul respirations, is confused, drowsy, and recently vomited. His glucose is 380 mg/dL, bicarbonate 14 mEq/L, pH 7.27, and has ketonuria. Other than tachypnea, vital signs are normal. What are essential components of initial therapy?

    1. Intravenous (IV) fluids, IV insulin infusion, potassium replacement.

    2. Immediate intubation, IV insulin infusion, IV fluids.

    3. Aggressive subcutaneous sliding scale insulin, IV fluids.

    4. IV fluids, bicarbonate replacement, IV insulin infusion.

14. A 60-year-old female patient with an established diagnosis of chronic autoimmune thyroiditis is seeing her nurse practitioner for routine follow-up of her thyroid labs, which are thyroid-stimulating hormone 7.0 units/mL (reference range 0.5–5.0) and free T4 0.5 ng/dL (0.7–1.4). She has been on levothyroxine 75 mcg by mouth daily for the last 2 months. What would you do with her levothyroxine dose?

    1. Keep it at 75 mcg.

    2. Decrease to 50 mcg.

    3. Increase to 100 mcg.

    4. Defer this decision, repeat labs, and schedule a follow-up visit.

15. A 55-year-old female patient with history of hypothyroidism and hyperlipidemia is admitted to a neuro floor after acute ischemic stroke. Her thyroid labs are thyroid-stimulating hormone 9.0 units/mL (reference range 0.5–5.0) and free T4 0.3 ng/dL (0.7–1.4). A review of her records reveals she is on levothyroxine 125 mcg by mouth daily and that her primary care provider adjusted the dose upward from 100 mcg 2 weeks before admission. What would you do with her levothyroxine dose?

    1. Keep it at 125 mcg.

    2. Decrease to 100 mcg.

    3. Increase to 150 mcg.

    4. Discontinue levothyroxine.

16. A 70-year-old male patient with idiopathic hypothyroidism is admitted to a med/surg floor with community-acquired pneumonia, hypoxia requiring 3 L of oxygen per nasal cannula, and several months of lethargy. His thyroid labs were obtained and are thyroid-stimulating hormone 15.0 units/mL (reference range 0.5–5.0) and free T4 0.2 ng/dL (0.7–1.4). He reports that over the last 6 months his primary care provider has increased his levothyroxine 4 times to a current dose of 250 mcg with the last dose adjustment 6 weeks ago. He denies medication nonadherence, and his spouse confirmed he takes it every morning with breakfast. Which of the following will properly address his thyroid function?

    1. Increase the levothyroxine dose to 275 mcg.

    2. Prescribe Synthroid 250 mcg "dispense as written."

    3. Change the time of day the current dose is taken.

    4. Place a referral for radioactive thyroid ablation.

17. A 58-year-old male patient is admitted to a cardiac unit following non-ST segment elevation myocardial infarction. He had cardiogenic shock and has been weaned off pressor and inotropic support. During his hospitalization, thyroid function tests were thyroid-stimulating hormone 6.5 units/mL (0.5–5.0), free T3 1.1 ng/dL (1.7–3.7), and free T4 0.6 ng/dL (0.7–1.4). How will the nurse practitioner address these thyroid function tests?

    1. Initiate levothyroxine 1.7 mcg/kg ideal body weight by mouth (PO) daily.

    2. Initiate levothyroxine 25 mcg PO daily.

    3. Initiate levothyroxine 50 mcg intravenously once, followed by 25 mcg PO daily.

    4. Instruct the patient to follow up with his primary care provider to have thyroid function rechecked in about 1 month.

18. A 50-year-old with type 2 diabetes was diagnosed with community-acquired pneumonia by his primary care provider 3 days ago and presents to the emergency department with a chief complaint of "not feeling well." He has a temperature of 96.5°F, heart rate 120 beats/min, and blood pressure 90/50 mmHg. Labs included white blood cells 14,000/μL, plasma glucose 650 mg/dL, and a urinalysis negative for infection or ketones. What is the diagnosis?

    1. Diabetic ketoacidosis.

    2. Hyperglycemic hyperosmolar state.

    3. Cannot make a diagnosis without a serum β-hydroxybutyrate.

    4. Hypoxic osmotic nonketosis.

19. The nurse practitioner has appropriately diagnosed a patient with hyperglycemic hyperosmolar state and has begun to correct the hyperglycemia with an intravenous insulin infusion. Which life-threatening laboratory abnormality should the nurse practitioner anticipate and closely monitor for?

    1. Elevated prothrombin time.

    2. Hypokalemia.

    3. Hypernatremia.

    4. Thrombocytopenia.

20. A patient was recently diagnosed with diabetes and was placed on an appropriate insulin regimen by another provider but is unable to articulate whether they have type 1 or type 2 diabetes mellitus. How can the nurse practitioner differentiate the two?

    1. Body mass index less than 30 is type 2.

    2. Age of symptom onset less than 30 years is type 1.

    3. C-peptide less than 0.2 nmol/L is type 1.

    4. Hemoglobin A1c greater than 11.5% is type 2.

21. How would the nurse practitioner respond to call from a nurse reporting severe metabolic acidosis with a critical pH of 7.1 in a patient who was appropriately diagnosed with diabetic ketoacidosis?

    1. Emergently administer 75 mEq sodium bicarbonate.

    2. Repeat the test as a pH this low is likely an error.

    3. Order a continuous infusion containing sodium bicarbonate.

    4. Continue hydration with 0.9% sodium chloride and repeat the labs within 2 to 4 hours.

22. A 65-year-old patient with history of type 2 diabetes, hypertension, hyperlipidemia, and early-onset Alzheimer disease who was admitted for urinary tract infection and mild sepsis is ready for discharge. When reconciling discharge medications for the patient, the nurse practitioner notices the patient was on an insulin pump. What is the most salient item the nurse practitioner should assess before instructing him to continue this diabetes regimen?

    1. Efficacy of prior glucose control with this method (e.g., hemoglobin A1c).

    2. Insurance coverage to pay for the pump supplies.

    3. Family support.

    4. Cognitive function.

23. Which of the following is diagnostic for diabetes mellitus?

    1. Hemoglobin A1c 7.2%.

    2. Fasting plasma glucose 120 mg/dL.

    3. Glucose 185 mg/dL 2 hours following a 75-g glucose load.

    4. Polyuria (greater than 2 mL/kg/hr) and body mass index greater than 40.

24. A 55-year-old female patient has been newly diagnosed with type 2 diabetes mellitus and has a hemoglobin A1c of 7.9%. What is the most appropriate initial glucose management strategy?

    1. Insulin aspart sliding scale and carbohydrate coverage.

    2. Metformin monotherapy.

    3. Metformin and sitagliptin dual therapy.

    4. Recommendation for 150 minutes of aerobic activity per week, dietician consult for low-carbohydrate diet counseling, and a goal of 2% to 3% weight loss over the next 12 months.

25. An 85-year-old male patient with well-controlled type 2 diabetes complains to the nurse practitioner about the cost of his current oral antihyperglycemic regimen and asks if metformin would be a reasonable option. The next course of action for the nurse practitioner is:

    1. Request a prior authorization for metformin from the insurance company and then prescribe it.

    2. Check serum creatinine and prescribe if less than 1.25 mg/dL.

    3. Check creatinine clearance.

    4. Check blood urea nitrogen.

26. A patient with well-controlled type 2 diabetes who was on metformin 1350 mg twice per day is recovering from sepsis with mild acute kidney injury and a current glomerular filtration rate of 50 mL/min/1.73 m². The metformin was held during his acute illness. What is an appropriate consideration when addressing restarting home medications?

    1. Do not restart metformin and counsel the patient that metformin is contraindicated.

    2. If you anticipate his renal function not to worsen, restart metformin but at a lower dose of 1000 mg twice per day.

    3. Check lactate and if less than 5 mmol/L; restart metformin 1350 mg twice per day.

    4. Restart metformin 1350 mg twice per day and anticipate titrating up to 1500 mg in 2 weeks.

27. A patient presenting to the emergency department with altered mental status, bradycardia, bradypnea, and hypothermia may have which endocrine diagnosis?

    1. Diabetic ketoacidosis.

    2. Thyroid storm.

    3. Myxedema coma.

    4. Pheochromocytoma.

28. Hypoglycemia can be associated with all the following *except*:

    1. Thyrotoxicosis.

    2. Myxedema coma.

    3. Adrenal crisis.

    4. Cushing syndrome.

29. Proptosis, goiter, diaphoresis, tremors, thin hair, hyperreflexia, fever, wide pulse pressures, signs of congestive heart failure, and atrial fibrillation are signs of:

    1. Thyroid storm.

    2. Myxedema coma.

    3. Pheochromocytoma.

    4. Diabetic ketoacidosis.

30. A 75-year-old female patient with a history of type 2 diabetes on sitagliptin and insulin glargine, hypothyroidism, and recently diagnosed mild cognitive impairment which, according to her daughter, worsened yesterday presented in a stupor and a core body temperature of 94°F presents to the emergency department after taking her dog for a 20-minute walk in 25°F weather. A top item for her differential diagnosis is:

    1. Insulin overdose.

    2. Exposure-related hypothermia.

    3. Acute addisonian crisis.

    4. Myxedema coma.

31. A 40-year-old with chronic adrenal insufficiency following resection of a pituitary macroadenoma 3 years ago is being admitted to the hospital with community-acquired pneumonia and mild sepsis. How should the practitioner manage the patient's steroid dose while the patient is admitted?

    1. Continue home prednisone 5 mg daily.

    2. Hold home prednisone to prevent immunosuppression.

    3. Administer hydrocortisone 50 mg intravenously every 6 hours.

    4. Administer a cosyntropin stimulation test.

32. A 28-year-old with no past medical history presents with headache, chest pain, hypertension, palpitations, and pallor. In addition to excluding cardiac etiologies, what endocrine abnormality could be the etiology of this clinical constellation?

    1. A new diagnosis of type 1 diabetes and ketoacidosis.

    2. Thyroid storm.

    3. Pheochromocytoma.

    4. Addison disease.

33. A patient treated with hydrocortisone (total daily dose = 30 mg) for chronic adrenal insufficiency has normal blood pressures and no current or recent acute illnesses. Current chemistry panel reveals serum sodium 148 mEq/L and potassium 3.3 mEq/L. What treatment modifications should the nurse practitioner make?

    1. Reduce the daily dose of hydrocortisone to 20 mg and obtain follow-up electrolytes and blood pressure.

    2. Double the daily dose of hydrocortisone and obtain follow-up electrolytes and blood pressure.

    3. Admit the patient to the hospital, place an arterial line, and start intravenous stress dose steroids.

    4. Continue current plan and schedule a follow-up visit in 4 to 6 weeks.

34. A 33-year-old male patient was diagnosed with antiphospholipid syndrome 3 months ago after developing an unprovoked deep vein thrombosis and had been started on warfarin. He was admitted 2 days ago with myocardial infarction and was started on intravenous heparin after a cerebral venous sinus thrombus was discovered earlier today after he began complaining of a severe headache. He has developed hypotension, nausea, and vomiting, and a stat echocardiogram shows normal ventricular function. What endocrine problem may be contributing this problem?

    1. Pituitary apoplexy.

    2. Diabetes insipidus.

    3. Parathyroid infarct.

    4. Hypoglycemia.

35. A 40-year-old patient with antiphospholipid syndrome presented with hemoptysis, cough, and shortness of breath. She had a 4-month history of progressive darkening of the skin and generalized weakness, nausea, anorexia, and a 7-pound weight loss over 1 month. A deep vein thrombosis, pulmonary embolism, and connective tissue disorder were ruled out. The patient's body mass index was 19 kg/m2, heart rate was 112 beats/min, and blood pressure was 108/76 mm Hg with a postural drop of 26. Pallor was also noted. What endocrine problem is causing this patient's symptoms?

    1. Pancreas infarct.

    2. Adrenal infarct.

    3. Thyroid infarct.

    4. Pineal infarct.

36. A 55-year-old with type 1 diabetes and chronic kidney disease stage 3 was admitted to the med/surg floor yesterday by a colleague and was started on a regular insulin sliding scale every 6 hours and a low-carbohydrate diet was ordered. The nurse practitioner notes that the blood glucose is inadequately controlled (range 180–250). To rectify your colleague's mismanagement, you would:

    1. Add insulin glargine and oral pioglitazone.

    2. Increase the amount of coverage on the sliding scale.

    3. Stop the sliding scale and schedule NPH insulin.

    4. Add insulin glargine and change the sliding scale to insulin lispro.

37. A patient with type 2 diabetes was admitted to the intensive care unit 3 days ago after acute coronary syndrome.

She was placed on an insulin infusion for glucose control that has been running at 2 to 2.5 units/hr for the last 24 hours with glucoses ranging from 145 to 178 mg/dL. Which plan to transition to subcutaneous insulin is appropriate?

    1. Start a regular insulin sliding scale with 2 units of coverage for each 50 mg/dL of blood glucose over 150 mg/dL.

    2. Follow hourly glucoses for the next 24 hours before converting to subcutaneous.

    3. Give half the daily insulin requirement as glargine once every day and split the remaining requirement as insulin lispro with meals.

    4. Start metformin 1000 mg twice per day and use regular insulin 8 units with each meal.

38. A female patient admitted to the floor with pneumonia and mild hypoxia is transferred to the intensive care unit with worsening sepsis. She was adequately fluid resuscitated and then started on norepinephrine with a current dose of 0.08 mcg/kg/min. Her blood glucose is 210 mg/dL. How should the nurse practitioner manage her glucose?

    1. Start a regular insulin subcutaneous sliding scale with a goal of 100 to 180 mg/dL.

    2. Start a regular insulin infusion with a goal of 140 to 180 mg/dL.

    3. Start insulin aspart subcutaneously with correction factor and sliding scale.

    4. Start a regular insulin infusion with a goal of 90 to 140 mg/dL.

39. The nurse practitioner is preparing the hospital discharge plan for a male patient with type 2 diabetes who typically drinks 10 to 15 cans of beer per day and has alcoholic cirrhosis. His prior regimen included metformin. The nurse practitioner should:

    1. Continue metformin because it is inexpensive and has good glucose-lowering effects.

    2. Reduce the dose of the metformin by 50% in the setting of cirrhosis.

    3. Discontinue the metformin because of a risk of lactic acidosis in cirrhosis.

    4. Discontinue the metformin because of the risk of potentiating ethanol's effect resulting in alcohol poisoning.

4 Endocrine Answers & Rationales

1. Answer: 2

Rationale: This scenario suggests a diagnosis of diabetes insipidus, for which serum sodium and urine specific gravity will aid in the diagnosis.

2. Answer: 1

Rationale: This patient has central diabetes insipidus from pituitary compression. Treatment involves urgent administration of desmopressin and fluids to attenuate the hypernatremia.

3. Answer: 3

Rationale: The syndrome of inappropriate antidiuretic hormone is commonly caused by pulmonary disease and malignancy. First-line treatment is a fluid restriction in the absence of symptoms such as seizure, mental status change, and falls.

4. Answer: 4

Rationale: Preferred insulin route in the intensive care unit setting is intravenous infusion with a target of 140 to 180 mg/dL to avoid hypoglycemic complications. Vasoconstriction and edema of subcutaneous tissue can alter absorption.

5. Answer: 1

Rationale: This patient had adequate glucose control and can be safely transitioned back to her home regimen in the absence of other contraindications.

6. Answer: 2

Rationale: Hospitalized patients with new hyperglycemia should be managed with basal, prandial, correction.

7. Answer: 1

Rationale: If you are unable to ensure that the patient comprehends her insulin administration regimen, then it is not safe, despite being the preferred initial treatment. Therefore the next most reasonable option is an oral agent with follow-up.

8. Answer: 2

Rationale: A cortisol level should be checked at 8 a.m.; a level less than 165 nmol/L is consistent with adrenal insufficiency (AI). Urinary cortisol is not helpful in diagnosis and the cortisol level after corticotropin test less than 500 nmol/L is diagnostic of AI.

9. Answer: 4

Rationale: Abrupt cessation of steroids after greater than 2 to 3 weeks can result in adrenal insufficiency. Signs of adrenal insufficiency include hypotension and fatigue.

10. Answer: 1

Rationale: Vomiting, abdominal pain, myalgia, joint pains, and severe hypotension are hallmark features of adrenal insufficiency. Additionally, recent surgical manipulation of the pituitary is the likely etiology of low corticotropin secretion leading to adrenal insufficiency.

11. Answer: 1

Rationale: Kussmaul respirations, confusion, drowsiness, and vomiting are suggestive of diabetic ketoacidosis. Diagnostic criteria for diabetic ketoacidosis are serum glucose greater than 200 to 300, bicarbonate less than 15 to 18, pH less than 7.3, and ketones present in the blood or urine.

12. Answer: 2

Rationale: Mortality is most common in diabetic ketoacidosis from the precipitating illness (e.g., myocardial infarct or sepsis), but in the absence of a precipitating illness, hypokalemia can be fatal.

13. Answer: 1

Rationale: Urgent initial therapy consists of intravenous fluids, insulin, and potassium and close monitoring of blood glucose and potassium levels to avoid hypoglycemia and hypokalemia.

14. Answer: 3

Rationale: High thyroid-stimulating hormone and low free T4 are consistent with undertreated hypothyroidism.

15. Answer: 1

Rationale: Although these labs would generally indicate undertreated hypothyroidism, thyroxine (T4) has a serum half-life of 1 week and dose adjustments are typically made no more frequently than every 4 to 6 weeks.

16. Answer: 3

Rationale: Levothyroxine absorption is altered when coadministered with food, supplements, and some medications and should be taken on an empty stomach 1 hour before or 4 hours after a meal.

17. Answer: 4

Rationale: During critical illness, the normal negative feedback loop is altered, resulting in nonthyroidal illness syndrome or euthyroid sick syndrome, especially in patients with cardiac illness. There is scant evidence to support starting thyroid replacement in the acute setting.

18. Answer: 2

Rationale: Absence of ketones rules out diabetic ketoacidosis and glucose greater than 600 mg/dL, hypovolemia, and hypothermia point to hyperosmolar hyperglycemic syndrome (synonymous with and formerly referred to as hyperosmolar nonketotic coma and hyperglycemic hyperosmolar nonketotic coma).

19. Answer: 2

Rationale: Administration of insulin forces extracellular potassium into the cell, which can result in hypokalemia.

20. Answer: 3

Rationale: C-peptide is a measure of pancreatic beta-cell function and is a part of proinsulin, is cosecreted with endogenous insulin, has a much longer half-life, and negligible hepatic clearance level. As such, it is a better marker than measuring insulin levels. A level less than 0.2 nmol/L is associated with type 1 diabetes mellitus.

21. Answer: 4

Rationale: Bicarbonate therapy is usually only recommended when the pH is less than 7.0 because of the concern for decreased cardiac contractility and arrhythmias.

22. Answer: 4

Rationale: Patients with insulin pumps must be able to intellectually and technically manage the device, count carbohydrates, self-bolus insulin, and check blood glucose. If cognitive function is impaired because Alzheimer disease prevents this, lethal hypoglycemia may occur.

23. Answer: 1

Rationale: Hemoglobin A1c greater than 7.0 is diagnostic of diabetes.

24. Answer: 2

Rationale: Patients with a hemoglobin A1c of 7% to 9% are appropriate for monotherapy; less than 7% is appropriate for lifestyle modifications.

25. Answer: 3

Rationale: Metformin should not be initiated in patients over 80 years of age without verifying that creatinine clearance is adequate.

26. Answer: 2

Rationale: Metformin can be used cautiously in chronic kidney disease stage 3a (glomerular filtration rate 45–60) with a maximum daily dose of 2000 mg. Monitor renal function closely to ensure stability following an acute illness.

27. Answer: 3

Rationale: Myxedema coma is associated with altered mental status, bradycardia, bradypnea, and hypothermia.

28. Answer: 4

Rationale: Thyrotoxicosis, myxedema coma, pheochromocytoma, and adrenal crisis can all be associated with hypoglycemia, but Cushing is a syndrome resulting from excess glucocorticoids, which can result in hyperglycemia.

29. Answer: 1

Rationale: Proptosis, goiter, diaphoresis, tremors, thin hair, hyperreflexia, fever, wide pulse pressures, signs of congestive heart failure, and atrial fibrillation are signs of thyroid storm.

30. Answer: 4

Rationale: A textbook scenario of myxedema coma is an elderly woman with hypothyroidism who presents with stupor after cold exposure. Additional common triggers to myxedema are myocardial infarction, sepsis, and trauma.

31. Answer: 3

Rationale: Patients on chronic steroids need stress dose steroids during an acute illness to prevent adrenal crisis. Concern for immunosuppression is secondary.

32. Answer: 3

Rationale: Pheochromocytoma causes abnormal endogenous catecholamine production from a benign, though biologically active, adrenal tumor and can be characterized by the five Ps: pressure (hypertension), pain (headache and chest pain), palpitations, perspiration, and pallor (caused by vasoconstriction).

33. Answer: 1

Rationale: Hydrocortisone can cause water and sodium retention and hypokalemia. With normal blood pressure, trialing a lower dose of steroids could normalize the electrolytes and this patient could potentially tolerate a lower dose.

34. Answer: 1

Rationale: Pituitary apoplexy (hemorrhage into the pituitary) can cause reduced adrenocorticotropic hormone and thus cortisol production. Low cortisol results in hypotension, nausea, and vomiting.

35. Answer: 2

Rationale: The conditions described suggest catastrophic antiphospholipid syndrome (APS) with multiple infarcts (coronaries, cerebral sinus). APS can cause venous, arterial, and small-vessel infarcts, including the adrenal glands, which release cortisol. Cortisol deficiency can cause hypotension, nausea, and vomiting. The other endocrine glands do not contribute to cortisol production.

36. Answer: 4

Rationale: Patients with type 1 diabetes need long-acting or continuous insulin in addition to correction factor.

37. Answer: 3

Rationale: Regular insulin is more appropriate for patients taking nothing by mouth or on tube feeding. Twenty-four hours on a stable insulin infusion typically provides sufficient data to determine the daily insulin requirement, and this strategy is supported in the literature.

38. Answer: 2

Rationale: Target glucose levels should be 110 or 140 to 180 mg/dL in critically ill patients: a goal this high lowers the risk of severe hypoglycemia. In patients with hypotension requiring pressor support, hyperglycemic crises, sepsis, or shock, insulin is best delivered via intravenous infusion to allow flexibility in dose given the unpredictability in nutrition and health status.

39. Answer: 3

Rationale: Metformin may be used in carefully selected cases of cirrhosis, but concomitant alcohol use increases the risk of lactic acidosis.

Musculoskeletal

5

1. A 25-year-old man was brought to the emergency department after a motor vehicle collision. He had an open fracture in the left femur that needed internal fixation, so he was admitted to the orthopedic unit. Hours later, he became confused and in respiratory distress; his blood pressure was 120/80 mmHg and his pulse 120 beats/min. There are multiple nonpalpable petechial rashes on the whole body. What most likely happened to this patient?

   1. Fat embolism.

   2. Aspiration pneumonia.

   3. Pulmonary edema.

   4. Lung contusion.

2. A 55-year-old woman presented to the emergency department with left shoulder pain after she fell down on her arm. On exam, there is obvious swelling over the right shoulder with ecchymosis and crepitus. What is the diagnosis of this patient?

   1. Rotator cuff tear.

   2. Humeral neck fracture.

   3. Upper brachial plexus injury.

   4. Clavicle fracture.

3. A 35-year-old man underwent surgery for fixation of a femur fracture. Three hours later, the patient started complaining of severe pain in his thigh that was not relieved by acetaminophen. The pain is worse when stretching his leg, and he has a pins-and-needle sensation in his thigh. There is also swelling in his thigh. Which is the next step in the management of this patient?

   1. Fasciotomy.

   2. Morphine.

   3. Thigh x-ray.

   4. Electromyography.

4. A 20-year-old man presented with left leg pain that started 2 weeks ago, and the pain has increased in the last days. He is training for the Olympics as a runner, and he just started stringent training for time trials. On exam, there are many tender points in the posterior part of the leg. X-ray was normal. Which of the following is the best test to determine the patient's problem?

   1. Electromyography.

   2. Leg Doppler.

   3. Lower limb magnetic resonance imaging.

   4. Lower limb computed tomography.

5. A 25-year-old man was brought to the emergency department after a motor vehicle collision. He had an open fracture of the left femur and had an internal fixation, so he was admitted to the orthopedic unit. Hours later, he became confused and had respiratory distress, his blood pressure was 120/80 mmHg, and his pulse 120 beats/min. There are multiple nonpalpable petechial rashes on the whole body. Which is the next step in the management of this patient?

   1. Antibiotics.

   2. Alteplase.

   3. Respiratory support.

   4. Furosemide.

6. A 55-year-old woman presented to the emergency department with left shoulder pain after she fell on her arm. On exam, there is obvious swelling over the right shoulder with ecchymosis and crepitus. Which of the following nerves can be injured in this patient?

   1. Median.

   2. Ulnar.

   3. Radial.

   4. Axillary.

7. A 35-year-old man underwent surgery for fixation of a femur fracture. Three hours later, the patient started complaining of severe pain in his thigh that was not relieved by acetaminophen. The pain is aggravated by stretching his leg, and he has a pins-and-needles sensation in his thigh. There is also swelling in his thigh. Which of the following is the most likely diagnosis?

   1. Rupture of the popliteal artery aneurysm.

   2. Compartment syndrome.

   3. Deep vein thrombosis.

   4. Cellulitis.

8. A 19-year-old man presented with left leg pain that started 1 week ago, and this pain has increased in the last few days. He is a college basketball player. On exam, there are many tender points in the Achilles tendon area. X-ray was normal. Which is the next step in the management of this patient?

   1. Rest.

   2. Bone cast.

   3. Physiotherapy.

   4. Antibiotic.

9. A 22-year-old female patient presents with right wrist pain after she fell on her outstretched arm. On exam, there is tenderness in the snuffbox region. X-ray was unremarkable. What is the most likely diagnosis in this patient?

   1. Distal ulnar fracture.

   2. Scaphoid fracture.

   3. Carpel tunnel syndrome.

   4. Metacarpal fracture.

10. A 66-year-old woman was brought to the emergency department after falling in the bathroom. She had left groin pain aggravated by movement of her leg. On exam, the left leg appeared shorter than the right and externally rotated. Which of the following types of fracture increases the risk of avascular necrosis of the head of the femur?

    1. Intracapsular.

    2. Subtrochanteric.

    3. Intertrochanteric.

    4. Midshaft femur.

11. A 17-year-old girl is brought to the emergency department after falling on her outstretched arm. Her arm is too painful to move. The x-ray showed a supracondylar fracture. Which of the following complications can happen in this patient?

    1. Median nerve injury.

    2. Axillary nerve injury.

    3. Brachial plexus injury.

    4. Axillary artery injury.

12. A 60-year-old female patient presented with knee pain on the right side that started a couple of weeks ago. This pain is aggravated by exercise and relieved by rest. She had stiffness in the morning for 10 minutes. She denies any history of fever, recent trauma, or swelling. She has a history of diabetes mellitus. On exam, there is decreased range of motion. Which of the following is the most like diagnosis in this patient?

    1. Gout.

    2. Osteoarthritis.

    3. Rheumatoid arthritis.

    4. Septic arthritis.

13. A 66-year-old male patient presented with left-sided knee pain that started 1 month ago. The pain is aggravated by exercise and relieved by rest. He denies any history of fever, recent trauma, or swelling. He has a history of diabetes mellitus. On exam, there is decreased range of motion. Knee x-ray showed a narrow joint space and osteophyte formation. Which of the following is *not* a risk factor for this condition?

    1. Aging.

    2. Obesity.

    3. Previous knee trauma.

    4. Hypertension.

14. A 55-year-old female patient presented with knee pain on the right side that started 2 months ago. The pain is aggravated by exercise and relieved by rest. She has stiffness in the morning for 10 minutes. She denies any history of fever, recent trauma, or swelling. She has a history of diabetes mellitus and hyperlipidemia. On exam, there is decreased range of motion. Her body mass index was 35 km/m^2. What does the nurse practitioner think will be found on the knee x-ray?

    1. Decrease joint space.

    2. Punched out erosions of the bone.

    3. Chondrocalcinosis.

    4. Soft tissue swelling.

15. A 62-year-old woman presented with chronic bilateral knee pain; the pain is aggravated by exercise and relieved by rest. She denies any history of fever, recent trauma, or swelling. She has a history of diabetes mellitus. Her body mass index was 36 kg/m^2. On exam, there is decreased range of motion. Knee x-ray showed a narrow joint space and osteophyte formation. Which of the following can decrease the progression of this disease?

    1. Acetaminophen.

    2. Ibuprofen.

    3. Weight reduction.

    4. Physiotherapy.

16. A 60-year-old man presented with groin pain that started 2 months ago. The pain radiates to his lower thigh. The pain is aggravated by movement and relieved by rest. He complains of morning stiffness that lasts for 15 minutes. He has a history of diabetes and his body mass index is 30 kg/m^2. On exam, there is decreased internal and external rotation. Which of the following is the cause of the patient's condition?

    1. Compression of the nerve root.

    2. Progressive destruction of articular cartilage.

    3. Neck femur fracture.

    4. Trochanteric bursitis.

17. A 56-year-old female patient presents with left-sided knee pain that started 1 month ago. The pain is aggravated by exercise and relieved by rest. She denies any history of fever, recent trauma, or swelling. She has a history of diabetes mellitus. On exam, there is decreased range of motion. Knee x-ray showed a narrow joint space and osteophyte formation. Which of the following is the first line of management in this patient?

    1. Intraarticular cortisol.

    2. Acetaminophen.

    3. Nonsteroidal antiinflammatory drugs.

    4. Colchicine.

18. A 55-year-old female patient presents with finger pain that started 2 months ago. The pain is aggravated by movement and relieved by rest. Her fingers are stiff in the morning for 10 minutes. She denies any history of fever, recent trauma, or swelling. She has a history of hyperlipidemia. On exam, there is decreased range of motion. Which of the following can be found in this patient?

    1. Dupuytren contracture.

    2. Swan neck deformity.

    3. Heberden nodes.

    4. Charcot joint.

19. A 20-year-old man presented with right leg pain that started 1 day ago but is getting worse. He has a fever and a history of sickle cell anemia. There is no history of recent trauma. On exam, his temperature was 101.2°F. He has decreased range of movement of his leg. Which of the following is the next step in the management of this patient?

    1. Palin x-ray.

    2. Magnetic resonance imaging.

    3. Complete blood count.

    4. Computed tomography scan.

20. A 22-year-old-man presented with left knee pain that started 2 days ago. He now has pain in his right ankle. He also has a history of dysuria and frequency. On exam, his conjunctiva appeared red. Which of the following is the most likely diagnosis in this patient?

    1. Lyme disease.

    2. Reactive arthritis.

    3. Tuberous arthritis.

    4. Septic arthritis.

21. A 25-year-old-female patient presented with joint pain that started 2 weeks ago. The pain mainly occurs in the knee and ankle joints. She also has a history of fever and dysuria. She has had multiple sexual partners in the last 6 months. On exam, there were multiple pustular rashes on her foot. Which of the following is the cause of the patient's symptoms?

    1. Viral infection.

    2. Tuberculosis.

    3. *Borrelia burgdorferi.*

    4. *Neisseria gonorrhoeae.*

22. A 60-year-old man presented with right knee pain that started 1 week ago. He has a history of right knee replacement 3 months ago. He has a fever. On exam, there is obvious swelling in the right knee with signs of inflammation with decreased range of movement. Which of the following is the next step in the management of this patient?

    1. Empirical antibiotics.

    2. Knee computed tomography.

    3. Synovial fluid analysis.

    4. Knee x-ray.

23. A 30-year-old man presents with left leg pain that started 2 days ago; the pain has been getting progressively worse. He has a fever and a history of sickle cell anemia. No history of recent trauma. On exam, his temperature was 101.0°F. He has decreased range of motion. Which of the following is the most likely diagnosis in this patient?

    1. Stress fracture.

    2. Osteomyelitis.

    3. Bursitis.

    4. Compartment syndrome.

24. A 50-year-old man presented with dull leg pain associated with a low-grade fever. He has a long history of uncontrolled diabetes mellitus and he underwent transmetatarsal amputation 3 months ago. On exam, his temperature is 100°F and there is tenderness over the left leg with erythema. The leg x-ray showed patchy osteopenia with periosteal reaction. Which of the following is the most likely diagnosis in this patient?

    1. Osteomyelitis.

    2. Cellulitis.

    3. Septic arthritis.

    4. Erysipelas.

25. A 55-year-old female patient presented with shoulder and pelvic pain that started 1 month ago. She has a history of fever and generalized fatigue. She cannot stand up without support. Her temperature was 99.9°F. Erythrocyte sedimentation rate was 60 mm/hr. Which of the following complications is this patient at risk for?

    1. Malignancy.

    2. Giant cell arteritis.

    3. Ischemic heart disease.

    4. Seizure.

26. A 60-year-old female patient presents with difficulty standing that started 1 month ago, but it has become more difficult over the last several days. She has a history of difficulty swallowing. She denies any history of fever, neurological deficit, or weight loss. Which of the following suggests this patient has polymyositis?

    1. Elevated muscle enzyme.

    2. Normal electromyography.

    3. Proximal muscle stiffness.

    4. Rash.

27. A 40-year-old man presented with low back pain that started 2 months ago. This pain was associated with morning stiffness and improved with activity. He has a history of ankle pain. On exam, there was tenderness over the iliac crest with limited mobility of the spine. Which of the following can be found in this patient?

    1. Swan neck deformity.

    2. Subcutaneous nodule.

    3. Rash.

    4. Bilateral sacroiliitis.

28. A 30-year-old woman presented to the outpatient clinic with progressive muscle weakness. She cannot stand or do many activities of daily living. On exam, there was a heliotrope rash with Gottron papules on her elbow. Her creatine phosphokinase test was elevated. Which of the following is the most likely diagnosis?

    1. Polymyositis.

    2. Dermatomyositis.

    3. Rheumatoid arthritis.

    4. Systemic lupus erythematosus.

29. A 50-year-old man presented with severe pain in the big toe. He has a history of gout on allopurinol. On exam, there is podagra in the right big toe with swelling and sign of inflammation. Which of the following is the next step in the management of this patient?

    1. Colchicine.

    2. High-dose allopurinol.

    3. Plasmapheresis.

    4. Prednisone.

30. A 40-year-old man presented with severe pain in the big toe that started a couple of hours ago. He denies any history of fever. On exam, there was swelling in the big toe surrounded by erythema and other signs of inflammation. Which of the following can be used to exclude septic arthritis?

    1. Plain x-ray.

    2. Synovial fluid aspiration.

    3. Lower limb computed tomography.

    4. Blood culture.

31. A 30-year-old man presented to the orthopedic clinic with right knee pain that started 3 weeks ago after he twisted his leg during a football game. He has a history of joint swelling that started gradually after the game. On exam, there was an obvious swelling in the right knee with joint line tenderness, decreased joint movement, and positive Apley test. Which of the following is the next step in the management of this patient?

    1. Knee x-ray.

    2. Knee magnetic resonance imaging.

    3. Synovial fluid aspiration.

    4. Physiotherapy.

32. A 40-year-old woman presented with progressive muscle weakness. She cannot stand and she is also having trouble doing activities of daily living. On exam, there was a malar rash with Gottron papules on her elbow. Her creatine phosphokinase was elevated and anti-Jo1 was positive. Which of the following is the next step in the management of this patient?

    1. Plasmapheresis.

    2. Levothyroxine.

    3. Prednisone.

    4. Edrophonium.

33. A 60-year-old female patient presented with shoulder and pelvic pain that started 3 weeks ago. She has a fever, generalized fatigue, and weight loss. She complains of lower extremity weakness and has difficulty standing up. Her temperature is 100.5°F. Which of the following lab results will be found in this patient?

    1. Normal C-reactive protein.

    2. Raised erythrocyte sedimentation rate.

    3. Hypochromic anemia.

    4. Low platelets.

34. A 66-year-old female patient visited her nurse practitioner for routine follow-up. She is concerned she may have osteoporosis. She reports that her sister was diagnosed with osteoporosis after fracturing a vertebra. Which of the following is the most accurate test for osteoporosis?

    1. Plain x-ray.

    2. Alkaline phosphatase.

    3. Dual-energy x-ray absorptiometry scan.

    4. Hip computed tomography.

35. A 60-year-old female patient presented with right leg swelling in the region that surrounds the knee. She has a history of severe osteoarthritis. On exam, there is a tender and palpable mass in the right popliteal fossa that is not pulsatile. Which is the next step in the management of this patient?

    1. Synovial fluid analysis.

    2. Knee ultrasound.

    3. Knee x-ray.

    4. Knee arthroscopy.

36. A 42-year-old woman presented with right hip pain that started 1 week ago. She denies any history of trauma, fever, or back pain. She has a history of systemic lupus for 10 years and is on prednisone. On exam, there was tenderness on the hip joint line with decreased range of movement. Which of the following is the gold standard for this patient's diagnosis?

    1. Plain x-ray.

    2. Hip magnetic resonance imaging.

    3. Synovial fluid analysis.

    4. Computed tomography angiogram.

37. A 30-year-old woman presented to the outpatient clinic with progressive muscle weakness in her lower extremities. On exam, there was a heliotrope rash with Gottron papules on her elbow. Her creatine phosphokinase was elevated. Which of the following will be positive in this patient?

    1. Anti-Jo1 antibody.

    2. Antihistone antibody.

    3. Rheumatoid factor.

    4. Anti–double-stranded DNA antibody.

38. A 60-year-old female patient presented with shoulder and pelvic pain that started 3 weeks ago. She has a fever, generalized fatigue, and weight loss. She is having trouble standing independently. Her temperature is 99.8°F. Which of the following can confirm the patient's diagnosis?

    1. Response to steroids.

    2. Raised erythrocyte sedimentation rate.

    3. Elevated creatine phosphokinase.

    4. Positive Jo1 antibody.

39. A 30-year-old man presented with low back pain that started 1 month ago. This pain was associated with morning stiffness and improved with activity. He has a history of shoulder pain. On exam, there was tenderness over the iliac crest with limited mobility of the spine. A pelvic x-ray showed bilateral sacroiliitis. Which of the following is the most likely diagnosis in this patient?

    1. Systemic lupus erythematosus.

    2. Rheumatoid arthritis.

    3. Ankylosing spondylitis.

    4. Systemic sclerosis.

40. A 66-year-old man presents with back pain that started 2 months ago. The pain is associated with calf pain mainly on the left side that is relieved by leaning forward. He has a history of leg numbness. He has no history of trauma or other chronic disease. Which of the following is the most likely diagnosis?

    1. Spinal stenosis.

    2. Compress fracture.

    3. Ankylosing spondylitis.

    4. Osteomyelitis.

41. A 45-year-old man presented with severe pain in the knee. He has a history of gout and is on allopurinol. He has a history of surgery 1 month ago because of duodenal ulcer perforation. On exam, there is a swelling in the joint with signs of inflammation. The synovial fluid analysis showed a white blood cell count of 20×10^3 per micrograms with needle-shaped crystals. Which is the next step in the management of this patient?

    1. Ibuprofen.

    2. High dose allopurinol.

    3. Plasmapheresis.

    4. Intraarticular methylprednisolone.

42. A young man presented with left knee pain that started 3 weeks ago after he twisted his leg during a basketball game. He has a history of joint swelling that started gradually after a recent game. On exam, there was an obvious swelling in the left knee with joint line tenderness, decrease of joint movement, and positive Apley test. Which of the following is the most likely diagnosis?

    1. Meniscal tear.

    2. Cruciate ligament injury.

    3. Bursitis.

    4. Tibial stress fracture.

43. A 30-year-old woman presented to the outpatient clinic with progressive muscle weakness in her lower extremities. On exam, there was a heliotrope rash with Gottron papules on her elbow. Her creatine phosphokinase was elevated. Anti-Jo1 antibody was positive. Which of the following should be *excluded* in this patient?

    1. Giant cell arteritis.

    2. Aortic aneurysm.

    3. Malignancy.

    4. Mesenteric ischemia.

Musculoskeletal Answers & Rationales   5

1. Answer: 1

Rationale: This patient has symptoms of fat embolism, which include altering the conscious level, respiratory distress, and petechial rash. Fat embolism mainly happens after long bone fractures such as of the tibia, femur, and humerus. Treatment of fat embolism includes respiratory support.

2. Answer: 2

Rationale: This patient has shoulder pain, swelling, ecchymosis, and crepitus, which happen when the humeral neck is fractured. Fracture in this site can lead to axillary nerve injury, which presents with weakness in the adduction of the arm.

3. Answer: 1

Rationale: This patient has compartment syndrome, which can happen after trauma or prolonged compression of an extremity. Compartment syndrome is characterized by new pain not related to previous pain and is aggravated by passive stretching. The treatment of compartment syndrome is a fasciotomy, which should be done without delay.

4. Answer: 3

Rationale: This patient is a runner and he just started training for the Olympic time trials and now he presents with leg pain, which is consistent with a stress fracture. Stress fractures are common in dancers and sports that require excessive training. The most common site for a stress fracture is the tibia. The x-ray may appear normal, but magnetic resonance imaging or bone scans can define this problem. The treatment for this is rest.

5. Answer: 3

Rationale: This patient has symptoms of fat embolism, which includes alteration in consciousness, respiratory distress, and petechial rash. A fat embolism mainly happens after long bone fractures such as in the tibia, femur, and humerus. Treatment of fat embolism includes respiratory support.

6. Answer: 4

Rationale: This patient has shoulder pain, swelling, ecchymosis, and crepitus, which happen when the humeral neck is fractured. Fracture in this site can lead to axillary nerve injury, which presents with weakness in the adduction of the arm.

7. Answer: 2

Rationale: This patient has compartment syndrome, which can happen after trauma or prolonged compression of an extremity. Compartment syndrome is characterized by new pain not related to previous pain and is aggravated by passive stretching. The treatment of compartment syndrome is a fasciotomy, which should be done without delay.

8. Answer: 1

Rationale: This patient is a college basketball player, so he is in good physical shape. He now presents with leg pain which mainly consistent with a strain of the Achilles tendon. Strains are common in dancers and athletes that do excessive training. The treatment of this is rest.

9. Answer: 2

Rationale: This patient presented with symptoms and signs of a scaphoid fracture, which happens after falling down on an outstretched hand. A scaphoid fracture is the most common carpal bone fracture, which mainly does not appear in the x-ray. The treatment of the scaphoid fracture includes spica cast to prevent thumb mobility for 10 days.

10. Answer: 1

Rationale: This patient has a left hip fracture, which is common in elderly people. The most common type of hip fracture is femoral neck fracture. There are several types of fractures according to the anatomical position of the fracture. Intracapsular fractures have a high chance of avascular necrosis of the head of the femur.

11. Answer: 1

Rationale: Supracondylar fracture of the humerus is one of the most common fractures in kids; it happens mainly after falling on an outstretched hand. This fracture has some complications, including brachial artery injury, median nerve injury, and compartment syndrome, so after reduction a neurovascular exam should be done.

12. Answer: 2

Rationale: This patient presented with symptoms of osteoarthritis. Osteoarthritis is noninflammatory arthritis that affects the knee joint in most cases. An x-ray revealed a narrow joint space with osteophyte formation.

13. Answer: 4

Rationale: This patient presented with symptoms of osteoarthritis. Osteoarthritis is noninflammatory arthritis that affects the knee joint in most cases. An x-ray revealed a narrow joint space with osteophyte formation. There are many risk factors for osteoarthritis, including obesity, overuse of the joint, previous injury, and aging.

14. Answer: 1

Rationale: This patient presented with symptoms of osteoarthritis. Osteoarthritis is noninflammatory arthritis that affects the knee joint in most cases. An x-ray revealed a narrow joint space with osteophyte formation.

15. Answer: 3

Rationale: This patient presented with symptoms of osteoarthritis. Osteoarthritis is noninflammatory arthritis that affects the knee joint in most cases. An x-ray revealed a narrow joint space with osteophyte formation. There are many risk factors for osteoarthritis, including obesity, overuse of the joint, previous injury, and aging. Weight loss is the only measure that can decrease the progression of osteoarthritis.

16. Answer: 2

Rationale: This patient presents with symptoms of osteoarthritis. Osteoarthritis is noninflammatory arthritis that affects weight-bearing joints and causes the destruction of articular cartilage. An x-ray revealed a narrow joint space with osteophyte formation.

17. Answer: 2

Rationale: This patient presents with symptoms of osteoarthritis. Osteoarthritis is noninflammatory arthritis that affects weight-bearing joints and causes the destruction of articular cartilage. The first line of management of osteoarthritis includes acetaminophen, which can relieve the pain but cannot prevent the progression of the disease.

18. Answer: 3

Rationale: This patient presents with symptoms of osteoarthritis. Osteoarthritis is noninflammatory arthritis. An x-ray revealed a narrow joint space with osteophyte formation. Prominent osteophytes can present in a distal pharyngeal joint like the Heberden and Bouchard nodes.

19. Answer: 2

Rationale: This patient has symptoms of osteomyelitis. Sickle cell is a risk factor of osteomyelitis, and the most common organism in those patients is *Salmonella*. The treatment of this condition in sickle cell patients is the same as in a healthy patient. The most sensitive test for osteomyelitis is magnetic resonance imaging.

20. Answer: 2

Rationale: This patient has symptoms of reactive arthritis, which include arthritis, conjunctivitis, and infection. This condition is an autoimmune disease that happens as a response to an infection, mainly in the gastrointestinal tract, the genitals, or the urinary tract. The most common organisms behind this condition are *Salmonella* and *Shigella*.

21. Answer: 4

Rationale: This patient has symptoms of disseminated gonorrhea, which include rash and arthritis but mainly oligoarthritis and urethritis. *Neisseria gonorrhoeae* is the second most common disease of sexually transmitted disease in the population. In the primary infection, the patient has no symptoms, but after dissemination to the entire body, symptoms began to appear.

22. Answer: 3

Rationale: This patient has symptoms and signs of septic arthritis. Also, he had one of the risk factors for developing it (knee replacement). *Staphylococcus aureus* is the most common organism in the early presentation after knee replacement. Septic arthritis is confirmed by synovial fluid analysis, which shows high white blood cells.

23. Answer: 2

Rationale: This patient has symptoms of osteomyelitis. Sickle cell is a risk factor of osteomyelitis, and the most common organism in those patients is *Salmonella*. The treatment of this condition in sickle cell patients is the same in a healthy patient. The most sensitive test for osteomyelitis is magnetic resonance imaging.

24. Answer: 1

Rationale: This patient has symptoms of osteomyelitis, which is infection in the bone. There are many risk factors for osteomyelitis, including diabetic foot, drug abuse, and a history of open fracture. In the acute stage, the x-ray will appear normal and magnetic resonance imaging has a high sensitivity, but in the late stage bone destruction and periosteal reaction will appear.

25. Answer: 2

Rationale: This patient has symptoms of polymyalgia rheumatica, which is an inflammatory disease presenting with pain and stiffness and with muscle weakness in some cases. Pain happens mainly in the shoulder and pelvic girdle muscles. One of the complications of this disease is giant cell arteritis, which happens in more than 30% of patients.

26. Answer: 1

Rationale: Polymyositis presents with progressive muscle weakness with dysphagia. The diagnosis of polymyositis is confirmed by elevated muscle enzymes, electromyography findings, and muscle biopsy. Most of the time the weakness is painless.

27. Answer: 4

Rationale: This patient has many symptoms of ankylosing spondylitis, which include back pain, enthesitis, morning stiffness, and bilateral sacroiliitis. This disease is one of HLA-B27; it mainly causes inflammation in the spine, which leads to chronic pain and decreased mobility.

28. Answer: 2

Rationale: This patient has symptoms of dermatomyositis, which includes proximal muscle weakness and rash with elevated creatine phosphokinase. In one-third of patients, this disease presents with hidden malignancy. Anti-Jo1 antibody will be positive in this patient.

29. Answer: 1

Rationale: This patient, with a history of gout, presents with symptoms of an acute attack of gout. According to the guidelines of the American College of Physicians, the drug of choice in acute attacks is colchicine or any type of nonsteroidal antiinflammatory drug (NSAID), but if the patient has any contraindication to NSAIDs intraarticular methylprednisolone is preferred.

30. Answer: 2

Rationale: Acute joint pain with swelling and erythema can be presented with acute arthritis. Acute arthritis has many differential diagnoses, including septic arthritis, an acute attack of gout, or pseudogout. These diseases can be differentiated by synovial fluid aspiration and analysis of the fluid.

31. Answer: 2

Rationale: This patient presented with features of meniscal tear, which presents a couple of days after the injury. Meniscal tear happened after the patient twisted his leg during a football game. The most sensitive and specific test for meniscal tear is magnetic resonance imaging.

32. Answer: 3

Rationale: This patient has symptoms of dermatomyositis, which include proximal muscle weakness and rash with elevated creatine phosphokinase. In one-third of patients, this disease presents with hidden malignancy. Anti-Jo1 antibody will be positive in this patient. The treatment of dermatomyositis includes a corticosteroid.

33. Answer: 2

Rationale: This patient has symptoms of polymyalgia rheumatica (PMR), which is an inflammatory disease presenting with pain and stiffness, with muscle weakness in some cases. Pain happens mainly in the shoulder and pelvic girdle muscles. One of the complications of this disease is giant cell arteritis, which happens in more than 30% of patients. In PMR, the erythrocyte sedimentation rate and C-reactive protein are usually elevated.

34. Answer: 3

Rationale: Osteoporosis is one of the most common diseases in elderly people. Many risk factors increase the possibility of osteoporosis, such as age, poor nutrition, sedentary life, and low weight. The most sensitive test for osteoporosis is a dual-energy x-ray absorptiometry scan, which measures bone density.

35. Answer: 2

Rationale: This patient presents with signs and symptoms of a Baker cyst, which is a collection of fluid in one of the bursae that surround the knee. This condition is common in the patient who suffers from osteoarthritis, rheumatoid arthritis, and other joint diseases. The diagnosis of this cyst can be done by knee ultrasound.

36. Answer: 2

Rationale: This patient, who is a known case of systemic lupus erythematosus, presented with symptoms of femoral head necrosis, which is one of the long-term steroid intake complications. This disease needs high suspicion and early diagnosis to avoid complications The gold standard for diagnosis of femoral head necrosis is a magnetic resonance imaging scan, which can detect the changes early.

37. Answer: 1

Rationale: This patient has symptoms of dermatomyositis, which include proximal muscle weakness and rash with elevated creatine phosphokinase. In one-third of patients, this disease presents with hidden malignancy. Anti-Jo1 antibody will be positive in this patient.

38. Answer: 1

Rationale: This patient has symptoms of polymyalgia rheumatica (PMR), which is an inflammatory disease presenting with pain and stiffness and with muscle weakness in some cases. Pain happens mainly in the shoulder and pelvic girdle muscles. In PMR, erythrocyte sedimentation rate and C-reactive protein are usually elevated, but diagnosis can be confirmed by response to prednisone.

39. Answer: 3

Rationale: This patient has many symptoms of ankylosing spondylitis, which include back pain, enthesitis, morning stiffness, and bilateral sacroiliitis. This disease is one of HLA-B27; it mainly causes inflammation in the spine, which leads to chronic pain and decreased mobility.

40. Answer: 1

Rationale: This patient presents with low back pain, pseudo-claudication, and leg numbness, which is the triad of spinal canal stenosis. In this disease back pain and claudication are aggravated by extension and relieved by flexion. It is mainly diagnosed by spinal magnetic resonance imaging.

41. Answer: 4

Rationale: This patient, who has a history of gout, presents with symptoms of an acute attack of gout. According to the guidelines of the American College of Physicians, the drug of choice in acute attacks is colchicine or any type of nonsteroidal antiinflammatory drug (NSAID), but if the patient has any contraindication to NSAIDs then intraarticular methylprednisolone is preferred.

42. Answer: 1

Rationale: This patient presented with features of meniscal tear and presents a couple of days after the injury. Meniscal tear happened after he twisted his leg during a basketball game. The most sensitive and specific test for meniscal tear is magnetic resonance imaging scan.

43. Answer: 3

Rationale: This patient has symptoms of dermatomyositis, which include proximal muscle weakness and rash with elevated creatine phosphokinase. In one-third of patients, this disease presents with hidden malignancy. Anti-Jo1 antibody will be positive in this patient.

Hematology/Immunology/Oncology

Acquired Immunodeficiency Syndrome (AIDS)/Human Immunodeficiency Virus (HIV)

1. A 28-year-old male patient presents to his infectious disease specialist with complaint of headaches, malaise, fever, and night sweats for the past week. He is homosexual and has one monogamous partner. He believes his partner is monogamous as well. He has been diagnosed with HIV in the past 6 months and his last CD4 count was 400 cells/μL 3 months prior. His current treatment includes dolutegravir, abacavir, and lamivudine. On exam, he is found to have nontender skin lesions with firm, nodular, purplish appearance. His labs reveal a CD4 count of 85 cells/μL. Which of the following is the diagnosis of his skin lesion?

   1. Kaposi sarcoma.

   2. Erythema multiform.

   3. Seborrheic dermatitis.

   4. Drug reaction.

2. A 45-year-old female patient was diagnosed with HIV by her primary care provider 2 weeks ago. She is waiting to see the infectious disease specialist and presents to the emergency department with a 2-day history of headache, fever, and confusion. At diagnosis, her CD4 count was 68 cells/μL. In the emergency department, computed tomography scan of the head shows multiple ring enhancing lesions. Which is the most likely etiology of these findings?

   1. *Bartonella henselae.*

   2. Cytomegalovirus encephalopathy.

   3. HIV encephalopathy.

   4. *Toxoplasma gondii.*

3. A 54-year-old male patient with a known history of HIV presents to the emergency department. He has been well controlled on highly active antiretroviral therapy and follows regularly with his infectious disease specialist. Over the past 2 weeks, he has noticed development of cough that has gradually worsened. He now has fever, night sweats, and weight loss. His chest imaging reveals a cavitary lesion in the right upper lobe with associated hilar adenopathy. His CD4 count is 356 cells/μL. What is the likely etiology of his presentation?

   1. *Pneumocystis jiroveci* pneumonia.

   2. *Mycobacterium tuberculosis* infection.

   3. Kaposi sarcoma.

   4. Bacterial pneumonia.

4. A 32-year-old male patient with a new diagnosis of HIV has begun highly active antiretroviral therapy in the past 1 week. He calls with complaint of increased nausea over the past week since starting therapy. He reports a long history of gastroesophageal disease (GERD) and remains on chronic proton-pump inhibitor therapy. He underwent upper endoscopy approximately 2 months prior to evaluate his GERD and found no concerns. He denies any other symptoms and otherwise is feeling well. What is most likely the cause of his new-onset symptoms?

   1. *Candida* esophagitis.

   2. Cytomegalovirus esophagitis.

   3. Herpes simplex virus esophagitis.

   4. Drug side effect.

5. You are providing education to a newly diagnosed HIV patient in your clinic. The patient is a pet lover and has numerous cats. Which bacteria are you concerned with and educate the patient about in changing the litter box?

   1. *Toxoplasma gondii.*

   2. *Bartonella henselae.*

   3. *Salmonella* species.

   4. *Francisella tularensis.*

6. The diagnostic criteria for AIDS is an HIV patient with which of the following?

    1. CD4+ T-cell count less than 500 cells/µL.

    2. CD4+ T-cell percentage of total lymphocytes greater than 14%.

    3. CD4+ T-cell count less than 200 cells/µL.

    4. CD4+ T-cell count between 200 and 500 cells/µL.

7. For HIV-infected patients, what should the CD4+ T-cell count be before initiation of antiretroviral therapy?

    1. CD4+ T-cell count less than 350 cells/µL.

    2. CD4+ T-cell count less than 200 cells/µL.

    3. CD4+ T-cell count less than 500 cells/µL.

    4. Should be started regardless of CD4+ T-cell count.

8. Your HIV patient presents to the clinic not feeling well. The patient complains of headache and dizziness that started a few days after initiation of dapsone for *Pneumocystis* pneumonia prophylaxis. While in the office you notice the patient has become cyanotic with tachypnea. What is the most likely differential based on the patient's recent initiation of dapsone?

    1. Pulmonary embolism.

    2. Pulmonary obstruction.

    3. Methemoglobinemia.

    4. Airway obstruction.

9. In assessing an HIV patient's susceptibility to opportunistic infections, which peripheral blood assay should be utilized?

    1. Absolute neutrophil count.

    2. CD4+ lymphocyte count.

    3. Cytomegalovirus status.

    4. CD20 B-cell count.

Autoimmune Disease

10. A 67-year-old female patient with a known history of Hashimoto thyroiditis has been followed for routine lab work including thyroid-stimulating hormone (TSH) and ultrasound for the past 2 years. She has remained on low-dose thyroid replacement for this time and TSH has remained in therapeutic range. She presents to your office with a 15-pound weight loss in the past 2 months with associated night sweats and enlarging, firm thyroid gland. In the past few weeks, she has noticed some hoarseness and in the past couple of days noticed difficulty swallowing. Repeat labs at the office visit reveal a TSH of 10 International Units/mL and a lactate dehydrogenase of 2500 units/L. What is the likely diagnosis of her condition?

    1. Primary thyroid lymphoma.

    2. Thyroid goiter.

    3. Acute thyroiditis.

    4. Papillary thyroid carcinoma.

11. A 54-year-old female patient with history of rheumatoid arthritis has been working with her specialist to adjust her hydroxychloroquine (Plaquenil) to an appropriate dose. She is currently at 400 mg daily dosing and has remained on therapy for the past 5 years. What recommendation should be made regarding the screening testing based on her current treatment?

    1. Audiology evaluation.

    2. Colonoscopy.

    3. Ophthalmology evaluation.

    4. Repeat rheumatoid factor assay.

12. When working up a patient for a diagnosis of sarcoidosis, which blood test can aid in this evaluation?

    1. Eosinophil sedimentation rate.

    2. Antinuclear antibody.

    3. Serum angiotensin-converting enzyme.

    4. C-reactive protein.

13. Before initiation of therapy for rheumatoid arthritis with disease-modifying antirheumatic drugs, what testing is *not* recommended?

    1. Ophthalmic examination.

    2. Tuberculosis screening.

    3. Hepatitis B and C screening.

    4. Baseline bone scan.

14. A 24-year-old male patient presents with ongoing low back pain for the past 3 months. Symptoms seem to improve with exercise but not rest. He reports feeling very stiff on waking in the morning. You are concerned with a possible diagnosis of ankylosing spondylitis. What specific testing would be diagnostic?

    1. Bilateral grade 2 sacroiliitis on imaging with positive human leukocyte antigen (HLA)-B27.

    2. No sacroiliitis on imaging with positive HLA-B27.

    3. Positive rheumatoid factor and negative HLA-B27.

    4. Negative rheumatoid factor and negative HLA-B27.

15. You are treating a patient who is anemic and has vitamin B$_{12}$ deficiency. You have noted the patient to be positive for antiparietal cell and intrinsic factor antibodies. What is the patient's diagnosis?

    1. Aplastic anemia.

    2. Fanconi anemia.

    3. Pernicious anemia.

    4. Sideroblastic anemia.

16. What findings are the hallmark of Hashimoto thyroiditis?

    1. Goiter.

    2. Circulating thyroid antibodies.

    3. Lack of thyroid antibodies.

    4. Lack of goiter.

17. You are working up a patient with known rheumatoid arthritis. What is a common clinical feature found in this patient population?

    1. Thyroiditis.

    2. Exophthalmia.

    3. Lymphadenopathy.

    4. Thrombocytopenia.

Blood Group Incompatibilities

18. If you are ordering a red blood cell transfusion for a patient and they need to receive cytomegalovirus-negative product, what is the best way to minimize this risk?

    1. Order irradiated blood product.

    2. Order leukocyte reduced product.

    3. Order washed red blood cells.

    4. Order frozen red blood cells.

19. Your patient with immune thrombocytopenia presents to the clinic. She has been taking dexamethasone 40 mg daily for the past 4 days for initial treatment. Her platelet count is 2000 and she has vaginal spotting. She is known to be platelet refractory on two separate occasions. Which of the following is a technique to improve platelet transfusion counts?

    1. Irradiated platelets.

    2. Human leukocyte antigen matching.

    3. Consecutive platelet transfusions.

    4. Nothing can be done if platelet refractory.

20. Pretransfusion testing includes ABO blood type, rhesus, and antibody screen to determine whether a patient has an unexpected red blood cell antibody. Positive antibodies can be clinically significant during transfusion of blood red blood cells because they can lead to

    1. Acute or delayed hemolytic reaction.

    2. Transmission of infection.

    3. Thrombophlebitis.

    4. Clotting abnormalities.

21. A 28-year-old female patient returns to postoperative care after emergency cesarean section. She is being transfused type A-positive packed red blood cells. As you review her records, you realize that her blood type noted before cesarean section was O negative. Your concerns regarding incompatible red blood cell transfusion would be validated by your understanding of which of the following?

    1. The patient's immunoglobulin (Ig)M anti-A can activate complement leading to intravascular hemolysis.

    2. The patient's IgM anti-A can activate complement leading to extravascular hemolysis.

    3. There are no concerns for transfusion, but the patient should receive anti-RhD immunoglobulin to prevent development of rhesus antibodies for future pregnancies.

    4. The patient's IgM anti-B can activate complement leading to intravascular hemolysis.

22. You are explaining ABO incompatibility to your patient and you let them know that a patient with ABO blood type "A" will have which antigens expressed on the surface of the red blood cell and which antibodies in the plasma?

    1. B antigens, anti-B antibodies.

    2. AB antigens, no antibodies.

    3. A antigens, anti-B antibodies.

    4. A antigens, anti-A antibodies.

23. You are working trauma in the emergency department and a patient known to your facility arrives with a gunshot wound to the chest. He is losing blood and you are tasked with ordering a blood transfusions for the patient. He is ABO blood type O negative. Which packed red blood cell transfusion can be given safely?

    1. B positive.

    2. A negative.

    3. AB negative.

    4. O positive.

24. You are evaluating a patient for hemolytic anemia. You are explaining a direct antibody test to your patient. What is this test looking for on the surface of the red blood cells?

    1. Immunoglobulin (Ig)M or complement.

    2. IgA or complement.

    3. ABO-specific antigens.

    4. IgG or complement.

25. Which is the most important factor in determining whether blood from a specific donor can be transfused to a specific recipient?

    1. Rh compatibility.

    2. ABO compatibility.

    3. Kell, Kidd, and Duffy antigen evaluation.

    4. Human leukocyte antigen typing.

Coagulopathies

26. A 50-year-old female patient with known history of type 1 von Willebrand disease presents for her screening colonoscopy. She has history of bleeding with procedures and will require what treatment preprocedure to reduce risk of bleeding?

    1. Fresh frozen plasma.

    2. Platelet transfusion.

    3. Desmopressin.

    4. Aminocaproic acid.

27. A patient with known protein C deficiency presents to your clinic with complaints of abnormal bruising/petechiae to the extremities. History reveals rectal bleeding for past 2 days as well as shortness of breath that started this morning. Which lab results would be consistent with acute disseminated intravascular coagulation?

    1. Normal platelet function, prolonged prothrombin time, normal D-dimer.

    2. Reduced platelet function, elevated D-dimer, reduced plasma fibrinogen.

    3. Reduced platelet function, elevated D-dimer, reduced thrombin time.

    4. Reduced platelet function, normal prothrombin time, normal thrombin time.

28. A 23-year-old male patient presents with known history of hemophilia. He is bleeding from the gums and bright red blood per rectum. Which product would be initially recommended?

    1. Factor VIII infusion.

    2. Cryoprecipitate.

    3. Desmopressin (DDAVP).

    4. Aminocaproic acid.

29. You have been managing an obese male patient in his 50s who presented to his primary care provider with easy bruising. You know he was recently hospitalized and was on heparin therapy for deep vein thrombosis prophylaxis. His platelets were normal with his admission and he is now 5 days from receiving heparin. Repeat of the platelet count shows platelets at 30 K/μL. You suspect heparin-induced thrombocytopenia. For future management, which anticoagulant would be an appropriate alternative to therapy?

    1. Heparin.

    2. Low-molecular-weight heparin.

    3. Fondaparinux.

    4. No alternative is indicated.

30. You are in the emergency department caring for a 55-year-old male patient with a history of uncontrolled diabetes and chronic renal disease. He reports recent travel for vacation with his family. He noted some shortness of breath toward the end of the trip as he returned home. On exam, he is noted to have a heart rate of 110 beats/min and oxygenation is 92% on room air. Electrocardiogram is normal sinus rhythm. Your primary concern is possible pulmonary embolism (PE). Initial labs are unremarkable except you note his creatinine is 2.7. What testing method would be safest and provide the most reliable result for identification of PE?

    1. Venous duplex of bilateral lower extremities.

    2. Chest x-ray.

    3. Ventilation perfusion scintillation scan.

    4. Computed tomography pulmonary angiogram.

31. You are currently managing a 64-year-old male patient with significant medical history. He is known to you for his history of atrial fibrillation and is currently managed with warfarin therapy. He has had stable international normalized ratio (INR) monthly and his warfarin dose has not needed to be adjusted for over 6 months. He calls your clinic after being seen in a local urgent care for a sinus infection. He reports new-onset bruising to his arms. You suspect his INR is elevated and have him come to the clinic. His INR returns at 4. Which of the following medications for treatment of acute sinusitis would you consider as contributing to the elevation of his INR?

    1. Trimethoprim/sulfamethoxazole.

    2. Cephalexin.

    3. Fluticasone.

    4. Cetirizine.

32. In a known hemophilia patient, which parameters would be consistent with the diagnosis?

    1. Prothrombin time (unaffected), activated partial thromboplastin time (prolonged), bleeding time (unaffected), platelet count (unaffected).

    2. Prothrombin time (unaffected), activated partial thromboplastin time (unaffected), bleeding time (unaffected), platelet count (unaffected).

    3. Prothrombin time (prolonged), activated partial thromboplastin time (prolonged), bleeding time (prolonged), platelet count (unaffected).

    4. Prothrombin time (prolonged), activated partial thromboplastin time (prolonged), bleeding time (unaffected), platelet count (unaffected).

33. Which condition would have the greatest risk for development of a blood clot?

    1. A 22-year-old female patient on oral contraceptive.

    2. A 22-year-old female patient with history of heterozygous factor V Leiden mutation.

    3. A 22-year-old female patient with homozygous factor V Leiden mutation.

    4. A 22-year-old female patient with homozygous factor V Leiden mutation on oral contraceptives.

34. You are evaluating a 28-year-old female patient with a history of multiple miscarriages for new lower extremity, unprovoked deep venous thrombosis. What diagnosis would be at the top of your list?

    1. Hemophilia.

    2. Sickle cell disease.

    3. Heterozygous Leiden factor V mutation.

    4. Antiphospholipid syndrome.

Leukemia and Tumors

35. A 43-year-old Hispanic male patient presents with increased fatigue, bleeding gums, and shortness of breath. He is noted, on admission, to have a white blood cell count of 9.8 K/µL, hemoglobin of 6.8 g/dL, platelets 38 K/µL, blasts noted on peripheral smear, lactate dehydrogenase of 460 units/L, D-dimer of 550 ng/mL, and fibrinogen of 88 mg/dL. Based on available results, what is your most likely diagnosis?

    1. Thrombotic microangiopathy.

    2. Acute promyelocytic leukemia with disseminated intravascular coagulation.

    3. Hemolytic anemia.

    4. Multiple myeloma.

36. A 74-year-old white male patient presents for annual follow-up. He reports no complaints. Routine screening labs show white blood cell count of 30,900 K/µL, hemoglobin 14.8 g/dL, and platelets 387 K/µL. Differential shows an increase in absolute metamyelocytes and absolute myelocytes. Absolute segmented neutrophils were increased at 19.6 K/µL and absolute banded neutrophils were increased at 0.87 K/µL. No blasts were noted by the pathologist. Further testing revealed no monoclonal protein and vitamin B_{12} and folate were normal. Genetic test was positive for translocation in BCR/ABL. What is your diagnosis?

    1. Chronic myelogenous leukemia.

    2. Chronic lymphocytic leukemia.

    3. Non-Hodgkin lymphoma.

    4. Lymphoproliferative disorder.

37. A 52-year-old African American presents for his first screening colonoscopy. He denies any complaints and has unknown family history. Colonoscopy reveals a 2-cm tubular adenoma with high-grade dysplasia. What is the interval for follow-up colon cancer screening?

    1. 1 year.

    2. 3 years.

    3. 5 years.

    4. 10 years.

38. You have been asked to evaluate a patient with polycythemia. Your workup reveals he has been dealing with ongoing fatigue and was started on testosterone replacement by his primary care provider for low testosterone levels. He presents to your clinic with a hemoglobin of 16.6 g/dL and hematocrit of 56%. Your workup reveals no abnormalities consistent with a myeloproliferative neoplasm. Your diagnosis is secondary polycythemia related to testosterone supplementation. What is your treatment recommendation?

    1. 500-mL phlebotomy.

    2. Discontinue testosterone.

    3. 250-mL phlebotomy.

    4. Repeat complete blood count in 4 weeks.

39. You are caring for a new diagnosed patient with diffuse large B-cell lymphoma. He reports to your nurse that he has experienced shortness of breath for the last week as well as facial swelling, headache, and right arm swelling. Based on your knowledge of his disease, which diagnosis would you suspect most?

    1. Acute deep venous thrombosis.

    2. Superior vena cava syndrome.

    3. Lymphedema.

    4. Bacteremia.

40. What is the chromosomal abnormality noted in a patient with chronic myelogenous leukemia who presents to your clinic for workup and management?

    1. Philadelphia chromosome (BCR/ABL fusion oncogene).

    2. FLT3 gene mutation.

    3. PML-RARA translocation, t(15,17).

    4. Normal cytogenetics.

41. What would be the initial treatment for tumor lysis syndrome prophylaxis for a newly diagnosed acute leukemia patient with a white blood cell count of 22,000 cells/μL, lactate dehydrogenase level of 980 units/L, and uric acid level of 5 mg/dL?

    1. Rasburicase.

    2. Allopurinol.

    3. Febuxostat.

    4. No prophylaxis is required.

42. You are caring for a 52-year-old female patient with a new diagnosis of acute leukemia. Her initial white blood cell count was 130×10^9 cells/L. She is actively receiving her induction chemotherapy. Her scheduled labs return abnormal. Her uric acid level is 12 mg/dL, potassium 5.8 mEq/L, phosphorus 4.6 mg/dL, and calcium 6 mg/dL. You recognize that her labs are consistent with tumor lysis syndrome. What management modality is key to stabilizing this patient?

    1. Hydration, rasburicase, cardiac monitoring, repeat lab work in 4 to 6 hours.

    2. Hydration, allopurinol, phosphate binder.

    3. Hydration and repeat labs in 12 hours.

    4. Hydration, allopurinol, Kayexalate, phosphate binder, repeat labs in 12 hours.

43. Your non–small cell lung cancer (NSCLC) patient calls the clinic saying he has profuse diarrhea. He reports onset over the past few days. He denies any recent changes to diet and no new medications for the past month. He continues on active treatment for his lung cancer and has remained on the same treatment for the past 2 months. Which therapy would cause you to be most concerned with this phone call?

    1. Platinum-based therapy.

    2. Immunotherapy.

    3. Radiation therapy.

    4. Surgical therapy.

Anemia

44. The patient is a 64-year-old Caucasian female patient who presented to the emergency department with ongoing fatigue, shortness of breath, weakness, and occasional palpitations. She reports symptoms have worsened over the past 2 to 3 months. She denies any unexplained weight loss, night sweats, cough, or bleeding. Her medical history is positive for hypertension controlled on lisinopril. She denies any other known medical complications. She reports endometrial ablation years previously related to abnormal menses and has been without a period for over 15 years. She denies any other surgeries. Her last colonoscopy was noted 2 years previously and reports tubular adenoma without other complications. She reports previous smoking history with an approximately 30 pack-year history but stopped smoking about 5 years ago. Her exam is only remarkable for diminished breath sounds on auscultation. Vitals are unremarkable. Laboratory examination reveals white blood count 5400/mm³, hemoglobin 9.8 g/dL (low), platelets 375,000 mm³, mean corpuscular volume 92 fL, mean corpuscular hemoglobin concentration 31 g/dL, and red blood cell distribution width 14. Normal differential was sodium 135 mEq/L, potassium 4.1 mEq/L, creatinine 1.6 mg/dL (elevated), calcium 10.1 mg/dL, estimated creatinine clearance 44.5 mL/min, glucose 98 mg/dL, total bilirubin 0.7 mg/dL, aspartate aminotransferase 28 units/L, and alanine aminotransferase 21 units/L. Urinalysis is unremarkable. Chest x-ray is consistent with emphysema. No other abnormalities are noted. Electrocardiogram is normal sinus rhythm. What is your working diagnosis?

    1. Normocytic normochromic anemia.

    2. Anemia unspecified.

    3. Iron-deficiency anemia caused by chronic blood loss.

    4. Macrocytic anemia.

45. The patient is a 64-year-old Caucasian female patient who presented to the emergency department with ongoing fatigue, shortness of breath, weakness, and occasional palpitations. She reports symptoms have worsened over the past 2 to 3 months. She denies any unexplained weight loss, night sweats, cough, or bleeding. Her medical history is positive for hypertension controlled on lisinopril. She denies any other known medical complications. She reports endometrial ablation years previously related to abnormal menses and has been without a period for over 15 years. She denies any other surgeries. Her last colonoscopy was noted 2 years previously and reports tubular adenoma without other complications. She reports previous smoking history with an approximately 30 pack-year history but stopped smoking about 5 years ago. Her exam is only remarkable

for diminished breath sounds on auscultation. Vitals are unremarkable. Laboratory examination reveals white blood count 5400/mm³, hemoglobin 9.8 g/dL (low), platelets 375,000 mm³, mean corpuscular volume 92 fL, mean corpuscular hemoglobin concentration 31 g/dL, and red blood cell distribution width 14. Normal differential was sodium 135 mEq/L, potassium 4.1 mEq/L, creatinine 1.6 mg/dL (elevated), calcium 10.1 mg/dL, estimated creatinine clearance 44.5 mL/min, glucose 98 mg/dL, total bilirubin 0.7 mg/dL, aspartate aminotransferase 28 units/L, and alanine aminotransferase 21 units/L. Urinalysis is unremarkable. Chest x-ray is consistent with emphysema. No other abnormalities are noted. Electrocardiogram is normal sinus rhythm. What lab testing should be obtained next?

    1. Ferritin, transferrin, folate, total iron binding, iron, vitamin B_{12}, reticulocyte count.

    2. Methylmalonic acid, homocysteine, vitamin B_{12}, folate, ferritin.

    3. Reticulocyte count, vitamin B_{12}, folate, serum protein electrophoresis (SPEP).

    4. SPEP, urine protein electrophoresis, vitamin B_{12}, folate, ferritin, lactic acid dehydrogenase, haptoglobin, blood smear.

46. A 44-year-old male patient presents with pneumocystis pneumonia for his 6-month follow-up. His workup reveals hemoglobin 11.8 g/dL, mean corpuscular volume 101, ferritin 128 ng/mL, folate 15 ng/mL, iron saturation 22.5%, vitamin B_{12} 420 pg/mL, and reticulocyte count 3.2%. What additional testing would be advised?

    1. Methylmalonic acid.

    2. Thyroid function testing.

    3. Intrinsic factor antibody.

    4. Lactate dehydrogenase.

47. A 34-year-old female patient is receiving a blood transfusion for anemia after childbirth. She has no other known medical history and had a normal pregnancy. Pretransfusion, her vitals were normal. After 1 hour of the transfusion, she developed symptoms consistent with transfusion-related acute lung injury (TRALI). Which of these symptoms are consistent with TRALI?

    1. Dyspnea, hypoxemia, tachycardia, fever, hypotension, and cyanosis.

    2. Dyspnea, hypoxemia, acute-onset rash, bradycardia, and hypertension.

    3. Dyspnea, hypoxemia, bradycardia, and hypotension.

    4. Dyspnea, hypoxemia, tachycardia, and hypertension.

48. You are managing a young man with history of sickle cell disease. He has classic signs of splenic sequestration and you have been asked to provide blood transfusion support because his hemoglobin has decreased by 2 g/dL. You are concerned about the effect of the blood transfusion due to which possibility?

    1. Hemolysis.

    2. Transfusion reaction.

    3. Fluid overload.

    4. Hyperviscosity syndrome.

49. A 56-year-old male patient with chronic kidney disease stage IV related to anemia of chronic kidney disease follows in your clinic. You would like to start him on therapy with darbepoetin. What blood test result would cause you to use alternative treatment before considering erythropoietin stimulating agent?

    1. Hematocrit 55%.

    2. Hemoglobin 8.5 g/dL.

    3. Erythropoietin 25 mIU/mL.

    4. Ferritin 10 ng/mL.

50. You are covering on call for the hematology division. You are called regarding a patient of the practice with known warm antibody autoimmune hemolytic anemia, and recent labs reveal hemoglobin is decreased from 10 to 8 g/dL. Lactate dehydrogenase is elevated at 450 units/L and haptoglobin is 5 mg/dL. What is the first-line treatment for this patient in hemolytic anemia?

    1. Blood transfusion support.

    2. Prednisone 1 mg/kg.

    3. Intravenous immune globulin.

    4. Rituximab.

51. A 64-year-old male patient presents to the emergency department with a 1-week history of worsening fatigue and shortness of breath. His symptoms started after upper respiratory symptoms including cough and persistent fever, which he felt was a chest cold. He also noted mild itching and on exam appears slightly jaundiced. His workup is positive for anemia with a hemoglobin of 9.8 g/dL, total bilirubin of 3.5 mg/dL, lactate dehydrogenase of 889 units/L, haptoglobin of 15 mg/dL, direct antiglobulin test positive for immunoglobulin G, and complement. What is your likely diagnosis?

    1. Autoimmune hemolytic anemia associated with *Mycoplasma pneumoniae.*

    2. *Streptococcal viridans* associated anemia.

    3. Microangiopathic hemolytic anemia.

    4. Disseminated intravascular coagulation.

52. Which condition would increase your risk of hemolytic anemia?

    1. Glucose-6-phosphate dehydrogenase deficiency.

    2. β thalassemia.

    3. Polyneuropathy, organomegaly, endocrinopathy/edema, monoclonal protein, skin changes (POEMS) syndrome.

    4. Polycythemia vera.

53. Which blood test is not important when initially working up a patient for anemia?

    1. Complete blood count.

    2. Reticulocyte count.

    3. Peripheral blood smear.

    4. Methylmalonic acid.

Hematology/Immunology/Oncology Answers & Rationales 6

Acquired Immunodeficiency Syndrome (AIDS)/Human Immunodeficiency Virus (HIV)

1. Answer: 1

Rationale: Kaposi sarcoma is related to human herpesvirus 8. The rash is characterized by nontender skin lesions with firm, nodular, purplish appearance. It is usually found when the CD4 count falls below 200 cells/µL.

2. Answer: 4

Rationale: Toxoplasma encephalitis can present in days to weeks. Patients may present with fever, headache, altered mental status, focal neurological changes, and seizures. Imaging can show ring enhancing lesions in approximately 90% of cases with edema and mass effect. The CD4 count is often less than 100 cells/µL.

3. Answer: 2

Rationale: HIV patients' risk of tuberculosis (TB) doubles within the first year after HIV seroconversion. Classic presenting symptoms of pulmonary TB with HIV patients are similar to non-HIV patients. These can include fever, cough, weight loss, malaise, and night sweats. Typical radiographic findings include cavitary lesions found in the upper lung fields.

4. Answer: 4

Rationale: Antiretroviral therapy side effects are extremely common and can contribute to poor compliance with therapy. Protease inhibitors can cause significant nausea and diarrhea and are the likely culprit. Other significant potential side effects of highly active antiretroviral therapy can include pancreatitis, hepatitis, hepatic necrosis, and self-limited neuropsychiatric problems.

5. Answer: 1

Rationale: To reduce risk of infection, it is important to educate HIV-infected patients about their surrounding risks. They should learn to avoid activities that might increase risk of exposure to opportunistic infections. Cleaning out a cat litter box increases risk for toxoplasmosis.

6. Answer: 3

Rationale: A patient is confirmed to have AIDS if the CD4 cell count is less than 200 cells/µL or less than 14% of total lymphocyte in the presence of proven HIV infection.

7. Answer: 4

Rationale: The Department of Health and Human Services Guidelines advise active antiretroviral therapy be started regardless of the CD4 cell count. Individuals with CD4 cell counts less than 200 are at increased risk for infections and should be advised to start therapy as soon as possible.

8. Answer: 3

Rationale: Methemoglobinemia is caused by an abnormal amount of methemoglobin. Methemoglobin is unable to release oxygen to body tissues effectively. Acquired methemoglobinemia is most commonly caused by two medications, dapsone and benzocaine.

9. Answer: 2

Rationale: CD4+ T cells continue to be a good indicator for susceptibility for HIV patients. A count less than 200 cells/µL correlates with increased susceptibility.

Autoimmune Disease

10. Answer: 1

Rationale: Primary thyroid lymphoma is four times more likely to be seen in women than in men. Approximately half of all primary thyroid lymphomas are seen in patients diagnosed with Hashimoto thyroiditis. Thyroid lymphoma can contribute to worsening hypothyroidism related to lymphoma infiltrating the thyroid gland.

11. Answer: 3

Rationale: Hydroxychloroquine is an antimalarial drug is beneficial in the treatment of rheumatoid arthritis. Hydroxychloroquine does not require monitoring of blood tests. Patients should be advised to schedule a yearly evaluation with ophthalmology after at least 5 years of therapy to detect signs of retinal toxicity associated with therapy.

12. Answer: 3

Rationale: Angiotensin-converting enzyme (ACE) is produced within cells of the sarcoid granuloma. The level may reflect the total disease burden. However, an ACE level alone is inadequate for diagnosis. The likelihood of sarcoidosis increases with higher ACE levels.

13. Answer: 4

Rationale: Baseline testing for initiation of disease-modifying antirheumatic drugs (DMARDS) includes ophthalmic examination because of the potential effects of hydroxychloroquine. Latent tuberculosis testing is indicated as many of the DMARDS are shown to increase risk of mycobacterium infection. Hepatitis B and C screening are advised because of the potential to reactivate the hepatitis virus. Baseline bone scan is not indicated.

14. Answer: 1

Rationale: Ankylosing spondylitis (AS) occurs more predominately in men ranging from 2.5:1 to 5:1. AS is considered to be one of the most common inflammatory disorders of the axial skeleton and typically begins in young adulthood. Classic symptoms consist of low back pain that persists for more than 3 months with associated early-morning stiffness, and is it typically improved by exercise but not by rest. The modified New York criteria for AS identify specific criteria for definitive diagnosis for AS. This includes imaging showing sacroiliitis (grade greater than or equal to 2 bilateral or grade 3 or 4 unilateral) with at least one clinical variable. These variables include low back pain and stiffness for greater than 3 months that improve with exercise but are not relieved by rest, limitation of motion of the lumbar spine in both sagittal and frontal planes, and limitation of chest expansion. Human leukocyte antigen B27 is rarely the definitive factor for diagnosis but in the setting of characteristic back symptoms, the test has reasonably high sensitivity and specificity.

15. Answer: 3

Rationale: Pernicious anemia is an autoimmune-derived anemia associated with vitamin B_{12} deficiency. Autoantibodies can be found to gastric parietal cells as well as intrinsic factor.

16. Answer: 2

Rationale: Hashimoto thyroiditis patients generally have subclinical hypothyroidism and are found to be euthyroid. The presence of circulating antibodies is the hallmark of the disease.

17. Answer: 3

Rationale: Patients with autoimmune disorders, such as rheumatoid arthritis, are often found to have associated lymphadenopathy. The lymph node histology generally is consistent with follicular hyperplasia.

Blood Group Incompatibilities

18. Answer: 2.

Rationale: Leukocyte-reduced red blood cells are considered cytomegalovirus (CMV) safe. Red blood cell products that are from seronegative donors or leukocyte reduced are associated with 1% to 1.5% CMV-transmission failure rates.

19. Answer: 2

Rationale: With the immune thrombocytopenia patient, one could assume she has developed alloantibodies. To try to overcome this effect, human leukocyte antigen–matched platelets can be attempted. Another option would include cross-matched platelets.

20. Answer: 1

Rationale: Pretransfusion testing allows for identification of antibodies to red blood cells. If positive, further identification is warranted to identify the specific antibody and reduce risk of complications. Complications can include acute or delayed hemolytic reaction, graft-versus-host affect, and it may contribute to transfusion-related acute lung injury.

21. Answer: 1

Rationale: If red blood cells of an incompatible ABO group are transfused a cascade of events can unfold. The patient is O negative, and the donor is A positive. The patient's immunoglobulin M anti-A may bind to the red blood cell surface and activate the complement cascade. This can lead to red blood cell lysis (intravascular hemolysis). Approximately 20% to 30% of ABO-incompatible transfusions may lead to some degree of morbidity, and approximately 5% to 10% contribute to death.

22. Answer: 3

Rationale: Red blood cell surface antigens indicate blood type. ABO blood type A will have A antigens on the surface of the red blood cell and will have anti-B circulating plasma antibodies.

23. Answer: 4

Rationale: Patients with ABO type O blood produce antibodies to both blood type A (anti-A) and B (anti-B). They may only receive blood transfusion from an O donor. Rh negative patients do not express the D antigen. On a routine basis, Rh negative patients should receive Rh negative blood. In cases of emergency or low inventory, Rh negative patients can receive Rh positive blood (women not of childbearing potential and men).

24. Answer: 4

Rationale: Direct antiglobulin test (DAT) uses reagents to detect the presence of immunoglobulin (Ig)G or complement on the surface of red blood cells. In hemolytic anemia cold agglutinin disease mediated by IgM, DAT would be positive for complement only. In warm autoimmune hemolytic anemia mediated by IgG, DAT would be positive for IgG or IgG plus complement.

25. Answer: 2

Rationale: ABO compatibility is the most important factor. Anti-A and anti-B antibodies are predominately immunoglobulin M and fix complement, which can cause acute intravascular hemolysis if ABO-incompatible red blood cells are transfused.

Coagulopathies

26. Answer: 3

Rationale: Desmopressin is indicated in von Willebrand type 1 to reduce risk of bleeding by administering prophylactically for minor procedures.

27. Answer: 2.

Rationale: Thrombocytopenia, decreased fibrinogen, and increased D-dimer are considered to be sensitive for the diagnosis but not specific. We consider the diagnosis of acute disseminated intravascular coagulation to be established if the patient has laboratory evidence of thrombocytopenia, coagulation factor consumption (e.g., prolonged prothrombin time, activated partial thromboplastin time; low fibrinogen), and fibrinolysis (e.g., increased D-dimer). With other differentials excluded, the triad of thrombocytopenia, coagulation factor consumption (decreased fibrinogen), and fibrinolysis (elevated D-dimer) can be diagnostic. Bleeding or thrombosis is supportive of the diagnosis.

28. Answer: 1

Rationale: Although all choices are appropriate in treatment of hemophilia patients with bleeding, factor VIII infusion provides the most appropriate replacement of clotting factor therapy in life-threatening bleeding.

29. Answer: 3

Rationale: Fondaparinux has shown to be used safely in patients with heparin-induced thrombocytopenia. There have been reports of what appears to be fondaparinux-induced thrombocytopenia, but this is extremely rare.

30. Answer: 3

Rationale: The ventilation perfusion (V/Q) scintillation scan offers an alternative to the computed tomography pulmonary angiogram when the patient has an allergy to contrast medium or renal disease that may be worsened because of contrast. A high probability result on V/Q scan confirms pulmonary embolus (PE), and normal V/Q scan excludes PE. A moderate or indeterminate probability result is not helpful, and the patient would need further pulmonary testing.

31. Answer: 1

Rationale: Sulfa antibiotics are known to interact with warfarin and increase the risk of bleeding/elevation of the international normalized ratio.

32. Answer: 1

Rationale: Hemophilia A and B are clinically very similar. Specific factor assays are used to differentiate and confirm diagnosis. The following criteria differentiate hemophilia from von Willebrand disease. The prothrombin time, bleeding time, and fibrinogen are normal. The activated partial thromboplastin time (aPTT) is prolonged when the factor levels are less than 30%. The aPTT measures the intrinsic clotting factor pathway and is prolonged associated with lack of clotting factors (hemophilia A, lack of factor VIII; hemophilia B, lack of factor IX).

33. Answer: 4

Rationale: Factor V Leiden (FVL) mutation is the leading cause of activated protein C resistance. Homozygous patients for FVL have an increased risk over heterozygous patients. Heterozygous patients have a 7-fold increased relative risk of vascular thromboembolism, whereas homozygous patients have an 80-fold increase in relative risk of vascular thromboembolism. Oral contraceptives further increase this risk.

34. Answer: 4

Rationale: Antiphospholipid syndrome is characterized by one or more unexplained venous thromboembolisms and poor adverse outcomes related to pregnancy. Antiphospholipid syndrome is an autoimmune thrombophilic condition and should be considered in this patient.

Leukemia and Tumors

35. Answer: 2

Rationale: Acute promyelocytic leukemia (APL) is a form of acute leukemia. Manifestations of acute leukemias are abnormalities in the myeloid lineage of cells. Decreased or increased white blood cells accompanied by normal or low hemoglobin and platelets can be characteristic. Peripheral smear can reveal leukemic cells and can be diagnostic. Prolonged prothrombin, thrombin, and partial thromboplastin times, as well as decreased fibrinogen levels, can be seen in patients with APL. The case illustrates evidence of bleeding, thrombocytopenia, elevated D-dimer, and decreased fibrinogen. These criteria are consistent with disseminated intravascular coagulation, and further workup should be pursued.

36. Answer: 1

Rationale: Chronic myelogenous leukemia presents with a hallmark. The predominance of granulocytes in all phases of differentiation is suggestive of the diagnosis. The preliminary diagnosis is made on abnormal myeloid lineage with confirmation obtained with the presence of translocation at chromosomes 9 and 22 (BCR/ABL).

37. Answer: 2

Rationale: Current evidence shows screening for colorectal cancer in asymptomatic patients can significantly reduce both incidence and mortality. The American Gastroenterology Society guidelines for colonoscopy surveillance after screening and polypectomy were updated in 2012. The 2012 consensus concluded that patients with one or more adenomas with high-risk features were at increased risk of advanced neoplasia during surveillance. Current recommendation is for a 3-year follow-up.

38. Answer: 2

Rationale: The most common cause of polycythemia is acquired secondary polycythemia. Some of the most frequent causes can be found in smokers with lung disease or obstructive sleep apnea patients. Testosterone (androgens) can have an exogenous erythropoietin effect contributing to polycythemia. In this case the testosterone dose can be lowered or discontinued.

39. Answer: 2

Rationale: Superior vena cava (SVC) syndrome is commonly seen in lung cancer and non-Hodgkin lymphoma patients. Obstruction of the SVC may occur acutely or over a few weeks. Symptoms can vary but commonly associated symptoms can consist of shortness of breath, facial edema, dilation of the neck veins, headaches, blurred vision.

40. Answer: 1

Rationale: Chronic myelogenous leukemia is considered a myeloproliferative disorder and is the most common. The Philadelphia chromosome (translocation between chromosome 9 and 22) is consistent with the diagnosis. The chromosome is named after its city of discovery.

41. Answer: 2

Rationale: Acute leukemia with a white blood cell count less than 25×10^9/L, lactate dehydrogenase less than 2× upper limit of normal, and uric acid level less than 8 mg/dL would be at intermediate risk for tumor lysis. Appropriate prophylaxis for this group would include hydration and allopurinol.

42. Answer: 1

Rationale: Tumor lysis syndrome is caused by massive tumor lysis and release of potassium, phosphorous, and uric acid. Uric acid and/or calcium phosphate crystals in the renal tubules can result in acute kidney injury. High-risk patients for tumor lysis include acute leukemia patients with white blood cell counts over 100×10^9 cells/L. Rasburicase is a recombinant urate-oxidase enzyme that converts uric acid to allantoin. Allantoin is an inactive and soluble metabolite of uric acid. Hydration, rasburicase, and appropriate management/monitoring of other electrolytes is mainstay therapy. Patients also may need dialysis to help with ongoing management.

43. Answer: 2

Rationale: Immune-related adverse events are associated with immune activation in checkpoint inhibitors. Patients may experience mucocutaneous and extracutaneous side effects. These effects can be delayed and severe. Early diagnosis with prompt treatment of diarrhea associated with enteritis/colitis should be recognized and treated accordingly for patients on immune therapy.

Anemia

44. Answer: 1

Rationale: Normocytic anemia by definition is the mean red blood cell volume is normal. (mean corpuscular volume [MCV] between 80 and 100 fL). Microcytic anemia is associated with an MCV less than 80 fL, and macrocytic anemias are characterized by an MCV greater than 100 fL. Findings are consistent with normocytic anemia if the MCV is between 80 and 100 fL.

45. Answer: 1

Rationale: Normocytic anemias are often caused by acute hemorrhage, hemolytic anemia, marrow hypoplasia, renal disease, and anemia of chronic disease. A useful tool to determine etiology is to check the reticulocyte count. Reticulocytes are newly formed red blood cells from the marrow. An elevated or decreased reticulocyte count can provide further insight into bone marrow response to anemia. With normocytic anemia, you may have an underlying macrocytosis with microcytosis and resulting mean corpuscular volume is in the normal range. As a result, it is imperative to evaluate for etiologies of both microcytosis as well as macrocytosis. The most common cause of macrocytic anemias is generally considered to be related to nutritional deficiency, such as vitamin B_{12} and/or folate deficiency. Microcytic anemia is generally felt to be related to iron-deficiency anemia, thalassemia, and hemoglobinopathies and anemia of chronic disease.

46. Answer: 2

Rationale: With diagnosis of macrocytic anemia, vitamin B_{12} and folic acid deficiencies are first considerations. If these results are within normal parameters, then further evaluation should be pursued. Consideration for hypothyroidism should be part of the further investigation because hypothyroidism is a cause of macrocytosis.

47. Answer: 1

Rationale: Transfusion-related acute lung injury can present during or within hours of a blood transfusion. Symptoms are generally dyspnea, hypoxemia, tachycardia, fever, hypotension, and cyanosis. Chest x-ray is generally consistent with pulmonary edema.

48. Answer: 4

Rationale: Red blood cell transfusion support is indicated in sickle cell crisis with splenic sequestration. The spleen can become engorged leading to decrease in hemoglobin. Patients can experience hypovolemic shock and cardiovascular collapse. Red blood cell transfusion support can correct this, but caution is advised because it can lead to hyperviscosity once splenic sequestration resolves.

49. Answer: 4

Rationale: Alternative causes other than anemia of chronic kidney disease should be evaluated and treated first. A ferritin of 10 is consistent with iron-deficiency anemia and should be treated before initiation of erythropoietin-stimulating agents.

50. Answer: 2

Rationale: For patients with warm antibody autoimmune hemolytic anemia, corticosteroids are considered to be first-line therapy in moderate to severe cases.

51. Answer: 1

Rationale: Most cases of autoimmune hemolytic anemia (AIHA) occur sporadically. Clinical manifestations often identified include elevated serum levels of indirect bilirubin, lactate dehydrogenase, and reduced serum haptoglobin concentration, and a positive direct antiglobulin test. Unlike microangiopathic hemolytic anemia, the direct antiglobulin test is positive in AIHA because most hemolysis is an extravascular process. Infections can be contributing factors, and a serious complication associated with *Mycoplasma pneumoniae* is cold autoimmune hemolytic anemia.

52. Answer: 1

Rationale: Glucose-6-phosphate dehydrogenase (G6PD) deficiency is an inherited disorder caused by a genetic defect in the red blood cell enzyme G6PD. G6PD is involved in protecting red blood cells from oxidative injury. With low levels of G6PD, red blood cells are more prone to hemolysis and can lead to a chronic hemolytic state.

53. Answer: 4

Rationale: Methylmalonic acid is not indicated when initially evaluating a patient for anemia. Initial testing should encompass a complete blood count, reticulocyte count, and peripheral blood smear. If vitamin B_{12} is evaluated after initial testing and found to be low, methylmalonic acid may be ordered to confirm vitamin B_{12} deficiency.

Neurology

7

1. A 25-year-old female patient visited her nurse practitioner for a follow-up. She has a history of epilepsy and is on a therapeutic dose of sodium valproate, but she still has a seizure every week. What is the next step of management in this patient?

   1. Add lamotrigine.

   2. Add gabapentin.

   3. Stop sodium valproate and start lamotrigine.

   4. Start electroconvulsive therapy.

2. A 30-year-old woman visited her nurse practitioner for a routine follow-up. She has a history of epilepsy on sodium valproate and she wants to have a baby. What is the appropriate next step for this patient?

   1. Stop all her medications now.

   2. Take 5 mg of folic acid daily and continue her medication.

   3. Switch to lamotrigine.

   4. Tell the patient that she cannot get pregnant.

3. A 22-year-old man is brought to the emergency department after a seizure. He had no history of seizures before and he does not have any chronic illnesses. On exam, he appeared confused, his blood pressure was 110/75 mmHg, his pulse was 80 beats/min, his temperature was 98.6°F, and his pupils were reactive. Which of the following is an indication to start an antiepileptic drug now?

   1. Normal electroencephalography.

   2. Patient has a neurological deficit.

   3. Normal brain computed tomography.

   4. Absence of family history of seizure.

4. A 25-year-old female patient presented to the outpatient clinic after she missed her period for 3 months. She has a history of epilepsy on carbamazepine. Her pregnancy test was positive. Which of the following is the appropriate next step for this patient?

   1. Stop carbamazepine immediately.

   2. Continue the carbamazepine.

   3. Provide advice to abort the fetus.

   4. Switch to lamotrigine.

5. A 26-year-old woman visited her nurse practitioner for a routine follow-up. She has a history of epilepsy and is on sodium valproate. Her last seizure was 2 years ago. What is the appropriate next step for this patient?

   1. Stop her medication suddenly.

   2. Taper her medication gradually.

   3. Continue the same treatment long term.

   4. Continue the treatment for 2 years.

6. A 25-year-old female patient presented to the outpatient clinic complaining of a repetitive movement of her left hand that happens multiple times throughout the day. This movement spread to involve the entire arm and left side of the face. She had no history of head trauma or loss of consciousness. Which of the following is the drug of choice for this patient?

   1. Sodium valproate.

   2. Carbamazepine.

   3. Diazepam.

   4. Ethosuximide.

7. A 30-year-old man presented with a visual field defect. He has a history of epilepsy and is on antiepileptic medication, but he cannot remember the name of it. He does not have any history of trauma, head injury, or neurological deficit. Which of the following drugs is the cause of the patient symptom?

    1. Vigabatrin.

    2. Midazolam.

    3. Phenobarbital.

    4. Lamotrigine.

8. A 35-year-old male alcoholic decided to suddenly quit drinking alcohol. Hours later, he had a seizure, so he was brought to the emergency department. On exam, he was conscious but confused. His blood pressure was 130/75 mmHg and he had no neurological deficits. Which of the following is true about the patient's condition?

    1. A seizure usually develops after 48 hours from alcohol abstinence.

    2. No need for a lifelong antiepileptic drug in this patient.

    3. Carbamazepine is the drug of choice for his seizures.

    4. Phenytoin is the drug of choice for his seizures.

9. A 17-year-old girl was brought by her family to the nurse practitioner after a drop in her grades over the past few months. She states she has periods throughout the day when she just "zones out" and does not remember what happens. Her electrocardiogram showed a bilateral symmetrical 3-Hz spike. Which of the following is the drug of choice for this patient?

    1. Ethosuximide.

    2. Carbamazepine.

    3. Phenytoin.

    4. Lamotrigine.

10. A young man complained of repetitive movement of his left hand, which happens many times throughout the day. This movement spreads to involve the entire arm and left side of the face. He has no history of head injury. What is the most likely diagnosis in this patient?

    1. Absent seizure.

    2. Simple partial seizure.

    3. Complex partial seizure.

    4. Myoclonic seizure.

11. A 35-year-old male patient was recently diagnosed with polycystic kidney disease, and he is now on an antihypertensive management. His brother died 2 years ago from hemorrhagic stroke. Which of the following is an appropriate test for this patient?

    1. Magnetic resonance arteriography.

    2. Kidney biopsy.

    3. Echocardiography.

    4. Urinalysis.

12. A 25-year-old female patient presented with progressive periorbital swelling on the left side that started a couple of days ago. The only medicine she takes is an oral contraceptive. On exam, she had ptosis on the left side with conjunctival injection and diplopia when looking upward. Which of the following is the most likely diagnosis?

    1. Subarachnoid hemorrhage.

    2. Cavernous sinus thrombosis.

    3. Myasthenia gravis.

    4. Posterior cerebral artery stroke.

13. A 25-year-old man presented with severe neck pain that started suddenly. Two hours later he started feeling weak in his left leg and had left facial paralysis. Strength was 2/5 in the left arm and 3/5 in his left leg. Which of the following is the most likely diagnosis?

    1. Multiple sclerosis.

    2. Meningitis.

    3. Carotid artery dissection.

    4. Rupture of aneurysm.

14. A 25-year-old male patient presented with progressive periorbital swelling on the left side that started a couple of days ago. He has a history of chronic sinusitis. On exam, he had ptosis on the left side with conjunctival injection and diplopia when looking upward. Which of the following nerves will not be affected in this case?

    1. Third cranial nerve.

    2. Abducent nerve.

    3. Facial nerve.

    4. Maxillary branch of the trigeminal nerve.

15. A 25-year-old male patient is complaining of frequent urination. He states he urinated over 5 L/day. He reports that 1 month ago he was discharged from the hospital after a brain injury caused by a car accident. Which of the following will be found on the evaluation of this patient?

    1. Low urine osmolality.

    2. High protein in the urine.

    3. Hematuria.

    4. Low plasma osmolality.

16. A 40-year-old female patient is complaining of frequent large-volume urination. She is urinating more than 5 L/day. One month ago, she was discharged from the hospital after she underwent craniotomy because of epidural hematoma after a car accident. Which of the following tests will confirm the patient's diagnosis?

    1. Brain computed tomography.

    2. Water deprivation test.

    3. Urinalysis.

    4. Abdominal ultrasound.

17. A 55-year-old woman presented with sudden onset of severe headache that started 1 hour ago. She also complains of nausea. She does not have any chronic disease and has no history of recent trauma. On exam, there was neck rigidity but no muscle weakness. Brain computed tomography was normal. Which of the following is the next step in the patient's management?

    1. Lumbar puncture.

    2. Discharge on acetaminophen.

    3. Carotid Doppler.

    4. Electroencephalography.

18. A 55-year-old man presents to the emergency department with uncontrolled hypertension and a headache that started 3 months ago. He has nausea and blurred vision. On exam, his blood pressure is 162/95 mmHg and his pulse is 55 beats/min. Brain computed tomography shows intracerebral and intraventricular hemorrhage. Which of the following is true?

    1. Increased intracranial pressure (ICP) less than 20 mmHg.

    2. Normal ICP between 20 and 30 mmHg.

    3. There is no cause for increased ICP.

    4. Cushing syndrome is the early manifestation of increased ICP.

19. A 55-year-old man presents to the emergency department with uncontrolled hypertension and a headache that started 3 months ago. He also complains of nausea and blurred vision. On exam, his blood pressure 157/95 mmHg and his pulse is 53 beats/min. Which of the following is the next step in the patient's management?

    1. Lumbar puncture.

    2. Electroencephalography.

    3. Brain computed tomography.

    4. Carotid Doppler.

20. A 62-year-old man presented to the outpatient clinic for evaluation of his progressive memory loss. This problem began 2 months ago. He also has urinary incontinence that started at the same time. On exam, he appears in good general health, his blood pressure is 120/90 mmHg, but he has a broad-based gait. Computed tomography of the brain showed an enlarged ventricle. Which of the following can present in this patient?

    1. Papilledema.

    2. Facial nerve palsy.

    3. Stiff neck.

    4. Loss of smell sensation.

21. A 35-year-old man presents to the emergency department after a motor vehicle accident. He was conscious and oriented with Glasgow Coma Scale score of 15. On exam, he has facial paralysis on the right side that started after the accident. Which of the following tests is the next step in the patient's management?

    1. Physiotherapy.

    2. Electromyography.

    3. Brain magnetic resonance imaging.

    4. Head computed tomography.

22. A 70-year-old male patient presented with vertigo and has difficulty sitting upright. He has a history of prolonged hypertension. On exam, he appears confused, but his vital signs are stable. He also has hiccups and ptosis of his left eyelid and horizontal nystagmus. Which part of the brain is affected in this patient?

    1. Lateral medulla.

    2. Cerebellum.

    3. Frontal lobe.

    4. Internal capsule.

23. A 45-year-old man with uncontrolled hypertension presented to the emergency department (ED) with sudden onset of headache that started 1 hour ago. His level of consciousness started to deteriorate on arrival to the ED. Head computed tomography showed intracerebral and intraventricular hemorrhage. Which of the following is a part of the Cushing triad?

    1. Hypotension.

    2. Dilated pupils.

    3. Tachycardia.

    4. Irregular breathing.

24. A 30-year-old male patient presents to the emergency department after a motor vehicle accident. At the time of presentation, he was conscious but had a headache. One hour later, he became unconscious and his right pupil was dilated, but his left pupil was normal. What is the most likely diagnosis?

    1. Epidural hematoma.

    2. Subdural hematoma.

    3. Intracranial hemorrhage.

    4. Subarachnoid hemorrhage.

25. A 50-year-old woman presented with sudden onset of severe headache that started 45 minutes ago. She also has nausea. She reports no chronic illnesses and no history of recent trauma. On exam, there was neck rigidity. Head computed tomography showed a hyperdense lesion in the sulci and interhemispheric fissure. What is the most likely diagnosis?

    1. Epidural hematoma.

    2. Subdural hematoma.

    3. Subarachnoid hemorrhage.

    4. Brain abscess.

26. A 60-year-old man, who is a heavy smoker, complains of headache for the past month. He also reports a history of significant weight loss; he denies fevers or night sweats. A head computed tomography showed two small heterogeneous cerebral masses. Which of the following is *most* likely the primary tumor in this patient?

    1. Lung.

    2. Melanoma.

    3. Stomach.

    4. Kidney.

27. A 65-year-old woman, with a history of diabetes and hypertension presented with right arm weakness that started 1 hour ago. She has a history of dysarthria. On exam, her blood pressure is 200/110 mmHg, strength in the right arm is 1/5 with right facial paralysis, and the strength in the right leg is 4/5. Head computed tomography showed no intracerebral hemorrhage. What is the mechanism behind the patient's symptoms?

    1. Occlusion of the right anterior cerebral artery.

    2. Occlusion of the right middle cerebral artery.

    3. Occlusion of the left middle cerebral artery.

    4. Occlusion of the left posterior cerebral artery.

28. A 40-year-old man is evaluated for back pain that started more than 2 months ago. It is associated with lower limb weakness with numbness. Spine magnetic resonance imaging showed an intramedullary mass at level L1. What is the most common intramedullary tumor?

    1. Glioblastoma.

    2. Osteoblastoma.

    3. Ependymoma.

    4. Hemangioma.

29. A 35-year-old man presents to the emergency department after a motorcycle accident. He was conscious, oriented with a Glasgow Coma Scale score of 15. On exam, he had facial paralysis on the right side, which started after the accident. Which of the following findings will most likely be seen on his head computed tomography (CT)?

    1. Temporal skull fracture.

    2. Parietal skull fracture.

    3. Occipital skull fracture.

    4. Normal CT.

30. A 60-year-old man presented to the outpatient clinic for evaluation of his progression of memory loss. He lives alone in his home and he works as an accountant. He reports that his memory loss happened about 2 months ago, and he states he has some urinary incontinence that started about the same time. On exam, he appears in good general health, his blood pressure was 120/90 mmHg, but he had a broad-based gait. Computed tomography of the head showed an enlarged ventricle. Which of the following is the next step of management for this patient?

    1. Acetazolamide.

    2. Ventriculoperitoneal shunt.

    3. Furosemide.

    4. Mannitol.

31. A 70-year-old woman with a history of diabetes and hypertension presented with sudden onset of right-sided weakness. She has no history of trauma and she states this has not happened before. On exam, her blood pressure is 200/110 mmHg, and her muscle strength in the right lower limb is 1/5 with positive Babinski reflex. What is the next step in this patient's management?

    1. Order a brain magnetic resonance imaging scan.

    2. Order a head computed tomography.

    3. Give alteplase.

    4. Order a carotid Doppler.

32. A 34-year-old man presented to the emergency department after a motorcycle accident. He was conscious and oriented, but his skull x-ray showed a skull fracture. Half an hour later, he lost consciousness and his right pupil became dilated, but the left pupil is normal. What is the next step in the patient's management?

    1. Admit the patient to the intensive care unit.

    2. Craniotomy.

    3. Head computed tomography.

    4. Funduscopy.

33. A 67-year-old woman with a history of diabetes and hypertension presented to the emergency department with sudden onset of right-sided weakness. On exam, her strength is 1/5 in both the right arm and leg and sensation is diminished. What is the most likely diagnosis?

    1. Anterior cerebral artery occlusion.

    2. Lacunar infarction.

    3. Posterior cerebral artery occlusion.

    4. Right middle cerebral artery occlusion.

34. A 60-year-old male patient presented with vertigo and difficulty sitting upright. He has a history of long-standing hypertension. On exam, he appeared confused, but his vital signs are stable. During evaluation he lost pain sensation on his right side and he had ptosis of the left eyelid with horizontal nystagmus. What is the mechanism behind the patient's condition?

    1. Occlusion of the anterior cerebral artery.

    2. Occlusion of the posterior cerebral artery.

    3. Occlusion of the middle cerebral artery.

    4. Occlusion of vertebral artery.

35. A 55-year-old female patient presented with a headache that has been present for the last 2 months. She reports that she also has right-sided weakness that started 1 week ago. On exam, her strength is 2/5. Head computed tomography showed left cerebral irregular lesion and hypodense central necrosis surrounded by edema. Which of the following is true about the patient's condition?

    1. Management includes surgical resection and chemotherapy and radiotherapy.

    2. No need for radiotherapy.

    3. It is a benign lesion.

    4. Median survival is 5 years without treatment.

36. A 22-year-old man presented to the emergency department after a motorcycle accident. He was conscious and oriented with a Glasgow Coma Scale score of 15, but he had clear fluid discharge from his nose. What is the most appropriate next step?

    1. Head computed tomography.

    2. Brain magnetic resonance imaging scan

    3. Fluid analysis.

    4. Lumbar puncture.

37. A 20-year-old female patient presents with limb weakness and diplopia. Her symptoms are worse at night and improve with rest. She has no history of illicit drug use. On exam, she is conscious and oriented, but she had ptosis. After putting an ice bag on her eye her ptosis was improved. What is the most likely diagnosis in this patient?

    1. Organophosphate poising.

    2. Myasthenia gravis.

    3. Systemic lupus erythematosus.

    4. Drug-induced myopathy.

38. A 25-year-old female patient presents to her nurse practitioner with complaints of a chronic headache that has been present for more than 6 months. The headache is worse at night and when wakes her up. She also has occasional nausea. She has no history of trauma or neurological deficit. Her body mass index was 34 kg/m². Her head computed tomography was normal and lumbar puncture showed high opening pressure with normal cerebral spinal fluid analysis. What is the next step in the patient's management?

    1. Ventriculoperitoneal shunt.

    2. Mannitol.

    3. Acetazolamide.

    4. Cortisol.

39. A 20-year-old female patient presented with limb weakness and diplopia. Her symptoms are worse at night and improve with rest. She has no history of illicit drug use or history of drug intake. On exam, she is conscious and oriented, but she had ptosis that resolved after putting an ice bag on her eye. What is the best treatment for this patient?

    1. Atropine.

    2. Pyridostigmine.

    3. Edrophonium.

    4. Steroid.

40. A 70-year-old woman with a history of uncontrolled hypertension suddenly lost consciousness. In the emergency department, she was in a coma with a Glasgow Coma Scale score of 3 with pinpoint pupils but reactive to light. What would you expect to find on the head computed tomography?

    1. Subarachnoid hemorrhage.

    2. Pontine hemorrhage.

    3. Cerebellar hemorrhage.

    4. Intracerebral hemorrhage.

41. A 65-year-old man presented to the outpatient clinic for evaluation of his progressive memory loss, which began 2 months ago. He lives alone in his home and he works as a teacher. He has a history of urinary incontinence that also started about 2 months ago. On exam, he appears in good health. His blood pressure is 120/90 mmHg, but he had a broad-based gait. Head computed tomography showed an enlarged ventricle. Which of the following is the cause of the patient's condition?

    1. Impairment of cerebral spinal fluid absorption.

    2. Obstruction of Sylvian duct.

    3. Rupture of bridging vein.

    4. Arteriovenous malformation.

42. A 60-year-old woman presented with sudden onset of severe headache and nausea that started 1 hour ago. She has no previous medical history and no history of trauma. On exam, there was neck rigidity. Head computed tomography showed a hyperdense lesion in the sulci and interhemispheric fissure. What is the most likely cause of this patient's findings?

    1. Rupture of the meningeal artery.

    2. Rupture of berry aneurysm.

    3. Sagittal sinus thrombosis.

    4. Arteriovenous malformation.

43. A 35-year-old homeless man presented to the nurse practitioner with complaints of a headache that started 2 days ago. He is also having projectile vomiting and photophobia. On exam, he had a stiff neck. Head computed tomography was normal, and lumbar puncture showed a high opening cerebrospinal fluid pressure with low glucose and high protein. What is the patient's diagnosis?

    1. Viral meningitis.

    2. Bacterial meningitis.

    3. Brain tumor.

    4. Benign intracranial hypertension.

44. A 30-year-old female patient is evaluated for complaints of a chronic headache that has been present for more than 6 months. The headache is worse at night and wakes her up. She also has associated nausea. No history of trauma or neurological deficit. Her body mass index is 30 kg/m². Her head computed tomography was normal, but her lumbar puncture showed a high opening pressure with normal cerebrospinal fluid analysis. What other assessment finding would the nurse practitioner expect in this patient?

    1. Seizure.

    2. Papilledema.

    3. Hyperreflexia.

    4. Neck rigidity.

45. A 30-year-old man was brought to the emergency department after he had a seizure. His wife reports that he has been complaining of a headache that started 2 days ago associated with projectile vomiting and photophobia. On exam, his temperature was 101.9°F. He also has a stiff neck. Which of the following can aid in the definitive diagnosis for this patient?

    1. Cerebrospinal fluid analysis.

    2. Funduscopy.

    3. Carotid angiography.

    4. Blood culture.

46. A 30-year-old female patient presented with limb weakness and diplopia. Her symptoms were worse at night but improved with rest. She has no history of illicit drug use. On exam, she was conscious and oriented, but she had ptosis. After putting an ice bag on her eyelid the ptosis improved. Which of the following is true about the patient's condition?

    1. It did not involve bulbar muscle.

    2. The defect in this disease is at a level of muscle.

    3. Body formed antibodies against the acetylcholine receptor.

    4. Patient symptoms usually improve by exercise.

47. A 50-year-old woman presented with sudden onset of severe headache that started 1 hour ago. She has no history of chronic disease and no history of recent trauma. On exam, there was neck rigidity. What would the nurse practitioner expect to find on the head computed tomography?

    1. Enlarged ventricle.

    2. Hyperdense lesion in the interhemispheric fissure.

    3. Depressed skull fracture.

    4. Intracerebral mass.

48. A 67-year-old woman with a history of diabetes and hypertension presented to the emergency department with right-sided weakness that started suddenly. On exam, her strength was 1/5 in both right arm and leg, and sensation was intact. Head computed tomography showed a small infarction in the internal capsule. Which of the following is a major risk factor that can cause this condition?

    1. Nephrotic syndrome.

    2. Previous history of meningitis.

    3. Chronic sinusitis.

    4. Diabetes mellitus.

49. A 70-year-old woman with a history of hypertension presented with right arm weakness that started 1 hour ago. She has a history of dysarthria. On exam, her blood pressure is 160/90 mmHg. Strength in the right arm is 1/5 with right facial paralysis and the strength in the right leg is 4/5. Head computed tomography showed no intracerebral hemorrhage. What is the best management option?

    1. Alteplase.

    2. Heparin.

    3. Warfarin.

    4. Clopidogrel.

50. A 70-year-old man, with diabetes and hypertension presents with right arm weakness that started 1 hour ago. He has a history of dysarthria and history of a previous hemorrhagic stroke 1 year ago. On exam, his blood pressure is 160/90 mmHg. His strength in the right arm is 1/5 with right facial paralysis, and the strength in the right leg is 4/5. Head computed tomography showed no intracerebral hemorrhage. Which of the following is an appropriate management option?

    1. Alteplase.

    2. Aspirin.

    3. warfarin.

    4. Heparin.

51. A 45-year-old female patient presents to the emergency department with limb weakness and diplopia. Her symptoms are worse at night, but they improve with rest. There is no history of illicit drug use. On exam, she had ptosis of her left eyelid. Of note, her Tensilon test was positive. Which of the following should be excluded in this patient?

    1. Breast cancer.

    2. Thymoma.

    3. Multiple sclerosis.

    4. Brain tumor.

52. A 65-year-old man presented with weakness and fatigue. He was recently diagnosed with small cell carcinoma. On exam, his blood pressure was 120/80 mmHg and his pulse was 80 beats/min. There is an obvious weakness in his proximal muscles with loss of deep tendon reflexes. His serum chemistry test is within normal limits. Which of the following is the most likely diagnosis?

    1. Hyperthyroidism.

    2. Lambert–Eaton syndrome.

    3. Brain metastasis.

    4. Parkinson disease.

53. A 65-year-old woman with diabetes and hypertension presented with right arm weakness that started 1 hour ago. She has a history of dysarthria. On exam, her strength in the right arm is 1/5 with right facial paralysis, and the strength in the right leg is 4/5. Head computed tomography showed no intracerebral hemorrhage. What is the contraindication for thrombolytic therapy?

    1. Surgery before 6 months.

    2. Platelet count is 110,000/mm^3.

    3. Blood pressure is 220/130 mmHg.

    4. Patient with a history of coffee ground vomiting 1 year ago.

54. A 22-year-old female patient who was 9 months pregnant was brought to the emergency department after a seizure. She was admitted to the obstetrical department after normal vaginal delivery 4 hours ago. On exam she appeared tired and confused; her blood pressure was 185/110 mmHg. She was transferred to the intensive care unit and intravenous magnesium sulfate was begun. Which of the following needs frequent monitoring in this patient?

    1. Central venous pressure.

    2. Heart rhythm.

    3. Reflexes.

    4. Intracranial pressure.

55. A 60-year-old male patient presents with vertigo and difficulty in sitting upright. He has a history of uncontrolled hypertension. On exam, he appears confused, his vital signs are stable, and he has lost pain sensation on his right side. He has a drooping of the eyelid on the left side with horizontal nystagmus. Which of the following is the most likely diagnosis?

    1. Medial medullary syndrome.

    2. Pontine hemorrhage.

    3. Wallenberg syndrome.

    4. Lacunar infarction.

56. A 50-year-old woman presents with sudden onset of severe headache that started 2 hours ago. She states that it felt like a "thunderclap." She has no medical history or recent trauma. On exam, there was neck rigidity. What is the next step in the patient's management?

    1. Head computed tomography.

    2. Lumbar puncture.

    3. Electroencephalography.

    4. Brain magnetic resonance imaging.

57. A 40-year-old female patient presented with bilateral leg weakness and diplopia. Her symptoms are worse at night, but they improve with rest. She has no history of illicit drug use. On exam, she had ptosis and her Tensilon test was positive. What is the next step in the patient's management?

    1. Chest computed tomography (CT).

    2. Head CT.

    3. Breast mammogram.

    4. Atropine.

58. A 40-year-old male patient arrives in the emergency department after a traffic accident. At the time of arrival, the patient was unconscious, his pupils were reactive but unresponsive to painful stimuli; he made a guttural sound. What is the Glasgow Coma Scale score in this patient?

    1. 5.

    2. 8.

    3. 7.

    4. 3.

59. A 55-year-old woman is brought to the emergency department after a seizure. She did not have any history of seizure before, but she was diagnosed with breast cancer 4 years ago and was treated surgically. The head computed tomography showed a 2.5 × 2.5–cm mass in the right temporal region surrounded by edema. Which of the following is suitable management for this patient?

    1. Chemotherapy.

    2. Surgical resection.

    3. Palliative care.

    4. Whole-brain radiation.

60. An 18-year-old woman was brought to the emergency department after she fainted during her chemistry lab at school. On arrival, she was conscious and oriented. Her pupils are reactive, but she did not remember what happened to her. Which of the following symptoms usually occurs with a pure syncopal episode?

    1. The patient bites their tongue.

    2. The patient is in a postictal state.

    3. The patient will have an aura.

    4. The patient will become conscious immediately.

61. A 30-year-old man was brought to the emergency department after a seizure; he did not have any history of seizures before and did not have any chronic illnesses. On exam, he appeared confused, his blood pressure was 110/75 mmHg, his pulse was 80 beats/min, and his temperature was 98.6°F. His pupils are reactive and there are no neurological deficits. What is the most appropriate next step in the patient's management?

    1. Head computed tomography.

    2. Lumbar puncture.

    3. Seizure prophylaxis.

    4. Electroencephalogram.

62. A 60-year-old man, who lives in an extended care facility, presented to the outpatient clinic for evaluation of his progressive memory loss. The problem began 2 months ago and is having a tremendous effect on his life. He also has a history of urinary incontinence that started at the same time. On exam, he appears in good general condition, his blood pressure was 120/90 mmHg, but he had a broad-based gait. What is the next step in this patient's management?

    1. Head computed tomography.

    2. Vitamin B_{12} level.

    3. Thyroid-stimulating hormone level.

    4. Urinalysis.

63. A 70-year-old man presented with weakness and fatigue. He has a history of small cell carcinoma treated by surgical resection 2 years ago. On exam, his vital signs are stable. There is an obvious weakness in his proximal muscles with loss of deep tendon reflexes. A chest x-ray showed a right lung mass. His serum chemistry test is within normal limits. Which of the following is the cause of the patient's symptoms?

    1. Autoantibodies against presynaptic Ca^{2+} channels.
    2. Autoantibodies against presynaptic acetylcholine channels.
    3. Demyelination of gray matter in the brain.
    4. Degeneration of lower motor neurons.

64. A 55-year-old man presented with complaints of a headache for the past 2 months. He also has a history of right-sided weakness that started 1 week ago. On exam, strength on the right is 2/5. Head computed tomography showed a left cerebral irregular lesion hypodense central necrosis surrounded by edema. What is this patient's diagnosis?

    1. Meningioma.
    2. Brain abscess.
    3. Glioblastoma.
    4. Ependymoma.

65. A 66-year-old woman with a history of hypertension and diabetes presented to the emergency department with left-sided weakness that started suddenly. On exam, her strength is 1/5 in both left arm and leg and the sensation was diminished. Head computed tomography shows intracerebral hemorrhage. Which of the following is the most common site for intracranial hemorrhage?

    1. Thalamus.
    2. Pons.
    3. Basal ganglion.
    4. Cerebellum.

66. A 30-year-old man presented with headache that started 2 days ago that is associated with photophobia. On exam, he had a stiff neck. Head computed tomography was normal and lumbar puncture was done. Which of the following results is present in viral meningitis?

    1. Cerebral spinal fluid (CSF) protein is greater than 250 mg/dL.
    2. CSF glucose is 50 mg/dL.
    3. CSF with white blood cell count of 5 cells/mL.
    4. The polymorphic nuclear cell is the main cell in the CSF.

67. A 60-year-old woman visited her nurse practitioner for evaluation of her headache, which started 3 weeks ago. She had a history of head trauma 1 month ago. On exam, she appeared conscious; her blood pressure was 120/80 mmHg, with no neck stiffness or neurological deficit. Head computed tomography showed chronic subdural hematoma. Which of the following is the mechanism of injury?

    1. Rupture of the middle meningeal artery.
    2. Rupture of berry aneurysm.
    3. Arterial venous malformation.
    4. Tearing of bridging vein.

68. A 25-year-old female patient is being evaluated for a chronic headache that has been present for 6 months. The headache is worse at night and often wakes her up. She also states that she has nausea when she has the headache. There is no history of trauma or neurological deficits. Her body mass index was 34 kg/m^2. Her head computed tomography was normal, and lumbar puncture showed high opening pressure with normal cerebral spinal fluid analysis. What is the diagnosis?

    1. Pseudotumor cerebri.
    2. Subarachnoid hemorrhage.
    3. Chronic sinusitis.
    4. Giant cell arteritis.

69. A 30-year-old woman was brought to the emergency department after a seizure. She has no previous history of seizures. She also has a headache that started 1 day ago. On exam, she appeared confused, and her temperature was 101.5°F. There is slight neck rigidity. Lumbar puncture was done and the cerebral spinal fluid analysis showed lymphocytosis with a protein level of 90 mg/dL. Which of the following is a suitable treatment for this patient?

    1. Intravenous (IV) steroids.
    2. Ventriculoperitoneal shunt.
    3. IV acyclovir.
    4. Do nothing.

70. A 22-year-old female patient was brought to the emergency department after a seizure. She is 2 days postpartum with her first baby. On exam, she appeared tired and confused; her blood pressure was 190/100 mmHg. Which of the following is the next step in the patient's management?

    1. Lorazepam.
    2. Magnesium sulfate.
    3. Phenytoin.
    4. Lumbar puncture.

71. A 60-year-old man presented to the outpatient clinic for evaluation of his progressive memory loss and urinary incontinence. On exam, he appears in good general health, his blood pressure is 120/90 mmHg, but he had a broad-based gait. If lumbar puncture showed normal opening pressure, what will be present on the head computed tomography?

    1. Sagittal venous thrombosis.

    2. Large ventricle.

    3. Chronic subdural hematoma.

    4. Pituitary macroadenoma.

72. A 40-year-old man was referred to the neurological clinic after he was diagnosed with third nerve palsy and after he presented with diplopia and headache. He does not have any past medical history. On exam, he has a stiff neck but no fever and his vital signs are within normal limits. Which of the following should be excluded in this patient?

    1. Multiple sclerosis.

    2. Intracerebral hemorrhage.

    3. Posterior communicating artery aneurysm.

    4. Carotid artery dissection.

73. A 20-year-old man was brought to the emergency department after a tonic-clonic seizure. His past medical history is noncontributory, but his mother has epilepsy. On exam, he appears confused and he does not remember what happened to him. His vital signs are within normal limits. Which of the following is considered the first line of management in this patient?

    1. Diazepam.

    2. Phenobarbital.

    3. Gabapentin.

    4. Sodium valproate.

74. A 25-year-old female patient presented to the outpatient clinic with complaints of loss of peripheral vision that started 1 month ago. She has no past medical history or reports of recent trauma. On exam, she appears well and her vital signs are stable. Visual exam revealed bitemporal hemianopia mainly in the upper quadrant. Which of the following is the most likely diagnosis?

    1. Pituitary macroadenoma.

    2. Left occipital infarction.

    3. Meningioma.

    4. Third nerve palsy.

75. A 25-year-old female patient visited her nurse practitioner for follow-up. She has a history of epilepsy and is on a therapeutic dose of sodium valproate, but she is still having at least one seizure every week. What is the next step in the patient's management?

    1. Add lamotrigine.

    2. Add gabapentin.

    3. Stop sodium valproate and start lamotrigine.

    4. Start electroconvulsive therapy.

76. A 30-year-old woman visited her nurse practitioner for routine follow-up. She has a history of epilepsy, is on sodium valproate, and she wants to get pregnant. What is the appropriate next step for this patient?

    1. Stop all her medication now.

    2. Take 5 mg of folic acid daily and continue her medication.

    3. Switch to lamotrigine.

    4. This patient cannot be pregnant.

77. A 25-year-old male patient visited his nurse practitioner for routine follow-up for his epilepsy. He is on lamotrigine after sodium valproate failed to control his seizures. However, he is still having at least 1 seizure a week, so sodium valproate was added to his regimen. Which of the following is an increased risk for this patient?

    1. Myocardial infarction.

    2. Addiction.

    3. Pancreatitis.

    4. Steven–Johnson syndrome.

78. A 22-year-old man is brought to the emergency department after a new-onset seizure. He had no previous history of seizure or any other chronic illnesses. On exam, he appeared confused, his blood pressure was 110/75 mmHg, his pulse was 80 beats/min, his temperature was 98.6°F, and his pupils were reactive. Which of the following is an indication to start an antiepileptic drug?

    1. Normal electroencephalography.

    2. Patient has a neurological deficit.

    3. Normal head computed tomography.

    4. No family history of seizure.

79. A 25-year-old female patient presented to the outpatient clinic after she missed her period for months. Her only medical history is epilepsy, which is treated with carbamazepine. Her pregnancy test was positive. Which of the following is the appropriate next step in the management of this patient?

    1. Stop carbamazepine immediately.

    2. Continue the treatment.

    3. Provide advice to abort the fetus.

    4. Switch to lamotrigine.

80. The AGACNP is examining a 55-year-old female patient with complaints of fever, generalized weakness, and abdominal pain for 4 days. For 2 weeks, the patient has noted a yellowish tinge to her skin but has ignored it. The patient also reports black-colored stool. Her son says she has been mildly confused. The patient has taken paracetamol for her fever. The patient's temperature is 101.0°F, and her blood pressure is 140/100 mmHg. Based on this history, the AGACNP suspects the patient has what?

    1. Hepatic encephalopathy.

    2. Post-seizure encephalopathy.

    3. Toxic encephalopathy from drugs.

    4. Toxic encephalopathy from alcohol intake.

81. A concussion is a type of traumatic brain injury in which sudden movement from a jolt or blow to the head causes the brain to bounce around in the skull, causing damage to the brain cells. Which of the following is a dangerous sign after a blow to the head that warrants going to the emergency department?

    1. Clumsy movements.

    2. One pupil larger than the other.

    3. Feeling dazed.

    4. Headache.

82. The AGACNP is examining a 65-year-old male patient whose wife has started to notice changes in his behavior after he bumped his head on a car door roughly 8 weeks ago. The patient is increasingly forgetful, according to the wife. She also reports he has an odd style of walking, with unduly small steps (shuffling). The patient has had a couple of episodes of urinary incontinence in the past 2 months. Based on this history, the AGACNP suspects the patient has what?

    1. Parkinson disease.

    2. Alzheimer disease.

    3. Normal pressure hydrocephalus.

    4. Congenital hydrocephalus.

83. Which of the following is a high-risk factor for increased intracranial pressure caused by idiopathic intracranial hypertension?

    1. Obesity.

    2. Young age.

    3. Male gender.

    4. Low vitamin A level.

84. The AGACNP is examining a 35-year-old pediatric nurse who complains of an upset stomach, vomiting, terrible headache, and lack of energy. The patient seems disoriented and confused, and some of what she says does not make sense. There is no report of a fever or rash. The patient says she has been feeling unwell since yesterday and has spent most of the day in bed. The AGACNP suspects stroke or meningitis and sends the patient to the emergency department. Which of the following tests and treatments is NOT recommended to manage the patient?

    1. CT scan.

    2. Lumbar puncture.

    3. Gastric lavage.

    4. Steroids and antibiotics.

85. A 40-year-old male alcoholic was brought to the emergency department with an ataxic gait and a decreased level of consciousness. On exam, he was confused and disoriented with slurred speech; his pupils are reactive to light. Which of the following would you expect to find in this patient?

    1. Pinpoint pupils.

    2. Nystagmus.

    3. Elevated blood pressure.

    4. Fever.

86. A 35-year-old male patient was recently diagnosed with polycystic kidney disease; he is now on antihypertensive management. His brother died 2 years ago from a hemorrhagic stroke. Which of the following is an appropriate test for this patient?

    1. Magnetic resonance arteriography.

    2. Kidney biopsy.

    3. Echocardiography.

    4. Urinalysis.

87. A 25-year-old female patient presented with progressive periorbital swelling on the left side that started a couple of days ago. The only medication she is on is oral contraceptives. On exam, she had ptosis on the left side with conjunctival injection and diplopia when looking upward. Which of the following is the most likely diagnosis?

    1. Subarachnoid hemorrhage.

    2. Cavernous sinus thrombosis.

    3. Myasthenia gravis.

    4. Posterior cerebral artery stroke.

88. A 25-year-old man presented with severe neck pain that started suddenly. Two hours later he started feeling weak in his left limb and he had left facial paralysis. Strength was 2/5 in the left arm and 3/5 in his left leg. Which of the following is the most likely diagnosis?

    1. Multiple sclerosis.

    2. Meningitis.

    3. Carotid artery dissection.

    4. Rupture of aneurysm.

89. A 40-year-old female patient who was diagnosed with polycystic kidney disease 1 year ago was seen by her nurse practitioner for follow-up. Her brother died 2 years ago from hemorrhagic stroke. If the patient underwent computed tomographic angiography, what would you expect to find?

    1. Posterior communication artery aneurysm.

    2. Chronic subdural hematoma.

    3. Berry aneurysm.

    4. Hydrocephalus.

90. A 25-year-old male patient presented with progressive periorbital swelling on the left side that started a couple of days ago. He has a history of chronic sinusitis. On exam, he had ptosis on the left side with conjunctival injection and diplopia when looking upward. Which of the following nerves is *not* affected in this patient?

    1. Third cranial nerve.

    2. Abducent nerve.

    3. Facial nerve.

    4. Maxillary branch of the trigeminal nerve.

91. A 50-year-old homeless man presents with a headache that started 2 days ago and is associated with projectile vomiting and photophobia. He has no history of any chronic disease. On exam, he has a stiff neck. Head computed tomography was normal and lumbar puncture showed high opening cerebral spinal fluid pressure with low glucose, high protein, and leukocytosis. What is the most likely the organism causing the patients symptoms?

    1. *Escherichia coli.*

    2. *Streptococcus pneumoniae.*

    3. *Proteus.*

    4. *Staphylococcus aureus.*

92. A 55-year-old man presented with headache that started 2 days ago associated with projectile vomiting. He has a history of diabetes mellitus for 10 years. On exam, he had a stiff neck and nystagmus with an ataxic gait. Head computed tomography was normal, and lumbar puncture showed high opening cerebrospinal fluid pressure with low glucose and high protein. What is the primary organism responsible for these symptoms?

    1. Meningococcus.

    2. *Mycobacterium tuberculosis.*

    3. *Listeria monocytogenes.*

    4. Herpes zoster virus.

93. A 25-year-old male patient is complaining of frequent urination. He is urinating more than 5 L/day. One month ago, he was discharged from the hospital after brain injury caused by a motor vehicle accident. Which of the following would you expect to find on evaluation of this patient?

    1. Low urine osmolality.

    2. High protein in the urine.

    3. Hematuria.

    4. Low plasma osmolality.

94. A 30-year-old male patient presented with polyuria. He states that he is urinating more than 4 L/day. He was recently discharged from the hospital after admission for a traumatic brain injury after a fall. Which of the following is the most likely diagnosis?

    1. Syndrome of inappropriate antidiuretic hormone secretion.

    2. Diabetes insipidus.

    3. Polycystic kidney disease.

    4. Urinary tract infection.

95. A 40-year-old female patient is complaining of frequent urination. She measured her urine and reports that she is urinating more than 5 L/day. One month ago, she was discharged from the neurosurgery unit after she underwent craniotomy because of an epidural hematoma after a motor vehicle accident. Which of the following tests will confirm the patient's diagnosis?

    1. Head computed tomography.

    2. Water deprivation test.

    3. Urinalysis.

    4. Abdominal ultrasound.

96. A 50-year-old male patient is complaining of urinary incontinence that began 2 days ago. He also has had severe back pain for the past 2 days. On exam, there was a significant weakness in the patient's right lower limb associated with hyporeflexia. Which of the following would also be present in this patient?

    1. Scrotal swelling.

    2. Nystagmus.

    3. Positive Babinski sign.

    4. Loss of bowel control.

97. A 55-year-old female patient presented with sudden onset of severe headache that started 4 hours ago. She also has complaints of nausea. She has no past medical history and no history of recent trauma. On exam, there was neck rigidity but no muscle weakness. Head computed tomography was normal. Which of the following is the next step in the management of this patient?

    1. Lumbar puncture.

    2. Discharge on nonsteroidal antiinflammatory drugs.

    3. Carotid Doppler.

    4. Electroencephalography.

98. A 55-year-old male patient presented to the emergency department with sudden severe back pain that started 1 day ago; he also reports urinary and fecal incontinence. On exam, he had bilateral lower limb weakness and hyperreflexia with positive Babinski. Which of the following is the site of the patient's lesion?

    1. Cervical spinal cord.

    2. Conus medullaris.

    3. Cauda equina.

    4. Lumbar spinal cord.

99. A 55-year-old man with uncontrolled hypertension presents with a persistent headache that started 3 months ago. He also is having nausea and blurry vision. On exam, his blood pressure is 150/95 mmHg and his pulse is 55 beats/min. Head computed tomography showed intracerebral and intraventricular hemorrhage. Which of the following is true?

    1. Intracranial pressure (ICP) is greater than 20 mmHg.

    2. Normal ICP is between 20 and 30 mmHg.

    3. There is no cause for increased ICP.

    4. Cushing syndrome is the early manifestation of increased ICP.

100. A 55-year-old man with uncontrolled hypertension presents with a persistent headache that started 3 months ago. He also is having nausea and blurry vision. On exam, his blood pressure is 150/95 mmHg and his pulse is 55 beats/min. Which of the following is the next step in the management of this patient?

    1. Lumbar puncture.

    2. Electroencephalography.

    3. Head computed tomography.

    4. Carotid Doppler.

101. A 62-year-old man presented to the outpatient clinic for evaluation of his progressive memory loss. This problem began 2 months ago. He has a history of urinary incontinence that started at the same time. On exam, he appears to be in good general condition. His blood pressure is 120/90 mmHg, but he has a broad-based gait. Computed tomography of the head showed an enlarged ventricle. Which of the following symptoms also may be present in this patient?

    1. Papilledema.

    2. Facial nerve palsy.

    3. Stiff neck.

    4. Loss of smell sensation.

102. A 45-year-old male patient is being evaluated for chronic headache that has been present for more than 3 months. He states it is worse when he leans forward. He is also having nausea and blurred vision. There is no history of trauma or neurological deficit. On exam, he appears confused, his blood pressure is 150/95 mmHg, and his pulse is 55 beats/min. Which of the following is the most likely diagnosis?

    1. Increased intracranial pressure.

    2. Ischemic stroke.

    3. Pontine hemorrhage.

    4. Chronic sinusitis.

103. A 45-year-old female alcoholic is brought to the emergency department because of a decreased level of consciousness. On exam, she was confused and disoriented with slurred speech. Her pupils are reactive to light, but she has nystagmus. Her symptoms are relieved after receiving thiamin. Which of the following signs would you expect to find in this patient?

    1. Ataxic gait.

    2. Wide-based gait.

    3. Cautious gait.

    4. Hemiparetic gait.

104. A 65-year-old man presented to the outpatient clinic for evaluation of his progressive memory loss. This problem began 4 months ago. He also has a history of urinary incontinence that started at the same time. On exam, he appears in good general health. His blood pressure is 120/90 mmHg. A head computed tomography showed an enlarged ventricle. Which of the following symptoms would also be expected in this patient?

    1. Wide-based gait.

    2. Scissor gait.

    3. Trendelenburg gait.

    4. Waddling gait.

105. A 67-year-old woman, with a history of diabetes, hypertension, dyslipidemia, and multiple small strokes presents with an infected pressure ulcer. On exam, she is bedridden and there are many grade III pressure ulcers on the right buttock and lower legs. Which of the following is the main risk factor for pressure ulcer formation?

    1. Immobility.

    2. Diabetes mellitus.

    3. Hypertension.

    4. Vascular disease.

7 Neurology Answers & Rationales

1. Answer: 3

Rationale: This patient has uncontrolled seizures on sodium valproate, which is the first line of management of generalized seizures. In uncontrolled seizure, despite monotherapy of antiepileptic drugs, the next step is to switch to another antiepileptic drug such as lamotrigine, phenytoin, or carbamazepine.

2. Answer: 2

Rationale: All the antiepileptic drugs have a teratogenic effect, but the risk of seizure is more than the risk of teratogenic effect, so the patient should continue her treatment and she should take folic acid to reduce the risk of spina bifida.

3. Answer: 2

Rationale: A provider usually starts antiepileptic drugs after the second seizure, but there are some patients who need an antiepileptic drug started immediately (e.g., in the patient with a strong family history of seizure, or in the patient with neurological deficit or structural abnormality on brain computed tomography). Also, patients with an abnormal electroencephalography can take the antiepileptic drug after one seizure.

4. Answer: 2

Rationale: All the antiepileptic drugs have a teratogenic effect, but the risk of seizure is more than the risk of teratogenic effect, so the patient should continue her treatment and she should take folic acid to reduce the risk of spina bifida.

5. Answer: 2

Rationale: Antiepileptic drugs should continue in this patient for at least 2 years from the last seizure, so any patient without seizures for 2 years can stop the medication. The medicine should be tapered off gradually over at least 6 months, except if the patient has a structural brain abnormality. In this case the patient should receive antiepileptic drugs for life.

6. Answer: 2

Rationale: A simple partial seizure can cause sensory or motor symptoms. An abnormal movement that happens can spread from the thumb to include the entire arm. The drug of choice in this case is carbamazepine.

7. Answer: 1

Rationale: Antiepileptic drugs can cause many side effects, and visual field defect is one of them. The most common medication that causes visual field defects is vigabatrin, which can be irreversible in 40% of patients. Because of this routine follow-up should be done every 6 months in these patients.

8. Answer: 2

Rationale: Any patient with a history of alcohol abuse is at risk for developing seizures when he or she decides to quit drinking. This seizure mainly happens within 24 hours after stopping the intake of alcohol. The patient will not need long-term antiepileptic medications. If this patient has a history of brain trauma, a brain computed tomography should be done.

9. Answer: 1

Rationale: This patient has symptoms of an absence of seizure. The drug of choice in the treatment of this patient is ethosuximide or sodium valproate. Carbamazepine can exaggerate the patient's symptoms.

10. Answer: 2

Rationale: A simple partial seizure can cause sensory or motor symptoms. One example is abnormal movement that can spread from the thumb to include the entire arm. The drug of choice in this case is carbamazepine.

11. Answer: 1

Rationale: Any patient diagnosed with polycystic kidney disease with a family history of hemorrhagic stroke or intracranial aneurysm is at risk for an intracranial or berry aneurysm.

12. Answer: 2

Rationale: This patient has symptoms of cavernous sinus thrombosis, which usually include headaches with third and fourth cranial nerve paralysis associated with periorbital swelling. Several factors that can increase the risk of cavernous sinus thromboses include thrombophilia, oral contraceptives, sinus infection, and head injury.

13. Answer: 3

Rationale: This patient has symptoms of stroke, which is uncommon in this age. There are two causes that can lead to stroke at a young age. One of them is carotid artery dissection that happens spontaneously or after trauma. The second cause for young-onset stroke is embolism from the heart.

14. Answer: 3

Rationale: This patient has symptoms of cavernous sinus thrombosis, which usually include headaches with third and fourth cranial nerve paralysis associated with periorbital swelling. There are many structures that pass through the cavernous sinus such as the third and fourth nerves and maxillary and ophthalmic branch of the trigeminal nerve. Several factors that can increase the risk of cavernous sinus thromboses include thrombophilia, oral contraceptives, sinus infection, and head injury.

15. Answer: 1

Rationale: One of the complications of traumatic brain injury is diabetes insipidus, which is characterized by urine osmolality less than 200 mOsm/kg or high or normal plasma osmolality with polyuria more than 3 L/day. Diabetes insipidus is mainly diagnosis by a water deprivation test.

16. Answer: 2

Rationale: One of the complications of traumatic brain injury is diabetes insipidus. It is characterized by urine osmolality less than 200 mOsm/kg or high or normal plasma osmolality with polyuria more than 3 L/day. Diabetes insipidus is mainly diagnosed by a water deprivation test.

17. Answer: 1

Rationale: This patient presents with a sudden severe headache, which is a typical presentation of subarachnoid hemorrhage. Subarachnoid hemorrhage appears on a brain computed tomography (CT) as a hyperdense lesion in the interhemispheric fissure, Sylvian fissures, and in the ambient cistern, which are typical sites of subarachnoid hemorrhage. If the CT was normal, then a lumbar puncture should be done.

18. Answer: 1

Rationale: The normal range of intracranial pressure (ICP) is between 7 and 15 mmHg. It is greater than 20 mmHg, so it is increased ICP. The symptoms of ICP include headache, nausea, and vomiting. The Cushing triad is the classical presentation of increased ICP, which includes hypertension, bradycardia, and irregular breathing. In most cases, the Cushing triad is a late symptom.

19. Answer: 3

Rationale: The normal range of intracranial pressure (ICP) is between 7 and 15 mmHg. If it is greater than 20 mmHg, it is considered increased. The symptoms of increased intracranial pressure include headache, nausea, and vomiting. The approach to management includes brain computed tomography then a lumbar puncture if there is no mass.

20. Answer: 1

Rationale: This patient has symptoms of normal pressure hydrocephalus, which is the triad of progressive memory loss, urinary incontinence, and abnormal gait. Also, this patient will have papilledema and signs of sixth nerve palsy. This diagnosis is confirmed by brain computed tomography, which showed an enlarged ventricle. A lumbar puncture will reveal normal opening pressure.

21. Answer: 4

Rationale: Fracture of the skull base is very common in a head injury, and it indicates a significant impact that needs evaluation by a head computed tomography. Fracture of the temporal bone can damage the facial nerve, which leads to facial paralysis. It also can cause vestibulocochlear injury. On the other hand, fractures of anterior skull bone can cause Battle sign or raccoon eyes.

22. Answer: 1

Rationale: This patient has symptoms of lateral medullary infarction or Wallenberg syndrome. This condition is caused by occlusion of the vertebral artery inside the cranium. Usually, patients with this syndrome will have a contralateral loss of pain and temperature with ipsilateral Horner syndrome.

23. Answer: 4

Rationale: This patient presented with signs of increased intracranial pressure (ICP), which include headache, nausea, and vomiting. The Cushing triad is the classical presentation of increased ICP, which includes hypertension, bradycardia, and irregular breathing. Sometimes this triad can present late.

24. Answer: 1

Epidural hematoma is characterized by a lucid interval. At presentation, the patient appears conscious and in good general condition, but then the patient's condition suddenly deteriorates. An epidural hematoma can be caused by rupture of the middle meningeal artery, whereas a subdural hematoma is mainly from rupture of an intracranial vein. Rupture of an aneurysm can cause an intracerebral hemorrhage.

25. Answer: 3

Rationale: This patient presents with a sudden severe headache, which is a typical presentation of subarachnoid hemorrhage. Subarachnoid hemorrhage typically appears on head computed tomography as a hyperdense lesion in the interhemispheric fissure, Sylvian fissures, and in the ambient cistern.

26. Answer: 1

Rationale: The most common source of cerebral metastases is the lung. Space-occupying lesions present mainly with signs of increased intracranial pressure, which include headache, vomiting, and seizures. The most common site of metastatic tumor in the brain is a gray-white junction.

27. Answer: 3

Rationale: The middle cerebral artery (MCA) supplies the parietal and temporal lobe and a lateral part of the frontal lobe. If an MCA stroke happens, the patient will have a contralateral face and arm weakness with a language deficit. Anterior cerebral artery occlusion causes contralateral leg weakness, whereas the posterior cerebral artery will cause ataxia with Horner syndrome.

28. Answer: 3

Rationale: Ependymoma is the primary central nervous system tumor, is the most common intramedullary tumor, and it has a good prognosis. Hemangioma and glioblastoma are extramedullary tumors.

29. Answer: 1

Rationale: Fracture of the skull base is very common in a head injury; it indicates a significant impact that needs evaluation by head computed tomography. Fracture of the temporal bone can damage the facial nerve leading to facial nerve paralysis or vestibulocochlear injury. On the other hand, fractures of the anterior skull bone can cause a Battle sign or raccoon eye.

30. Answer: 1

Rationale: This patient has symptoms of normal pressure hydrocephalus, which is the triad of progressive memory loss, urinary incontinence, and abnormal gait. This diagnosis is confirmed by head computed tomography, which showed an enlarged ventricle. A lumbar puncture will reveal normal opening pressure. The treatment of normal pressure hydrocephalus includes recurrent lumbar puncture or ventriculoperitoneal shunt.

31. Answer: 2

Rationale: This patient presented with an acute neurological deficit with a history of diabetes and hypertension, which raised suspicion of stroke. The first step after stabilizing the patient's condition is to do a head computed tomography (CT) to exclude intraventricular hemorrhage or other causes of the neurological deficit. Head CT is more available and more reliable in diagnosing a hemorrhage than magnetic resonance imaging.

32. Answer: 3

Rationale: Epidural hematomas are characterized by a lucid interval at presentation, but then the patient will suddenly deteriorate. An epidural hematoma is caused by rupture of the middle meningeal artery. The first step in diagnosing an epidural hematoma is a head computed tomography, and then the patient needs to have a craniotomy to evacuate the hematoma.

33. Answer: 2

Rationale: Lacunar infarction is caused by occlusion of the penetrating branch of the cerebral artery, mainly in the posterior limb of the internal capsule. Lacunar infarction presents with well-recognized symptoms such as pure motor hemiparesis, pure sensory deficit, dysarthria, or ataxic gait. With a lacunar infarction, all parts of the body are equally affected and there is no sign of cortical involvement.

34. Answer: 4

Rationale: This patient has symptoms of lateral medullary infarction, or Wallenberg syndrome. This condition is caused by occlusion of the vertebral artery inside the cranium. Usually, patients with this syndrome will have a contralateral loss of pain and temperature with ipsilateral Horner syndrome.

35. Answer: 1

Rationale: Glioblastoma is the most common primary intracranial tumor and is mainly found in the cerebral hemisphere in the patient in his or her fifth decade of life. Glioblastoma appears on head computed tomography as an irregular hyperdense area with a central necrotic lesion. The curative treatment of this tumor includes surgical resection with chemotherapy and radiotherapy. Median survival is 1 year without treatment.

36. Answer: 1

Rationale: This patient has a cerebrospinal fluid leak from his nose, which happens if there is a fracture in the area of the paranasal sinus, the mastoid air cell, or the middle ear. Head computed tomography is the best investigation to diagnose a skull fracture. With evidence of a depressed fracture, surgery intervention to repair the dura is needed immediately to prevent other sequels like meningitis. Fluid analysis is only indicated if the patient has signs of meningitis.

37. Answer: 2

Rationale: Myasthenia gravis is a neuromuscular disease that causes skeletal muscle weakness, ptosis, double vision, and limb weakness. These symptoms improve with rest and are aggravated by exercise. It is diagnosed by an edrophonium test and treated with oral anticholinesterase agents that prevent acetylcholine receptor antibodies from destroying acetylcholine.

38. Answer: 3

Rationale: The patient has symptoms of increased intracranial pressure (ICP), which include headache, nausea, and high opening cerebrospinal fluid pressure. On the other hand, there is no abnormality in the investigation and no neurological deficit to suggest idiopathic intracranial hypertension or pseudotumor cerebri. The treatment goal includes decreasing ICP. The first line of management includes acetazolamide and possibly furosemide. Reducing weight will reduce the symptoms in obese patients. A ventriculoperitoneal shunt is used only in refractory cases.

39. Answer: 2

Rationale: Myasthenia gravis is a neuromuscular disease that causes skeletal muscle weakness, ptosis, double vision, and limb weakness. These symptoms improve with rest and are aggravated by exercise. It is diagnosed by an edrophonium test and treated with oral anticholinesterase agents that prevent acetylcholine receptor antibodies from destroying acetylcholine.

40. Answer: 2

Rationale: Pontine hemorrhage is present in 12% of all intracranial hemorrhages. The patient is also in a coma with total paralysis in all limbs caused by disruption of the reticular system. The patient will have pinpoint pupils that sometimes react to light.

41. Answer: 1

Rationale: This patient has symptoms of normal pressure hydrocephalus, which include the triad of progressive memory loss, urinary incontinence, and abnormal gait. This diagnosis is confirmed by head computed tomography, which showed an enlarged ventricle. This condition mainly is caused by a decrease in cerebrospinal fluid production, which happens gradually so the brain will adapt with a gradual increase of hydrocephalus. A lumbar puncture will reveal normal opening pressure.

42. Answer: 3

Rationale: This patient presented with a sudden severe headache, which is a typical presentation of subarachnoid hemorrhage (SAH). It appears on head computed tomography as a hyperdense lesion in typical sites such as the interhemispheric fissure, Sylvian fissures, and in the ambient cistern. The most common cause of SAH is the rupture of a berry aneurysm, whereas arteriovenous malformation is associated with intracerebral and intraventricular hemorrhage.

43. Answer: 2

Rationale: This patient has symptoms of meningitis. The characteristic cerebrospinal fluid (CSF) findings in bacterial meningitis were found in this patient, including high protein, increased polymorphonuclear cells, and low glucose. In benign intracranial hypertension, CSF analysis will be normal but with high opening pressure.

44. Answer: 2

Rationale: The patient has symptoms of increased intracranial pressure (ICP), which include headache, nausea, papilledema, and high opening cerebrospinal fluid pressure. There is no abnormality in the investigation and no neurological deficit. All this points to idiopathic intracranial hypertension or pseudotumor cerebri. The treatment goal includes decreasing the ICP. The first line of management includes acetazolamide and possibly furosemide. Reducing weight will reduce the symptoms in obese patients.

45. Answer: 1

Rationale: This patient has symptoms of meningitis. Meningitis is best diagnosed by lumbar puncture and cerebrospinal fluid analysis, which helps us to know which organism is causing the infection. Funduscopy is used to discover if the patient has papilledema, which is a sign of increased intracranial pressure.

46. Answer: 2

Rationale: Myasthenia gravis is a neuromuscular disease that causes skeletal muscle weakness, ptosis, double vision, and limb weakness. The symptoms improve with rest and are aggravated by exercise. It is diagnosed by an edrophonium test and treated by oral anticholinesterase agents that prevent acetylcholine receptor antibodies from destroying acetylcholine.

47. Answer: 2

Rationale: This patient presented with a sudden severe headache, which is a typical presentation of subarachnoid hemorrhage. It appears on head computed tomography as a hyperdense lesion in the interhemispheric fissure, which is a typical site of subarachnoid hemorrhage.

48. Answer: 4

Rationale: Lacunar infarction is caused by occlusion of the penetrating branch of the cerebral artery mainly in the posterior limb of the internal capsule. Lacunar infarction presents with well-recognized symptoms such as pure motor hemiparesis, pure sensory deficit, dysarthria, or ataxic gait. In lacunar infarction, all parts of the body are equally affected and there are no signs of cortical involvement. Diabetes mellitus and hypertension are the major risk factors for lacunar infarction.

49. Answer: 1

Rationale: The patient presented with symptoms of acute ischemic stroke, and head computed tomography showed no intracerebral hemorrhage. Because of this, the next step of management is alteplase, which is a thrombolytic therapy that can be used for ischemic stroke within 3 hours from symptom initiation. There is no role for heparin or warfarin in treating ischemic stroke, and the only antithrombotic agent that can be used is aspirin.

50. Answer: 2

Rationale: The patient presented with symptoms of an acute ischemic stroke and head computed tomography showed no intracerebral hemorrhage. The next step of management is alteplase, but this patient has a history of hemorrhagic stroke, which is a contraindication for alteplase. Because alteplase is contraindicated, the next step is aspirin.

51. Answer: 2

Rationale: Myasthenia gravis is a neuromuscular disease that causes skeletal muscle weakness, ptosis, double vision, and limb weakness. These symptoms improve with rest and are aggravated by exercise. It is diagnosed by an edrophonium test and treated by oral anticholinesterase agents that prevent acetylcholine receptor antibodies from destroying acetylcholine. All patients who are newly diagnosed with myasthenia gravis should undergo chest computed tomography to exclude thymoma.

52. Answer: 2

Rationale: The patient has a history of small cell carcinoma and presented with proximal muscle weakness. This suggests he has Lambert–Eaton, which is a paraneoplastic syndrome. In this syndrome, the body attacks the calcium channels on nerve endings that are required to trigger the release of chemicals (acetylcholine). Treatment for this disease includes plasmapheresis and immunosuppression drugs.

53. Answer: 3

Rationale: The patient presented with symptoms of acute ischemic stroke and head computed tomography showed no intracerebral hemorrhage. The next step of management is alteplase, which is a thrombolytic therapy that can be used in ischemic stroke within 3 hours from symptom initiation. There are several contraindications for thrombolytic therapy including previous hemorrhagic stroke, systolic blood pressure over 180 mmHg, previous surgery, or gastrointestinal bleeding within 3 months.

54. Answer: 3

Rationale: This patient has eclampsia, which happens most commonly within 6 to 12 hours after delivery. The first line of treatment for eclampsia after securing the airway is magnesium sulfate. Magnesium sulfate needs close monitoring of the reflexes to avoid toxicity.

55. Answer: 3

Rationale: This patient has symptoms of lateral medullary infarction, or Wallenberg syndrome. This condition is caused by occlusion of the vertebral artery inside the cranium. Usually, patients with this syndrome will have a contralateral loss of pain and temperature with ipsilateral Horner syndrome.

56. Answer: 1

Rationale: This patient presented with a sudden severe "thunderclap" headache, which is a typical presentation of subarachnoid hemorrhage (SAH). It appears on head computed tomography (CT) as a hyperdense lesion in the interhemispheric fissure. A lumbar puncture can be used to aid in the diagnosis of an SAH, but a head CT or funduscopy should be done first to exclude any other lesion that causes increased intracranial pressure.

57. Answer: 1

Rationale: Myasthenia gravis is a neuromuscular disease that causes skeletal muscle weakness, ptosis, double vision, and limb weakness. These symptoms improve with rest and are aggravated by exercise. It is diagnosed by an edrophonium test and treated by oral anticholinesterase agents that prevent acetylcholine receptor antibodies from destroying acetylcholine. All patients newly diagnosed with myasthenia gravis should undergo a chest computed tomography to exclude thymoma.

58. Answer: 1

Rationale: The Glasgow Coma Scale is a measure of the patient's the best response for each group. The groups include a motor score that ranges from 1 to 6, a verbal category that ranges from 1 to 5, and an eye category that ranges from 1 to 4. When these scores are added together the range should be between 3 and 15.

59. Answer: 2

Rationale: The most common causes of brain metastases in the female patient are lung cancer and then breast cancer. This patient has a history of breast cancer and now presents with a single mass in the brain. The treatment of choice in the patient with single brain metastases is surgical resection of the mass.

60. Answer: 4

Rationale: A seizure is characterized by an aura, tongue laceration, and a loss of autonomic function. Syncopal attacks present with loss of consciousness with loss of posture and motor tone for a moment, after which the patient immediately returns to baseline neurological function.

61. Answer: 1

Rationale: This patient with no significant history presented with an unprovoked first seizure. Any patient with a first-time seizure should undergo head computed tomography to exclude any structural abnormalities such as a mass or any acute neurological event such as a subarachnoid hemorrhage.

62. Answer: 1

Rationale: This patient has symptoms of normal pressure hydrocephalus, which is the triad of progressive memory loss, urinary incontinence, and abnormal gait. This diagnosis is confirmed by head computed tomography, which showed an enlarged ventricle. A lumbar puncture will reveal normal opening pressure.

63. Answer: 1

Rationale: The patient has a history of small cell carcinoma and presented with proximal muscle weakness, suggesting the Lambert–Eaton syndrome, which is a paraneoplastic syndrome. In this syndrome, the body develops an antibody against presynaptic calcium channels. The treatment of this disease includes plasmapheresis and immunosuppression drugs.

64. Answer: 3

Rationale: Glioblastoma is the most common primary intracranial tumor, and it is mainly found in the cerebral hemisphere of the patient in his or her fifth decade of life. Glioblastoma appears on head computed tomography as an irregular hyperdensity with a central necrotic lesion. The curative treatment of this tumor includes surgical resection with chemotherapy and radiotherapy. The median survival is 1 year without treatment.

65. Answer: 3

Rationale: Hypertension is the most common risk factor for an intracranial hemorrhage (ICH). The most common site for ICH is the basal ganglion, especially in an internal capsule, and then the thalamus. In cerebral lesions, the patient usually suffers from a motor deficit on the opposite side of the lesion.

66. Answer: 2

Rationale: This patient has symptoms of meningitis. Characteristic cerebrospinal fluid findings of viral meningitis were found in this patient, which include protein less than 100 mg/dL, increased lymphatic cells, and normal glucose levels.

67. Answer: 4

Rationale: Subdural hematomas can happen in elderly people with a minimal head injury. It results from rupture of an intracranial vein or bridging vein. Epidural hematomas result from rupture of the middle meningeal artery. Rupture of an aneurysm can cause an intracerebral hemorrhage.

68. Answer: 1

Rationale: The patient has symptoms of increased intracranial pressure (ICP), which include headache, nausea, and high opening cerebrospinal fluid pressure. There is no abnormality in the exam and no neurological deficits. The symptoms and exam suggest idiopathic intracranial hypertension or pseudotumor cerebri. The treatment goal includes a decrease in ICP. The first line of management includes acetazolamide and possibly furosemide. Weight loss can decrease the symptoms in obese patients.

69. Answer: 3

Rationale: This patient has symptoms of meningitis. Cerebrospinal fluid analysis shows parameters of viral meningitis including lymphocytosis with high protein. The most common virus for meningitis is the *Enterovirus* family. There is no treatment, and most cases resolve on their own.

70. Answer: 2

Rationale: This patient has eclampsia, a rare but serious condition in which high blood pressure results in seizures during pregnancy or soon after pregnancy. Eclampsia affects about 1 in every 200 women with preeclampsia. You can develop eclampsia even if you do not have a history of seizures. The first line of treatment for eclampsia after securing the airway is magnesium sulfate. Magnesium sulfate needs close monitoring of the reflexes to avoid toxicity.

71. Answer: 2

Rationale: This patient has symptoms of normal pressure hydrocephalus, which include the triad of progressive memory loss, urinary incontinence, and abnormal gait. This diagnosis is confirmed by head computed tomography, which showed an enlarged ventricle. A lumbar puncture will reveal normal opening pressure.

72. Answer: 3

Rationale: Third nerve palsy can present with ptosis, dilated pupil, and diplopia. There are several comorbid conditions that can cause third nerve palsy including diabetes, vasculitis, and posterior communicating artery aneurysm. If the patient presented with painful third nerve palsy, the posterior communicating artery should be excluded.

73. Answer: 4

Rationale: Treatment of epilepsy usually starts after two seizures if the patient has no history of structural abnormality. The first line of management in tonic-clonic seizure is sodium valproate, whereas lamotrigine and carbamazepine are considered as second-line management.

74. Answer: 1

Rationale: There are several causes of bitemporal hemianopia, but the cause will depend on which area is more affected. If the upper quadrant is affected more than the lower quadrant, then inferior chiasmal compression is suspected. The most common cause of inferior chiasmal compression is pituitary macroadenoma.

75. Answer: 3

Rationale: This patient has uncontrolled epilepsy while on sodium valproate, which is the first line of management for generalized seizures. In the patient with uncontrolled epilepsy, despite the monotherapy of antiepileptic drugs, the next step is to switch to another antiepileptic drug such as lamotrigine, phenytoin, or carbamazepine.

76. Answer: 2

Rationale: All the antiepileptic drugs have a teratogenic effect, but the risk of seizure on the fetus is more than the risk of teratogenic effect. The patient should continue her treatment and she should take folic acid to reduce the risk of spina bifida.

77. Answer: 4

Rationale: In the treatment of epilepsy, monotherapy is preferred, and the first line of management is sodium valproate. If sodium valproate fails to control the epilepsy, then we can switch to lamotrigine. If the seizure is still uncontrolled, we can use both drugs together, but these should be used cautiously because of the risk of Steven–Johnson syndrome.

78. Answer: 2

Rationale: An antiepileptic drug should be started after the second seizure, but if the patient has a structural abnormality on the head computed tomography, neurological deficit, and/or a strong family history of seizure, then an antiepileptic drug should be started immediately.

79. Answer: 2

Rationale: All the antiepileptic drugs have a teratogenic effect, but the risk of seizure on the fetus is more than the risk of teratogenic effect. The patient should continue her treatment and she should take folic acid to reduce the risk of spina bifida.

80. Answer: 1

Rationale: Hepatic encephalopathy is a condition in which the brain and nervous system suffer damage caused by liver dysfunction. Toxic substances that are normally removed from the body by the liver build up in the blood and reach the brain. The yellowish skin and black stools point to liver dysfunction. The history does not suggest toxic encephalopathies or post-seizure encephalopathy.

81. Answer: 2

Rationale: One pupil larger than the other is a dangerous sign that can indicate the formation of a hematoma (collection of blood) on the brain. The other three are signs and symptoms of concussion that warrant an emergency department visit if they are getting progressively worse.

82. Answer: 3

Rationale: Normal pressure hydrocephalus (NPH) can be the result of infection, tumor, or head trauma. The history of bumping the head and the gradual onset of progressive symptoms after the incident point to NPH. Features of Parkinson disease, such as tremor, and Alzheimer disease, such as aphasia, are not reported. Congenital hydrocephalus is present at birth or develops shortly after birth.

83. Answer: 1

Rationale: Obesity/weight gain is a high-risk factor for increased intracranial pressure. The condition is common among obese women of childbearing age. Idiopathic intracranial hypertension (IIH) is less frequent in children and the elderly. Less than 10% of patients with IIH are male. Hypervitaminosis A (high levels of vitamin A) is a risk factor for IIH.

84. Answer: 3

Rationale: Gastric lavage is not recommended based on the patient's symptoms. All the other answers are recommended investigative and treatment measures. A CT scan can help identify brain infarcts. A lumbar puncture can help detect bacterial meningitis. Steroids and antibiotics can be instituted if investigations point to bacterial meningitis.

85. Answer: 2

Rationale: A patient with Wernicke encephalopathy will have an ataxic gait, slurred speech, confusion, dilated pupils, and nystagmus. All these signs raise suspicion for Wernicke encephalopathy, which happens in alcoholics, especially those who are malnourished. The treatment for this is thiamine, which can reverse and prevent Wernicke encephalopathy.

86. Answer: 1

Rationale: Any patient diagnosed with polycystic kidney disease with a family history of hemorrhagic stroke or intracranial aneurysm should have a magnetic resonance angiography for further evaluation.

87. Answer: 2

Rationale: This patient has symptoms of cavernous sinus thrombosis, which usually include headaches with third and fourth cranial nerve paralysis associated with periorbital swelling. There are several factors that can increase the risk of cavernous sinus thromboses such as thrombophilia, oral contraceptives, sinus infection, and head injury.

88. Answer: 3

Rationale: This patient has symptoms of stroke, which rarely happens at this age. There are two causes that can lead to stroke at a young age. One of them is carotid artery dissection that happens spontaneously or after trauma, and the second cause for young-onset stroke is embolism from the heart.

89. Answer: 3

Rationale: Any patient diagnosed with polycystic kidney disease with a family history of hemorrhagic stroke or intracranial aneurysm who develops symptoms suggesting an intracranial aneurysm has a high likelihood of having a berry aneurysm.

90. Answer: 3

Rationale: This patient has symptoms of cavernous sinus thrombosis, which usually include headaches with third and fourth cranial nerve paralysis associated with periorbital swelling. There are many structures that pass through the cavernous sinus that can be affected such as the third and fourth nerves and maxillary and ophthalmic branch of the trigeminal nerve. Thrombophilia, oral contraceptive pills, sinus infection, and head injury are several factors that can increase the risk of cavernous sinus thromboses.

91. Answer: 2

Rationale: This patient had symptoms of meningitis. The characteristic cerebrospinal fluid findings of bacterial meningitis were found in this patient including high protein, increased polymorphonuclear cells, and low glucose. The most common organism causing bacterial meningitis is *Streptococcus pneumoniae*.

92. Answer: 3

Rationale: This patient had symptoms of meningitis. The characteristic cerebrospinal fluid findings of bacterial meningitis were found in this patient including high protein, increased polymorphonuclear cells, and low glucose. The most common cause of meningitis in the immunocompromised patient is *Listeria*.

93. Answer: 1

Rationale: One of the complications of traumatic brain injury is diabetes insipidus. It is characterized by urine osmolality less than 200 mOsm/kg and high or normal plasma osmolality with polyuria more than 3 L/day. Diabetes insipidus is mainly diagnosed by a water deprivation test.

94. Answer: 2

Rationale: One of the complications of traumatic brain injury is diabetes insipidus, which is caused by decreased release of antidiuretic hormone from the pituitary gland. Diabetes insipidus is characterized by urine osmolality less than 200 mOsm/kg and high or normal plasma osmolality with polyuria more than 3 L/day. Diabetes insipidus is mainly diagnosed by a water deprivation test.

95. Answer: 2

Rationale: One of the complications of traumatic brain injury is diabetes insipidus, which is characterized by urine osmolality less than 200 mOsm/kg and high or normal plasma osmolality with polyuria more than 3 L/day. Diabetes insipidus is mainly diagnosed by a water deprivation test.

96. Answer: 4

Rationale: This patient has the symptoms of cauda equine syndrome, which can be caused by trauma that leads to the rupture of a disc or caused by inflammatory conditions. This is an emergent situation that needs rapid intervention to release the compression before ischemia happens.

97. Answer: 3

Rationale: This patient presented with a sudden severe headache, which is a typical presentation of subarachnoid hemorrhage (SAH). It appears on head computed tomography (CT) as a hyperdense lesion typically seen in the interhemispheric fissure, Sylvian fissures, and in the ambient cistern. If CT is normal, then lumbar puncture should be done 6 hours after onset of symptoms.

98. Answer: 2

Rationale: This patient has the symptoms of conus medullaris syndrome, which can present with symmetrical motor weakness and early bladder and bowel dysfunction with hyperreflexia and sudden back pain. Conus medullaris syndrome is an emergency that needs urgent surgical decompression.

99. Answer: 1

Rationale: The normal range of intracranial pressure (ICP) is between 7 and 15 mmHg. If it is greater than 20 mmHg, then it is considered increased. The symptoms of increased ICP include headache, nausea, and vomiting. The Cushing triad is the classical presentation of increased intracranial pressure, which includes hypertension, bradycardia, and irregular breathing. In most cases, this triad can present late.

100. Answer: 3

Rationale: The normal range of intracranial pressure (ICP) is between 7 and 15 mmHg. If it is greater than 20 mmHg, it is considered increased. The symptoms of increased intracranial pressure include headache, nausea, and vomiting. Evaluating the patient with increased intracranial hypertension includes a head computed tomography. A lumbar puncture can be performed if there is no mass.

101. Answer: 1

Rationale: This patient has symptoms of normal pressure hydrocephalus, which is the triad of progressive memory loss, urinary incontinence, and abnormal gait. This patient will have papilledema and signs of sixth nerve palsy. This diagnosis is confirmed by head computed tomography, which showed an enlarged ventricle. A lumbar puncture will reveal normal opening pressure.

102. Answer: 1

Rationale: The patient has symptoms of increased intracranial pressure (ICP), which include headache, nausea, papilledema, and high opening cerebrospinal pressure. There are many causes that lead to increased ICP including a space-occupying lesion, intracerebral hemorrhage, and idiopathic reasons.

103. Answer: 1

Rationale: A patient with Wernicke encephalopathy will have an ataxic gait, slurred speech, confusion, dilated pupils, and nystagmus. All these signs raise suspicion for Wernicke encephalopathy, which happens in alcoholics, especially those who are malnourished. The treatment of this condition is thiamine, which can reverse and prevent Wernicke encephalopathy.

104. Answer: 1

Rationale: This patient has symptoms of normal pressure hydrocephalus, which is the triad of progressive memory loss, urinary incontinence, and wide-based gait. This patient also will have papilledema and signs of sixth nerve palsy. Diagnosis is confirmed by a head compute tomography, which showed an enlarged ventricle. A lumbar puncture will reveal normal opening pressure.

105. Answer: 1

Rationale: Pressure ulcers occur at sites overlying bony structure. The most common cause of these ulcers is pressure as a result of immobility. A pressure ulcer can extend to involve skin, soft tissue, and muscle.

Gastrointestinal

1. A 50-year-old Asian American patient presents to the hospital with a 1-month history of burning epigastric pain with difficulties in swallowing. The pain is not relieved by eating, and he tried famotidine 20 mg/day tablets when symptoms occur, but there is a minimal relief. The patient's medication is lisinopril 5 mg/day for hypertension. Which is the best action for this patient?

   1. Initiate calcium carbonate 500-mg tablet.

   2. Refer for endoscopic evaluation.

   3. Change Lisinopril to amlodipine.

   4. Initiate omeprazole 20 mg twice daily.

2. A 59-year-old woman (height 65 inches, weight 77 kg) with a history of heart failure and myocardial infarction is admitted to the intensive care unit with severe community-acquired pneumonia. Five hours after admission she develops acute respiratory failure, hypotension, and acute kidney injury from sepsis. Mechanical ventilation is implanted, and a nasogastric (NG) tube is placed. She currently takes ramipril 10 mg/day, carvedilol 12.5 mg/twice daily, levothyroxine 125 mcg/day, and aspirin 75 mg. Her white blood cell count is 25×10^3 cells/mm^3, platelet count is 170,000/mm^3, serum creatinine is 3.7 mg/dL (baseline 1.27 mg/dL), potassium is 4.5 mEq/L, international normalized ratio is 1.1, aspartate aminotransferase is 30 international units/mL, and alanine aminotransferase is 45 international units/mL. Which approach is the most appropriate for preventing stress-related mucosal disease in this patient?

   1. Pantoprazole 40 mg intravenous (IV) once daily.

   2. Cimetidine 8 mg/hr IV infusion.

   3. Sucralfate 1 mg four times daily by NG tube.

   4. Magnesium hydroxide 30 mL daily by NG tube.

3. A 45-year-old woman complains of severe pain related to the swelling of three metacarpophalangeal joints on her right hand. She has suffered for 2 weeks and cannot perform her usual household activities. Radiograms reveal bone decalcifications and erosions. A serum rheumatoid factor is obtained that is elevated. Her medical history includes hypertension and dyslipidemia. Her medication is ramipril 10 mg/day, aspirin 81 mg/day, and atorvastatin 40 mg/day. The physician would like to initiate systemic antiinflammatory drugs for her rheumatoid arthritis with high-dose nonsteroidal antiinflammatory therapy; however, the physician is worried about potential gastrointestinal toxicity. What is the best recommended regimen for treating the patient's pain?

   1. Indomethacin 75 mg/day.

   2. Piroxicam 20 mg/day plus misoprostol 600 mcg three times daily.

   3. Naproxen 500 mg twice daily plus omeprazole 20 mg/day.

   4. Celecoxib 400 mg twice daily.

4. The patient is a 79-year-old man with a history of type 2 diabetes, anemia, and chronic low back pain admitted to the hospital for abdominal pain lasting 3 days. His last bowel movement was 4 days ago. The physician examined him and found moderate left upper quadrant tenderness. An abdominal radiograph reveals a large amount of stool in the colon with no signs of obstruction. His current medications are glipizide 5 mg twice daily, iron supplement, acetaminophen 500 mg four times daily, and oxycodone/acetaminophen 5/375 mg as needed for pain. His serum creatinine is 1.8 mg/dL. Which therapy would be the best management for the patient's constipation?

   1. Bisacodyl suppositories.

   2. Methylnaltrexone injection.

   3. Psyllium or inulin.

   4. Linaclotide.

5. A 63-year-old African American woman is assessed in the emergency department for a 48-hour history of black stool, dizziness, confusion, and vomiting a substance resembling coffee grounds. Her medical history is myocardial infarction, hypertension, and seasonal allergies. She has taken naproxen 500 mg twice daily for 3 years, lisinopril 20 mg/day, aspirin 325 mg/day, and loratadine 10 mg/day. Nasogastric aspiration (NG) is positive for blood, and endoscopic evaluation reveals a 2.5-cm antral ulcer. A rapid urease test is negative for *Helicobacter pylori*. What recommendation is best for this patient?

   1. Pantoprazole 80 mg intravenous (IV) bolus followed by an 8-mg/hr infusion.

   2. IV famotidine 20 mg/hr for 5 days.

   3. Oral lansoprazole 15 mg/day by NG tube.

   4. Magnesium hydroxide 30 mL daily by NG tube.

6. The patient is a 43-year-old man with a history of bipolar disorder for 3 years, chronic angina, and recurrent urinary tract infection, and he is admitted to the emergency department with severe nausea, vomiting, fever, and back pain. On exam, he has a dry mucous membrane and right-sided costovertebral tenderness. A urinalysis is obtained and is positive for leukocyte esterase. His serum creatinine is 1.2 mg/dL and blood urea nitrogen is 30 mg/dL. His current medications are risperidone 6 mg twice daily and sertraline 100 mg/day. He reports that he has an allergy to sulfamethazine/trimethoprim. Which drug would be the best treatment for the patient's vomiting?

   1. Diphenhydramine 50 mg intravenously (IV) three times daily.

   2. Ondansetron 4 mg IV three times daily.

   3. Haloperidol 5 mg IV once daily.

   4. Prochlorperazine 10 mg tablet orally twice daily.

7. The patient is a 35-year-old Hispanic woman admitted to the hospital who complains of new-onset abdominal pain for 9 weeks together with two to three bloody stools per day and weight loss. She reports an allergy to "sulfa-containing medication." Colonoscopy reveals diffuse superficial colonic inflammation consistent with ulcerative colitis. The inflammation is continuous and extends to the hepatic flexure. Which is the best drug regimen for this patient?

   1. Infliximab 5 mg/kg as a single dose.

   2. Hydrocortisone enema 100 mg every day.

   3. Mesalamine 1.6 g orally three times daily.

   4. Sulfasalazine extended-release tablet 1 g orally three times daily.

8. A 25-year-old white woman with a history of Crohn disease comes in the clinic with a chief concern of mucopurulent drainage from an erythematous region on her abdomen. On exam, colonoscopy reveals a moderate-sized enterocutaneous fistula in the right upper abdomen area. Her medications are mesalamine 1.6 mg orally three times daily and azathioprine tablet 75 mg twice daily. Her physician wants to prescribe infliximab. What is the best recommendation before the initiation of therapy?

   1. Rule out tuberculosis by purified protein derivative or QuantiFERON-TB test.

   2. Obtain an echocardiogram to assess cardiac function.

   3. Administer a test dose before the initial infusion.

   4. Obtain liver function tests before the initial infusion.

9. The patient is a 50-year-old African American man seen in the clinic for follow-up. He has a history of alcoholic cirrhosis. His endoscopy from 1 month ago revealed some large esophageal varices without any history of bleeding. At that time, the vital signs included heart rate 87 beats/min, respiratory rate 15 breaths/min, and blood pressure 135/80 mmHg. The physician recommended propranolol 10 mg orally three times daily. At his evaluation today, he does not complain of any new concerns from propranolol dose. His vital signs now include heart rate 73 beats/min, respiratory rate 16 breaths/min, and blood pressure 120/75 mmHg. What is the best management for this case?

   1. Increase propranolol dose to 20 mg three times per day.

   2. Change propranolol to carvedilol 2.5 mg orally once daily.

   3. Add isosorbide dinitrate 10 mg orally three times daily.

   4. Continue the current regimen with a close following up after 4 weeks.

10. A 56-year-old Asian woman (height 70 inches, weight 75 kg) with a history of alcohol abuse and chronic hepatitis C virus (HCV; genotype 2) started taking sofosbuvir 400 mg daily and ribavirin 600 mg twice daily 2 weeks ago. She returns to the clinic today with a complaint of fatigue, scleral icterus, and pallor. There is no clinical evidence of bleeding. Laboratory values reveal the following: hematocrit 30% (baseline 39%), total bilirubin 3.2 mg/dL, aspartate aminotransferase 148 international units/mL (baseline 300 international units/mL), alanine aminotransferase 175 international units/mL (baseline 400 international units/mL), serum creatinine 0.8 mg/dL, HCV RNA 1×10^6 copies/mL (baseline 2.5×10^6 copies/mL), white blood cell count 7.8×10^3 cells/mm^3, and platelet count 170,000/mm^3. What is the most likely cause of the patient's symptoms?

    1. Systemic manifestations of chronic HCV disease.
    2. Worsening of her liver disease secondary to inadequate treatment.
    3. An adverse effect secondary to treatment with sofosbuvir.
    4. An adverse effect secondary to treatment with ribavirin.

11. The patient is a 20-year-old man seeking advice about a possible exposure to hepatitis A virus (HAV). He saw reports on a website that a chef at a local restaurant where he dined 4 weeks earlier had active HAV. He heard that HAV could have been transmitted through the food. He does not have any vaccination documentation, and he does not remember receiving an HAV vaccine in the past. Which is the best recommendation for this patient?

    1. Initiate HAV vaccine.
    2. Recommend HAV immune globulin.
    3. Continue to observe the patient for symptoms.
    4. Administer HAV vaccine and immune globulin.

12. A woman and her 15-year-old son present to the nurse practitioner's office for consultation. Her son ate a meal that was prepared by his friend, who was known to have hepatitis A virus (HAV) infection. The mother was afraid that her son might have contracted HAV because he has never been vaccinated against it. What is the best consultation you can provide to the mother?

    1. The son should receive HAV vaccine today.
    2. The son should wait for more than 14 days then receive the vaccine.
    3. Advise the mother that her son does not need any intervention.
    4. Because the son is not showing any symptoms, he could not have HAV.

13. A 35-year-old Asian woman presents to the general medicine floor with abdominal pain, severe nausea and vomiting, and abdominal distention secondary to alcoholic hepatitis. She has a history of alcohol abuse for 15 years and osteoporosis for 2 years. Her current medications are alendronate 10 mg tablet once daily and calcium supplement 500 mg twice daily. Her serum creatinine is 0.6 mg/dL, aspartate aminotransferase is 250 international units/L, alanine aminotransferase is 65 international units/L, total bilirubin is 10.3 mg/dL, prothrombin time is 19 seconds (normal 12 seconds), and albumin is 2.1 g/L. Abdominal paracentesis shows no evidence of spontaneous bacterial peritonitis. What is the best therapy for the patient's alcoholic hepatitis?

    1. Octreotide 50 mcg/hr intravenously.
    2. Prednisone 40 mg/day.
    3. Midodrine 7.5 mg/day.
    4. Pentoxifylline 400 mg three times daily.

14. The patient is a 65-year-old African American man admitted to the emergency department with abdominal pain and severe nausea and vomiting. The patient history is alcoholic abuse for 20 years and he does not take any medication. The laboratory evaluation reveals serum creatinine is 0.5 mg/dL, alanine aminotransferase is 100 international units/L, aspartate aminotransferase is 270 international units/L, total bilirubin is 11.5 mg/dL, prothrombin time is 21 seconds (control 12 seconds), and albumin is 2.5 g/L. After the exam, there is no evidence of variceal bleeding or spontaneous bacterial peritonitis. Which is the best intervention for this patient?

    1. Naproxen 200 mg orally twice daily.
    2. Octreotide 50 mcg/hr intravenously.
    3. Prednisone 40 mg/day for 4 weeks followed by a 2-week taper.
    4. Ribavirin 600 mg twice daily.

15. A 70-year-old Hispanic man is assessed in the emergency department for a 36-hour history of black and tarry stools, dizziness and confusion, and vomiting a substance that looks like coffee grounds. The patient is healthy and does not take any medication except naproxen 500 mg for occasional back pain. Nasogastric aspiration (NG) is positive for blood, and subsequent endoscopy reveals a 3-cm antral ulcer with a visible vessel. The vessel was obliterated with an epinephrine solution, and a rapid urease test is positive for *Helicobacter pylori*. Which recommendation is best for this patient?

    1. Sucralfate 1 g four times daily by NG tube.

    2. Oral omeprazole 20 mg/day by NG tube.

    3. Pantoprazole 80 mg intravenous bolus followed by an 8 mg/hr infusion.

    4. Lansoprazole 30 mg twice daily plus amoxicillin 1000 twice daily plus clarithromycin 500 twice daily for 14 days.

16. The patient is a 70-year-old woman admitted to the clinic with a 3-month history of burning epigastric pain. The patient tried calcium carbonate 500-mg chewable tablet, but the pain was not relieved. Her friend, who suffered from the same symptoms, told her to take ranitidine 20 mg daily, but the symptoms were only partially relieved. She denies any other symptoms. She has a history of stroke 1 year ago; her current medication includes aspirin 81 mg once daily. Which is the best recommended therapy for the patient?

    1. Initiate omeprazole 20-mg tablet daily.

    2. Refer for possible endoscopic therapy.

    3. Change ranitidine to cimetidine.

    4. Stop using aspirin 81 tablet.

17. A 50-year-old Asian woman with a 6-month history of gastroesophageal reflux disease presents to the clinic. She is taking lansoprazole 15-mg tablet once daily and ranitidine 20 mg for breakthrough symptoms. Her symptoms are still present 3 to 4 days per week, and it is interfering in her daily life. She denies drinking alcohol or eating spicy food; she was adherent to her medication. An endoscopy evaluation reveals no ulcers or erosion. What is the best drug regimen for the patient?

    1. Add metoclopramide 10 mg four times daily.

    2. Switch to pantoprazole 40 mg daily.

    3. Add sucralfate 1 g four times daily.

    4. Increase lansoprazole to 15 mg twice daily.

18. The patient is a 66-year-old man referred to your office for a 2-week history of abdominal pain with heme-positive stools. He has a history of diabetes type 2 and peripheral neuropathy. His current medication includes metformin 1000 twice daily, aspirin 325 mg daily, and gabapentin 600 mg three times daily. In addition, he takes over-the-counter ketoprofen daily for 3 months secondary to uncontrolled neck pain. After the exam, an endoscopy reveals a 1.5-cm gastric ulcer with an intact clot. The patient's rapid urease test for *Helicobacter pylori* is negative. What is the best treatment for the patient's ulcer?

    1. Pantoprazole 40 mg twice daily plus amoxicillin 1000 mg twice daily plus clarithromycin 500 mg twice daily for 10 days.

    2. Famotidine 40 mg twice daily for 4 weeks.

    3. Lansoprazole 30 mg twice daily for 8 weeks.

    4. Sucralfate 1 g daily for 8 weeks.

19. A 33-year-old woman is referred to the gastroenterologist with a 2-week history of chronic cough, noncardiac chest pain, acidic taste in the mouth, and heartburn. She was diagnosed with HIV 3 years ago. Her medications are atazanavir, tenofovir, and emtricitabine. Two months ago, her CD4 count was 550 cells/mm^3 and the viral load was 4000 copies/mL. She has tried over-the-counter aluminum hydroxide, but there was only partial relief for her symptoms. On exam, electrocardiogram is normal, serum creatinine is 0.8 mL/dL, CD4 is 450 cells/mm^3, and the viral load is 5500 copies/mL. What is the best management for the patient's symptoms?

    1. Refer for possible endoscopic evaluation.

    2. Screening for *Helicobacter pylori*.

    3. Initiate cimetidine 200 mg three times daily.

    4. Initiate rabeprazole 20 mg/day orally.

20. A 75-year-old Hispanic man is admitted to the clinic with upper abdominal pain that becomes worse when eating. His history includes myocardial infarction, hypertension, and diabetes type 2. His current medications are aspirin 325 mg daily, metformin 1000 mg twice daily, lisinopril 20 mg daily, and carvedilol 12.5 mg daily. On exam, there is no blood at the rectal area, and the patient denies any other symptoms. The result of colonoscopy is negative, but endoscopy revealed a 2-cm gastric ulcer. A rapid urease test was performed for *Helicobacter pylori* and the result was positive. Which treatment is best for the patient's ulcer?

    1. Misoprostol 200 mcg twice daily for 8 weeks.

    2. Omeprazole 40 mg daily for 8 weeks.

    3. Ranitidine 150 mg twice daily for 8 weeks.

    4. Lansoprazole 30 mg twice daily plus amoxicillin 1000 mg twice daily plus clarithromycin 500 mg twice daily for 14 days.

21. The patient is a 45-year-old African American man seen by the gastroenterologist with a concern of sharp epigastric pain for 5 weeks. He reports that the pain is often worse with eating, and it is present at least 4 days per week. He has tried over-the-counter antacids, but there was only minimal relief. The patient admits that he drinks one beer per a day; he currently takes no medications. He reports an allergy to penicillin (rash). The patient is diagnosed with *Helicobacter pylori*. What is the best treatment for *H. pylori*?

    1. Pantoprazole 40 mg twice daily plus amoxicillin 1000 mg twice daily plus clarithromycin 500 mg twice daily for 7 days.

    2. Omeprazole 20 mg twice daily plus cephalexin 1 g twice daily plus clarithromycin 500 mg twice daily for 14 days.

    3. Bismuth subsalicylate 525 mg four times daily plus tetracycline 500 mg four times daily plus metronidazole 500 mg three times daily plus omeprazole 20 mg twice daily for 14 days.

    4. Levofloxacin 500 mg daily plus metronidazole 500 mg twice daily plus omeprazole 20 mg twice daily for 21 days.

22. A 25-year-old white woman is admitted to the clinic with a 2-week history of bloody diarrhea and abdominal pain. The symptoms continue every day about four to six times a day; the patient takes loperamide, but it has a minimal effect. A colonoscopy evaluation revealed active ulcerative colitis affecting her descending colon and rectum. She has no known drug allergies. Which drug regimen is best?

    1. Mesalamine enema 1000 mg rectally once daily.

    2. Balsalazide 750 mg twice daily.

    3. Methotrexate 25 mg intramuscularly once weekly.

    4. Infliximab 5 mg/kg intravenously.

23. The patient is a 35-year-old African American man (height 70 inches, weight 65 kg) who presents to the hospital with a 12-week history of cramping abdominal pain, fever, and four or five bloody stools per day. A colonoscopy has revealed patchy inflammation in the colon and terminal ileum consistent with moderate active Crohn disease. Vital signs include body temperature is 98°F, heart rate is 110 beats/min, respiratory rate is 19 breaths/min, and blood pressure is 116/68 mmHg. Which therapeutic choice is the best?

    1. Mesalamine 1000 mg four times orally.

    2. Budesonide 9 mg orally once daily.

    3. Infliximab 325 mg intravenously and azathioprine 130 mg daily.

    4. Adalimumab 40 mg subcutaneously every 2 weeks.

24. A 65-year-old man comes with his wife to the clinic. His medical history includes diabetes type 2, peripheral neuropathy, and moderate to severe Crohn disease. He currently takes 18 units of glargine before bed, gabapentin 600 mg three times daily, a vitamin B_{12} tablet, and infliximab 5 mg/kg. After the evaluation, the laboratory values revealed serum creatinine is 1.3 mg/dL, body temperature is 100°F, blood pressure is 135/80 mmHg, respiratory rate is 16 breaths/min, and heart rate is 100 beats/min. Which is the best management for the patient's symptoms?

    1. Increase infliximab dose to 10 mg twice daily.

    2. Initiate mesalamine 1000 mg four times daily.

    3. Initiate budesonide 9 mg orally once daily.

    4. Stop infliximab.

25. A 40-year-old Hispanic man is admitted to the emergency department with new-onset speaking troubles, difficulty in walking, week muscle, and personality changes. The patient's medical history includes active severe ulcerative colitis (UC), hypertension, and previous stroke 3 years ago. He currently takes aspirin 81 mg daily, captopril 50 mg twice daily, vitamin supplements, and natalizumab. His UC symptoms were out of control, and his previous medication has failed to control his symptoms. He was then started on natalizumab 300 mg intravenously every 4 weeks. Which drug is causing the new-onset symptoms for this patient?

    1. Natalizumab.

    2. Aspirin 81 mg tablet.

    3. Vitamin supplements.

    4. Captopril.

26. A 38-year-old Hispanic woman with a history of Crohn disease (CD) presents to the clinic for follow-up. Her symptoms were diagnosed as moderate to severe active CD, and the gastroenterologist recommended infliximab 5 mg as a single dose, then at 2 and 6 weeks, then every 8 weeks as maintenance. The patient started the infusion of the medication at the clinic, then suddenly became hypotensive and her temperature has increased. Which management is the best to prevent infusion-related infliximab symptoms?

    1. Ketoprofen.

    2. Infuse over at least 30 minutes.

    3. Pretreatment with acetaminophen.

    4. Symptoms will disappear with time.

27. A 60-year-old Asian woman is admitted to a clinic with bloody stools three to four times per day and abdominal cramps 8 weeks ago. The patient history is heart failure New York Heat Association class III and hypertension. Her current medications are ramipril 10 mg daily, carvedilol 12.5 mg twice daily, and spironolactone 25 mg daily. A colonoscopy reveals active mild to moderate ulcerative colitis affecting her descending colon and rectal area. What drug will be the most appropriate for the patient's symptoms?

    1. Mesalamine enema 1000 mg rectally once daily.

    2. Budesonide 9 mg per day orally.

    3. Infliximab 5 mg/kg intravenously (IV).

    4. Natalizumab 300 mg IV.

28. A 44-year-old man with a history of alcoholic liver cirrhosis (Child–Pugh class C) is admitted to the emergency department with nausea, abdominal pain, and fever. Physical exam revealed distended abdomen with shifting dullness, a positive fluid wave, and the presence of diffuse rebound tenderness. His current medications include furosemide 80 mg twice daily and spironolactone 200 mg once daily. A paracentesis exam revealed turbid ascites fluid, which was sent for culture. Laboratory analysis for the fluid reveals albumin concentration of 0.9 g/dL and the presence of 1×10^3 white blood cells (48% polymorphonuclear neutrophils). Serum laboratory studies reveal serum creatinine 1.4 mg/dL, blood urea nitrogen 38 mg/dL, aspartate aminotransferase 70 international units/mL, alanine aminotransferase 30 international units/mL, serum albumin 2.5 mg/dL, and total bilirubin 3.2 mg/dL. What is the best management for the patient's symptoms?

    1. Initiate oral trimethoprim/sulfamethazine double strength.

    2. Initiate albumin and wait the culture result.

    3. Initiate intravenous (IV) vancomycin plus gentamycin.

    4. Initiate IV ceftriaxone plus albumin therapy.

29. A 30-year-old African American woman with a history of alcoholic liver cirrhosis (Child–Pugh class B) is admitted with a history of 3 days of confusion, disorientation, lethargy, and asterixis. On exam, she is afebrile, with abdominal tenderness, and dry mucous membranes. A paracentesis is performed and is negative for infection. Which recommendations are best for treating a patient with hepatic encephalopathy?

    1. Initiate lactulose 30 mL orally every 2 hours.

    2. Initiate rifaximin 600 mg orally once daily.

    3. Initiate cefotaxime 1 g intravenously once daily.

    4. Initiate polyethylene glycol 3350 15 g twice daily.

30. A 73-year-old woman with a history of hepatic cirrhosis secondary to alcohol abuse and ascites is admitted to the intensive care unit. On exam, the laboratory tests reveal serum creatinine is 2 mg/dL, blood urea nitrogen is 40 mg/dL, no current nephrotoxins, and absence of parenchymal kidney disease. There is no improvement in serum creatinine after withdrawal and administration of albumin, and a renal ultrasound is normal. Which treatment is best for the patient's symptoms?

    1. Stop albumin and initiate octreotide.

    2. Initiate a combination with albumin and octreotide 200 mcg subcutaneously three times daily.

    3. Initiate albumin with furosemide.

    4. Initiate pentoxifylline plus prednisolone.

31. A 55-year-old Asian woman with a history of hepatic cirrhosis, hepatic encephalopathy, and ascites presents to the clinic for follow-up. On exam, the laboratory tests reveal ascetic fluid protein concentration is 1.3 g/dL, serum creatinine is 2 mg/dL, blood urea nitrogen is 40 mg/dL, sodium is 125 mg/dL, prothrombin time is 5 seconds, and bilirubin is 3.5 mg/dL. There is no evidence for gastrointestinal bleeding. The nurse practitioner is concerned that the patient may have spontaneous bacterial peritonitis (SBP). What is the best drug for the prevention of SBP?

    1. Albumin 1.5 g/kg plus cefotaxime 2 g twice daily.

    2. Ceftriaxone 2 g intravenously once daily.

    3. Trimethoprim/sulfamethazine double strength for 5 days/week.

    4. Propranolol 50 mg twice daily.

32. A 66-year-old white man is admitted to the hospital with a 2-week history of protuberant abdomen, shifting dullness, abdominal pain, and fluid wave. The patient has a history of alcohol abuse of more than 15 years. The paracentesis for the ascites is done, and the result reveals serum-ascites albumin gradient 1.3. He currently takes naproxen 750 mg for occasional neck pain. The nurse practitioner advises him to stop drinking alcohol and taking naproxen immediately. Which next management is the best for this patient?

    1. Initiate furosemide 40 mg and spironolactone 100 mg daily.

    2. Initiate nadolol.

    3. Initiate albumin and cefotaxime 2 g intravenously.

    4. Initiate sulfamethazine/trimethoprim double strength.

33. A 40-year-old man with a history of intravenous drug abuse is evaluated in the clinic for chronic hepatitis B virus (HBV) infection. Although he received the diagnosis 7 months ago, he has not been treated. Laboratory values reported today include HBsAg positive, HBeAg positive, aspartate aminotransferase 600 international units/mL, alanine aminotransferase 900 international units/mL, HBV DNA is 10,000 international units/mL, serum creatinine 0.9 mg/dL, international normalized ratio 1.4, and albumin 4 g/dL. He has no evidence of ascites or encephalopathy. A liver biopsy reveals severe necroinflammation and fibrosis. Resistance testing reveals the presence of the *YMDD* mutation. What is the best course of action?

    1. Initiate pegylated interferon alfa-2a plus ribavirin.

    2. Withhold drug therapy and recheck HBV DNA in another 6 months.

    3. Initiate tenofovir 300 mg/day.

    4. Initiate lamivudine 100 mg/day.

34. A 33-year-old Hispanic woman (height 72 inches and weight 75 kg) is seen today for a new diagnosis of chronic hepatitis C virus (HCV) genotype 1a. Laboratory values reveal aspartate aminotransferase 400 international units/mL, alanine aminotransferase 450 international units/mL, HCV RNA 850,000 international units/mL, serum creatinine 1.2 mg/dL, hemoglobin 12.5 g/dL, and white blood cells 12×10^3 cells/mm^3. A liver biopsy reveals fibrosis. Further testing reveals the presence of the NS3Q80K polymorphism. Which option is best for the treatment of chronic HCV infection?

    1. Withhold therapy and wait 8 weeks.

    2. Initiate sofosbuvir and simeprevir.

    3. Initiate sofosbuvir and ledipasvir.

    4. Initiate pegylated interferon, ribavirin, and sofosbuvir.

35. A 25-year-old pregnant woman in her first trimester is seen in the emergency department. The patient has a 1-week history of nausea, vomiting, and drowsiness. On exam, her blood pressure is 135/80 mmHg and heart rate is 60 beats/min. The patient denies any alcohol or drug abuse. She is healthy and does not take any medication except folic acid 5 mg one tablet daily. Which treatment is best for this patient?

    1. Doxylamine.

    2. Aprepitant.

    3. Haloperidol.

    4. Ondansetron.

36. A 63-year-old woman with an 8-year history of diabetes type 2 and hypertension is seen in the hospital for follow-up. Her laboratory evaluation reveals blood pressure 138/78 mmHg, A1c 7.5, and heart rate 65 beats/min. Her current medications are lisinopril 10 mg daily, insulin glargine 9 units before bed, and glulisine 4 units three times daily. She suffers from nausea, vomiting, and abdominal pain. Which treatment is best for the patient's symptoms?

    1. Ondansetron.

    2. Metoclopramide.

    3. Meclizine.

    4. Scopolamine.

37. A 72-year-old white man is seen in the emergency department with a 5-day history of nausea, vomiting, abdominal pain, and jaundice. His past medical history includes chronic angina, hypertension, and epilepsy. His current medications are ramipril 20 mg twice daily, metoprolol succinate 100 mg twice daily, aspirin 81 mg once daily, nitroglycerin sublingual as needed, and valproic acid 50 mg twice daily. Abdominal ultrasonography has shown necrosis, hemorrhage at the pancreas, pseudocysts, and no gallstones were found. He denies any alcohol or drug abuse. Which drug can cause acute pancreatitis?

    1. Aspirin.

    2. Valproic acid.

    3. Ramipril.

    4. Metoprolol succinate.

38. A 48-year-old woman with a history of chronic alcohol abuse for 20 years is evaluated in the clinic for chronic pancreatitis. For the past month and half she has noticed an increase in the frequency of bowel movements to four or five times per day. She describes her stool as foul smelling and slimy. During this time, she had a 13-kg weight loss and has abdominal cramps. Quantification of fecal fat indicates an excretion of 20 g every 24 hours. Her albumin is 2.2 mg/dL, and her weight is 59 kg. She currently takes morphine controlled-release 45 mg twice daily and oxycodone 5 mg every 4 to 6 hours as needed. What is the best course of action for this patient?

    1. Initiate pancrelipase 30,000 units per meal.

    2. Add multivitamins to her regimen.

    3. Initiate dronabinol to improve appetite.

    4. Increase morphine controlled-release to 60 mg twice daily.

39. A 53-year-old Hispanic man (height 77 inches, weight 60 kg) is seen in the clinic for evaluation of chronic pancreatitis. He has a 25-year history of alcohol abuse and a 10-year history of marijuana abuse. For 3 months, he noticed an increase in frequency of bowel movements, and he describes his stool as foul smelling and slimy. He has had an unintentional 15-kg weight loss and has suffered from abdominal pain. On exam today, his abdominal pain is improved, and he has a 5-kg weight gain. He currently takes pancrelipase 35,000 units per meal, morphine controlled-release 60 mg twice daily, and oxycodone 5 to 10 mg every 4 to 6 hours as needed. Which answer is incorrect about pancrelipase?

    1. Causes fibrosing colonopathy.

    2. Contraindicates if pork allergy is present.

    3. Causes Hyperuricosuria and hyperuricemia.

    4. Pregnancy category B.

40. The patient is a 28-year-old woman who is 17 weeks' pregnant and presents with mild myalgias; a low-grade fever (temperature is 99.9°F); three or four loose, watery bowel movements; and two episodes of vomiting during the past 24 hours. She reports that her 2-year-old daughter and several children in the kindergarten had the same symptoms 4 days ago. The result of a rapid influenza test is negative; her white blood cell count is 8×10^3 cells/mm^3 and serum creatinine is 0.9 mg/dL. She reports no known drug allergies. She is given a diagnosis of a presumed viral gastroenteritis. What is the best treatment for this patient's diarrhea?

    1. Pyridoxine.

    2. Loperamide.

    3. Lactase.

    4. Bismuth subsalicylate.

41. A 44-year-old American African man (height 73 inches and weight 95 kg) presents to the clinic with a history of diabetes type 2, hypertension, and obesity. The patient's medications are metformin 1000 mg twice daily, captopril 50 mg twice daily, orlistat 120 mg three times daily, and mineral supplements. He reports an increase in stool output to four or five times per day for the past 2 weeks. He describes his stool as oily and loose and he reports flatulence. Which drug causes the patient's symptoms?

    1. Orlistat.

    2. Metformin.

    3. Mineral supplements.

    4. Captopril.

42. A 35-year-old woman has had intermittent crampy abdominal pain for 3 to 5 days per week, bloating, and reduced frequency of bowel movement for the past 7 months. Before this, she had a bowel movement once daily, but now, she reports a bowel movement every 2 to 3 days. She reports that the symptoms are not related to a specific food. The result of extensive diagnostic workup is negative, and she is given a diagnosis of irritable bowel syndrome with constipation. Which therapeutic intervention is best for this patient?

    1. Amitriptyline 50 mg/day.

    2. VSL #3 probiotics three capsules daily.

    3. Tegaserod 6 mg twice daily.

    4. Lubiprostone 8 mg twice daily.

43. A 27-year-old woman who is 20 weeks' pregnant came to the medical floor with a 2-week history of infrequent passage of stool, hard stool, and abdominal pain. The patient's only history is gestational diabetes; she currently takes insulin detemir. She reports no known allergies. The patient is diagnosed with constipation. Which drug regimen is best for the patient's symptoms?

    1. Senna.

    2. Polyethylene glycol.

    3. Linaclotide.

    4. Lubiprostone.

44. The patient is a 33-year-old woman seen on the medical floor with a 2-month history of bloating, abdominal cramps, and watery stool. The result of extensive diagnostic workup is negative. She is given a diagnosis of irritable bowel syndrome-diarrhea predominant (IBS-D). What is the best drug therapy for the patient's symptoms?

    1. Metronidazole.

    2. Linaclotide.

    3. Alosetron.

    4. Lubiprostone.

45. The patient is a 45-year-old woman with no significant medical history. She presents to the emergency department with fever and severe right lower quadrant pain. The pain has been dull for the last 3 days, but it suddenly becomes severe while she is in the emergency department. Her oral temperature is 102°F and she has rebound tenderness on abdominal exam. She is taken to surgery immediately, where a perforated appendix is diagnosed and repaired. Which antibiotic the best is for follow-up?

    1. No antibiotics are need after surgical repair of a perforated appendix.

    2. Ceftriaxone 1 g intravenously (IV) plus metronidazole 500 mg IV every 8 hours.

    3. Vancomycin 1 g IV every 12 hours plus metronidazole 500 mg IV every 8 hours.

    4. Cefazolin 1 g IV every 8 hours plus ciprofloxacin 400 mg IV every 12 hours.

46. A 64-year-old man presents to the emergency department with a 3-day history of redness and swelling of his upper right extremity. He scraped his arm while he was cleaning some brush in his yard. Although the scratch was initially healing, the area around the injury has become more painful and redness appears to be spreading. His medical history includes osteoarthritis, hypertension, and gastroesophageal reflux. His medications are omeprazole 20 mg once daily, captopril 50 mg once daily, and acetaminophen 500 mg oral tablet as needed. He is hospitalized and sent home after a few days with a prescription for oral clindamycin. Two weeks after the completion of his therapy, he has watery diarrhea and goes to the emergency department. The laboratory test revealed a positive *Clostridium difficile* result, white blood cells 25,000 cells/mm³, and serum creatinine 1.9 mg/dL. Which therapeutic drug regimen is the best for the patient's symptoms?

    1. Vancomycin 125 mg orally four times daily for 10 days.

    2. Metronidazole 500 mg orally three times daily for 5 days.

    3. Rifaximin 400 mg orally twice daily for 7 days.

    4. Fidaxomicin 200 mg orally twice daily for 14 days.

47. The patient is a 63-year-old African American woman who presents to the medical floor with a 3-day history of abdominal pain and watery diarrhea. Her medical history is positive for hypertension, gastroesophageal reflux, and osteoarthritis. She currently takes ramipril 20 mg orally once daily, pantoprazole 40 mg orally once daily, acetaminophen 500 mg orally twice daily, and calcium supplements. She reports no known drug allergies; she denies any alcohol or drug abuse history. Her laboratory tests reveal albumin 2.8 g/dL, white blood cell 30 × 10³ cells/mm³, and serum creatinine 1.7 mg/dL

(the baseline is 0.9 mg/dL). Which drug can cause the patient's symptoms?

    1. Calcium supplement.

    2. Acetaminophen.

    3. Pantoprazole.

    4. Ramipril.

48. A 47-year-old white woman is seen in the clinic for follow-up. Her medical history includes myocardial infarction 3 years ago, chronic angina, and peptic ulcer 2 years ago. Her medications are aspirin 81 mg once daily, clopidogrel 75 mg once daily, atenolol 50 mg twice daily, nitroglycerin sublingual as needed, and lansoprazole 15 mg twice daily. The laboratory results show sodium 140 mEq/L, potassium 3 mEq/L, and magnesium 1.2 mEq/L (baseline 1.9 mEq/mL). She was given 60 mEq of potassium intravenously, but 2 hours later the concentration of potassium and magnesium are still low. Which drug can cause hypomagnesemia?

    1. Lansoprazole.

    2. Aspirin.

    3. Clopidogrel.

    4. Nitroglycerin.

49. The patient is a 47-year-old Asian woman with a history of hepatitis B virus infection. She presents to the clinic to receive her chemotherapy dose for the breast cancer. Her laboratory tests reveal she is HBsAb positive, HBsAg negative, HBcAb positive, and HBeAg negative. Which of the following is the best option for this patient?

    1. Lamivudine daily during chemotherapy.

    2. Adefovir daily during chemotherapy.

    3. Lamivudine until 6 months' post chemotherapy.

    4. Entecavir daily until 6 months' post chemotherapy.

50. A 30-year-old white man presents to the medical floor with a 4-week history of abdominal tenderness, abdominal pain, and four to five bloody stools per day. His medical history is significant for major depression, which is treated with citalopram 20 mg daily. Colonoscopy reveals superficial ulceration and a visibly variable mucosa consistent with ulcerative colitis. The ulceration is continuous and extends distantly to the splenic flexure. No inflammation was seen in the descending or sigmoid colon. Which drug therapy would be best to initiate with this patient?

    1. Mesalamine enema 1 g four times daily.

    2. Mesalamine 1.6 orally three times daily.

    3. Methyl prednisone 125 mg daily.

    4. Azathioprine 75 mg orally one daily.

51. You are rounding with the inpatient teaching service and a nurse asks your opinion on the utility of pancreatic enzymes for patient with pancreatitis. Which statement would be appropriate regarding the usage of pancreatic enzyme supplementation?

    1. Recommended to control steatorrhea in patients with chronic pancreatitis.

    2. Improve the constipation symptoms for patient with chronic pancreatitis.

    3. Decrease the severity of disease for patients with acute pancreatitis.

    4. Decrease the frequency of the acute pancreatic exacerbations.

52. A 62-year-old woman with a history of hepatitis C cirrhosis (Child–Pugh class C) is admitted to the clinic for abdominal pain, jaundice, fever, chills, and confusion. On exam, there is abdominal distension that is painful on palpitation, oral temperature is 104°F, heart rate is 95 beats/min, and respiratory rate is 20 breaths/min. Abdominal ultrasonography is positive for ascites. Her laboratory results show white blood cells 19×10^3 cells/mm³, serum creatinine 0.8 mg/dL, ammonia level 65 mcg/dL, ascetic fluid positive for protein of 0.9 g/dL, and white blood cell count 3.8×10^3 cells/mm³ with 84% neutrophils. The cultures are pending. Which therapy would be best for this patient?

    1. Cefotaxime 1 g intravenously (IV) for 5 days and albumin IV on days 1 and 3.

    2. Trimethoprim/sulfamethazine IV for 5 days.

    3. Moxifloxacin 750 orally for 5 days and albumin IV on days 1 and 3.

    4. Vancomycin 1 g IV every 12 hours for 5 days.

53. A 45-year-old white man with a new diagnosis of cirrhosis (Child–Pugh class B) secondary to alcohol abuse presents to the medical floor for consultation. He was recently discharged from the hospital in which he completed a course therapy of spontaneous bacterial peritonitis. Abdominal ultrasonography reveals that he is positive for ascites, and the esophagogastroduodenoscopy reveals that there are no shown varices. On physical exam, the patient is positive for abdominal distention, blood pressure is 135/75 mmHg, and heart rate is 70 beats/min. The patient denies any shortness of breath, edema, or any mental changes. His laboratory results are serum creatinine 1.1 mg/dL, albumin 4.2 g/dL, and the serum ascites albumin gradient is 1.3. What medications should be initiated for this patient?

    1. Nadolol 20 mg daily.

    2. Furosemide 40 mg daily and spironolactone 100 mg daily.

    3. Furosemide 40 mg daily and spironolactone 100 mg daily and nadolol 20 mg daily.

    4. Furosemide 40 mg daily and spironolactone 100 mg daily and norfloxacin 400 mg daily.

54. A 27-year-old Hispanic woman is admitted to the clinic with concerns of a decreasing number of bowel movements. She used to go to the bathroom every day, but now she goes every 3 days. The patient has flatulence, and she describes the stool as hard. Her medical history includes osteoarthritis and hypothyroidism. She currently takes levothyroxine 90 mcg orally and alendronate 70 mg/week. What is the best therapy for the constipation?

    1. Psyllium 1 g teaspoonful orally three times daily.

    2. Methylnaltrexone 450 mg orally once daily.

    3. Lactulose 30 mg orally three times daily.

    4. Plecanatide 3 mg orally once daily.

55. A 42-year-old Hispanic man with a 2-month history of sore throat, metallic acid taste, epigastric pain, and stomach discomfort presents to the hospital. After the exam, he is diagnosed with gastroesophageal reflux disease and prescribed omeprazole 40 mg orally once daily. Today, the patient returns to his nurse practitioner with complaints of nighttime awakenings and feeling nauseous in the morning. Which treatment adjustment would be most appropriate to manage his symptoms?

    1. Change omeprazole to ranitidine 150 mg orally once daily.

    2. Change omeprazole to aluminum peroxide effervescence.

    3. Increase the omeprazole dose to 40 mg twice daily.

    4. Add famotidine 40 mg at bedtime to his regimen.

56. A 53-year-old woman presents to the clinic for consultation. Her medical history includes liver cirrhosis (Child–Pugh class B) secondary to alcohol abuse. The abdominal ultrasonography shows no ascites symptoms, but the esophagogastroduodenoscopy reveals medium to large esophageal varices without any signs of gastroesophageal bleeding. Which therapy is the best for this patient?

    1. Nadolol 40 mg orally once daily.

    2. Metoprolol 25 mg orally twice daily.

    3. Isosorbide mononitrate 60 mg daily.

    4. Pantoprazole 40 mg orally once daily.

57. A 65-year-old man comes with his wife to the clinic for follow-up. His medical history is positive for mild symptoms of Alzheimer disease. He complains of a sore throat and heartburn. The laboratory tests reveal serum creatinine 0.9 mg/dL, sodium 135 mEq/mL, and potassium 4 mEq/mL. He currently takes donepezil 5 mg daily. The patient has tried over-the-counter ranitidine 75 mg orally once daily, but he experienced only partial relief. You diagnose him with gastroesophageal reflux disease. Which drug therapy is the best for this patient?

    1. Metoclopramide 50 mg orally three times daily.

    2. Erythromycin 140 g orally three times daily.

    3. Increase ranitidine dose to 150 orally twice daily.

    4. Lansoprazole 30 mg orally once daily.

58. The patient is a 32-year-old African American man (height 65 inches, weight 105 kg) who presents to the emergency department with diffuse abdominal pain for the past 3 days. It has increased in intensity over the past 7 hours. He drinks about 15 beers daily. His vital signs include blood pressure 160/90 mmHg, respiratory rate 22 breaths/min, and heart rate 95 beats/min. His laboratory tests reveal serum creatinine is 1.8 mg/dL, blood glucose is 250 mg/dL, amylase is 400 international units/L, and lipase is 250 international units/L. What is the best intervention for acute pancreatitis?

    1. Hydromorphone 0.2 mg intravenously (IV) every 4 hours as needed.

    2. Octreotide 100 mcg subcutaneously every 8 hours.

    3. Parenteral nutrition to provide 2500 kcal/day.

    4. Imipenem 500 mg IV every 6 hours.

59. A 73-year-old white woman presents to the emergency department with an altered mental status and complains of diffuse pain. Her medical history includes hypertension, hyperlipidemia, alcoholic liver cirrhosis, and a gastrointestinal (GI) bleed 1 year ago. The emergency department intern reports that he wants to avoid opioids because of her altered mental status and avoid acetaminophen because of her liver disease. Moreover, the intern is concerned about using nonsteroidal antiinflammatory drugs (NSAIDs) because of the patient's history of GI bleeding. Which NSAIDs should be avoided in this patient?

    1. Ketorolac.

    2. Ibuprofen.

    3. Naproxen.

    4. Diclofenac.

60. A 53-year-old Asian man with a 25-year history of alcohol abuse and a 10-year history of drug abuse presents to the clinic complaining of oily stool and weight loss. His medical history includes chronic pancreatitis. Which condition is most likely present?

    1. Gastric ulcer.

    2. Steatorrhea.

    3. Dumping syndrome.

    4. Lactulose intolerance.

61. A 46-year-old man presents to the emergency department with several symptoms including abdominal pain, diarrhea, fatigue, and weight loss. His medical history is positive for Crohn disease with multiple small and large bowel resection surgeries. The surgical team is consulted and determines another intestinal resection surgery is needed. The patient tolerates surgery without any complications. He is transferred to the intensive care unit immediately. Parenteral nutrition is ordered given the nutritional requirements for the patient with short-bowel syndrome. Which supplement is not necessary for this patient?

    1. Vitamin K.

    2. Vitamin C.

    3. Omega-3 fatty acids.

    4. Vitamin E.

62. A 33-year-old woman presents to the hospital with a 2-week history of abdominal cramps that become worse after eating. An ultrasonography reveals a 2.5-cm gastric ulcer; there is no evidence of gastric bleeding. What is the preferred noninvasive test to confirm *Helicobacter pylori* eradication?

    1. Urea breath test.

    2. A serological antibodies detection test.

    3. A stool antigen test.

    4. A whole-blood antibody-detection test.

63. A 53-year-old woman comes the emergency department with pyrosis, regurgitation, and acid metallic taste in her mouth. After the exam, the patient is diagnosed with gastroesophageal reflux disease. The patient takes ibuprofen for neck pain, and the nurse practitioner prescribes omeprazole 40 mg orally once daily. What is the most important education information that should be provided to the patient?

    1. Take omeprazole at the same time as the nonsteroidal antiinflammatory drugs.

    2. Take omeprazole 30 to 60 minutes before breakfast.

    3. Take omeprazole at the bedtime.

    4. Take omeprazole after breakfast.

64. The patient is a 63-year-old woman admitted to the intensive care unit with acute respiratory failure and thrombocytopenia. She has a high risk for gastric bleeding because of stress-related mucosal disease. Which is the best proton-pump inhibitor therapy for gastric bleeding prophylaxis?

    1. Omeprazole.

    2. Lansoprazole.

    3. Pantoprazole.

    4. Esomeprazole.

65. A 73-year-old white man comes to the clinic with melena and lightheadedness. His medical history includes a low-dose aspirin for cardiovascular prophylaxis. Physical exam reveals normal blood pressure (135/80 mmHg) and heart rate (75 beats/min) without any signs of orthostatic changes. Melena is confirmed on rectal exam. Endoscopy evaluation reveals a 4.5-cm duodenal ulcer with a clear base. Which one of the following should be performed now?

    1. Perform a test to exclude *Helicobacter pylori* and continue with a high dose of proton-pump inhibitor therapy.

    2. Treat with misoprostol.

    3. Treat empirically with antibiotics for *H. pylori*.

    4. Obtain serum gastrin level to exclude Zollinger–Ellison syndrome.

1. Answer: 2

Rationale: This patient complained of signs of dysphagia, an alarming symptom associated with more complicated gastroesophageal reflux disease (GERD). The patient has tried a histamine 2 receptor antagonist with minimal relief. The patient is older than 45 years old, which increases his risk of developing gastric ulcers, so he should be referred for endoscopic evaluation. This will be not effective; therefore answer 1 is incorrect. Amlodipine (answer 3) reduce lower esophageal sphincter tone; therefore it is an appropriate recommendation for reducing GERD symptoms. This should be considered after invasive testing is performed. However, using proton-pump inhibitors (answer 4) will be appropriate after the evaluation. A twice daily dose is not as essential as initial dosing.

2. Answer: 1

Rationale: The patient complained of stress-related mucosal disease (SRMD), which has developed in critically ill patients and could lead to upper gastrointestinal bleeding. Therapy initiation to prevent SRMD is based on the presence of risk factors. The patient's risk factors are mechanical ventilation and coagulopathy; therefore she would meet the criteria for initiation of pharmacological therapy. Pantoprazole (answer 1) would be the best choice because it does not require renal adjustment. Cimetidine (answer 2) is suitable for SRMD prevention because it carries the U.S. Food and Drug Administration–approved indication, but the dosing provided is incorrect. The approved dose of cimetidine is 50 mg/hr. Cimetidine would be dose adjusted for the patient's creatinine clearance. Sucralfate (answer 3) is not the best choice because of the need for multiple dosing daily and the risk of aluminum accumulation for patients suffering from kidney disease. Magnesium hydroxide (answer 4) is not as effective as histamine 2 receptor antagonists and proton-pump inhibitors. Also, it can lead to electrolyte accumulation in a patient with a kidney injury.

3. Answer: 3

Rationale: Patients on long-term nonsteroidal antiinflammatory drug therapy may development of gastrointestinal (GI) toxicity; therefore assessment of patients and drug-related factors are necessary. This patient is considered to be at high risk of a cardiovascular event because she uses a low-dose aspirin. A GI agent should be included at the lowest effective therapeutic dose to avoid GI toxicity. Because of this, indomethacin (answer 1), piroxicam (answer 2) and celecoxib (answer 4) are not recommended. Indomethacin and piroxicam actually may increase the GI complication. Misoprostol is effective, but it is associated with a high incidence of diarrhea and abdominal pain.

4. Answer: 1

Rationale: This patient presents with acute constipation, and the contributing factors include the use of iron supplement and oxycodone without using a drug regimen for constipation prevention. Therapy should be instituted to provide a quick onset to initiate bowel movement and provide symptomatic relief. Bisacodyl suppositories (answer 1) can provide a rapid stimulation of the lower intestine tract without the risk of electrolyte absorption. The patient's creatinine clearance is low, so it will be the best choice for this case. Methylnaltrexone (answer 2) is indicated for opioid-induced constipation, and it would generally not be used as a first-line agent. The added cost for methylnaltrexone injection is higher than the traditional laxatives; therefore it is not the best drug regimen. Psyllium or inulin (answer 3) is a bulk-forming laxative that would not treat acute constipation. Linaclotide (answer 4) is approved by the U.S. Food and Drug Administration for inflammatory bowel syndrome treatment; therefore this answer is not suitable for this patient.

5. Answer: 1

Rationale: The patient presents with signs and symptoms of nonsteroidal antiinflammatory drug (NSAID)-induced upper gastrointestinal (GI) bleeding. She has several factors for NSAID-induced upper GI bleeding including age older than 60 years old, use of high-dose aspirin, and long duration of naproxen use. According to the recommendations of nonvariceal bleeding, the patient should receive intravenous proton-pump inhibitors (PPIs) by bolus, then subsequent continuous infusion for 72 hours; therefore answer 1 is the best recommendation for this patient. A histamine 2 receptor antagonist (answer 2) is less efficacious for the treatment and prevention of rebleeding for NSAID-induced ulcers. Oral PPIs (answer 3) are effective in preventing and healing NSAID-induced ulcer; however, the dose of lansoprazole is inadequate for the treatment of this patient. Oral PPIs should be used at an appropriate dose after finishing intravenous therapy for at least 8 weeks. Antacids (answer 4) are not effective for treatment of NSAID-induced ulcer.

6. Answer: 2

Rationale: This patient complains of pyelonephritis symptoms associated with nausea and vomiting. The nurse practitioner will prescribe the appropriate antibiotic therapy to treat the infection. However, the patient will need symptomatic relief until the antibiotics take effect. Diphenhydramine (answer 1) is effective for nausea associated with motion sickness, but it has no effect on severe vomiting cases. Ondansetron (answer 2) is a serotonin antagonist that is effective in the treatment of vomiting and nausea caused by a variety of medical conditions. Despite its effect on serotonin, it does not cause any drug interaction with the patient's sertraline dose. Haloperidol (answer 3) is not appropriate for this patient because of his cardiovascular history. Haloperidol can increase the risk of QTc prolongation and extrapyramidal adverse effect. Prochlorperazine (answer 4) is commonly used to treat vomiting symptoms, but the oral doses are not appropriate for a patient who suffers from severe vomiting. Moreover, prochlorperazine is a dopamine antagonist, and the patient is receiving a high dose of risperidone. Therefore the combination can lead to the development of extrapyramidal symptoms and QTc prolongation.

7. Answer: 3

Rationale: The patient's symptoms can be classified in the mild to moderate active disease category. Mesalamine (answer 3) is the first-line therapy for an active extensive disease at a dose equivalent of 4.8 g/day. Infliximab (answer 1) is not appropriate for this patient; using biological agents is required for moderate to severe active diseases. Moreover, infliximab has a long-term action, which that is why it can be used in a maintenance drug regimen. Hydrocortisone enema (answer 2) would be appropriate for patients with disease distal to the splenic flexure. Sulfasalazine tablets (answer 4) would be appropriate for this case, but the patient has reported an allergy to "sulfa-containing medication"; therefore sulfasalazine is incorrect.

8. Answer: 1

Rationale: Infliximab is an appropriate agent for treatment of fistulizing Crohn disease. Tumor necrosis factor agents can reactivate latent infections such as tuberculosis. Therefore patients should perform the purified protein derivative or QuantiFERON-TB test to rule out underlying tuberculosis infection before drug initiation. However, infliximab is associated with exacerbation of underlying heart failure and is contraindicated in patients with New York Heart Association class III or IV disease. A baseline echocardiogram is not necessary to assess the cardiac function for a healthy patient who does not complain of any clinical signs of the heart failure.

Therefore, answer 2 is incorrect. Although infliximab therapy is associated with infusion-related reaction, administering a test dose is not routinely recommended, so answer 3 is incorrect. The patient does not have any clinical signs of hepatitis B so liver function tests (answer 4) are not recommended.

9. Answer: 1

Rationale: Nonselective beta-blockers are appropriate as first-line therapy for large varices and liver cirrhosis. The therapy goal is to achieve a heart rate of 55 beats/min or a 25% reduction from the baseline. The patient seems to be tolerating the propranolol dose; therefore it is recommended to increase the propranolol dose to 20 mg three times per day (answer 1). Changing nonselective beta-blockers to a cardioselective agent (answer 2) is not preferred because propranolol can prevent splanchnic vasodilatation. Adding isosorbide dinitrate (answer 3) can lead to portal hypotension; however, nitrates have not been shown to improve the mortality rate. The patient did not achieve the therapy goal, and he should be observed to reassess the need for further dose adjustment; therefore answer 4 is incorrect.

10. Answer: 4

Rationale: Hepatitis C virus (HCV) genotype 2 responds well to the combination of sofosbuvir and ribavirin. The patient does not appear to have any symptoms consistent with extrahepatic manifestations of HCV (answer 1) like glomerulonephritis or rheumatological disorders. Although this patient appears to be responding to the treatment, as indicated by a reduction of aminotransferases and HCV RNA, the earliest that HCV RNA should be evaluated is 4 weeks, not 2 weeks (answer 2). The patient does not appear to have any adverse effect to sofosbuvir (answer 3). The patient has evidence of hemolysis, scleral icterus, rapid decline in hematocrit, and fatigue. These symptoms represent hemolytic anemia secondary to ribavirin (answer 4), which commonly occur in the first 2 weeks of the therapy.

11. Answer: 3

Rationale: Postexposure therapy for hepatitis A virus (HAV) can be offered to restaurant patrons if a food handler is documented to have HAV infection. The most effective therapies for the postexposure prophylaxis are administration of the HAV vaccine or immune globulin. The period of administration should be within 14 days of exposure. The patient does not meet the criteria because his exposure period was more than 14 days; therefore answers 1 and 2 are incorrect. He should be observed for signs and symptoms of active disease (answer 3). The combination of HAV vaccine and immune globulin for postexposure prophylaxis is unnecessary.

12. Answer: 1

Rationale: The patient needs a postexposure therapy because hepatitis A virus (HAV) infection could be transmitted by the contaminated food, and he was in close contact with a documented infected person. The most effective therapy for post-exposure HAV infection is HAV vaccine within 14 days from the exposure (answer 1). The patient should not wait more than 14 days because the virus incubation occurs between 14 and 50 days (answer 2). Answer 3 is incorrect because the son was in close contact with a colleague that has a documented HAV infection. It is unethical behavior when the health care member does not respond to the patient's consultation (answer 4).

13. Answer: 4

Rationale: The patient presents with elevated aminotransferases, consistent with alcoholic hepatitis. The prognosis of alcoholic hepatitis can be evaluated by the Maddrey discriminant function (MDF) score, calculated as $4.6 \times$ (patient's PT-control PT) + total bilirubin (milligrams per deciliter), where PT is prothrombin time. Patients who scored greater than 32 are believed to have a poor prognosis. This patient's MDF score is 42.5. Octreotide (answer 1) would be indicated for acute variceal bleeding. Prednisone 40 mg is indicated for treatment of alcoholic hepatitis, but the patient suffers from osteoporosis so corticosteroids would be contraindicated. Prednisone can increase the risk of bone fractures; therefore answer 2 is incorrect. Midodrine (answer 3) would be indicated for spontaneous bacterial hepatitis. Pentoxifylline (answer 4) is the best therapy for this patient because it can be used when prednisone is contraindicated. Also, pentoxifylline has shown to lower hepatic mortality by 14% compared with placebo.

14. Answer: 3

Rationale: The patient has a history of alcohol abuse for many years, and his exams have revealed an elevation of aminotransferase enzymes. The patient would suffer from alcoholic hepatitis. The prognosis of alcoholic hepatitis can be evaluated by the Maddrey discriminant function (MDF) score, which is calculated as $4.6 \times$ (patient's PT–control PT) + total bilirubin, where PT is prothrombin time. Patients who score more than 32 are believed to have a poor prognosis. This patient's MDF score is 52.9, therefore, he would qualify for treatment with 4 weeks of prednisone 40 mg daily follwer by a 2-week taper. Naproxen (answer 1) is not recommended for treatment of alcoholic hepatitis. In addition, nonsteroidal antiinflammatory drugs can lead to acute kidney injury in patients with liver disease. Octreotide (answer 2) is indicated for treatment of acute variceal bleeding, and the patient

has no variceal bleeding. Prednisone (answer 3) shows a 30% decrease in the risk ratio of short-term death, therefore, it is the correct answer. Ribavirin (answer 4) is indicated for treatment of hepatitis C virus, and this patient has no history of hepatic virus infection.

15. Answer: 3

Rationale: The patient presents with signs and symptoms consistent with *Helicobacter pylori*–induced upper gastrointestinal (GI) bleeding. According to the consensus recommendation for nonvariceal bleeding, he should receive an intravenous (IV) proton-pump inhibitor (PPI) bolus, followed by subsequent continuous infusion for 72 hours (answer 3). Sucralfate (answer 1) has minimal efficacy in the setting of acute GI bleeding. Oral omeprazole (answer 2) is effective in preventing and healing the GI ulcer. Oral PPIs should be used at an appropriate dose after finishing the intravenous therapy. Lansoprazole, amoxicillin, and clarithromycin (answer 4) are the triple therapy used in treatment of *H. pylori*. However, the patient should take the IV PPIs first.

16. Answer: 1

Rationale: The patient presents with symptoms of gastroesophageal reflux disease (GERD). She has tried antacids but had no relief. She then tried a histamine 2 receptor antagonist (H_2RA) with minimal relief. The best therapy for her is starting a treatment with proton-pump inhibitors for at least 4 weeks if no erosive esophagitis is present (answer 1). The patient does not complain of any other symptoms such as difficulty with swallowing, bleeding, or weight loss; therefore she does not need endoscopic intervention (answer 2). Changing ranitidine to another H_2RA like cimetidine is unnecessary for this patient (answer 3). The patient has a history of stroke 1 year ago and takes aspirin 81 mg as secondary prevention. We cannot advise her to stop using aspirin because it will increase the risk of mortality (answer 4).

17. Answer: 4

Rationale: Patients receiving proton-pump inhibitor (PPI) therapy for gastroesophageal reflux disease (GERD) should be reassessed for efficacy. This patient has partial improvement but is still not optimally controlled despite adherence and lifestyle modification. Adding metoclopramide (answer 1) would be inappropriate because there is no evidence for gastrointestinal dysmotility. Switching to another PPI such as pantoprazole (answer 2) could be tried when lansoprazole becomes intolerable. Sucralfate (answer 3) has no role in the treatment of GERD. The GERD guidelines endorse increasing the PPI frequency to twice daily in patients with continuing symptoms; therefore answer 4 is the best choice.

18. Answer: 3

Rationale: The two most common causes of peptic ulcer bleeding are presence of *Helicobacter pylori* and nonsteroidal antiinflammatory drug (NSAID) use. This patient has a gastric ulcer with evidence of a clot (indicating recent bleeding) because he uses high-dose aspirin plus ketoprofen. The patient is older than 60 years old, which is another risk factor for NSAID-induced gastric ulcer. His rapid urease test has shown a negative result so answer 1 is incorrect. Histamine 2 receptor antagonists (answer 2) are less efficacious than proton-pump inhibitors (PPIs) in the healing of gastric ulcers. PPIs (answer 3) are the most preferred drug for healing NSAID-induced gastric ulcer because of their excellent efficacy, and they are better tolerated. Sucralfate (answer 4) has not shown any role in healing NSAID-induced ulcers.

19. Answer: 4

Rationale: The patient presents with atypical symptoms of gastroesophageal reflux disease. She has taken over-the-counter aluminum hydroxide, which can decrease absorption of atazanavir because of an increase in pH; therefore the viral load increased and CD4 count decreased. Aluminum can cause accumulation, which can lead to toxicity in patients with renal disease. She does not complain of any complicated symptoms such as difficulty in swallowing, bleeding, or weight loss; therefore there is no indication for the endoscopy evaluation (answer 1). Endoscopy is recommended in the presence of alarm symptoms or in the screening of patients at high risk for complications. Screening of *Helicobacter pylori* (answer 2) is not recommended; however, it is recommended in patients with peptic ulcer disease. Initiating cimetidine (answer 3) would not be preferred because of its interactions with other drugs. Cimetidine inhibits cytochrome P450 enzymes 1A2, 2C9, 2D6, and 3A4, which can affect her HIV therapy. Initiating proton-pump inhibitors is preferred (answer 4) because there is no interaction or decrease in concentration of atazanavir with these drugs.

20. Answer: 4

Rationale: The most common causes of peptic ulcer disease are *Helicobacter pylori* infection and nonsteroidal antiinflammatory drug use. In addition, the patient is older than 60 years, which is another risk factor for *H. pylori*–induced ulcers. Misoprostol (answer 1) is effective in preventing and healing ulcers, but it is not preferred because of the need for several daily doses and it is poorly tolerated because of a high incidence of abdominal pain, cramping, and diarrhea. Omeprazole (answer 2) is the most preferred treatment for healing the ulcer, but *H. pylori* should be eradicated first, then proton-pump inhibitors (PPIs) are recommended. Histamine 2 receptor antagonists (answer 3) have fewer efficacies in healing and preventing ulcers than PPIs. The triple regimen for *H. pylori* eradication (answer 4) is the most appropriate treatment for the patient's ulcer. *H. pylori* is a known carcinogen; therefore it should be eradicated before the beginning of a PPI treatment course for 8 weeks. The general recommendation, based on the American College of Gastroenterology guidelines, is to include an antisecretory agent (PPI is preferred) plus at least two antibiotics (clarithromycin and amoxicillin or metronidazole) in the eradication regimen.

21. Answer: 3

Rationale: The test-and-treat approach is appropriate in patients with dysphagia through *Helicobacter pylori* infection. Patients who are older than 45 to 55 years or those with severe symptoms should be referred for endoscopic evaluation to rule out the possibility of complicated disease. Patients could be tested for *H. pylori* using various diagnostic approaches. The eradication of *H. pylori* leads to high rates of ulcer healing and minimizes ulcer recurrence. According to the treatment guidelines of the American College of Gastroenterology (ACG), the eradication regimen of *H. pylori* infection should include at least two antibiotics plus an antisecretory agent (proton-pump inhibitors [PPIs] preferred) given for 10 to 14 days. The triple-therapy regimen containing two antibiotics (clarithromycin and metronidazole) and a PPI is the most preferred regimen, and it is given within 10 to 14 days of diagnosis. Therefore answer 1 is incorrect because the duration is too short. Cephalosporins (answer 2) are not recommended for *H. pylori* treatment. Quadruple therapy with bismuth subsalicylate, tetracycline, metronidazole, and PPI (answer 3) could be used as a first-line treatment for patients with penicillin allergy or as a second-line treatment of initial failure of the triple-drug therapy. A fluoroquinolone-based regimen (answer 4) should be reserved as salvage therapy for patients who have failed triple and quadruple therapy. In answer 4, the duration of 21 days is too long.

22. Answer: 1

Rationale: Bloody diarrhea has continued for four to six times per day, so the patient has mild to moderate ulcerative colitis (UC). Her active UC is affecting the descending colon and rectum. Treatment with topical aminosalicylate therapy (answer 1) as suppositories or enema is a more effective option for patients with distal disease than oral therapies (answer 2). Methotrexate (answer 3) has a limited role in maintaining corticosteroid-induced remission in patients with Crohn disease but not UC. Infliximab (answer 4) would be appropriate for moderate to severe UC when the aminosalicylate therapy has failed.

23. Answer: 3

Rationale: The patient has moderate to severe Crohn disease (CD) that involves the terminal ileum and colon. Mesalamine (answer 1) is well tolerated but is minimally effective in moderate to severe CD. Budesonide (answer 2) is effective in mild to moderate CD affecting the terminal ileum and proximal colon; therefore the severity and the location of the disease would not fit this regimen. Combining infliximab and azathioprine has been shown to result in the highest rates of remission in moderate to severe CD compared with the use of either agent alone. The dose of infliximab is 5 mg/kg intravenously and the azathioprine dose is 2 to 2.5 mg/kg orally so answer 3 is correct. Adalimumab (answer 4) would be appropriate, but the dose is for maintenance and would need to be 160 mg initially for induction.

24. Answer: 1

Rationale: The patient is not responding to infliximab; therefore increasing the dose to 10 mg/kg would be appropriate to manage his active Crohn disease (CD) symptoms. Initiating mesalamine (answer 2) would not be recommended because aminosalicylate is more effective in mild to moderate disease. Budesonide (answer 3) is effective with mild to moderate CD affecting the terminal ileus and proximal colon. Infliximab has various adverse effects, but its benefits outweigh its risks; therefore, stopping infliximab (answer 4) is not appropriate.

25. Answer: 1

Rationale: The patient presents with a history of severe ulcerative colitis. All of his previous medications have failed to control his symptoms. The recommendation is for natalizumab 300 mg intravenously every 4 weeks. Natalizumab is associated with the development of progressive multifocal leukoencephalopathy. The patient should be monitored for mental status changes during treatment, and consider magnetic resonance imaging and lumbar puncture if mental status or weakness is observed. The patient must enroll in the TYSABRI Outreach: Unified Commitment to Health (TOUCH) program before the drug is dispensed because of its potential for serious adverse effects. TYSABRI® (natalizumab) is available only through the TOUCH Prescribing Program. Aspirin 81 mg (answer 2), vitamin supplements (answer 3), and captopril (answer 4) have not shown any association with the development of progressive multifocal leukoencephalopathy.

26. Answer: 3

Rationale: The patient complains of infusion-related infliximab symptoms, which lead to hypotension, fever, chills, urticaria, and pruritus. Using nonsteroidal anti-inflammatory drugs (answer 1) would be not preferred because they can lead to nephrotoxicity for patients with kidney disease. Infusion

should be over at least 2 hours to avoid the hypotension and urticarial symptoms, so answer 2 is incorrect. Pretreatment with acetaminophen or antihistamines would be preferred to avoid any infusion-related symptoms; therefore, answer 3 will be the best management strategy. Waiting until the infusion-related symptoms disappear with time (answer 4) is a tough choice for patients who have a history of severe disease.

27. Answer: 1

Rationale: The patient presents to the clinic with an 8-week history of bloody stool three to four times per day and abdominal cramps. The colonoscopy reveals mild to moderate ulcerative colitis (UC) affecting the descending colon and rectum. Aminosalicylate suppositories or enema (answer 1) are preferred for the patient's symptoms. Budesonide (answer 2) is appropriate for treatment and maintenance mild to moderate UC, but it would be more effective for patients with mild to moderate Crohn disease (CD) involving the terminal ileum and ascending colon. Infliximab (answer 3) is not indicated for patients with mild to moderate cases, but it is recommended for patients with moderate to severe UC. Infliximab is contraindicated for patients with a history of heart failure New York Heart Association class III and IV. Natalizumab (answer 4) would not be the best drug to manage the patient's symptoms. It is indicated for patients with severe cases of UC. The patient must enroll in the TYSABRI Outreach: Unified Committee to Health (TOUCH) program before the drug is dispensed because of its association with progressive multifocal leukoencephalopathy.

28. Answer: 4

Rationale: Patients with cirrhosis and ascites are at risk of developing spontaneous bacterial peritonitis (SBP), which is an infection of the ascetic fluid usually caused by an enteric gram-negative organism. Typical signs of infection include nausea, fever, abdominal cramps, and rebound tenderness. The paracentesis evaluation reveals more than $250/mm^3$ of polymorphonuclear neutrophils in the ascetic fluid, and the patient's value is $480/mm^3$. The use of oral antibiotics to treat SBP is not well studied (answer 1); however, some oral regimes (e.g., norfloxacin or trimethoprim/sulfamethazine) should be instituted and continued indefinitely after recovery to reduce the incidence of subsequent infection. If the clinical and laboratory signs and symptoms are present, antibiotic therapy should be initiated immediately to target gram-negative organisms, so answer 2 is incorrect. Aminoglycosides should be avoided because of their potential to cause nephrotoxicity (answer 3), and vancomycin should be reserved for resistant gram-positive organisms. The third-generation cephalosporin ceftriaxone or cefotaxime is preferred (answer 4). In addition to adding antibiotics, the use of intravenous albumin reduces the incidence of renal failure and improves 30-day mortality. Albumin is indicated for patients with serum creatinine more than 1 mg/dL and blood urea nitrogen more than 30 mg/dL.

29. Answer: 1

Rationale: Management of overt hepatic encephalopathy should initially involve removal of precipitating factors and the use of therapies aimed at reducing ammonia concentration. The guidelines of the American Association for the Study of Liver Diseases recommend using lactulose 30 mL every 2 hours (answer 1) to rapidly reduce ammonia concentration in the short term. Rifaximin (answer 2) is as effective as lactulose, and it may be better tolerated. The approved dose for reduction of an overt hepatic encephalopathy in patients 18 years and older is 550 mg twice daily. The drug cost may be greater, but this may be offset by a shorter length of treatment. Third-generation cephalosporins (answer 3) are not well studied in the treatment of hepatic encephalopathy, but other oral regimes such as neomycin and metronidazole are as effective as lactulose. However, polyethylene glycol 3350 (answer 4) has shown faster improvement than lactulose in treating patients with hepatic encephalopathy. The recommended dosage is 4 L given orally or by nasogastric tube over 4 hours.

30. Answer: 2

Rationale: The patient presents with hepatorenal syndrome, and she has no current kidney disease or nephrotoxins. The patient's serum creatinine would not improve by using albumin only (answer 1). The most preferred treatment for patients with hepatorenal syndrome is a combination of albumin and octreotide 200 mcg subcutaneously three times daily (answer 2). Using furosemide (answer 3) does not benefit patients with hepatorenal syndrome. The combination of pentoxifylline and prednisolone is indicated for treating patients with alcoholic liver disease.

31. Answer: 3

Rationale: The patient presents to the clinic with a history of cirrhosis, mild encephalopathy, and ascites. Her laboratory values reveal ascetic fluid protein concentration less than 1.5 g/dL and serum creatinine greater than 1.2 mg/dL, BUN greater than 25 mg/dL, sodium less than 125 mg/dL, and bilirubin greater than 3 mg/dL. Her values indicate prevention of spontaneous bacterial peritonitis. Albumin plus cefotaxime (answer 1) would be the preferred treatment for patients that have an infection caused by spontaneous bacterial peritonitis (SBP) and the patient has no signs or symptoms for the infection. Ceftriaxone (answer 2) would be indicated for the primary prevention of SBP, but it is more often preferred for patients who have acute upper gastrointestinal (GI) bleeding. The patient should be given a 7-day course of ceftriaxone during hospitalization. Using trimethoprim/sulfamethazine (answer 3) is the best choice for the primary prevention of SBP. It should be considered as an indefinite antibiotic prophylaxis in patients without GI bleeding. Nonselective beta-blockers (answer 4) are not appropriate for the prevention of SBP, but they are indicated for prevention of GI variceal bleeding.

32. Answer: 1

Rationale: The patient presents to the hospital with signs and symptoms of ascites. He has a long history of alcohol abuse. The paracentesis revealed serum-ascites albumin gradient greater than 1.1, which is an indication for ascites caused by portal hypertension. The patient should stop drinking alcohol immediately to prevent a prognosis of liver disease and stop taking nonsteroidal antiinflammatory drugs associated with sodium/water retention to prevent renal failure. The best next management for this patient is a combination of furosemide and spironolactone (answer 1). An appropriate starting regimen is 40 mg furosemide and 100 mg spironolactone. Nadolol (answer 2) is a nonselective beta-blocker therapy that is indicated in the prevention of GI variceal bleeding. Using albumin with cefotaxime (answer 3) would be preferred for patients who have signs and symptoms of infections caused by spontaneous bacterial peritonitis (SBP). Oral antibiotics (answer 4) sulfamethazine/trimethoprim or norfloxacin could be used as an indefinite prophylaxis for SBP.

33. Answer: 3

Rationale: This patient has strong evidence of a chronic hepatitis B virus (HBV) infection because of the elevation of alanine aminotransferase and aspartate transaminase, the presence of HBsAg and HBeAg, and the high concentration of HBV DNA. There is also necroinflammation and fibrosis in the biopsy and a *YMDD* mutation. He has compensated liver disease on the basis of his albumin concentration, international normalized ratio, and lack of ascites or encephalopathy. Initiating pegylated interferon alfa-2a and ribavirin (answer 1) are indicated for chronic hepatitis C virus treatment. Because of the elevation of liver function tests, biopsy result, and a high viral load, the patient should receive his therapy without any delay (answer 2). Tenofovir (answer 3) is recommended for treatment of patients with chronic HBV infection and *YMDD* mutation. Lamivudine (answer 4) is not appropriate for this patient because his resistance tests reveal *YMDD* mutation.

34. Answer: 3

Rationale: The patient has a new diagnosis of chronic hepatitis C virus (HCV). The patient needs the treatment because of elevated liver function tests, the biopsy result, and high viral load (answer 1). The guidelines of the American Association for the Study for Liver Diseases (AASLD) and the Infectious Diseases Society of America (IDSA) recommend treating all patients with chronic HCV, except those with short life expectancy that would not be altered by treatment. However, the combination of sofosbuvir and simeprevir (answer 2) is appropriate for chronic HCV infection, genotype 1a. It is not suitable for this patient because of the presence of NS3Q80K polymorphism, which significantly reduces the effectiveness of simeprevir. According to AASLD/IDSA guidelines, the most preferred regimen for genotype 1a is sofosbuvir and ledipasvir (answer 3). The drug regimen including pegylated interferon, sofosbuvir, and ribavirin was previously recommended, but direct-acting agents are now preferred (answer 4).

35. Answer: 1

Rationale: The patient presents with nausea and vomiting induced by pregnancy. The best choice is doxylamine (answer 1), which is approved for pregnant women who do not respond to conservative management. Doxylamine is considered a pregnancy category A. Aprepitant (answer 2) still has not been assigned a pregnancy category by the U.S. Food and Drug Administration. There are insufficient data available on the use of this drug in pregnancy to inform drug-related risk. Aprepitant should be used during pregnancy only if clearly needed. Use of haloperidol (answer 3) during pregnancy has been associated with withdrawal symptoms in the neonate and poor neonatal adaption syndrome. Also, it is associated with an increase of spontaneous abortion, congenital anomaly, or low birth weight. Ondansetron (answer 4) has a pregnancy category B, and it can be used if doxylamine treatment failed.

36. Answer: 2

Rationale: The patient presents with gastroparesis because of her history of diabetes type 2, which leads to diabetes complications. Serotonin antagonist (answer 1) is preferred to treat chemotherapy-induced nausea and vomiting. Metoclopramide (answer 2) is the best drug for treatment of gastroparesis induced by diabetes type 2. Antihistaminic agents (answer 3) and scopolamine (answer 4) are preferred to treat nausea and vomiting caused by motion sickness.

37. Answer: 2

Rationale: The patient presents with signs and symptoms of acute pancreatitis. He denies any alcohol or drug abuse, but he takes a medication that can cause these symptoms. Acute pancreatitis is often reversible once the underlying cause is addressed. The patient has a history of chronic angina; therefore it is important for him to take aspirin 81 mg daily to decrease the mortality. There are no reports showing that aspirin (answer 1) causes acute pancreatitis. Valproic acid (answer 2) induces severe acute pancreatitis with pseudocyst formation. The patient shows gastrointestinal symptoms so this complication may be difficult to diagnose. Raised pancreatic amylase and lipase would confirm clinical suspicion. Ramipril (answer 3) and metoprolol succinate (answer 4) are used for patients with a chronic angina and no reports show they can cause acute pancreatitis.

38. Answer: 1

Rationale: The patient has signs and symptoms for maldigestion and malabsorption secondary to the loss of pancreatic exocrine function. This is diagnosed by the presence of steatorrhea, weight loss, and an elevated fecal fat concentration. Management should include replacement of exogenous pancreatic enzymes to facilitate nutrition digestion and absorption (answer 1). Oral pancrelipase products are pork derived and contain amylase, lipase, and protease. A typical starting dose for adults should deliver 30,000 to 40,000 units per meal, with titration based on the reduction of steatorrhea and evidence of weight gain. Adding multivitamins (answer 2) would be beneficial; however, patients with chronic pancreatitis may need extra supplementation of fat-soluble vitamins after the enzyme therapy is initiated and increased caloric intake to facilitate weight gain. Using appetite stimulants like dronabinol (answer 3) will be not beneficial if enzyme therapy is not initiated. However, morphine relieves abdominal pain, but increasing the dose to 60 mg twice daily would not be useful without initiating the pancreatic enzymes (answer 4).

39. Answer: 4

Rationale: The patient has signs and symptoms for maldigestion and malabsorption secondary to the loss of pancreatic exocrine function. Management should include replacement of exogenous pancreatic enzymes to facilitate nutrition digestion and absorption. A typical starting dose of pancrelipase for an adult should deliver 30,000 to 40,000 units before each meal, with titration based on reduction of steatorrhea and evidence of weight gain. Fibrosing colonopathy (answer 1) is generally seen with doses greater than 10,000 units/kg/day. Pancrelipase products are pork derived and include lipase, amylase, and protease. These products are contraindicated if pork allergy is present (answer 2). High doses of exogenous pancreatic enzymes lead to hyperuricosuria and hyperuricemia as an adverse drug reaction (answer 3); therefore they should be used with caution for patients with renal impairment, gout, or hyperuricemia. Pancrelipase products should be prescribed to the pregnant woman only if needed. The risks and benefits of the product should be considered for the context of the need to provide adequate nutrition support to a pregnant woman with exogenous pancreatic enzyme insufficiency. Pancrelipase products are pregnancy category C (answer 4).

40. Answer: 2

Rationale: Diarrhea is caused by a variety of conditions, and viral pathogens are one of the most common causes. This patient's diarrhea is probably caused by contact with her small daughter, who is in kindergarten and had similar symptoms a few days earlier. A low-grade fever, myalgias, watery diarrhea, and vomiting refer to a potential viral cause. Antidiarrheal therapy should be selected according to patient preference and the presence of any precautions or contraindications. The patient is pregnant, so if the patient desired a therapy, it should be chosen to minimize risks to the patient and the fetus. However, pyridoxine (answer 1) is safe and it carries a U.S. Food and Drug Administration (FDA) pregnancy category A rating. It should be indicated for patients with nausea and vomiting who failed any conservative strategy. Loperamide (answer 2) is an effective agent for short-term relief of diarrhea, and it carries an FDA pregnancy category B rating. Lactase (answer 3) would be indicated only if the patient's diarrhea were secondary to lactose intolerance. Bismuth subsalicylate (answer 4) should be avoided in pregnant and nursing patients because of the risk of potential toxicity.

41. Answer: 1

Rationale: Drug-induced diarrhea can occur by a variety of mechanisms. The patient presents with symptoms of an oily and loose diarrhea. Orlistat (answer 1) is the correct answer because it has common adverse effects such as flatulence, oily and loose stool, and fecal incontinence. Metformin (answer 2) is the first line of treatment for diabetes type 2, and it can cause nausea and diarrhea when patients first start of taking it or the dose is raised, but it does not cause an oily diarrhea. Mineral supplements (answer 3) have not been shown to cause diarrhea, but an excessive amount of the mineral vitamins could cause it. Captopril (answer 4) has a common adverse effect of diarrhea, but there are no known reports that captopril can cause an oily stool.

42. Answer: 4

Rationale: The patient meets the criteria for irritable bowel syndrome with constipation (IBS-C) on the basis of a negative diagnostic workup, and the presence of abdominal pain, floating, and constipation for more than 3 months. Drug therapy should target the predominant symptoms. The most beneficial agents for IBS-C are bulk-forming laxatives, which improve the frequency of bowel movement and can reduce the floating, and selective serotonin reuptake inhibitors (SSRIs), which provide relief from abdominal pain, improve global symptoms, and improve the motility in most patients. Amitriptyline is tricyclic antidepressants (answer 1) and has a similar effect to SSRIs but are associated with an anticholinergic effect that may worsen constipation. Probiotics such as VSL #3 (answer 2) can improve the global symptoms, but they would not improve the bowel frequency. Tegaserod (answer 3) can be used in emergency cases only because of its association with development of cardiovascular events. Lubiprostone (answer 4) is approved for IBS-C in women older than 18 years. Because it improves motility and abdominal pain, it is the drug therapy most suitable for this patient.

43. Answer: 2

Rationale: The patient presents with a 2-week history of constipation. Her pregnancy is a common factor for causing constipation. Stimulant laxatives (answer 1) like senna do not appear to be associated with an increased risk of malformation. However, pregnant woman might experience unpleasant side effects such as abdominal cramps with the use of stimulant laxatives. Polyethylene glycol (answer 2) is an osmotic laxative could be preferred for a pregnant woman, and patients with renal and hepatic diseases. Linaclotide (answer 3) is approved by the U.S. Food and Drug Administration (FDA) for IBS-C and chronic idiopathic constipation (CIC). Lubiprostone (answer 4) is indicated an FDA pregnancy category C rating and needs a negative pregnancy test before using. In addition, it is FDA approved for CIC and irritable bowel syndrome with constipation (IBS-C) for women older than 18 years.

44. Answer: 3

Rationale: The patient presents with symptoms of irritable bowel syndrome-diarrhea predominant (IBS-D). Drug therapy should target the predominant symptoms. A short-course (10–14 days) of nonabsorbable antibiotic could improve the global symptoms of IBS, especially bloating in IBS-D. Rifaximin 550 mg three times daily for 14 days has U.S. Food and Drug Administration (FDA) approval for IBS-D, but there is limited data with metronidazole (answer 1). Linaclotide (answer 2) has FDA approval for IBS with constipation (IBS-C). Alosetron (answer 3) is a serotonin 3-antagonist that is approved by FDA for IBS-D. It improves the global symptoms and reduces motility. Lubiprostone (answer 4) is approved by the FDA for IBS-C in women older than 18 years.

45. Answer: 2

Rationale: A perforated appendix requires antibiotic therapy after surgery for an intraabdominal infection, so answer 1 is incorrect. Ceftriaxone plus metronidazole is the best drug regimen for the intraabdominal infection (answer 2). The combination of vancomycin and metronidazole does not have adequate activity against aerobics and gram-negative organisms (answer 3). The combination of cefazolin and ciprofloxacin does not have adequate activity against anaerobic organisms (answer 4).

46. Answer: 1

Rationale: The patient has a severe episode of *Clostridium difficile* diarrhea, as demonstrated by elevated white blood cell count and serum creatinine; therefore vancomycin (answer 1) for 10 days is the best drug regimen for this patient. Metronidazole (answer 2) is optimal for the patient's symptoms, but the duration is too short. Rifaximin (answer 3) is not a first-line agent, and the duration is too short. Fidaxomicin (answer 4) could be used as a first-line agent in patients who are at high risk of recurrence, but 14 days' duration is too long.

47. Answer: 3

Rationale: The patient presents with signs and symptoms of *Clostridium difficile* infection that is detected by the elevation of serum creatinine, albumin, and white blood cells. The patient has a history of gastroesophageal reflux disease (GERD) for which proton-pump inhibitors (PPIs) are the best drug therapy. PPIs (answer 3) are reported to induce *C. difficile* infection. The physician should reevaluate the need of PPI use and limit the dose and duration. Calcium supplement (answer 1) is associated with inducing constipation. Acetaminophen (answer 2) and angiotensin-converting enzyme inhibitors (answer 4) have not shown any relation with *C. difficile*-induced diarrhea.

48. Answer: 1

Rationale: The patient's laboratory test revealed hypokalemia and hypomagnesaemia. The potassium concentration level does not increase despite potassium infusion because of the decrease in magnesium concentration level. She is not taking diuretics or digoxin. Proton-pump inhibitors (PPIs; answer 1) have shown a major adverse effect like hypomagnesemia; it is rare, but it is a serious complication. The physician should reevaluate the need for PPIs or limit the dose and duration. Antiplatelet drugs (answers 2 and 3) could be used for cardiovascular management. Nitroglycerin (answer 4) is indicated for angina treatment.

49. Answer: 3

Rationale: Reactivation of hepatitis B virus (HBV) during periods of immunosuppression is an important consideration in the patient who has a previously resolved HBV infection. The laboratory test for the patient is positive for HBcAb, indicating that she is at risk for reactivation. It is believed that the risk of reactivation extends beyond the direct period of immunosuppression. Therefore the preventative antiviral therapy should extend 6 months after the cessation of the chemotherapy. Answers 1 and 2 are incorrect because the duration of the therapy is too short, so the development of resistance in the face of viral replication would be low. Because the patient is presumed to have resolved the infection with no viral replication, there is a minimal concern for resistance organisms or resistance development; therefore agents such as adefovir or entecavir (answer 4) should not be used.

50. Answer: 2

Rationale: The patient presents with mild disease activity because of his presenting symptoms. The ulceration is continuous and extends to the splenic flexure. Mesalamine enema (answer 1) is not appropriate for this patient because an enema could be used if the ulceration is descending. Oral mesalamine (answer 2) is the best option for this patient because of the disease location and its mild symptoms. Corticosteroid induction (answer 3) is appropriate for patients with severe disease or for those who do not respond to aminosalicylate medications. Azathioprine (answer 4) is indicated only for maintenance therapy.

51. Answer: 1

Rationale: Exogenous pancreatic enzymes are indicated for patients with exocrine pancreatic insufficiency. The exogenous pancreatic enzymes are recommended to improve the steatorrhea symptoms and malabsorption in patients with chronic pancreatitis (answer 1). They do not improve the constipation symptoms for patients with chronic pancreatitis (answer 2). Exogenous pancreatic enzymes have shown no benefits in the treatment of acute pancreatitis (answers 3 and 4 are incorrect).

52. Answer: 1

Rationale: The patient presents with signs and symptoms of spontaneous bacterial peritonitis (SBP) because her polymorphonuclear cell count is greater than 2.5×10^3 cells/mm^3. Cefotaxime with albumin should be initiated in all patients with SBP (answer 1). Although sulfamethazine/trimethoprim is beneficial as a preventative strategy for SBP, it is not indicated for treatment of acute management of SBP (answer 2). Moxifloxacin (answer 3) could not be used in the acute management of SBP. Vancomycin (answer 4) would not cover the organisms that are commonly associated with SBP, including *Escherichia coli* or *Klebsiella pneumoniae*.

53. Answer: 4

Rationale: The patient's esophagogastroduodenoscopy has not shown any varices; therefore there is no need for beta-blockers (answers 1 and 3 are incorrect). The abdominal ultrasonography reveals ascites and the serum-ascites albumin gradient is greater than 1.1, so the patient needs a diuretic combination of furosemide and spironolactone. He currently completed a course of therapy for SBP, so the patient needs a secondary prevention therapy and use norfloxacin indefinitely. Therefore answer 2 is incorrect and the most correct answer is 4.

54. Answer: 1

Rationale: The patient's medical history includes hypothyroidism, which is one of the most common causes for constipation. Psyllium (answer 1) is the best option because it is used for intermittent and chronic constipation, and it is safe for renal and hepatic disease and pregnant and geriatric patients. Methylnaltrexone (answer 2) has U.S. Food and Drug Administration approval for opioid-induced constipation (OIC) in palliative care patients and for OIC in adult patients with noncancer pain. Lactulose (answer 3) is preferred for the treatment of constipation for patients with chronic liver disease. Plecanatide (answer 4) is FDA approved for chronic idiopathic constipation for adults.

55. Answer: 3

Rationale: The most effective therapy regimen for the treatment of patients with gastroesophageal reflux disease (GERD) is the use of proton-pump inhibitors (PPIs). The patient has a partial response with PPIs; therefore changing the therapy regimen from PPIs to histamine 2 receptor antagonists (H_2RA) would be ineffective for treatment of GERD (answer 1). Changing of the therapy regimen from PPIs to antacids also would not be effective (answer 2). Increasing the PPI dose from an oral tablet once daily to twice daily is a strong recommendation, according to the guidelines. It is used to treat nighttime awakenings and the feeling of nausea in the morning (answer 3). Adding an H_2RA to the regimen would be effective, but this is a conditional recommendation with limited evidence according to the guidelines (answer 4).

56. Answer: 1

Rationale: The patient presents to the clinic with a history of liver cirrhosis. Her exam reveals medium to large esophageal varices without signs of gastrointestinal bleeding or ascites. The best drug therapy for this patient is a nonselective beta-blocker (answer 1) that decreases the portal pressure. Selective beta-blockers would not be indicated for treatment of esophageal varices (answer 2). Isosorbide mononitrate (answer 3) is not appropriate for treatment of esophageal varices. Adding proton-pump inhibitors (answer 4) has no benefits for varices treatment.

57. Answer: 4

Rationale: The patient presents to the medical floor with symptoms of gastroesophageal reflux disease (GERD). He takes over-the-counter ranitidine with only a partial response. Metoclopramide (answer 1) would be ineffective for this patient, but it is indicated for patients with diabetes type 2 suffering from gastroparesis. Metoclopramide could lead to extrapyramidal symptoms and QTc prolongation. Erythromycin (answer 2) is a promotility agent and is not indicated for GERD treatment. Increasing ranitidine dose to 150 mg twice daily (answer 3) would be a conditional recommendation according to the guidelines. The patient has Alzheimer disease and increasing the dose interval from once daily to twice daily would not be preferred for him. Proton-pump inhibitors (answer 4) are the most effective treatment for patients with GERD, according to the American College of Gastroenterology (ACG) guidelines.

58. Answer: 1

Rationale: The patient presents with signs and symptoms of acute pancreatitis, which is confirmed by the elevation of the pancreatic enzymes. Pain management is the cornerstone of treatment of patients with acute pancreatitis. Pain management involves the use of intravenous narcotics as hydromorphone (answer 1). Octreotide (answer 2) does not enough data to support its use. Parenteral nutrition is indicated for patients who were without nutrition for more than 7 days, and this patient is well-nourished (answer 3). Antibiotics, in general, are not recommended for treatment of acute pancreatitis cases, but it could be used in presence of extra pancreatic infections or any infected necrosis (answer 4).

59. Answer: 1

Rationale: Nonsteroidal antiinflammatory drugs (NSAIDs) should be stratified by gastrointestinal and cardiovascular risk. Ketorolac (answer 1) is used in short-term management of moderate and severe pain and is usually not prescribed for more than 5 days. Other NSAIDs (answers 2, 3, and 4) should be avoided but have minimal concerns compared with ketorolac.

60. Answer: 2

Rationale: Gastric ulcers (answer 1) are most often caused from long-term nonsteroidal antiinflammatory drug use or *Helicobacter pylori* infection, and they do not cause an oily stool. Steatorrhea (answer 2) is characterized by increased fecal fat excretion secondary to fat maldigestion and malabsorption; therefore it leads to weight loss and oily stool. Dumping syndrome (answer 3) is characterized by accelerated gastric emptying of hyperosmolar contents into the small bowel resulting in release of vasoactive hormone. Dumping syndrome could not cause an oily stool. Lactulose intolerance (answer 4) is caused by lactase deficiency, the enzyme required to absorb lactose found in dairy products. Lactulose intolerance also does not cause an oily stool.

61. Answer: 2

Rationale: The patient has a medical history of Crohn disease with multiple bowel resection surgeries. Patients with Crohn disease often have vitamin deficiencies, especially fat-soluble vitamins (A, D, E, and K) and essential fatty acids (omega-3 and omega-6); therefore answers 1, 3, and 4 are incorrect. Vitamin C deficiency (answer 2) would not be a common complication of short-bowel syndrome because vitamin C is a water-soluble vitamin.

62. Answer: 1

Rationale: There are two types of nonendoscopic tests available: tests that identify active infection and tests that detect antibodies. Antibody tests could not differentiate between the active infection or previously eradicated *Helicobacter pylori*; therefore answers 2 and 4 are incorrect. The nonendoscopic tests are noninvasive, more convenient, and less expensive than the endoscopic tests and include the urea breath test (answer 1). The urea breath test is more accurate than a stool antigen test (answer 3).

63. Answer: 2

Rationale: The patient has symptoms of gastroesophageal reflux disease and the best therapy for her are proton-pump inhibitors (PPIs). PPIs and nonsteroidal antiinflammatory drugs (NSAIDs) should not be taken together. NSAIDs increase the risk for gastric ulcers and bleeding (answer 1). Omeprazole becomes more effective when it is taken 30 to 60 minutes before breakfast (answer 2) instead of taking it at bedtime (answer 3) or after breakfast (answer 4).

64. Answer: 1

Rationale: Although all of these proton-pump inhibitors are considered for gastric bleeding prophylaxis caused by stress-related mucosal disease, only omeprazole (as a powder for oral suspension) is approved by the U.S. Food and Drug Administration for this indication.

65. Answer: 1.

Rationale: The patient presents with signs of mild bleeding without orthostatic changes and a duodenal ulcer with a clear base. He takes low-dose aspirin for cardiovascular prophylaxis; therefore he has many factors can lead to gastrointestinal ulcers. A test should be performed to exclude *Helicobacter pylori*, and the patient should stop their acid-suppressive medications for about 24 hours before administration of the test. The patient should take a high dose of proton-pump inhibitors (PPIs) for ulcer healing (answer 1). Misoprostol (answer 2) is as effective in treatment of ulcers as PPIs, but it has unpleasant complications such as abdominal cramps and diarrhea. The guidelines of the American College of Gastroenterology (ACG) do not recommend empiric antibiotic treatment for *H. pylori* without performing a test to exclude it (answer 3). The patient has no symptoms of Zollinger–Ellison syndrome, so obtaining a serum gastrin level would be beneficial (answer 4).

9

Renal and Genitourinary

1. The patient is a 64-year-old white woman (height 73 inches, weight 90 kg) who presents to the clinic with abdominal pain and dizziness. She reports that she did not eat or drink for 24 hours because she has a history of gastroenteritis. On exam, the blood pressure reading while sitting is 120/85 mmHg and drops to 90/60 mmHg when standing. Her heart rate is 95 beats/min. The laboratory tests reveal sodium (Na) is 140 mEq/L, potassium is 4 mEq/L, chloride (Cl) is 105 mEq/L, blood urea nitrogen is 42 mg/dL, serum creatinine is 1.3 mg/dL, and glucose is 190 mg/dL. What is the best action for this patient?

   1. Administer trimethoprim/sulfamethazine double strength orally for 3 days.

   2. Administer furosemide 40 mg intravenously.

   3. Administer Insulin lispro 5 units subcutaneously.

   4. Administer fluid bolus (500 mL of NaCl solution).

2. A 63-year-old Asian man has diabetes, hypertension, and estimated glomerular filtration rate of 40 mL/min/1.73 m². He takes simvastatin 40 mg daily, ramipril 10 mg daily, and metformin 1000 mg twice daily. Laboratory values reveal hemoglobin is 12 mg/dL, parathyroid hormone is 200 pg/mL, sodium is 135 mEq/L, potassium is 3.9 mEq/L, calcium is 8.9 mEq/dL, albumin is 3.5 g/dL, phosphorus is 5.9 mg/dL, and 25-hydroxyvitamin D is 50 ng/mL. Which therapy is the best to prevent chronic kidney disease-mineral and bone disorders?

   1. Cinacalcet.

   2. Ergocalciferol.

   3. Calcium carbonate.

   4. Calcitriol.

3. The patient is a 35-year-old African American woman who is admitted to the hospital with a 2-day history of nausea, vomiting, abdominal cramps, dysuria, and flank pain. She is diagnosed with pyelonephritis and is prescribed a 5-day course of parenteral aminoglycosides. The patient develops acute tubular necrosis. Antibiotic therapy is adjusted based on culture and sensitivity results. Which set of laboratory data is consistent with this presentation?

   1. Blood urea nitrogen (BUN)/serum creatinine ratio is 15:1, urinary sodium more than 40 mEq/L, fractional excretion of sodium (FENa) more than 2%, specific gravity is less than 1.015, and muddy casts are present.

   2. BUN/serum creatinine ratio is 15:1, urinary sodium is greater than 40 mEq/L, FENa greater than 2%, specific gravity is less than 1.015, no casts visible.

   3. BUN/serum creatinine ratio is greater than 20:1, urinary sodium is less than 20 mEq/L, FENa is less than 1%, specific gravity is more than 1.018, and hyaline casts are present.

   4. BUN/serum creatinine ratio is greater than 20:1, urinary sodium is less than 10 mEq/L, FENa is less than 1%, specific gravity is 1.010, muddy casts are present.

4. A 53-year-old Asian man presents to the emergency department with an 8-hour history of strong chest pain, diaphoresis, and dyspnea. His medical history includes diabetes type 2, and he takes metformin 1000 mg twice daily. The nurse practitioner is concerned about a possible myocardial infarction and recommends coronary angiography. The patient develops acute tubular necrosis after the procedure. Which set of laboratory data is consistent with this presentation?

   1. Blood urea nitrogen (BUN)/serum creatinine ratio is 20:1, urinary sodium is greater than 40 mEq/L, fractional excretion of sodium (FENa) is less than 1%, specific gravity is 1.018, and no visible casts.

   2. BUN/serum creatinine ratio is 15:1, urinary sodium is greater than 40 mEq/L, FENa is greater than 2%, specific gravity is 1.010, and no visible casts.

   3. BUN/serum creatinine ratio is 10:1, urinary sodium is greater than 40 mEq/L, FENa is greater than 2%, specific gravity is 1.015, and muddy casts are present.

   4. BUN/serum creatinine ratio 20:1, urinary sodium is less than 20 mEq/L, FENa is less than 1%, specific gravity is 1.018, and muddy casts are present.

5. A 67-year-old Asian man has an estimated glomerular filtration rate of 40 mL/min/1.73 m². His hemoglobin (Hgb) is 13.5 g/dL, with normal red blood cell indices without treatment. What is the recommended minimum frequency of Hgb monitoring for this patient?

   1. Monthly.

   2. Every 3 months.

   3. Every 6 months.

   4. Every 12 months.

6. The patient is a 59-year-old white woman who comes to the clinic for a follow-up. The patient's estimated glomerular filtration rate is 25 mL/min/1.73 m². Her hemoglobin (Hgb) is 10.5 g/dL, and the nurse practitioner recommends iron tablets once daily. The patient does not receive dialysis treatment. What is the recommended minimum frequently of Hgb monitoring for this patient?

   1. Not needed.

   2. Four times every year.

   3. Two times every year.

   4. Every 12 months.

7. A 54-year-old patient with chronic kidney disease stage 4 (estimated glomerular filtration rate is 20 mL/min/1.73 m²) has received a diagnosis of gram-negative bacteremia. The nurse practitioner prescribes drug X for him, but there are no published reports on how to adjust the dose of drug X in a patient with impaired kidney function. The package of drug X shows that it has significant renal elimination with 30% excreted unchanged in the urine. The usual dose of drug X is 400 mg/day intravenously and is provided as 100 mg/mL in a 6-mL vial. Which is the best dosage of drug X for this patient?

   1. 5.5 mg/mL.

   2. 4.1 mg/mL.

   3. 3.6 mg/mL.

   4. 3 mg/mL.

8. The patient is a 57-year-old white man who has a history of hypertension and currently takes ramipril 10 mg once daily. His estimated glomerular filtration rate is 35 mL/min/1.73 m² and albumin/creatinine ratio is 25 mg/g. According to the Kidney Disease Improving: Global Outcomes guidelines, what is the patient's blood pressure goal?

   1. 130/80 mmHg.

   2. 140/90 mmHg.

   3. 120/90 mmHg.

   4. 140/70 mmHg.

9. A 43-year-old woman presents to the clinic for follow-up. The patient's medical history is positive for diabetes type 2 and hypertension. On exam, her blood pressure is 145/88 mmHg, A1c is 7.5, albumin/creatinine ratio is 40 mg/g, and her estimated glomerular filtration rate is 45 mL/min/1.73 m². According to the Kidney Disease Improving: Global Outcomes guidelines, what is the patient's blood pressure goal?

   1. 130/80 mmHg.

   2. 140/90 mmHg.

   3. 150/90 mmHg.

   4. 130/70 mmHg.

10. A 54-year-old Hispanic man (height 73 inches, weight 53 kg) with a history of severe Crohn disease presents to the emergency department. The patient complains of severe vomiting and bloody diarrhea; therefore he is malnourished, and he is not able to tolerate anything by mouth. His serum creatinine is 0.6 mg/dL, and his estimated kidney function is critical. What is the best method for assessing kidney function for this patient?

    1. Iothalamate study.

    2. 24-hour urine collection.

    3. Cockcroft–Gault equation.

    4. Modification of Diet in Renal Disease study equation.

11. A 68-year-old woman presents to the hospital to evaluate her kidney function. Laboratory data show sodium 140 mEq/L, blood urea nitrogen 35 mg/dL, serum creatinine 1.8 mg/dL, urinary sodium 26 mEq/L, and urinary creatinine 15.3 mg/dL. What is the best estimation for the patient's fractional excretion of sodium?

    1. 4.3%.

    2. 1.2%.

    3. 3.5%.

    4. 2.1%.

12. A 68-year-old African American man (height 68 inches, weight 49 kg) is admitted in a long-term care facility with a 3-year history of advanced Alzheimer disease. The patient has confusion and is aggressive toward the facility staff. He refuses to take any food or his medications. His laboratory test shows serum creatinine is 0.5 mg/dL. The patient has oliguria, weight loss, and is malnourished. Which is the best equation for assessing kidney function?

    1. Chronic Kidney Disease Epidemiology Collaboration (CKD-EPI).

    2. Brater equation.

    3. Jelliffe equation.

    4. 24-hour urine collection.

13. A 57-year-old Asian woman is admitted to the intensive care unit after having a myocardial infarction 5 days ago; her New York Heart Association is class III and left ventricular ejection fraction is 35%. She currently has pneumonia and hypotension for 3 days despite the adequate hydration. Before her admission, her serum creatinine was 1.0 mg/dL; yesterday, the blood urea nitrogen (BUN) and serum creatinine were 33 mg/dL and 2.9 mg/dL, respectively. Today, her BUN and serum creatinine are 42 mg/dL and 4 mg/dL, respectively. Her urine osmolality is 285 mOsm/kg, and her sodium urine is 45 mEq/L; there are tubular cellular casts in the urine. Which is the most likely renal diagnosis?

    1. Prerenal azotemia.

    2. Functional-mediate acute kidney injury (AKI).

    3. Acute tubular necrosis.

    4. Postrenal AKI.

14. A 53-year-old man presents to the clinic with a history of dysuria and a burning sensation while urinating. The patient is diagnosed with benign prostatic hypertrophy. He currently takes tamsulosin 0.8 mg daily, tadalafil 5 mg daily, and finasteride 5 mg daily. His laboratory tests show blood urea nitrogen is 18 mg/dL, serum creatinine is 1.5 mg/dL, urinary sodium is 43 mg/dL, serum sodium is 135 mEq/mL, urinary osmolality is 285 mOsm/kg, and fractional excretion of sodium is 2.5%. What is the most likely renal diagnosis?

    1. Postrenal acute kidney injury (AKI).

    2. Chronic kidney disease.

    3. Functional-mediated AKI.

    4. Intrinsic AKI.

15. A 45-year-old Hispanic woman comes to the hospital for follow-up. Her medical history is positive for hypertension and diabetes type 2. She currently takes lisinopril 20 mg daily and glipizide 5 mg twice daily. Her urinalysis shows blood urea nitrogen and serum creatinine are 40 mg/dL and 1.5 mg/dL, respectively; urinary sodium is 15 mEq/mL; and no casts are visible. What is the most likely renal diagnosis?

    1. Postrenal acute kidney injury (AKI).

    2. Intrinsic AKI.

    3. Glomerular disease.

    4. Functional AKI.

16. A 35-year-old patient presents to the emergency department with a 10-day history of dysuria, abdominal pain, vomiting, and flank pain. He is diagnosed with pyelonephritis and is prescribed a 14-day course of trimethoprim/sulfamethazine tablet double strength. His medical history includes hypertension, osteoarthritis, and hypothyroidism. His medications are captopril 50 mg twice daily, acetaminophen 500 mg three times per day, and levothyroxine 105 mcg/day. Which drug can cause pseudonephrotoxicity?

    1. Captopril.

    2. Acetaminophen.

    3. Levothyroxine.

    4. Trimethoprim/sulfamethazine.

17. A 67-year-old white man who has had chronic kidney disease stage 4 for 7 years is maintained on chronic hemodialysis. His medical history includes hypertension, myocardial infarction, and mild congestive heart failure. His medications are epoetin 10,000 units intravenously three times weekly at dialysis, renal multivitamins, valsartan 80 mg twice daily, bisoprolol 5 mg once daily, aspirin 75 mg once daily, calcium acetate and 1334 mg three times daily with meals. Laboratory values show hemoglobin 9 g/dL, intact parathyroid hormone 300 pg/mL, sodium 135 mEq/mL, potassium 4.5 mEq/mL, phosphorus 4.7 mg/dL, calcium 9 mg/dL, serum creatinine 7 mg/dL, and albumin 3.5 g/dL. His ferritin concentration is 95 ng/mL, and his transferrin saturation is 18%. Which approach is the best way to manage the patient's anemia?

    1. Intravenous iron.

    2. Increase epoetin dosage.

    3. Oral iron.

    4. Maintain current regimen.

18. The patient is a 43-year-old woman (height 65 inches, weight 75 kg) who is admitted to the hospital with a history of chronic kidney disease stage 3. The patient does not receive hemodialysis treatment. She has a medical history that includes diabetes type 2; she reports an allergy from sulfa-containing medication (hives). On exam, the laboratory tests show hemoglobin concentration is 9.5 g/dL, ferritin concentration is 150 ng/dL, transferrin saturation is 25%, calcium is 9.5 mg/dL, potassium is 3.3 mEq/mL, phosphorus is 5 mg/dL, intact parathyroid hormone is 250 pg/mL, and serum creatinine is 3.5 mg/dL. Which approach is the best way to manage the patient's anemia?

    1. Adding epoetin 6500 units three times per week.

    2. Administer intravenous iron.

    3. The patient does not need medications.

    4. Administer oral iron.

19. The patient is a Hispanic man who comes to the health care facility with his 76-year-old grandmother for follow-up. The grandmother's medical history is positive for Alzheimer's disease and chronic kidney disease stage 4. She has not received dialysis treatment. The grandson reports that she takes her medication regularly. She takes memantine 5 mg once daily, rivastigmine 6 mg twice daily, epoetin 6500 units three times per week, and renal multivitamins. Her laboratory values reveal hemoglobin concentration is 9.3 g/dL, ferritin concentration is 100 ng/dL, transferrin saturation is 24%, sodium (Na) is 145 mEq/mL, potassium is 5 mEq/mL, chloride is 108 mEq/mL, calcium is 9.5 mg/dL, albumin is 3.4 g/dL and serum creatinine is 3.5 mg/dL. Which approach is the best and most useful for this patient?

    1. Adding intravenous iron.

    2. Administering red blood cells.

    3. Adding oral iron.

    4. Increasing the epoetin dose to 10,000 units three times per week.

20. The patient is a 47-year-old Asian man (weight 66 kg) who is admitted to the intensive care unit after an acute myocardial infarction and pulmonary edema. He has a history of hypertension and he smoked tobacco 15 years ago. He currently takes lisinopril 20 mg/day, nicotine patch 14 mg/day applied every morning, and aspirin 75 mg/day. Before this admission, his serum creatinine was normal (baseline is 0.9 mg/dL). After 24 hours, his kidney function had declined (blood urea nitrogen is 25 and serum creatinine is 2.1 mg/dL), despite receiving 4 L of intravenous fluid. Urinalysis shows muddy brown casts and the urinary volume is decreased to 250 mL over

the last 12 hours. What is the best assessment for kidney function for this patient?

    1. Creatinine clearance (CrCl) using Cockcroft equation.

    2. Estimated glomerular filtration rate using the Modification of Diet in Renal Disease study equation.

    3. CrCl using the Brater equation.

    4. Collection of urine over 24 hours.

21. The patient is a 47-year-old Asian man (weight 66 kg) who is admitted to the intensive care unit after an acute myocardial infarction and pulmonary edema. He has a history of hypertension and he has smoked 1 pack of cigarettes a day for the last 15 years. He currently takes lisinopril 20 mg/day, nicotine patch 14 mg/day applied every morning, and aspirin 75 mg/day. Before admission, his serum creatinine was normal (baseline is 0.9 mg/dL). After 24 hours, his kidney functions have declined (blood urea nitrogen is 25 and serum creatinine is 2.1 mg/dL), despite receiving 4 L of intravenous fluid. On urinalysis, muddy brown casts are present, and the urinary volume has decreased to 250 mL over the last 12 hours. What is the most likely cause of this patient's impaired kidney function?

    1. Chronic kidney disease.

    2. Acute tubular necrosis.

    3. Postrenal acute kidney injury.

    4. Prerenal azotemia.

22. The patient is a 47-year-old Asian man (weight 66 kg) who is admitted to the intensive care unit after an acute myocardial infarction and pulmonary edema. He has a history of hypertension and he has smoked 1 pack of cigarettes a day for the last 15 years. He currently takes lisinopril 20 mg/day, nicotine patch 14 mg/day applied every morning, and aspirin 75 mg/day. Before admission, his serum creatinine was normal (baseline is 0.9 mg/dL). After 24 hours, his kidney function has declined (blood urea nitrogen is 25 and serum creatinine is 2.1 mg/dL), despite receiving 4 L of intravenous fluid. On urinalysis, muddy brown casts are present, and the urinary volume has decreased to 250 mL over the last 12 hours. Which medication should be discontinued at this time because of its potential for adverse effects on kidney functions?

    1. Keep the current medications.

    2. Nicotine patch.

    3. Lisinopril.

    4. Aspirin.

23. The patient is a 47-year-old Asian man (weight 66 kg) who is admitted to the intensive care unit after an acute myocardial infarction and pulmonary edema. He has a history of hypertension and he has smoked 1 pack of cigarettes a day for the last 15 years. He currently takes lisinopril 20 mg/day, nicotine patch 14 mg/day applied every morning, and aspirin 75 mg/day. Before admission, his serum creatinine was normal (baseline is 0.9 mg/dL). After 24 hours, his kidney function has declined (blood urea nitrogen is 25 and serum creatinine is 2.1 mg/dL), despite receiving 4 L of intravenous fluid. On urinalysis, muddy brown casts are present, and the urinary volume has decreased to 250 mL over the last 12 hours. Which intervention is best to manage the patient's presentation?

    1. Furosemide.

    2. Hydrochlorothiazide.

    3. Water and sodium restriction.

    4. Intravenous 0.9% sodium chloride.

24. The patient is a 66-year-old American African woman (height 73 inches, weight 85 kg) who is admitted to the intensive care unit with a severe community-acquired pneumonia. Her vital signs are body temperature 103.5°F, respiratory rate 35 breaths/min, blood pressure 85/60 mmHg, and serum creatinine 2 mg/dL (baseline is 0.8 mg/dL). She received ceftriaxone 1 g intravenously and moxifloxacin 750 mg orally. According to RIFLE (risk, injury, failure, loss of kidney function, and end-stage kidney disease) classification, which stage is represented in this patient?

    1. Injury to kidney.

    2. Failure of kidney.

    3. Loss of kidney function.

    4. End-stage kidney disease.

25. A 56-year-old white woman is admitted to the intensive care unit for an angiography procedure. The patient has had severe chest pain, sweating, and shortness of breath for the past 3 hours. Her vital signs are blood temperature 150/90 mmHg, respiratory rate 30 breaths/min, heart rate 88 beats/min, and serum creatinine 4.3 mg/dL (baseline is 1.0 mg/dL). According the Acute Kidney Injury Network criteria, which stage is represented in this patient?

    1. Stage 1.

    2. Stage 2.

    3. Stage 3.

    4. Stage 4.

26. A 32-year-old woman in her first trimester presents to the emergency department with her husband with severe vomiting and nausea. She denies alcohol abuse; she reports allergy from pets (rhinitis). On physical exam, her vital signs show blood pressure is 94/65 mmHg, heart rate is 90 beats/min, respiratory rate is 35 breaths/min, blood urea nitrogen is 40 mg/dL, serum creatinine is 1.8 mL/dL, sodium is 129 mEq/mL, chloride is 108 mL/dL, potassium is 2.9 mEq/mL, and urinary sodium is 15 mEq/L. Which strategy is the best for management of this case?

    1. Adding furosemide.

    2. Intravenous 0.9% of sodium chloride.

    3. Fluid restriction.

    4. Oral hydration with water.

27. A 43-year-old man comes to the emergency department with severe pain in flank areas and back, dysuria, and vomiting. A computed tomography shows calcium stones in the urethra and the right kidney. The laboratory tests are obtained and reveal blood urea nitrogen is 25 ng/dL, serum creatinine is 2 mg/dL, urinary sodium is 50 mEq/L, and no casts are visible. The patient has postrenal acute kidney injury as a diagnosis. What is the best treatment for a patient with nephrolithiasis?

    1. Furosemide.

    2. Fluid restriction.

    3. Increase fluid intake.

    4. Spironolactone.

28. A 63-year-old man is admitted to the intensive care unit with a 3-day history of fever, flank pain, and vomiting. The patient is diagnosed with a complicated pyelonephritis. His medical history includes liver alcoholic cirrhosis and mild encephalopathy. After 2 days of admission, his blood urea nitrogen (BUN) is 100 mg/dL and serum creatinine is 4 mg/dL. the nurse practitioner recommends renal replacement therapy. Which of the following is incorrect regarding indications for renal replacement therapy?

    1. Blood urea nitrogen (BUN) is greater than 100 mg/dL.

    2. Refractory metabolic acidosis.

    3. Uremia and encephalopathy.

    4. Life-threatening hypomagnesemia.

29. A 57-year-old white woman presents to the hospital with intermittent chest pain. Her medical history includes hypertension, diabetes type 2, and chronic kidney disease (Kidney Disease Improving Global Outcomes stage 3). She currently takes captopril, hydrochlorothiazide, and metformin. Her laboratory values show serum creatinine 1.6 mg/dL, hemoglobin 13 g/dL, and hematocrit 39%. There is no evidence for edema. The patient is to undergo elective cardiac catheterization. Which medication should be interrupted before beginning cardiac catheterization?

    1. Captopril.

    2. Hydrochlorothiazide.

    3. Metformin.

    4. No medication should be stopped.

30. A 57-year-old white woman presents to the hospital with intermittent chest pain. Her medical history includes hypertension, diabetes type 2, and chronic kidney disease (Kidney Disease: Improving Global Outcomes stage 3). She currently takes captopril, hydrochlorothiazide, and metformin. Her laboratory values show serum creatinine 1.6 mg/dL, hemoglobin 13 g/dL, and hematocrit 39%. There is no evidence for edema. The patient is to undergo elective cardiac catheterization. Which approach is best for hydration?

    1. Oral hydration with water.

    2. 0.9% of sodium saline.

    3. 0.45% of sodium saline.

    4. 5% dextrose and 0.45% sodium saline.

31. A 57-year-old white woman presents to the hospital with intermittent chest pain. Her medical history includes hypertension, diabetes type 2, and chronic kidney disease (Kidney Disease: Improving Global Outcomes stage 3). She currently takes captopril, hydrochlorothiazide, and metformin. Her laboratory values show serum creatinine 1.6 mg/dL, hemoglobin 13 g/dL, and hematocrit 39%. There is no evidence for edema. The patient is to undergo elective cardiac catheterization. After the administration of contrast, what is the optimal time to reevaluate renal function to assess for the development of contrast-associated nephrotoxicity?

    1. 24 hours.

    2. 3 days.

    3. 7 days.

    4. 10 days.

32. A 52-year-old woman presents to an oncology facility to receive her chemotherapy course. She receives cisplatin. Her laboratory values include sodium 135 mEq/L, potassium 3 mEq/L, calcium 9 mg/mL, magnesium 1.7 mg/mL, and serum creatinine 1.8 mg/mL. Which of the following is *incorrect* for prevention of cisplatin-induced nephrotoxicity?

    1. Use the smallest dosage possible.

    2. Aggressive intravenous hydration within 24 hours.

    3. Adding amifostine.

    4. Increase frequency of administration.

33. A 38-year-old woman, who has had a history of bipolar disease for 15 years presents to the clinic for follow-up. She has taken lithium for the last 11 years. Her laboratory values show serum creatinine is 1.9 mg/dL and blood urea nitrogen is 23 mg/dL; she is admitted to the intensive care unit to treat lithium toxicity symptoms. Which strategy is *incorrect* for prevention of lithium-induced chronic interstitial nephritis?

    1. Maintaining a low lithium concentration.

    2. Monitoring the kidney function closely.

    3. Administration of furosemide.

    4. Oral hydration is beneficent.

34. A 57-year-old Hispanic man presents to the health care facility with a history of hypertension, previous myocardial infarction, chronic kidney disease, and diabetes type 1. He denies any drug allergies or history of drug abuse, but he smokes cigarettes (2 packs per day). His medications include metoprolol succinate 100 mg daily, aspirin 81 mg, candesartan 16 mg/day, and insulin glargine 16 units before bed. His vital signs reveal blood pressure is 194/85 mmHg, heart rate is 65 beats/min, and respiratory rate is 25 breaths/min. His laboratory values show albumin/creatinine ratio is 450 mg/g, serum creatinine is 1.8 mg/dL, and estimated glomerular filtration rate is 40 mL/min/1.73 m^2. According to his Kidney Disease Improving Global Outcomes (KDIGO) criteria, what is the best assessment for his kidney disease?

    1. Stage 1.

    2. Stage 2.

    3. Stage 3.

    4. Stage 4.

35. A 57-year-old Hispanic man presents to the health care facility with a history of hypertension, previous myocardial infarction, chronic kidney disease, and diabetes type 1. He denies any drug allergies or history of drug abuse, but he smokes cigarettes (2 packs per day). His medications include metoprolol succinate 100 mg daily, aspirin 81 mg, candesartan 16 mg/day, and insulin glargine 16 units before bed. His vital signs reveal blood pressure is 194/85 mmHg, heart rate is 65 beats/min, and respiratory rate is 25 breaths/min. His laboratory values show albumin/creatinine ratio is 450 mg/g, serum creatinine is 1.8 mg/dL, and estimated glomerular filtration rate is 40 mL/min/1.73 m². According to Kidney Disease Outcomes Quality Initiative stages, what is the best assessment for his kidney disease?

    1. Stage 1.

    2. Stage 2.

    3. Stage 3.

    4. Stage 4.

36. A 57-year-old Hispanic man presents to the health care facility with a history of hypertension, previous myocardial infarction, chronic kidney disease, and diabetes type 1. He denies any drug allergies or history of drug abuse, but he smokes cigarettes (2 packs per day). His medications include metoprolol succinate 100 mg daily, aspirin 81 mg, candesartan 16 mg/day, and insulin glargine 16 units before bed. His vital signs reveal blood pressure is 194/85 mmHg, heart rate is 65 beats/min, and respiratory rate is 25 breaths/min. His laboratory values show albumin/creatinine ratio is 450 mg/g, serum creatinine is 1.8 mg/dL, and estimated glomerular filtration rate is 40 mL/min/1.73 m². Using the Kidney Disease Improving Global Outcomes categorization, which assessment is best for this patient's albuminuria?

    1. Category A1.

    2. Category A2.

    3. Category A3.

    4. Nephrotic-range of proteinuria.

37. A 47-year-old Asian woman presents to the health care facility with a history of hypertension, chronic kidney disease, and diabetes type 1. She denies any drug allergies or history of drug abuse. Her medications include metoprolol succinate 100 mg daily, aspirin 81 mg, and insulin glargine 16 units before bed. Her vital signs reveal A1c is 7.5%, blood pressure is 194/85 mmHg, heart rate is 65 beats/min, and respiratory rate is 25 breaths/min. Her laboratory values show albumin/creatinine ratio is

250 mg/g, serum creatinine is 1.8 mg/dL, and estimated glomerular filtration rate is 40 mL/min/1.73 m². Which action is the best to limit the progression of her kidney disease?

    1. Add ramipril.

    2. Increase metoprolol succinate dosage.

    3. Add amlodipine.

    4. Add nifedipine.

38. A 43-year-old man comes to the health care facility for follow-up. His medical history includes hypertension, diabetes type 2, osteoarthritis, and chronic kidney disease. He currently takes atenolol 50 mg/day, acetaminophen 500 mg twice daily, and glipizide 5 mg daily. He does not smoke cigarettes and denies any drug abuse. Two months ago, his vital signs were blood pressure 143/93 mmHg, serum creatinine 1.8 mg/dL, A1c 7.3%, and albumin/creatinine ratio 400 mg/g. The nurse practitioner recommended the addition of enalapril. Today, his vital signs are blood pressure 135/85 mmHg, serum creatinine 2.1 mg/dL, and serum potassium 5.3 mEq/L. Which recommendation is the best for this patient?

    1. Change enalapril to valsartan and monitor serum potassium, serum creatinine, and blood pressure in 2 weeks.

    2. Change enalapril to diltiazem and monitor serum potassium, serum creatinine, and blood pressure in 2 weeks.

    3. Add chlorthalidone and monitor serum potassium, serum creatinine, and blood pressure in 2 weeks.

    4. Increase atenolol dosage and monitor serum potassium, serum creatinine, and blood pressure in 2 weeks.

39. The patient is a 35-year-old African American woman with chronic kidney disease and hypertension history she comes to the clinic for checkup. Her vital sighs reveal blood pressure 128/75 mmHg, serum creatinine 3 mg/dL (baseline 1.9 mg/dL), and albumin/creatinine ratio 35 mg/g. Her medications are enalapril 10 mg twice daily and metolazone 5 mg daily. Which action is the best for this patient?

    1. Stop enalapril.

    2. Continue the current regimen.

    3. Decrease enalapril dosage.

    4. Increase metolazone dosage.

40. A 59-year-old man is admitted to the hospital with a history of chronic kidney disease (stage 3), gout, and previous myocardial infarction. His medications include aspirin 81 mg daily, allopurinol 50 mg daily, and carvedilol 12.5 mg twice daily. The nurse practitioner is concerned about his lipid concentration; his laboratory values show low-density cholesterol is 200 mg/dL and triglycerides are 300 mg/dL. Which medication benefits the patient the most?

    1. Pravastatin 20 mg/day.

    2. Niacin 1000 mg daily.

    3. Ezetimibe.

    4. Lifestyle modification only.

41. The patient is a 57-year-old woman who is admitted to the hospital for dialysis treatment. She has a history of hypertension and osteoarthritis. She is being assessed for hemodialysis access. Which hemodialysis access is the best for this patient?

    1. Arteriovenous fistula.

    2. Arteriovenous graft.

    3. Tenckhoff catheter.

    4. Subclavian catheter.

42. A 70-year-old man is undergoing long-term hemodialysis and has several episodes of hypotension during hemodialysis. After the nonpharmacological approach is optimized, which medication is best to manage his low blood flow?

    1. Fludrocortisone.

    2. Midodrine.

    3. Sodium chloride tablets.

    4. Levocarnitine.

43. A 73-year-old Hispanic man comes to the clinic for his dialysis treatment. He has a 10-year history of cigarette smoking and a 5-year history of marijuana use. His medical history includes hypertension, previous myocardial infarction, and heart failure New York Heart Association class II. He has an episode of hypotension during his dialysis. Which choice is the *incorrect* approach and should be avoided?

    1. Increase of ultrafiltration rate.

    2. Decrease of ultrafiltration rate.

    3. Administer saline boluses.

    4. Trendelenburg position.

44. A 63-year-old woman comes to the health care facility with a history of chronic kidney disease and receives peritoneal dialysis. She has a fever and abdominal pain. She notes her abdominal dialysate has become cloudy. Her laboratory values of the dialysate reveal many white blood cells, primarily neutrophils. Gram stain and culture of the fluid are obtained. What is the best empiric therapy for this patient, according to the International Society for Peritoneal Dialysis guidelines?

    1. Cefazolin and ceftazidime instilled intraperitoneally.

    2. Vancomycin instilled intraperitoneally.

    3. Clindamycin plus vancomycin intravenously.

    4. Metronidazole plus gentamicin intravenously.

45. The patient is a 56-year-old Asian man who presents to the health care facility with chronic kidney disease receiving peritoneal dialysis. The patient read several websites about peritoneal dialysis complications, and he has concerns about it. Which complication of peritoneal dialysis would be *incorrect*?

    1. Dialysis-related peritonitis.

    2. Fluid overload.

    3. Hyperglycemia.

    4. Hypercalcemia.

46. A 70-year-old white man receiving hemodialysis treatment who has had end-stage kidney disease for 7 years comes to the clinic. His hemodialysis access is an arteriovenous fistula. The patient's medical history includes hypertension, mild congestive heart failure, atrial fibrillation, and epilepsy. He takes aspirin 81 mg daily, metoprolol succinate 100 mg/day, ramipril 20 mg daily, epoetin alfa 10,000 units three times every week, calcium acetate 2 g three times daily after meals, and renal multivitamins daily. Laboratory values show hemoglobin is 10.5 g/dL, parathyroid hormone is 650 pg/mL, sodium is 143 mEq/L, potassium is 4.9 mEq/L, calcium is 9 mg/dL, serum creatinine is 7.5 mg/dL, albumin is 2.5 g/dL, phosphorus is 7.9 mg/dL, serum ferritin is 600 ng/mL, and transferrin saturation is 33%. His red blood cells and white blood cells are normal. The patient is afebrile. What is the most likely cause of this patient's relatively epoetin resistance?

    1. Infection.

    2. Iron deficiency.

    3. Phenytoin.

    4. Hyperparathyroidism.

47. A 70-year-old white man receiving hemodialysis treatment with end-stage kidney disease for 7 years comes to the clinic. His hemodialysis access is an arteriovenous fistula. The patient's medical history includes hypertension, mild congestive heart failure, atrial fibrillation, and epilepsy. He takes aspirin 81 mg daily, metoprolol succinate 100 mg/day, ramipril 20 mg daily, epoetin alfa 10,000 units three times every week, calcium acetate 2 g three times daily after meals, and renal multivitamins daily. Laboratory values show hemoglobin is 10.5 g/dL, parathyroid hormone is 650 pg/mL, sodium is 143 mEq/L, potassium (is 4.9 mEq/L, calcium is 9 mg/dL, serum creatinine is 7.5 mg/dL, albumin is 2.5 g/dL, phosphorus is 7.9 mg/dL, serum ferritin is 600 ng/mL, and iron saturation is 33%. His red blood cells and white blood cells are normal. The patient is afebrile. What is the best to manage this patient's hyperparathyroidism?

    1. Change calcium acetate to calcium carbonate.

    2. Change calcium acetate to sevelamer and cinacalcet.

    3. Add intravenous vitamin D analog.

    4. Increase calcium acetate dosage.

48. A 55-year-old man with chronic kidney disease and hypertension presents to the clinic for consultation. His medications are epoetin alfa 14,000 units three times every week, renal multivitamins daily, and ramipril 10 mg daily. Which of the following is NOT true regarding erythropoiesis-stimulating agents?

    1. Erythropoiesis-stimulating agents (ESAs) are under the U.S. Food and Health Administration Risk Evaluation and Mitigation Strategies program.

    2. ESA dosage should be decreased to 50% if hemoglobin increases to greater than 1 g/dL in 2 weeks.

    3. ESA resistance is caused by iron deficiency, infection, hyperparathyroidism, and folate deficiency.

    4. Monitor hemoglobin every 2 to 4 weeks.

49. A 73-year-old man with stage 5 chronic kidney disease who receives dialysis treatment presents to the health care facility for follow-up. The laboratory values show calcium 9.8 mg/dL, phosphorus 7 mg/dL, sodium 145 mEq/L, potassium 4.5 mEq/L, parathyroid hormone (PTH) 800 pg/dL, and 25-hydroxyvitamin D 10 ng/mL. What is the frequency of laboratory monitoring for this patient, according to the Kidney Disease Improving Global Outcomes guidelines?

    1. No need for frequent laboratory monitoring for grade 5 chronic kidney disease.

    2. Calcium every 6 to 12 months, phosphorus every 6 to 12 months, intact PTH, and 25-hydroxyvitamin D is in baseline.

    3. Calcium every 3 to 6 months, phosphorus every 3 to 6 months, intact PTH every 6 to 12 months, and 25-hydroxyvitamin D is in baseline.

    4. Calcium every 1 to 3 months, phosphorus every 1 to 3 months, intact PTH every 3 to 6 months, and 25-hydroxyvitamin D is in baseline.

50. The patient is a 37-year-old white man with stage 4 chronic kidney disease who presents to the health care facility for follow-up. He currently takes epoetin alfa 14,000 units three times every week, renal multivitamins, ergocalciferol, and cinacalcet. His laboratory tests show serum creatinine is 6.5 mg/dL, intact parathyroid hormone is 550 pg/mL, 25-hydroxyvitamin D is 15 ng/mL, and serum ferritin is 550 mg/dL. Which statement is *incorrect* about cinacalcet?

    1. Cinacalcet has drug interaction with ketoconazole, which may increase cinacalcet concentration by up to twofold.

    2. Cinacalcet inhibits CYP2D6.

    3. Cinacalcet is safe for patients with seizure disorders.

    4. Cinacalcet could cause hypocalcemia.

51. A 66-year-old Hispanic woman with end-stage kidney disease for 10 years is admitted to the health care facility for dialysis treatment. Her nurse practitioner prescribed for her etelcalcetide because of her elevated intact parathyroid hormone and calcium. According to the guidelines, which statement is *false* for the etelcalcetide medication?

    1. The initial dose of etelcalcetide is 5 mg intravenously three times weekly after hemodialysis.

    2. Use etelcalcetide with caution for patients with seizure disorders.

    3. Etelcalcetide could cause QT prolongation and may worsen heart failure.

    4. Discontinue cinacalcet for at least 14 days before initiation of etelcalcetide.

52. The patient is a 73-year-old woman with chronic kidney disease stage 3 who is admitted to the emergency department with a 3-day history of abdominal pain, vomiting, and flank pain. The laboratory evaluation reveals that there is an infection in her urinary tract; she is diagnosed with pyelonephritis. Which medication should not be adjusted for patients with decreased kidney function?

    1. Metronidazole.

    2. Meperidine.

    3. Spironolactone.

    4. Rosuvastatin.

Renal Genitourinary Answers & Rationales

1. Answer: 4

Rationale: The patient presents with acute kidney injury (AKI) symptoms, and the initial treatment of AKI is identifying and reversing the insult to the kidney if possible. This patient has prerenal azotemia caused by hypotension and increased heart rate. Adding sulfa antibiotics would not have any benefits for this patient because she does not have any signs for urinary tract infections (answer 1). Administering diuretics such as furosemide (answer 2) could worsen her volume depletion and probably further impair her kidney function. Although the glucose level is elevated, adding insulin units is unnecessary at this time (answer 3). Fluid management is critical to managing AKI; therefore administration of a fluid bolus with normal saline would be the best choice for this patient.

2. Answer: 3

Rationale: There are many factors that can contribute to the development of chronic kidney disease-mineral and bone disorders such as hypocalcemia, hyperparathyroidism, hyperphosphatemia, decrease of vitamin D, and decreased production of 1.25-dihydroxyvitamin D. The patient's laboratory values reveal hyperparathyroidism, which may be related to an increasing phosphorus concentration. The first approach is to administer a phosphate binder. Knowing the corrected calcium concentration is necessary for this patient. The [measured Ca + (0.8) (4 − serum albumin) = 8.9 + (0.8) (4 − 3.5) = 8.9 + 0.4 = 9.3 mEq/dL]; therefore this patient has hypocalcemia. Cinacalcet (answer 1) is reserved for patients with hyperparathyroidism despite the normalization of phosphate in patients with hypercalcemia. Ergocalciferol (answer 2) is unnecessary for this patient because his 25-hydroxyvitamin D concentration is greater than 30 ng/mL. Calcium carbonate (answer 3) is the best phosphate binder for this case because the patient has hypocalcemia, and it is acceptable with a corrected serum calcium concentration. An active vitamin D medication such as calcitriol (answer 4) could be added if the parathyroid concentration remains elevated, despite normalization of serum phosphate.

3. Answer: 1

Rationale: The patient develops acute tubular necrosis (ATN), so she has an intrinsic acute kidney injury (AKI). Aminoglycosides can cause direct damage to the tubules. In ATN, the blood urea nitrogen/serum creatinine ratio could be normal (between 10 and 15:1), but it is greater than 20:1, so it is reflecting hypovolemia, which is common in prerenal azotemia. Urinary sodium less than 20 mEq/L is a marker of hypovolemia. The fractional excretion of sodium (FENa) value could distinguish between prerenal and intrinsic AKI. A low FENa (less than 1%) in a patient with oliguria suggests that the tubular function is still intact, but a FENa greater than 2% refers to intrinsic AKI. The specific gravity is normal in intrinsic AKI and is elevated (greater than 1.018) in prerenal azotemia. Muddy casts are often present in intrinsic AKI because of the renal tubule cell damage. Therefore answers 2, 3, and 4 are incorrect.

4. Answer: 4

Rationale: The patient develops acute tubular necrosis (ATN); therefore, he has an intrinsic acute kidney injury. Coronary angiography can cause nephrotoxicity because of the use of intravenous contrast. Metformin should be stopped about 24 hours before the coronary angiography procedure because the iodinated contrast dye can increase the nephrotoxicity risk. Blood urea nitrogen/serum creatinine ratio could be normal (10 to 15:1) in ATN, but it becomes greater than 20:1 in prerenal azotemia. Urinary sodium greater than 40 mEq/L is an indication of ATN, but when it becomes less than 20 mEq/L, it reflects hypovolemia. A fraction excretion of sodium (FENa) less than 1% is an indication of intact tubular function, but a FENa greater than 2% refers to an intrinsic AKI. The specific gravity is normal in ATN, and it is greater than 1.018 in prerenal azotemia. The presence of casts is a strong marker for ATN. Therefore, answers 1, 2, and 3 are incorrect.

5. Answer: 4

Rationale: This patient has stage 3 chronic kidney disease (CKD) because his estimated glomerular filtration rate is less than 60 mL/min/1.73 m². His hemoglobin (Hgb) concentration is greater than 13 g/dL, so he does not have anemia. Hgb concentration should be monitored according to the CKD stage. Monthly monitoring is never recommended for a patient who does not have anemia (answer 1). Monitoring Hgb every 3 months should occur for patients with stage 5 CKD and receiving dialysis (answer 2). Monitoring of Hgb concentration is recommended every 6 months for patients with stages 4 and 5 CKD who have not received dialysis treatment (answer 3). Monitoring Hgb every 12 months should be recommended for patients with stage 3 CKD (answer 4).

6. Answer: 3

Rationale: The patient has stage 4 chronic kidney disease (CKD) because her estimated glomerular filtration rate (eGFR) is less than 30 mL/min/1.73 m² and greater than 15 mL/min/1.73 m². Her hemoglobin (Hgb) is less than 13 g/dL; therefore she is diagnosed with anemia and the nurse practitioner recommends iron tablets. The patient has anemia and should monitor her Hgb according to her eGFR; therefore answer 1 is incorrect. Monitoring of hemoglobin concentration four times per year should be recommended for patients with stage 5 CKD who are receiving dialysis (answer 2). The Hgb should be monitored at least two times per year for patients with stage 4 CKD or stage 5 CKD and who do not receive dialysis treatment (answer 3). Monitoring hemoglobin concentration once yearly should be recommended for patients with stage 3 CKD (answer 4).

7. Answer: 4

Rationale: The fraction of drug excreted in the urine can determine the proper dose of a drug when specific dosing guidelines are not available. The Rowland–Tozer equation can determine the percentage of the usual dosage to give a patient with known kidney disease (Q), considering the ratio of the patient's renal function to normal.

$$Q = 1 - [Fe(1 - KF)] = 1 - [0.3(1 - 20/120)] = 1 - 0.25$$
$$= 0.75 \text{ or } 75\% \text{ of usual dosage}$$

If the usual dose of drug X is 400 mg/day, so the adjusted dose will be 300 mg/day (400 × 0.75) = 300. Thus the patient should receive 3 mL of the 100 mg/mL preparation (300 mg/100 mg/mL). Therefore answers 1, 2, and 3 are incorrect.

8. Answer: 2

Rationale: The Kidney Disease: Improving Global Outcomes guidelines provide recommendations for blood pressure goals for patients with chronic kidney disease according to the severity of proteinuria. The patient's albumin/creatinine ration (ACR) is less than 30 mg/g; therefore he is considered to have normal to mildly elevated albuminuria. According to the guidelines, patients with albuminuria in this stage (1) should have a goal blood pressure less than 140/90 mmHg (answer 2 is correct). When the patient's ACR is greater than 30 mg/g, he is considered to have a moderate to severe elevated albuminuria, and according to the guidelines, the goal of the blood pressure should be less than 130/80 mmHg (answer 1 is incorrect). Answer 3 is incorrect because the systolic blood pressure is too low (less than 130 mmHg), and answer 4 is incorrect because the diastolic blood pressure is too low (less than 80 mmHg).

9. Answer: 1

Rationale: The Kidney Disease Improving Global Outcomes (KDIGO) guidelines provide recommendations for blood

pressure goals for patients with chronic kidney disease. The patient's medical history includes diabetes type 2 and the albumin/creatinine ratio is greater than 30 mg/g; therefore she is considered to have a moderate to severe elevated albuminuria. According to the KDIGO guidelines, the goal blood pressure should be less than 130/80 mmHg (answer 1 is correct) for patients with chronic kidney disease (CKD) and moderate to severe elevated albuminuria. The goal blood pressure of less than 140/90 mmHg is preferred for patients with CKD and normal to mildly elevated albuminuria (answer 2) is incorrect. Answer 3 is incorrect because the systolic blood pressure goal is too high, and answer 4 is incorrect because the diastolic blood pressure is too low.

10. Answer: 2

Rationale: This patient is significantly below his ideal body weight and has malnutrition. An iothalamate study (answer 1) will measure glomerular filtration rate (GFR), but it is not used clinically. A timed urine collection (answer 2) is best to assess the kidney function for this patient. However, the urine collection must be complete to ensure an accurate measurement of renal function. Cockcroft–Gault equation (answer 3) and Modification of Diet in Renal Disease study equation (answer 4) are incorrect because these equations would likely overestimate his renal function. Although these equations are the most appropriate for estimating kidney functions, it is better to use them on the intact kidney.

11. Answer: 4

Rationale: Calculation of fractional excretion of sodium (FENa) is necessary for estimating acute kidney injury (AKI) and to differentiate between the prerenal azotemia and the intrinsic AKI. When FENa is calculated and the result is greater than 2%, the patient has an intrinsic AKI.

$$FENa = [(\text{urinary sodium/serum sodium})/$$
$$(\text{urinary creatinine/serum creatinine})] \times 100$$
$$= [(26/140)/(15.3/1.8)] \times 100$$
$$= [0.18/8.5] \times 100 = 2.1\%$$

12. Answer: 4

Rationale: The patient is malnourished and refuses food and medications; therefore he has oliguria. The chronic kidney disease epidemiology collaboration (CKD-EPI) equation is based on stable serum creatinine, so it is difficult to use where there is an unstable serum creatinine (answer 1). Brater (answer 2) and Jelliffe (answer 3) equations are probably more accurate than Cockcroft and CKD-EPI, but they have not been rigorously tested. If the patient is nonoliguric, creatinine clearance can be calculated according to a timed urine collection and by using the average of serum creatinine samples obtained before and after the urine collection (answer 4).

13. Answer: 3

Rationale: The patient has hypotension despite adequate hydration. The blood urea nitrogen and serum creatinine are between 10 and 15:1, urinary sodium is greater than 40 mEq/L, and there is low urinary osmolality and cellular casts. All these signs refer to intrinsic acute kidney injury (AKI); therefore answer 3 is correct. Prerenal azotemia (answer 1) is considered when the urinary sodium is less than 20 mEq/L, high urinary osmolality, absence of casts, and the blood urea nitrogen/serum creatinine ratio is greater than 20:1. Functional AKI would look similar to prerenal AKI on urinalysis with no presence of casts and low urinary sodium (answer 2). Postrenal AKI (answer 4) occurs when the patient has kidney stones or cancers.

14. Answer: 1

Rationale: Bladder outlet obstruction is the most common cause of postrenal acute kidney injury (AKI) (answer 1). The patient suffers from benign prostatic hypertrophy because the laboratory tests reveal blood urea nitrogen (BUN)/creatinine ratio is between 10 and 15:1, urinary sodium is greater than 40 mEq/mL, there is a low urine osmolality, and fractional excretion of sodium is greater than 2%. Chronic kidney disease (answer 2) is kidney damage for more than 3 months, as defined by structural or functional abnormality of the kidney, with or without decreased glomerular filtration rate. Functional-mediated acute kidney injury (AKI) (answer 3) is determined when the serum BUN/creatinine ratio is greater than 20:1, urinary sodium is less than 20 mEq/mL, there is a high urine osmolality, and the fractional excretion of sodium is less than 1%. Intrinsic AKI (answer 4) would look similar to postrenal AKI on urinalysis. In addition, the cellular tubular casts are a marker of the intrinsic AKI.

15. Answer: 4

Rationale: The patient does not have any signs or symptoms of postrenal acute kidney injury (AKI). Postrenal AKI is related to presence of kidney stones, cancers, or benign prostatic hypertrophy for men (answer 1). The muddy brown granular casts, urinary sodium greater than 40 mEq/mL, and a blood urea nitrogen/serum creatinine ratio between 10 and 15:1 are markers for intrinsic AKI (answer 2). Glomerular disease (answer 3) occurs with or without a decrease in glomerular filtration rate (GFR), and proteinuria is the hallmark of glomerular disease. Lisinopril is an angiotensin-converting enzyme inhibitor that causes a vasodilatation of efferent arterioles and leads to a decrease in glomerular hydrostatic pressure and resultant decrease in GFR; this occurs in a functional AKI (answer 4).

16. Answer: 4

Rationale: Captopril (answer 1) is an angiotensin-converting enzyme inhibitor (ACEi) that can cause vasodilatation of efferent arterioles and lead to decrease of glomerular hydrostatic pressure; thus an ACEi can cause functional acute

kidney injury (AKI). Acetaminophen (answer 2) is metabolized by *N*-acetyl-p-benzoquinone, which is produced by liver. Levothyroxine (answer 3) has not been shown to have any nephrotoxicity symptoms. Trimethoprim/sulfamethazine (answer 4) could inhibit the tubular secretion of creatinine and leads to pseudonephrotoxicity.

17. Answer: 1

Rationale: The hemoglobin concentration of the patient is not at goal; it should be greater than 10 g/dL. Iron studies show that the patient is iron deficient because the ferritin concentration is less than 500 ng/mL and transferrin saturation is less than 30%. Intravenous iron (answer 1) is the most appropriate approach for patients with chronic kidney disease (CKD) who are receiving hemodialysis. Increasing the epoetin dosage (answer 2) would not increase red cell production with the absence of adequate iron. Oral iron (answer 3) is recommended for patients with nondialysis CKD. The patient is not at goal, which makes answer 4 incorrect.

18. Answer: 1

Rationale: The patient has anemia of chronic kidney disease (CKD). She suffers from CKD stage 3, and the hemoglobin concentration is lower than 10 g/mL; therefore adding epoetin doses would be recommended for this patient, according to Kidney Disease Improving Global Outcomes guidelines (answer 1). Administering intravenous iron (answer 2) would be appropriate for patients with CKD who are receiving dialysis treatment. In addition, iron should be added after administering epoetin doses if the iron stores are still insufficient. The patient is not at goal; therefore she needs to manage her anemia, which is related to the CKD (answer 3). Administering oral iron (answer 4) would be appropriate for patients with nondialysis CKD. Moreover, iron supplements should be added after administering epoetin dosages if the hemoglobin concentration is still low.

19. Answer: 3

Rationale: The patient presents with chronic kidney disease (CKD) stage 4 and she has not received dialysis. Her hemoglobin concentration (Hgb) is lower than 10 g/dL and she receives epoetin doses without any increase in the hemoglobin concentration. Adding intravenous iron (answer 1) is not recommended for patients with non-dialysis CKD. Administering red blood cells (answer 2) would not be preferred for this patient. The patient does not have coronary heart disease, which could prevent her from taking epoetin doses; however, epoetin administration reduces the need for red blood transfusion. Adding oral iron (answer 3) is the most preferred strategy for managing the patient's anemia with non-dialysis CKD because the ferritin concentration is less than 300 ng/mL and transferrin saturation is less than 30%, according to the KDIGO guidelines. Increasing epoetin dosage (answer 4) would not be beneficial because the iron stores are still deficient. Moreover, the epoetin would not increase the red blood cell production with the absence of adequate iron.

20. Answer: 4

Rationale: The patient presents with acute kidney injury (AKI) stage 2 because of an increasing serum creatinine of 2 to 2.9 times greater than baseline and a urinary volume less than 0.5 mL/kg/hr for the last 12 hours; therefore the kidney function is unstable. The Cockcroft equation (answer 1) and the Modification of Diet in Renal Disease study equation (answer 2) are incorrect because they are preferred in patients with stable kidney functions. The Brater equation would be preferred over the other methods, but it overestimates the kidney functions because the patient is anuric (answer 3). A 24-hour urine collection (answer 4) would be recommended for patients with unstable serum creatinine and anuria.

21. Answer: 2

Rationale: The patient presents with acute kidney injury (AKI) stage 2 caused by an increasing serum creatinine 2 to 2.9 times greater than baseline and a urinary volume less than 0.5 mL/kg/hr over the last 12 hours. Chronic kidney disease (CKD) (answer 1) is kidney damage for more than 3 months, as defined by structural and functional abnormality of the kidney with or without decreased of glomerular filtration rate, according to The National Kidney Foundation Kidney Disease Outcome Quality Initiative. The patient has muddy brown casts in his urine, and his blood urea nitrogen (BUN)/serum creatinine ratio is between 10 and 15:1; these are markers of acute tubular necrosis (answer 2). Postrenal AKI (answer 3) occurs in patients with benign prostatic hyperplasia, some kinds of cancers, and in the presence of nephrolithiasis. Prerenal azotemia occurs for patients with BUN/serum creatinine ratio greater than 20:1 and there is no presence of visible casts (answer 4).

22. Answer: 3

Rationale: The strategy of managing acute kidney injury (AKI) is to remove any potentially nephrotoxic drugs, direct toxins, or medications that alter intrarenal hemodynamics; therefore staying at the current regimen (answer 1) is incorrect. Nicotine patches (answer 2) do not have an adverse effect on kidney function, so they should be continued. Lisinopril is an angiotensin-converting enzyme inhibitor, which is one of the most nephrotoxic drugs and could impact kidney function (answer 3). Although, nonsteroidal antiinflammatory drugs are a nephrotoxic drug that should be discontinued to manage AKI, using a low dose of aspirin is acceptable and could be used without adversely effecting kidney function (answer 4).

23. Answer: 1

Rationale: The patient presents with intrinsic acute kidney injury (AKI), anuria, and pulmonary edema. Although loop diuretics such as furosemide have not been shown to improve clinical outcomes for patients with acute tubular necrosis (ATN), they may increase the urinary output, which will improve the fluid and electrolyte balance. Thus adding furosemide would be appropriate for this patient (answer 1). Thiazide diuretics (answer 2) are not appropriate for patients who have AKI or if the creatinine clearance is less than 30 mL/min/1.73 m². Water and sodium restriction (answer 3) would be beneficial for management of this patient, but this restriction cannot be used if loop diuretics have failed. Administering intravenous 0.9% sodium chloride could worsen the case because the patient has hypervolemia.

24. Answer: 1

Rationale: To stratifying acute kidney injury (AKI) you can use the RIFLE (risk, injury, failure, loss, and end-stage kidney disease) criteria. The patient presents with severe community-acquired pneumonia and has an increasing serum creatinine two times the baseline. According to RIFLE classification, increasing serum creatinine two times the baseline is classified as an injury to the kidney (answer 1). When the serum creatinine is increased more than 4 mg/dL or serum creatinine is increased to three times the baseline, it is classified as failure of the kidney (answer 2). Loss of kidney function occurs when there is a complete loss of kidney function for greater than 4 weeks (answer 3). End-stage kidney disease (answer 4) happens when there is a complete loss of kidney function for greater than 3 months.

25. Answer: 3

Rationale: The patient presents with acute kidney injury. Acute Kidney Injury Network (AKIN) is a diagnostic criteria and requires one of the following with 48 hours: an absolute increase in serum creatinine greater than 0.3 mg/dL or 1.5 to 1.9 × baseline (stage 1) (answer 1 is incorrect), increase in serum creatinine 2–2.9 mg/dL × baseline (stage 2) (answer 2 is incorrect), or increase in serum creatinine greater than 3 × baseline, which means serum creatinine more is increased than 4 mg/dL (stage 3) (answer 3 is correct). AKIN criteria involve three stages only; therefore (answer 4) is incorrect.

26. Answer: 2

Rationale: The patient presents with signs of volume depletion because of her pregnancy, which leads to acute kidney injury. From her values, the blood urea nitrogen (BUN)/serum creatinine ratio is greater than 20:1 and urinary sodium is lower than 20 mEq/L; therefore there are signs for prerenal azotemia. Adding loop diuretics (answer 1) could worsen the case. The best strategy for management of this patient is fluid resuscitation with intravenous 0.9% sodium chloride solution (answer 2). The patient does not have any signs of edema; therefore the fluid restriction would not beneficial (answer 3). The patient has severe vomiting and is intolerant of oral hydration with water (answer 4).

27. Answer: 3

Rationale: The patient presents with nephrolithiasis and signs of acute kidney injury (AKI). The blood urea nitrogen/serum creatinine ratio is 10 to 15:1 and urinary sodium is greater than 40 mEq/L. These are markers for postrenal AKI. Adding furosemide could lead to volume depletion and worsen the case (answer 1). Fluid restriction (answer 2) is not beneficial for this patient. For removing kidney stones, increasing hydration is the best strategy for management of this case (answer 3). Spironolactone (answer 4) would not be appropriate for this case because it is not preferred for patients with creatinine clearance less than 30 mL/min/1.73 m^2.

28. Answer: 4

Rationale: Renal replacement therapy is indicated for acute kidney injury for the following reasons: blood urea nitrogen (BUN) is greater than 100 mg/dL (answer 1), treatment of refractory metabolic acidosis has failed with pharmacological treatment (answer 2), uremia and encephalopathy, and life-threatening electrolyte imbalance, such as hyperkalemia but not hypomagnesemia (answer 4 is incorrect).

29. Answer: 3

Rationale: The patient has chronic kidney disease history with an elevated serum creatinine. Metformin should be interrupted for two reasons. One reason is that metformin is historically contraindicated for patient with serum creatinine is greater than 1.5 mg/dL in men and 1.4 mg/dL in women because it would increase the risk of lactic acidosis. Metformin also should be interrupted if the patient is to undergo procedures using iodinated contrast dye in 24 hours because of the risk of nephrotoxicity. It should then reinitiated after 48 hours. Therefore answers 1, 2, and 4 are incorrect.

30. Answer: 2

Rationale: The patient has chronic kidney (CKD) disease and is going to have elective cardiac catheterization. Intravenous contrast use could cause direct tubular toxicity and could decrease tubular flow rates. The patient has risk factors for nephrotoxicity such as preexisting CKD and diabetes type 2. Oral hydration with water (answer 1) would not be effective hydration for preventing contract induced nephrotoxicity. The intravenous 0.9% of saline solution is considered the most effective hydration for preventing contrast-induced nephrotoxicity (answer 2). Therefore answers 3 and 4 are incorrect.

31. Answer: 1

Rationale: The contrast could increase the serum creatinine and the blood urea nitrogen (BUN) within 24 hours and peak 2 to 5 days after the procedure. Monitoring of serum creatinine

at 24 hours will help identify the development of contrast-associated nephrotoxicity; therefore (answer 1) is correct. Waiting for more than 48 hours would delay the detection of renal damage, so answers 2, 3, and 4 are incorrect.

32. Answer: 4

Rationale: The patient receives cisplatin and it could increase serum creatinine peaks 10 to 12 days after therapy starts and may continue to increase with subsequent cycles of therapy. There are many risk factors of toxicity, which should not be avoided, whereas cisplatin administration includes using the smallest dosage possible (answer 1 is correct), administering an aggressive intravenous hydration (answer 2 is correct), adding a cisplatin-chelation as amifostine (answer 3 is correct), and decreasing the frequency of administration (answer 4 is incorrect).

33. Answer: 3

Rationale: Long-duration of lithium (more than 10 years) could lead to worsening kidney function, which is often asymptomatic. There are many strategies that should be taken to decrease the risk of lithium-induced chronic interstitial nephritis, which include maintaining the lowest lithium concentration (answer 1), monitoring the kidney function closely (answer 2), and avoiding dehydration (answer 4). Adding loop diuretics could worsen the case and leads to volume depletion; therefore it could increase the risk of nephrotoxicity (answer 3).

34. Answer: 3

Rationale: The patient's estimated glomerular filtration rate is 40 mL/min/1.73 m^2; therefore according to the Kidney Disease Improving Global Outcomes stages, his chronic kidney disease would be classified as stage 3 (answer 3 is correct).

35. Answer: 3

Rationale: According to the National Kidney Foundation Kidney Disease Outcomes Quality Initiative (KDOQI), chronic kidney disease (CKD) is kidney damage for greater than 3 months, as defined by structural or functional abnormalities of the kidney, with or without decreased glomerular filtration rate (GFR). The patient's estimated GFR (eGFR) is 40 mL/min/1.73 m^2; therefore according to KDOQI stages, he is in stage 3 (eGFR is between 30 and 59 mL/min/1.73m^2) (answer 3 is correct). A patient's GFR would be classified as stage 1 when the GFR is less than 90 mL/min/1.73 m^2 (answer 1 is incorrect). A patient's GFR would be classified as stage 2 when the GFR is between 60 and 89 mL/min/1.73 m^2 (answer 2 is incorrect). Also, a patient's GFR could be classified as stage 4 when the GFR is between 15 and 29 mL/min/1.73 m^2 (answer 4 is incorrect).

36. Answer: 3

Rationale: The Kidney Disease Improving Global Outcomes guidelines provide guidance on categorization of albuminuria according to the albumin/creatinine ratio (ACR). Category A1 is an ACR less than 30 mg/g (answer 1 is incorrect). Category A2 is a moderate increase of albuminuria with an ACR of 30 to 300 mg/g (answer 2 is incorrect). Category A3 is a severe increase of albuminuria with an ACR greater than 300 mg/g (answer 3 is correct). Nephrotic-range proteinuria is a protein excretion exceeding 3000 mg/g (answer 4 is incorrect).

37. Answer: 1

Rationale: The patient presents with diabetic nephropathy because of her diabetes mellitus and the presence of moderate albuminuria. Progression could be accelerated by poor blood pressure control and poor blood glucose control. In patients with diabetic nephropathy, the A1c goal should be less than 7%, and the blood pressure goal should be less than 130/80 mmHg to limit the progression of the kidney disease. Adding angiotensin-converting enzyme inhibitors (ACEis) would reduce the mortality and chronic kidney disease progression, so (answer 1) is the best choice. Increasing the metoprolol succinate dosage could control the blood pressure, but it would not limit the kidney progression (answer 2). Adding nondihydropyridine calcium channel blockers might be initiated in patients who cannot tolerate ACEis or angiotensin receptor blockers (answer 3). Adding dihydropyridine as nifedipine (answer 4) is not recommended in diabetic nephropathy because of the conflicting literature on its efficacy.

38. Answer: 3

Rationale: This patient has diabetic nephropathy based on his laboratory values, which include elevation in blood pressure, serum creatinine, and albumin/creatinine ratio. The blood pressure goal for patients with diabetic nephropathy should be less than 130/80 mmHg. The increase is serum creatinine is less than 30%; therefore enalapril should be continued without change. That makes answers 1 and 2 incorrect. Adding chlorthalidone (answer 3) is the best choice to achieve the blood pressure goal and monitoring of serum creatinine and potassium are appropriate for this patient (answer 3). Increasing the beta-blockers would not be beneficial for limiting his kidney function prognosis (answer 4).

39. Answer: 1

Rationale: The patient has moderately increased albuminuria, chronic kidney disease, and elevation of the serum creatinine from the baseline. Hold angiotensin-converting enzyme inhibitors if serum potassium is greater than 5.6 mEq/L and serum creatinine is greater than 30% after the

initiation; therefore (answer 1) would be the best action for this patient and answers 2 and 3 are incorrect. Metolazone is a thiazide diuretic that will not add any benefits if the dosage is increased for patients with elevated serum creatinine more than 30% (answer 4 is incorrect).

40. Answer: 1

Rationale: The patient has a history of chronic kidney disease (CKD), myocardial infarction (MI), and elevation of low-density cholesterol; therefore he needs lifestyle modification with a pharmacological treatment (answer 4 is incorrect). Adding statins is recommended for patients with CKD who are older than 50 years. In addition, pravastatin is safer than other statins for patients with kidney disease (answer 1). Niacin (answer 2) would be an acceptable regimen for treatment the hyperlipidemia, but it is contraindicated for patients with a history of gout. Using ezetimibe alone would not have the same benefits as using it with statins (answer 3).

41. Answer: 1

Rationale: The best access for this patient is the arteriovenous fistula (answer 1) because it is natural and formed by the anastomosis of an artery and vein. In addition, it has the lowest incidence of infection and thrombosis, lower cost, and longest survival. Arteriovenous graft (answer 2) is the second choice, which is usually preferred for patients with vascular diseases. Tenckhoff catheter (answer 3) is a catheter for peritoneal dialysis. A subclavian catheter (answer 4) is commonly used if permanent access is unavailable, but it is not preferred because it has high infection and thrombosis rates, and low blood flow leads to inadequate analysis.

42. Answer: 2

Rationale: Fludrocortisone (answer 1) is a synthetic mineralocorticoid that is used for hypertension in other situations. The best-studied agent is midodrine, an α_1 agonist, 2.5 to 10 mg orally before dialysis. Sodium chloride tablets (answer 3) would not work acutely and should be avoided. Levocarnitine (answer 4) has been tried, but there are insufficient data for its benefits.

43. Answer: 1

Rationale: The patient has hypotension during his dialysis treatment. The hypotension should be prevented by midodrine before the dialysis. When hypotension occurs during a hemodialysis treatment, the nonpharmacological approaches should be tried such as decreasing the ultrafiltration rate (answer 2), administering saline boluses (answer 3), and Trendelenburg position (answer 4). Therefore increasing the ultrafiltration rate would be an incorrect answer (answer 1).

44. Answer: 1

Rationale: This patient presents with peritonitis, which is the most common cause peritoneal dialysis failure. The empiric treatment should cover the gram-positive and gram-negative bacteria. The intraperitoneal administration is preferred more than the intravenous administration. According to the International Society for Peritoneal Dialysis guidelines, the best empiric therapy is the intraperitoneal administration of a first-generation cephalosporin or vancomycin *plus* intraperitoneal administration of a third-generation of cephalosporin or aminoglycosides; therefore answer 1 is the best choice, and answer 2 is incorrect. In addition, cefazolin could provide activity against staphylococcus unless an area has a high rate of methicillin-resistant organisms. The third-generation cephalosporin or aminoglycosides has activity against *Pseudomonas*. In a patient with dialysis-related peritonitis, empiric anaerobic coverage is unnecessary, so answers 3 and 4 are inappropriate.

45. Answer: 3

Rationale: Peritoneal dialysis often is less preferred than hemodialysis because of its complications, which include the peritonitis (answer 1 is correct), fluid overload (answer 2 is correct), hypoglycemia (answer 3 is incorrect), and hypercalcemia or hypocalcemia (answer 4 is correct).

46. Answer: 4

Rationale: Infection and inflammation are the most common causes for epoetin resistance (answer 1), but the patient is afebrile and nothing in his presentation suggests an infection or inflammatory process. The patient does not have iron deficiency because his serum ferritin is greater than 500 ng/mL and transferrin saturation is greater than 30% (answer 2). Phenytoin (answer 3) has been associated with anemia in other patient population, but not in patients receiving hemodialysis treatment. The patient has hyperparathyroidism, which is one of the most common causes for epoetin resistance (answer 4).

47. Answer: 2

Rationale: The patient needs to treat his hyperparathyroidism, which places him at high risk of renal osteodystrophy and vascular calcification. Although his measured calcium is normal, the corrected calcium concentration is elevated, and he has a high phosphorus concentration. Therefore changing to calcium carbonate (answer 1) or increasing the calcium acetate dosage (answer 4) are incorrect. Changing calcium acetate to sevelamer is the best choice to avoid the increase in calcium concentration. In addition, adding cinacalcet will lower the intact parathyroid hormone (PTH) and potentially serum calcium (answer 2). Adding intravenous vitamin D analog can worsen hypercalcemia, and it has no impact on reducing the intact PTH (answer 3).

48. Answer: 2

Rationale: Patients who are receiving erythropoiesis-stimulating agents (ESAs) should be under the U.S. Food and Drug Administration Risk Evaluation and Mitigation Strategies program (answer 1). If the hemoglobin increase is greater than 1 g/dL in 2 weeks, ESAs should be decreased to 25% only (answer 2). There are many reasons contributing to ESA resistance such as iron deficiency, folate and vitamin B_{12} deficiency, infection and inflammation, hyperparathyroidism, vitamin C deficiency, and other factors (answer 3). Hemoglobin should be monitored every 2 to 4 weeks during initiation, and at least monthly in dialysis patients and at least 3 months in nondialysis patients with chronic kidney disease (answer 4).

49. Answer: 4

Rationale: According to the Kidney Disease Improving Global Outcomes guidelines, there is laboratory frequency monitoring in chronic kidney disease (CKD) stages 3 to 5, and this patient presents with CKD stage 5; therefore answer 1 is incorrect. At CKD stage 3 calcium should be monitored every 6 to 12 months, phosphorus every 6 to 12 months, intact parathyroid hormone (PTH) and 25-hydroxycitamin D are at baseline (answer 2). At CKD stage 4, calcium should be monitored every 3 to 6 months, phosphorus every 3 to 6 months, intact PTH every 6 to 12 months, and 25-hydroxyvitamin D is at baseline (answer 3). At CKD stage 5, calcium should be monitored every 1 to 3 months, phosphorus every 1 to 3 months, intact PTH every 3 to 6 months, and 25-hydroxyvitamin D is at baseline (answer 4).

50. Answer: 3

Rationale: Cinacalcet is a calcimimetic that attaches to the calcium receptor on the parathyroid gland and increases the sensitivity of receptors to serum calcium concentration, reducing parathyroid hormone (PTH). Cinacalcet is metabolized primarily by CYP3A4; thus ketoconazole (CYP3A4 inhibitor) could increase the cinacalcet concentration by up to twofold (answer 1). Cinacalcet could inhibit CYP2D6, inhibiting the metabolism of cytochrome CYP2D6 substrates such that dosage reduction in drugs with narrow therapeutic indices may be required (e.g., tricyclic antidepressants) (answer 2). Cinacalcet can be used cautiously in patients with seizure disorders (answer 3 is incorrect). Cinacalcet could cause hypocalcemia as an exacerbation (answer 4).

51. Answer: 4

Rationale: Etelcalcetide is a synthetic peptide calcimimetic that activates the calcium-sensing receptor on the parathyroid gland, reducing parathyroid hormone (PTH). The initial dose is 5 mg intravenously three times weekly after hemodialysis, and the dosage could be titrated in 2.5- to 5-mg increments at intervals of at least every 4 weeks (answer 1). Etelcalcetide could be used with caution for patients with seizure disorders and may cause hypocalcemia (answer 2). Etelcalcetide has an adverse effect of QT prolongation, worsening heart failure, nausea, diarrhea, and hypocalcemia (answer 3). Cinacalcet should be discontinued for at least 7 days before initiation of etelcalcetide; thus, answer 4 is incorrect.

52. Answer: 1

Rationale: Almost all antibiotics require dosage adjustment exception ceftriaxone, metronidazole, clindamycin, nafcillin, and macrolides (answer 1). Meperidine should be avoided for patients with decreased kidney function because it may accumulate (answer 2). Potassium-sparing diuretics such as spironolactone should be avoided for patients with creatinine clearance less than 30 mL/min/1.73 m^2 (answer 3). Almost all statins, particularly rosuvastatin, should be adjusted for patients with decreased kidney function (answer 4).

Integumentary

10

1. A 20-year-old female patient presents to your clinic complaining of 10 comedones on her face and 12 inflammatory lesions. She is obese and likes to eat chocolate every day. She is healthy and denies any drug abuse, but she drinks vodka when she is out with friends. Which of the following is *not* a cause for her acne problem?

   1. Cosmetics.

   2. Menstruation.

   3. Fatty meals.

   4. Vegetables.

2. A 20-year-old female patient presents to your clinic complaining of 10 comedones on her face and 12 inflammatory lesions. She is obese and likes to eat chocolate every day. She is healthy and denies any drug abuse, but she drinks vodka when she is out with friends. Which classification is correct for her presentation?

   1. Mild acne.

   2. Moderate acne.

   3. Severe acne.

   4. Psoriasis.

3. A 20-year-old female patient presents to your clinic complaining of 10 comedones on her face and 12 inflammatory lesions. She is obese and likes to eat chocolate every day. She is healthy and denies any drug abuse, but she drinks vodka when she is out with friends. Which treatment is best for her?

   1. Topical retinoid.

   2. Topical clindamycin.

   3. Oral isotretinoin.

   4. Benzoyl peroxide.

4. A 23-year-old male patient who has approximately 45 pustular lesions on his face, shoulder, and back, which increase during the autumn months, visits his nurse practitioner. He reports that he has seasonal rhinitis and he has a penicillin allergy (anaphylactic shock). Which classification is the appropriate for this presentation?

   1. Mild acne.

   2. Moderate acne.

   3. Severe acne.

   4. Stevens–Johnson syndrome.

5. A 23-year-old male patient who has approximately 45 pustular lesions on his face, shoulder, and back, which increase during the autumn months, visits his nurse practitioner. He reports that he has seasonal rhinitis and he has a penicillin allergy (anaphylactic shock). Which therapy is the best for this patient?

   1. Topical retinoid.

   2. Topical retinoid plus benzoyl peroxide.

   3. Topical retinoid plus benzoyl peroxide plus oral clindamycin.

   4. Oral isotretinoin.

6. A 23-year-old male patient who has approximately 45 pustular lesions on his face, shoulder, and back, which increase during the autumn months, visits his nurse practitioner. He reports that he has seasonal rhinitis and he has a penicillin allergy (anaphylactic shock). The nurse practitioner prescribed a topical retinoid and oral tetracycline. He was researching about how oral vitamins can worsen his acne. Which vitamin is the best for him?

   1. Vitamin B_1.

   2. Vitamin B_6.

   3. Vitamin B_{12}.

   4. Vitamin A.

7. A 27-year-old Hispanic female patient presents to her nurse practitioner with complaints of facial acne. The nurse practitioner prescribes a topical retinoid. When the patient puts the topical retinoid on her face, she feels a slight burning sensation. What should the nurse practitioner advise the patient to do?

    1. Stop topical retinoid.

    2. Initiate oral isotretinoin.

    3. Administer topical retinoid in the morning.

    4. Administer topical retinoid in the evening.

8. A 26-year-old female patient, who is currently taking multiphasic birth control pills, presents to her nurse practitioner with complaints of 10 inflammatory comedones on her face. The nurse practitioner recommends a topical retinoid and topical clindamycin. The nurse practitioner educates the patient about the topical medications and birth control pills. Which of the following states is correct?

    1. There are no adverse drug interactions with the birth control and the topical medications.

    2. She should use one method for contraception while using the topical medications.

    3. She should use two methods for contraception while using the topical medications.

    4. She will need to discontinue her birth control pills while using the topical medications.

9. A 17-year-old male patient comes to your health care facility with inflammatory nodular acne on his face, back, and shoulders. His current medications are topical retinoid, topical benzoyl peroxide, and oral tetracycline. The nodular acne has become unresponsive to his medications, and he has started to develop scarring because of increasing irritation. Which therapy is the best alternative drug for this patient?

    1. Continue his regimen.

    2. Oral isotretinoin.

    3. Topical retinoid plus topical azelaic acid.

    4. Oral drospirenone.

10. A 17-year-old male patient comes to your health care facility with inflammatory nodular acne on his face, back, and shoulders. His current medications are topical retinoid, topical benzoyl peroxide, and oral tetracycline. The nodular acne has become unresponsive to his medications, and he has started to develop scarring because of increasing irritation. The nurse practitioner recommends isotretinoin, and he and his family have agreed to start this medication after they are educated about potential adverse effects. Which additional measure is best before the patient initiates his medication?

    1. Enroll the patient in the iPledge program to avoid teratogenicity.

    2. Have the patient obtain clearance from a mental health provider to begin using the agent because it has been associated with suicidal ideations.

    3. Remain diligent to testing hepatic transaminases every other week until therapy is discontinued; discontinue the medication if the patient does not adhere to testing.

    4. Have the patient agree to avoid driving after sunset for 6 months secondary to vision changes associated with the drug.

11. A 39-year-old Asian male patient presents to his nurse practitioner with itchy and painful skin lesions on his knees. He smokes 1 pack of cigarettes a day and has hypertension that is controlled with diltiazem. The nurse practitioner diagnosed him with psoriasis. Which of the following does not contribute to psoriasis?

    1. Smoking.

    2. Genetic factors.

    3. Ibuprofen.

    4. Diltiazem.

12. A 63-year-old African American female patient presents with a history of bipolar disorder and resistant hypertension. She comes to the primary care office complaining of itchy and painful skin lesions on her back and neck. The lesions cover about 7% of the total body surface area. She is diagnosed with psoriasis. What is the classification of the severity of her psoriasis?

    1. No psoriasis.

    2. Mild psoriasis.

    3. Moderate psoriasis.

    4. Severe psoriasis.

13. A 63-year-old African American female patient presents with a history of bipolar disorder and resistant hypertension. She comes to the primary care office complaining of itchy and painful skin lesions on her back and neck. The lesions cover about 7% of the total body surface area. She is diagnosed with psoriasis. Her current medications include hydrochlorothiazide 50 mg daily, verapamil 240 mg daily, lithium 900 mg daily, and valproic acid 50 mg daily. Which medication is most likely contributing to psoriasis?

    1. Hydrochlorothiazide.

    2. Verapamil.

    3. Lithium.

    4. Valproic acid.

14. A 52-year-old male patient with a 25-year history of hypertension and 10-year history of type 2 diabetes presents to his nurse practitioner with itchy and painful lesions on his arms. He denies any alcohol or drug abuse. He currently takes lisinopril 20 mg daily, hydrochlorothiazide 50 mg daily, carvedilol 25 mg daily, and metformin 500 mg twice daily. Which medication is most likely contributing to this presentation?

    1. Lisinopril.

    2. Hydrochlorothiazide.

    3. Carvedilol.

    4. Metformin.

15. A 35-year-old Hispanic male patient presents to his nurse practitioner with lesions covering his face, legs, and arms. The lesions are painful and itchy. These lesions cover 12% of the total body surface area. He has a long history of type I bipolar disorder. The nurse practitioner is concerned that he may have psoriasis. Which classification is correct to help in the treatment of this patient?

    1. Mild psoriasis.

    2. Moderate psoriasis.

    3. Severe psoriasis.

    4. Stevens–Johnson syndrome.

16. A 65-year-old male patient comes to your clinic with itchy and burning lesions on his back. After the exam, the nurse practitioner diagnosed him with psoriasis. His medical history includes hypertension and osteoarthritis. His current medications are acetaminophen and captopril. He reports that his father had psoriasis, too. Which medication is most likely appropriate for this patient?

    1. Topical corticosteroids.

    2. Ultraviolet radiation.

    3. Topical calcipotriene.

    4. Azathioprine.

17. A 65-year-old Asian male patient comes to your clinic with itchy and burning lesions on his back. After the exam, the nurse practitioner diagnosed him with psoriasis. His medical history includes hypertension and osteoarthritis. His current medications are acetaminophen and captopril. He reports that his father had psoriasis too. His nurse practitioner prescribes topical corticosteroids, but his lesions have not healed. Which medication should be added for this patient?

    1. Continue at the current medication.

    2. Initiate topical calcipotriene.

    3. Administer ultraviolet radiation.

    4. Change to infliximab.

18. A 65-year-old Asian male patient comes to your clinic with itchy and burning lesions on his back. After the exam, the nurse practitioner diagnosed him with psoriasis. His medical history includes hypertension and osteoarthritis. His current medications are acetaminophen and captopril. He reports that his father had psoriasis, too. His nurse practitioner prescribes topical corticosteroids, but his lesions have not healed. Then the nurse practitioner added topical vitamin D. The symptoms started to heal, but some lesions started to appear on his scalp. Which treatment is best for his new symptoms?

    1. Antidandruff shampoo and steroid lotion.

    2. Azathioprine.

    3. Infliximab.

    4. Adalimumab.

19. A 56-year-old male patient with a 9-year history of psoriasis on his face and neck visits his nurse practitioner for routine follow-up. His medications are topical corticosteroids and topical vitamin D. His symptoms were treated with these medications, but the lesions have returned again and are not responsive to his previous regimen. Which therapy should be added to this case?

    1. Oral corticosteroids.

    2. Oral calcipotriene.

    3. Azathioprine.

    4. Phototherapy.

20. A 35-year-old female patient presents to the nurse practitioner with fever and necrotic lesions that began on her neck but are spreading to her back and legs. The nurse practitioner diagnosed her with Stevens–Johnson syndrome. Her lesions cover 24% of the total body surface area. What is the best treatment for this patient?

    1. Topical corticosteroids.

    2. Prednisone 1 to 2 mg/kg/day for 3 to 5 days.

    3. Oral vitamin D and topical corticosteroids.

    4. Methotrexate and topical vitamin D and topical corticosteroids.

21. A 45-year-old female patient presents to her nurse practitioner at her primary care office with painful lesions on her neck and back. Her lesions cover 10% of the total body surface area. She is healthy and denies any other medical problems. The nurse practitioner diagnosed her with eczema. What is the best treatment for the patient?

    1. Topical corticosteroids.

    2. Methotrexate.

    3. Initiate infliximab.

    4. Oral vitamin D.

22. A 63-year-old woman presents with a long-standing history of type 2 diabetes and hypertension. She reports that she had tonsillitis 2 weeks ago and was on amoxicillin for treatment. She presents to the emergency department with a papular erythematous rash scattered on her back and several bullae on her fingers. She currently takes metformin 500 mg twice daily, sitagliptin 100 mg daily, hydrochlorothiazide 50 mg daily, and lisinopril 10 mg daily. The nurse practitioner (NP) is concerned that the patient has Stevens–Johnson syndrome, so the NP consulted the intensive care unit. Which agent is most likely responsible for this adverse drug reaction?

    1. Metformin.

    2. Sitagliptin.

    3. Hydrochlorothiazide.

    4. Amoxicillin.

23. A 35-year-old white male patient presents to the emergency department with a severe cutaneous hypersensitivity reaction. He reports that 3 days ago he went to his primary care provider with symptoms of a urinary tract infection and he had been taking sulfamethazine/trimethoprim double strength. The nurse practitioner thinks the patient has toxic epidermal necrosis. Which agent could *not* cause this adverse drug reaction?

    1. Phenytoin.

    2. Sulfa drugs.

    3. Piroxicam.

    4. Lisinopril.

24. A 43-year-old African American female patient presents with a 5-year history of gout, osteoarthritis, and hypothyroidism. Her medications include allopurinol 100 mg daily, acetaminophen 1000 mg three times daily, levothyroxine 125 mcg/day, and calcium supplements daily. She comes to the emergency department with several bullae on her fingers and sloughing of skin on her abdomen and back. She is transferred to the intensive care unit for treatment of Stevens–Johnson syndrome. Which medication is the most likely to induce Stevens–Johnson syndrome?

    1. Acetaminophen.

    2. Allopurinol.

    3. Levothyroxine.

    4. Calcium supplements.

25. A 43-year-old African American female patient presents with a 5-year history of gout, osteoarthritis, and hypothyroidism. Her medications include allopurinol 100 mg daily, acetaminophen 1000 mg three times daily, levothyroxine 125 mcg/day, and calcium supplements daily. She comes to the emergency department with several bullae on her fingers and sloughing of skin on her abdomen and back. She is transferred to the intensive care unit for treatment of Stevens–Johnson syndrome. Which therapy is the first to be initiated for this patient?

    1. Initiate supportive care.

    2. Discontinue allopurinol.

    3. Administer intravenous immunoglobulin.

    4. Initiate cyclosporine.

26. A 56-year-old woman with a history of seizures presents to the clinic for consultation. She has also been experiencing fatigue, sensitivity to sunlight, and hair loss. She is on phenytoin for seizures. The nurse practitioner diagnosed her with systemic lupus erythematous (SLE). Which agents will *not* induce SLE?

    1. Phenytoin.

    2. Carbamazepine.

    3. Isoniazid.

    4. Hydralazine.

27. A 56-year-old woman with a history of seizures presents to the clinic for consultation. She has been experiencing fatigue, sensitivity to sunlight, and hair loss. She is on phenytoin for seizures. The nurse practitioner diagnosed her with systemic lupus erythematous. Which therapy is the best for this patient?

    1. Nonsteroidal antiinflammatory agents.

    2. Topical corticosteroids.

    3. Oral corticosteroids.

    4. Azathioprine.

28. A 35-year-old female patient with a history of systemic lupus erythematous (SLE) presents to her nurse practitioner with concerns about her SLE. She is currently on hydroxychloroquine 200 mg per day and it does not seem to be helping. What treatment should the nurse practitioner initiate next?

    1. Increase hydroxychloroquine dose to achieve serum concentration greater than 1000 ng/mL.

    2. Add infliximab 5 mg/kg/day.

    3. Add omega-3 fatty acids.

    4. Add azathioprine 2 mg/kg/day.

29. A 35-year-old female patient with a history of systemic lupus erythematous (SLE) presents to her nurse practitioner with concerns about her SLE. She is currently on hydroxychloroquine 200 mg/day, and she is concerned about potential adverse drug reactions. Which adverse reaction is *not* associated with hydroxychloroquine?

    1. Migraine.

    2. Myopathy.

    3. Aplastic anemia.

    4. Decreased of visual acuity.

30. A 35-year-old female patient with a history of systemic lupus erythematous (SLE) presents to her nurse practitioner with concerns about her SLE. She is currently on hydroxychloroquine 200 mg/day, and she is concerned about potential adverse drug reactions. Which screening test is most recommended for patients treated with hydroxychloroquine?

    1. Hypersensitivity test.

    2. Kidney function tests.

    3. Liver enzymes tests.

    4. Ophthalmological tests.

31. A 75-year-old male patient presents to the emergency department with scald burns covering 15% of his total body surface after talking a hot bath. Wound biopsy reveals gram-negative rods. He reports the he has penicillin and sulfa allergies. Which topical antimicrobial is the best for this presentation?

    1. Silver sulfasalazine.

    2. Silver nitrate.

    3. Nystatin.

    4. Gentamycin.

32. An 18-year-old female patient presents to the dermatology clinic with a history of rash with pruritus. The nurse practitioner has diagnosed her with urticaria. The patient reports that she has no known food or drug allergies, but she did go to a new neighborhood swimming pool. What should the nurse practitioner recommend for the patient?

    1. Famotidine.

    2. Cyclosporine.

    3. Montelukast.

    4. Cetirizine.

33. An 18-year-old female patient presents to the dermatology clinic with a history of rash with pruritus. The nurse practitioner has diagnosed her with urticaria. The patient reports that she has no known food or drug allergies, but she did go to a new neighborhood swimming pool. The nurse practitioner recommends loratadine. After 1 week, she returned to the clinic because the symptoms are not any better. Which medication should the nurse practitioner recommend for this patient?

    1. Famotidine.

    2. Cetirizine.

    3. Corticosteroids.

    4. Montelukast.

10 | Integumentary Answers & Rationales

1. Answer: 4

Rationale: The patient presents with mild acne. Cosmetics can block skin pores and lead to acne (answer 1 is incorrect). Menstruation leads to the development of hormonal acne (answer 2 is incorrect). Fatty meals and chocolate should be avoided because they could develop acne (answer 3 is incorrect). Vegetables and fruits are healthy food full of vitamins and minerals that do not cause acne. There also are nonpharmacological treatments for acne cases (answer 4 is correct).

2. Answer: 1

Rationale: This patient has fewer than 15 comedones and fewer than 15 inflammatory lesions, so her presentation is classified as mild acne (answer 1). Psoriasis is another skin condition that has no relation to this presentation (answer 4).

3. Answer: 1

Rationale: This patient presents with signs and symptoms of mild acne. She has fewer than 15 comedones and fewer than 15 inflammatory lesions. The best treatment for her is topical retinoid, which reduces the presence of mild to moderate noninflammatory lesions (answer 1). Topical antibiotics (answer 2) should not be used alone, but they could be combined with a topical retinoid if there is a presence of pus; therefore this choice is incorrect. Oral isotretinoin (answer 3) is appropriate only for treatment of severe cases because of its potential adverse effects. Benzoyl peroxide (answer 4) is inappropriate for this presentation because it is preferred for moderate cases. It should be combined with topical retinoid and not used alone.

4. Answer: 2

Rationale: The patient presents with more than 30 and fewer than 125 lesions; thus moderate acne (answer 2) is the correct choice.

5. Answer: 3

Rationale: This patient is classified as moderate acne because he has more than 30 inflammatory lesions and fewer than 125 total lesions. Topical retinoid (answer 1) is the best choice for treatment of mild acne. Benzoyl peroxide could be added to the topical retinoid for treatment of moderate acne, but this regimen is not the optimal treatment without adding oral antibiotics. Thus answer 2 is incorrect and answer 3 is the best choice. Oral isotretinoin (answer 4) is restricted only for severe cases because of its severe adverse effects.

6. Answer: 4

Rationale: There are vitamins that can help with acne. Vitamin A is a powerful antioxidant that helps prevent acne by reducing the amount of sebum in the skin. So answers 1, 2, and 3 are incorrect.

7. Answer: 4

Rationale: The patient has acne, and the nurse practitioner recommends a topical retinoid. The patient starts to feel some irritation and burning sensation, but it usually resolves within 2 to 4 weeks. Stopping topical retinoid (answer 1) would be an unsuccessful strategy because the topical retinoid could reduce the presence of mild to moderate noninflammatory lesions. Initiating oral isotretinoin (answer 2) would be inappropriate because it is recommended for severe cases only because of its potential severe risk for patients who use it. Administering topical retinoid in the morning could increase the burning sensation when she goes outside as well as photosensitivity and sunburns (answer 3). Administering topical retinoid in the evening (answer 4) would be appropriate to avoid the burning sensation.

8. Answer: 3

Rationale: The patient is of childbearing age and sexually active. Topical retinoid should be avoided during pregnancy because it has adverse effects on the fetus, and therefore answer 1 is incorrect. A woman of childbearing age should use two different methods for contraception, such as barrier and hormonal therapy (answers 2 and 4 are incorrect).

9. Answer: 2

Rationale: The patient has nodular acne on his face, back, and shoulders that has become unresponsive to the medications he is taking (answer 1 is incorrect). Oral isotretinoin (answer 2) is appropriate for severe cases. This patient needs it because he is unresponsive to the first-line treatment, so isotretinoin is the best alternative drug in this case. Topical retinoid and topical azelaic acid (answer 3) would be inappropriate without using oral antibiotics. Oral drospirenone (answer 4) is an antiadrenergic progesterone agent and is unadvised.

10. Answer: 1

Rationale: Patients who take oral isotretinoin must be enrolled in the iPledge program to avoid teratogenicity during or before pregnancy (answer 1). A patient taking oral isotretinoin should be counseled on the potential increased risk of depression and suicidal thoughts, but they do not need a mental health provider to sign off on therapy (answer 2). Routine monitoring for hepatic transaminase should be recommended until the patient reaches the effective dose, but nonadherence to testing is not an indication to stop the therapy (answer 3). No reports have shown any night vision problems (answer 4).

11. Answer: 4

Rationale: There are many risk factors associated with the development of psoriasis. Smoking is a predisposing factor to developing psoriasis (answer 1). Genetic factors (answer 2) are evidenced by the higher incidence reported between first- and second-degree relatives and monozygotic twins. Ibuprofen is a nonsteroidal antiinflammatory drug that induces psoriasis (answer 3). There are no reports related to the development of psoriasis with calcium channel blockers (answer 4).

12. Answer: 3

Rationale: The classification of psoriasis is based on the percentage of body involvement. The patient has a spreading psoriasis on her back and neck, so answer 1 is incorrect. Mild psoriasis (answer 2) should be less than 3% of the total body surface area. Moderate psoriasis (answer 3) is 3% to 10% of the total body surface area. Severe psoriasis (answer 4) should be greater than 10% of total body surface area.

13. Answer: 3

Rationale: The patient has psoriasis, which was induced by medication. The acronym NAILS is a helpful reminder for an agent that could cause psoriasis: nonsteroidal antiinflammatory drugs, antimalarial, angiotensin-converting enzyme inhibitors, Inderal (β-receptor antagonist), lithium, and/or salicylates or steroid withdrawal. Thus answer 3 is correct, and answers 1, 2, and 4 are incorrect.

14. Answer: 1

Rationale: The patient presents with itchy lesions and has a history of hypertension. She has psoriasis and the acronym NAILS is a helpful reminder for an agent could cause psoriasis: nonsteroidal antiinflammatory drugs, antimalarial, angiotensin-converting enzyme inhibitors, Inderal (β-receptor antagonist), lithium, and/or salicylates or steroid withdrawal. Therefore answer 1 is correct, and answers 2, 3, and 4 are incorrect.

15. Answer: 3

Rationale: Psoriasis is classified according to the percentage of body involvement. Mild psoriasis (answer 1) is less than 3% of the total body surface area. Moderate psoriasis (answer 2) is between 3% to 10% of total body surface area. Severe psoriasis (answer 3) is greater than 10% of the total body surface area. Stevens–Johnson syndrome (answer 4) is severe cutaneous hypersensitivity reactions.

16. Answer: 1

Rationale: This patient has mild to moderate psoriasis. Topical corticosteroids (answer 1) are considered as a first-line treatment of psoriasis. Ultraviolet radiation (answer 2) should be added as third-line treatment if the psoriasis is not relieved with the topical corticosteroids and topical calcipotriene. Topical calcipotriene (answer 3) should be added to the topical corticosteroids if the corticosteroid treatment failed. Azathioprine (answer 4) is considered for treatment of moderate to severe psoriasis, so this choice is incorrect.

17. Answer: 2

Rationale: The patient has mild to moderate psoriasis, and his psoriasis is not resolved with topical corticosteroids, so continuing at the same medication without adding another drug will be inappropriate (answer 1). Adding topical calcipotriene (answer 2) is the best choice. Administering ultraviolet radiation (answer 3) would be appropriate if the topical corticosteroids and calcipotriene have failed. Infliximab (answer 4) is a biological treatment that is appropriate for treatment patients with moderate to severe psoriasis.

18. Answer: 1

Rationale: The patient's psoriasis starts to improve, but there is a new lesion on the scalp, so the best agents are antidandruff shampoo and intermittent steroid lotion (answer 1). Azathioprine and biological agents (answers 2, 3, and 4) are appropriate for severe psoriasis.

19. Answer: 4

Rationale: The patient has had a long history with psoriasis, and he is not responsive to his medications; thus he needs to begin with moderate to severe treatment. Oral corticosteroids (answer 1) and oral calcipotriene (answer 2) do not have any role in the treatment of patients with psoriasis. Azathioprine (answer 3) is the best choice for treating patients with moderate to severe cases, but phototherapy (answer 4) should be tried first before beginning systemic agents.

20. Answer: 2

Rationale: A large multicenter European study and a meta-analysis suggest that a short course of moderate to high dose of systemic corticosteroids (e.g., prednisone 1–2 mg/kg a day for 3–5 days) may not be harmful and may have a beneficial effect if given early in the course of the disease (answer 2 is correct).

21. Answer: 1

Rationale: For patients with mild atopic dermatitis, low potency corticosteroid cream or ointment (e.g., desonide 0.05%, hydrocortisone 2.5%) is the preferred treatment. Topical corticosteroids are applied one or two times per day for 2 to weeks. Emollients should be liberally used multiple times per day in conjunction with topical corticosteroids. Emollients can be applied before or after topical corticosteroids.

22. Answer: 4

Rationale: The patient has Stevens–Johnson syndrome. Drugs that could cause this syndrome include antibiotics such as penicillin, amoxicillin, and cephalosporin, so answer 4 is correct, and answers 1, 2, and 3 are incorrect.

23. Answer: 4

Rationale: Some antiepileptics such as phenytoin, carbamazepine, and lamotrigine could cause severe cutaneous hypersensitivity (answer 1). Trimethoprim/sulfamethazine (answer 2) could cause this dangerous adverse effect. Piroxicam (answer 3) is a nonsteroidal antiinflammatory drug that can also cause this adverse drug reaction. Lisinopril (answer 4) could induce angioedema only.

24. Answer: 2

Rationale: The patient has Stevens–Johnson syndrome, which can be induced by allopurinol (answer 2). Thus answers 1, 3, and 4 are incorrect.

25. Answer: 2

Rationale: The patient presents to the emergency department with severe cutaneous hypersensitivity that was induced by allopurinol. Initiating supportive care (answer 1) without stopping the agent that caused the reaction that would be an unsuccessful plan. The first step should be to discontinue allopurinol (answer 2). Administering intravenous (IV) immunoglobulin (answer 3) should be initiated after stopping the agent and initiating supportive care. Cyclosporine (answer 4) should be added after administering IV immunoglobulin.

26. Answer: 2

Rationale: Drugs that can induce systemic lupus erythematous include phenytoin, isoniazid, hydralazine, procainamide, and quinidine. Carbamazepine could induce Stevens–Johnson syndrome. Thus answers 1, 3, and 4 are incorrect choices, and answer 2 is the correct choice.

27. Answer: 2

Rationale: The patient presents with hair loss and skin rash. Nonsteroidal antiinflammatory drugs (answer 1) are appropriate for joint symptoms and pleurisy. Topical corticosteroids (answer 2) are the best choice for patients with mild cases of skin rash. Oral corticosteroids (answer 3) should be in higher doses and are appropriate for patients with severe cases. Azathioprine (answer 4) is appropriate for patients with severe systemic lupus erythematous.

28. Answer: 4

Rationale: The patient is not responsive to the hydroxychloroquine dose and increasing the dose to achieve a serum concentration greater than 1000 ng/mL does not reduce the likelihood of disease flare (answer 1). Adding biological agents such as infliximab (answer 2) would not be beneficial. Adding systemic agents such as azathioprine (answer 4) is appropriate to control the symptoms and limit the dose of systemic corticosteroids used by this patient.

29. Answer: 1

Rationale: Hydroxychloroquine has several adverse drug reactions such as myopathy, muscle weakness, agranulocytosis, aplastic anemia, decreased visual acuity, and pigment changes if the dose is greater than 6.5 mg/kg of lean body weight. Thus answers 2, 3, and 4 are incorrect, and answer 1 is the correct choice.

30. Answer: 4

Rationale: The American Academy of Ophthalmology recommends that patients have funduscopic and visual field exams within the first year of starting hydroxychloroquine; ophthalmological screening recommendations are based on the risk of drug-related disease. If the dose of hydroxychloroquine is greater than 6.5 mg/kg or 3 mg/kg for chloroquine for more than 5 years, the annual ophthalmological screening is recommended. Therefore answer 4 is correct, and answers 1, 2, and 3 are incorrect.

31. Answer: 2

Rationale: The patient presents with scald burns, and the wound biopsy Gram stain shows gram-negative rods. He is allergic to sulfa drugs and penicillin; therefore silver sulfasalazine (answer 1) would be inappropriate. However, silver sulfasalazine is used to prevent and treat infections of second- and third-degree burns. Silver nitrate (answer 2) would be the alternative treatment for patients with sulfa allergy. Nystatin (answer 3) is an antifungal drug, which cannot cover the bacterial infections. Gentamycin (answer 4) is an aminoglycoside, which is a broad-spectrum antibiotic that would not be preferred at this time.

32. Answer: 4

Rationale: The patient presents with urticaria, and according to the guidelines, a nonsedating histamine 1 antihistamine is the first-line therapy, so cetirizine (answer 4) is the best choice for this case. Famotidine (answer 1) is a histamine 2 receptor antagonist and is considered second-line therapy. Cyclosporine (answer 2) and montelukast (answer 3) are considered third- and fourth-line therapies for treatment of patients with urticaria.

33. Answer: 1

Rationale: The patient has had urticaria and the first-line therapy is a nonsedating histamine 1 antihistaminic agent. She has not experienced any response with loratadine, so a histamine 2 receptor antagonist is the best choice for this presentation (answer 1). Cetirizine (answer 2) is a nonsedating histamine 1 antihistaminic agent, so it is an incorrect choice. Corticosteroids (answer 3) and montelukast (answer 4) are appropriate if the histamine 2 receptor antagonist fails.

11

Multisystem

1. What is the key *early* sign or symptom of lower extremity compartment syndrome?

   1. Loss of distal pulses.

   2. Pain.

   3. Edema.

   4. Paralysis.

2. In an unconscious patient suspected of having lower leg compartment syndrome, what management strategy is most appropriate for evaluating the need for fasciotomy?

   1. Check the posterior tibialis pulses every hour and consult surgery for a fasciotomy when the pulse becomes thready.

   2. Obtain quantitative pressures in all four compartments and consult surgery for a fasciotomy if pressures are greater than 15 mmHg.

   3. Obtain quantitative pressures in all four compartments and consult surgery for a fasciotomy if tissue perfusion pressure (i.e., diastolic blood pressure minus compartment pressure) is less than 30 mmHg.

   4. Obtain quantitative pressures in the compartment of highest concern and consult surgery for a fasciotomy if the pressure is greater than 30 mmHg.

3. A 40-year-old patient is admitted to the hospital after a motorcycle crash 1 day ago. The patient suffered multiple injuries, including a nondisplaced fracture of the tibia. Verbal communication is unreliable because of a moderate traumatic brain injury, but he moans during routine care when his leg is manipulated despite receiving hydromorphone 1 mg intravenously 30 minutes ago. What exam technique could point toward compartment syndrome?

   1. Assess for pain with passive range of motion of the toes and ankle.

   2. Check for posterior tibialis and dorsal pedal pulses.

   3. Palpate the calf assessing for firmness and compare with the contralateral calf.

   4. Check for capillary refill greater than 2 seconds in the distal toes.

4. In a patient with intraabdominal pressure greater than 20, *initial* management strategies should include:

   1. Emergent laparotomy to decompress.

   2. Decompression of intraluminal components via nasogastric and/or rectal tubes.

   3. Administration of a 20-mL/kg bolus of crystalloids.

   4. Decrease ventilator minute volume.

5. In a patient with abdominal compartment syndrome, which of the following is likely unrelated to the syndrome?

   1. Acute renal failure.

   2. Reduced cardiac output.

   3. Reduced ventilator compliance.

   4. Elevated central venous pressure.

6. A patient with acute pancreatitis was aggressively fluid resuscitated and has developed acute renal failure and hypotension, which has become less fluid-responsive. An appropriate next step would be to:

   1. Check abdominal pressure.

   2. Increase the volume of the crystalloid boluses.

   3. Order a routine echocardiogram.

   4. Transfuse two units of packed red blood cells.

7. Immediately following decompression for abdominal compartment syndrome, what changes to ventilator settings should be anticipated in response to altered pulmonary physiology?

   1. Reduce positive end-expiratory pressure (PEEP) and tidal volume.

   2. Change to a spontaneous mode.

   3. Change to bilevel mode with short release times during low PEEP.

   4. Increase the fraction inspired oxygen (Fio_2).

8. An 18-year-old male patient acquired a tibial fracture while playing soccer, was appropriately splinted in the emergency department, and was discharged home with crutches and instructions to follow up with an orthopedic specialist in several days. He returned 12 hours later with worsened pain despite taking ibuprofen and oxycodone as prescribed. Which constellation of sign and symptoms are greater than 90% diagnostic of compartment syndrome?

   1. Pain out of proportion to the injury and loss of distal arterial pulses.

   2. Pain with passive range of motion, paresthesias, and decreased distal arterial pulses.

   3. Pain out of proportion to the injury, pain with passive range of motion, and paresis.

   4. Limb asymmetry, pain with passive range of motion.

9. Which statement is true?

   1. Muscle fascia is somewhat flexible to accommodate edema or bleeding.

   2. Myonecrosis occurs after approximately 6 to 8 hours of compartment pressure elevation.

   3. Intramuscular pressure is equal throughout an entire contiguous compartment.

   4. The diagnosis of compartment syndrome requires a high degree of clinical suspicion and rapid measurement of compartment pressures.

10. A farm worker is brought to the emergency department by a coworker who reports he was not feeling well, had a runny nose, was crying, and sweating profusely, and shortly before arriving developed cough and dyspnea, became lethargic, and urinated on himself. What diagnosis accounts for all these sign and symptoms and must be recognized emergently?

    1. Sepsis from influenza.

    2. Suicide attempt with tricyclic antidepressant overdose.

    3. Heart failure from atypical myocardial infarction.

    4. Organophosphate exposure.

11. A farm worker is brought to the emergency department by a coworker who reports he was not feeling well, had a runny nose, was crying, and sweating profusely, and shortly before arriving developed cough and dyspnea, became lethargic, and urinated on himself. He is noted to have copious respiratory secretions and dyspnea. What medication will be the mainstay of therapy for this patient's initial treatment?

    1. Glycopyrrolate.

    2. Albuterol.

    3. Atropine.

    4. Epinephrine.

12. A patient with a history of depression and suicide attempts is brought to the emergency department by family after reportedly taking an entire bottle of acetaminophen approximately 2 to 3 hours ago. What intervention is most likely to reduce mortality?

    1. Follow acetaminophen levels and escalating therapy decisions when levels exceed 200 mcg/mL.

    2. Administer activated charcoal orally or via nasogastric tube.

    3. Administer *N*-acetylcysteine.

    4. Emergent hemodialysis.

13. A 75-year-old female patient underwent right total knee replacement 2 weeks ago and returns for continued severe pain. After discussing current analgesic therapy with the patient, you ascertain she has been taking oxycodone/acetaminophen 5/325 mg every 4 hours around the clock and 1000 mg acetaminophen two to three times per day for breakthrough pain. Because of concern for liver injury, an aspartate aminotransferase (AST) was done and found to be 140 units/L. What is the most appropriate management plan?

    1. Educate the patient on acetaminophen dosing and instruct her to discontinue over-the-counter acetaminophen.

    2. Discontinue all acetaminophen, prescribe plain oxycodone, and repeat AST in 3 to 5 days.

    3. Discontinue all acetaminophen, administer activated charcoal.

    4. Discontinue all acetaminophen, administer *N*-acetylcysteine.

14. A patient with a history of depression and suicidality was brought to the emergency department by family after he started "not acting right." Earlier in the day he had difficulty urinating and was mumbling unintelligible words, then on the way to the hospital became unconscious and had a seizure. He is hypotensive, has rigidity, and has a QRS duration of 150 ms. What did this patient likely overdose on?

    1. Tricyclic antidepressant.

    2. Selective serotonin reuptake inhibitor.

    3. Monoamine oxidase inhibitor.

    4. Rubbing alcohol.

15. A patient with a history of depression and suicidality was brought to the emergency department by family after he started "not acting right." Earlier in the day he had difficulty urinating and was mumbling unintelligible words, then on the way to the hospital became unconscious and had a seizure. He is hypotensive, has rigidity, and has a QRS duration of 150 ms. Which answer describes appropriate medical management?

    1. Supportive care, cardiac monitoring.

    2. Administer pralidoxime (2-PAM).

    3. Physostigmine and phenobarbital.

    4. Sodium bicarbonate and lorazepam.

16. A 40-year-old male patient was brought to the emergency department by ambulance on a nonrebreather mask after being involved in an industrial explosion. He is unconscious, hypotensive, and having ventricular arrhythmias. While starting another intravenous catheter, the nurse notes that his venous blood looks arterial. Of the possible inhalations, which will require emergent treatment?

    1. Carbon monoxide.

    2. Ammonia.

    3. Methane.

    4. Cyanide.

17. You are called to see your patient who has an acutely altered level of consciousness, bradycardia, and reduced respiratory rate. He was admitted 2 days ago for intravenous antibiotics for an arm abscess and was recently alert and oriented. On exam, he moans with sternal rub and has pinpoint pupils. Which medication is most likely to reverse this syndrome?

    1. Albuterol.

    2. Naloxone.

    3. Romazicon.

    4. Sodium bicarbonate.

18. A 73-year-old female patient with a history of diabetes and depression, for which she takes sertraline, was started on metoclopramide for gastroparesis. She developed a fever of 102.5°F, agitation, dilated pupils, tremor, and diaphoresis. What is the likely diagnosis?

    1. Malignant hyperthermia.

    2. Meningitis.

    3. Sepsis.

    4. Serotonin syndrome.

19. A patient on venlafaxine for depression who was started on linezolid for an infected diabetic foot ulcer has developed delirium, diarrhea, and fever of 101.2°F. After stopping the offending medications, what other treatment should be initiated for serotonin syndrome?

    1. Rehydration with crystalloids.

    2. Administration of meperidine with titration of dose until cessation of diarrhea.

    3. Intubation and administration of deep sedation and paralytics for 24 to 48 hours.

    4. Administration of cyproheptadine.

20. In a patient with hypovolemic shock, what is the primary physiological goal of resuscitation?

    1. Maintain normal blood pressure.

    2. Restore intravascular oxygen-carrying capacity.

    3. Restore intravascular volume.

    4. Maintain normal platelet count and function.

21. A 21-year-old male patient sustained a penetrating injury to the medial proximal thigh and paramedics reported that he was found in a large pool of blood. They had a brief transport and have given 1 L of crystalloid and applied a tourniquet. His heart rate is 130 beats/min, respiratory rate is 25 breaths/min, and he is anxious and confused. He is normothermic. The next fluid administered should be:

    1. Isotonic crystalloid.

    2. Albumin.

    3. Blood.

    4. Hypertonic saline.

22. During massive transfusion, what electrolyte needs repletion?

    1. Sodium.

    2. Potassium.

    3. Calcium.

    4. Magnesium.

23. A 40-year-male patient was involved in a motor vehicle collision and sustained head and abdominal injuries. His Glasgow Coma Score is 7, and his systolic blood pressure (SBP) is 92 mmHg. How should this patient's blood pressure be managed?

    1. Permit hypotension, with a target SBP of 80 to 90 mmHg.

    2. Use blood transfusions and norepinephrine to achieve a target SBP of greater than 120 mmHg.

    3. Use normal saline and packed red blood cells with a target SBP of 80 to 90 mmHg.

    4. Use blood transfusions and norepinephrine with a target SBP of 80 to 90 mmHg.

24. How should life-threatening bleeding at a noncompressible site be stopped?

    1. Support the hemodynamic status with transfusions and increase the platelet count to 150 cells/mL.

    2. Permit hypothermia to promote coagulation.

    3. Administer large volumes of plasma, platelets, and saline.

    4. Via endovascular or open surgery, depending on the site and the nature of the bleeding.

25. A 45-year-old male patient involved in a high-velocity motor vehicle crash sustained a C4 fracture with loss of sensation and motor function below the C4 level. The secondary survey did not reveal any other major injuries. A neurosurgical consult is pending. What medical intervention has been shown to improve neurological outcomes after traumatic spinal cord injury?

    1. High-dose methylprednisolone.

    2. Fludrocortisone.

    3. Augment mean arterial pressure to greater than 85 mmHg.

    4. Keep Pao_2 greater than 200.

26. A 45-year-old male patient involved in a high-velocity motor vehicle crash sustained a C4 fracture with loss of sensation and motor function below the C4 level. The secondary survey did not reveal any other major injuries. A full exam is performed, and he has an American Spinal Injury Association impairment scale of A at the C4 level. His mean arterial pressure is 70 mmHg and heart rate is 50 beats/min. Which medication would you use to correct his vital signs?

    1. Phenylephrine.

    2. Norepinephrine.

    3. Milrinone.

    4. Isoproterenol.

27. A 45-year-old male patient involved in a high-velocity motor vehicle crash sustained a C4 fracture with loss of sensation and motor function below the C4 level. The secondary survey did not reveal any other major injuries. A full exam is performed, and he has an American Spinal Injury Association impairment scale of A at the C4 level. His mean arterial pressure is 55 mmHg and heart rate is 50 beats/min. The following laboratory results are available: sodium 142, hemoglobin 12.6, and lactate 1.3. He has warm dry skin. What type of shock is most likely?

    1. Septic.

    2. Hemorrhagic.

    3. Neurogenic.

    4. Spinal.

28. A 68-year-old male patient was riding a bicycle and was struck by a car. His spine was immobilized, and he was transported to the emergency department with neck pain. His Glasgow Coma Scale is 15, vital signs are normal, and he has no paralysis or paresthesias. Next steps in care of this patient include:

    1. Obtain a three-view C-spine x-ray.

    2. Obtain a cervical spine computed tomography.

    3. Discontinue cervical immobilization.

    4. Remove collar and rotate head 45 degrees left and right; obtain imaging if this induces pain.

29. A 60-year-old male patient was involved in an all-terrain vehicle rollover and was brought to the hospital by ambulance. There was a delay of 90 minutes because of the remote location of the crash. His injuries include a head injury (Glasgow Coma Scale 5), tension pneumothorax, and one femur fracture. His initial heart rate is 145 beats/min, blood pressure 70/30 mmHg, and temperature 94°F. What is the best treatment for this patient's hypothermia?

    1. Administer blood via a warming device and use a warming blanket to normalize body temperature.

    2. Continue mild hypothermia for neuroprotection.

    3. Apply ice packs to include moderate hypothermia for neuroprotection.

    4. Initiate venous–venous extracorporeal membrane oxygenation for rapid rewarming.

30. A 60-year-old male patient was involved in an all-terrain vehicle rollover and was brought to the hospital by ambulance. There was a delay of 90 minutes because of the remote location of the crash. His injuries include a head injury (Glasgow Coma Scale 5), tension pneumothorax, and one femur fracture. His initial heart rate is 145 beats/min, blood pressure 70/30 mmHg, and temperature 94°F. No laboratory results are initially available, and his family denies anticoagulant use. Which of the following should be considered to reduce the extent of hemorrhage?

    1. Tranexamic acid.

    2. Four-factor prothrombin complex concentrate.

    3. Recombinant factor VIIa.

    4. Protamine sulfate.

31. A 60-year-old male patient was involved in an all-terrain vehicle rollover and was brought to the hospital by ambulance. There was a delay of 90 minutes because of the remote location of the crash. His injuries include a head injury (Glasgow Coma Scale 5), tension pneumothorax, and one femur fracture. His initial heart rate is 145 beats/min, blood pressure 70/30 mmHg, and temperature 94°F. How should hypovolemia be corrected in this case of hemorrhagic shock?

    1. 1 L of lactated Ringer's, then packed red blood cells (PRBCs).

    2. Lactated Ringer's, PRBCs, plasma, and platelets in a 1:1:1:1 ratio.

    3. 1 L of lactated Ringer's, then PRBCs, plasma, and platelets in a 1:1:1 ratio.

    4. 3 to 4 L of lactated Ringer's, then PRBCs, plasma, platelets, and cryoprecipitate in a 1:1:1:1 ratio.

32. A 60-year-old male patient was involved in an all-terrain vehicle rollover and was brought to the hospital by ambulance. There was a delay of 90 minutes because of the remote location of the crash. His injuries include a head injury (Glasgow Coma Scale 5), tension pneumothorax, and one femur fracture. His initial heart rate is 145 beats/min, blood pressure 70/30 mmHg, and temperature 94°F. An arterial blood gas reveals a pH of 7.20, Pco_2 42, Pao_2 45, and bicarbonate 11. What additional laboratory test would confirm trauma's classic "lethal triad"?

    1. Direct and indirect bilirubin.

    2. Prothrombin time and international normalization ratio.

    3. Lactate.

    4. Venous oxygen saturation.

33. A 60-year-old male patient was involved in an all-terrain vehicle rollover and was brought to the hospital by ambulance. There was a delay of 90 minutes because of the remote location of the crash. His injuries include a head injury (Glasgow Coma Scale 5), tension pneumothorax, and one femur fracture. His initial heart rate is 145 beats/min, blood pressure 70/30 mmHg, and temperature 94°F. An arterial blood gas reveals a pH of 7.20, Pco_2 42, Pao_2 45, and bicarbonate 11. What blood pressure target do advanced trauma life support guidelines call for?

    1. Mean arterial pressure greater than 60 to 65.

    2. Systolic blood pressure greater than 80.

    3. Systolic blood pressure greater than 100.

    4. Mean arterial pressure greater than 85.

34. A 60-year-old male patient was involved in an all-terrain vehicle rollover and was brought to the hospital by ambulance. His injuries include a head injury (Glasgow Coma Scale 5), tension pneumothorax, and one femur fracture. His current heart rate is 115 beats/min, blood pressure 100/40 mmHg (mean arterial pressure [MAP] 60), and temperature 98.2°F. After initial stabilization, a head computed tomography did not reveal any hemorrhage amenable to surgical evacuation. An intraparenchymal intracranial pressure (ICP) monitor was placed and his ICP is 20 mmHg. Does this new data alter blood pressure management strategy?

    1. No, ICP less than 20 is acceptable.

    2. Yes, target a MAP of greater than 80 mmHg.

    3. Yes, target a systolic blood pressure of greater than 110 mmHg.

    4. Yes, target a systolic blood pressure of 160 to 180 mmHg.

35. A 19-year-old male patient who weighs 75 kg sustained full-thickness burns over 20% of his body. What volume of fluid is an approximation of how much fluid to administer over the first 24 hours?

    1. 1 L.

    2. 3 L.

    3. 6 L.

    4. 10 L.

36. A patient is brought to the emergency department via ambulance with severe burns and was intubated before arrival. The burns were sustained in a house fire and include circumferential burns around the torso. The patient is unconscious and has the following vital signs: heart rate 135 beats/min, blood pressure 90/38 mmHg, and oxygen saturation 96%. Which item is the highest priority for managing this patient?

    1. Calculate fluid requirement using the Parkland formula.

    2. Transfuse two units of packed red blood cells.

    3. Ensure adequate ventilation and check a carboxyhemoglobin.

    4. Consult surgery for an escharotomy.

37. A 24-year-old male patient was brought to the hospital by ambulance after being assaulted with a baseball bat. He has several facial lacerations and significant edema of the face, ear, and hands. His Glasgow Coma Score is 4 (eye opening 1 [E1]/verbal response 1 [V1]/ motor response 2 [M2]) and was intubated. After initial stabilization, a noncontrast head computed tomography (CT) revealed facial and basilar skull fractures. What additional urgent imaging should be obtained?

    1. Brain magnetic resonance imaging (MRI).

    2. Cervical spine MRI.

    3. CT angiography of the neck and brain arteries.

    4. Hand and wrist x-rays.

38. A 24-year-old male patient was brought to the hospital by ambulance after being assaulted with a baseball bat. He has several facial lacerations and significant edema of the face, ear, and hands. His Glasgow Coma Score is 4 (E1/V1/M2) and was intubated. After initial stabilization, a noncontrast head computed tomography revealed facial and basilar skull fractures. His pupillary exam is 3 mm and sluggish on the right and 8 mm and nonreactive on the left. Which of the following is an inappropriate action to take?

    1. Administer mannitol 20% 1 g/kg of body weight.

    2. Raise the head of bed to 30 to 45 degrees.

    3. Administer 500 mL of 3% sodium chloride.

    4. Adjust ventilator settings to target a $Paco_2$ of 45 to 50.

39. A 32-year-old male patient was a helmeted motorcycle driver and was involved in a low-velocity collision with a sport utility vehicle (SUV). Paramedics report that he needed to be extracted from underneath the SUV where his legs were pinned. The patient complains of severe bilateral leg pain but denies other injuries. On exam, he has multiple abrasions and lacerations on the thighs and an obvious bony deformity, and cool skin on his extremities. His heart rate is 115 beats/min, respiratory rate is 24 breaths/min, blood pressure is 120/60 mmHg, and his initial hemoglobin is 13.9. Which is the best treatment that the AGACNP should do at this time?

    1. Consult orthopedic surgery for surgical femur repair.

    2. Suture the thigh lacerations.

    3. Repeat hemoglobin in 1 hour.

    4. Transfuse uncrossed packed red blood cells.

40. A 40-year-old female patient with no past medical history presented to the emergency department with redness surrounding a minor abrasion she sustained a week before and was diagnosed with cellulitis. She was given cefazolin and admitted to a medical floor. On arrival to the floor her blood pressure was 100/50 mmHg, heart rate was 130 beats/min, oxygen saturation was 89%, and she was noted to have wheezing. Your first step in managing this patient is to:

    1. Administer a 2-L bolus of isotonic crystalloid.

    2. Administer epinephrine 0.01 mg/kg intramuscularly.

    3. Draw a venous blood sample and check the differential for eosinophilia.

    4. Administer diphenhydramine 25 mg intravenously.

41. An 85-year-old female patient with ischemic heart disease and congestive heart failure with a left ventricular ejection fraction of 20% to 25% presented to the emergency department with redness surrounding a minor abrasion she sustained a week before and was diagnosed with cellulitis. She was given cefazolin and admitted to a medical floor. On arrival to the floor her blood pressure was 100/50 mmHg, heart rate 130 beats/min, oxygen saturation 89%, and she was noted to have wheezing. Your first step in managing this patient is to:

    1. Draw an arterial blood gas.

    2. Electively intubate the patient.

    3. Order a chest x-ray.

    4. Transfer the patient to the intensive care unit.

42. A 40-year-old female patient with no past medical history presented to the emergency department with redness surrounding a minor abrasion she sustained a week before and was diagnosed with cellulitis. She was given cefazolin and admitted to a medical floor. On arrival to the floor her blood pressure was 80/30 mmHg (a decrease from 110/50 mmHg in the emergency department), heart rate 130 beats/min, oxygen saturation 89%, and she was noted to have stridor. After ordering epinephrine, your next priority in managing this patient is to:

    1. Administer ranitidine.

    2. Administer racemic epinephrine.

    3. Prepare for intubation, anticipating a difficult airway.

    4. Administer diphenhydramine.

43. An 85-year-old female patient with ischemic heart disease and congestive heart failure with a left ventricular ejection fraction of 20% to 25% for which she takes carvedilol, presented to the emergency department with redness surrounding a minor abrasion she sustained a week before and was diagnosed with cellulitis. She was given cefazolin and admitted to a medical floor. On arrival to the floor she was appropriately diagnosed with anaphylaxis, given intramuscular epinephrine twice, then was started on an epinephrine infusion and her heart rate decreased to 55 beats/min and she remained hypotensive. What adjunctive medication may help to restore hemodynamic stability in this case?

    1. Diphenhydramine.

    2. Glucagon.

    3. Ranitidine.

    4. Naloxone.

44. A 55-year-old patient with no significant past medical history is admitted with community-acquired pneumonia. She is confused, has a Glasgow Coma Score of 14, and mild hypoxia (Pao_2 80 on room air), and her mean arterial pressure is 60 mmHg. A lactate level was 2.8. The next step to manage this patient is to:

    1. Repeat and trend lactate.

    2. Order a 30-mL/kg bolus of crystalloids.

    3. Insert a central venous catheter for vascular access and to check central venous oxygen saturation.

    4. Order a 1-L bolus of 0.9% normal saline followed by norepinephrine to keep the mean arterial pressure greater than 65 mmHg.

45. A patient admitted to the intensive care unit 7 days ago with septic shock from infective endocarditis was resuscitated in the emergency department including appropriate fluid resuscitation, empiric broad-spectrum antibiotics (piperacillin/tazobactam and vancomycin), insertion of a femoral central venous catheter, and administration of norepinephrine. His blood cultures grew a strain of *Staphylococcus aureus* that was sensitive to both the piperacillin/tazobactam and vancomycin, but repeat blood cultures have failed to clear. What intervention may aid resolution of bacteremia?

    1. Inhaled nebulized tobramycin.

    2. Coronary angiography.

    3. Removal of central venous catheter.

    4. Penicillin G.

46. A 49-year-old immunocompetent male patient presented to the emergency department with headache for 8 hours, nuchal rigidity, and photophobia; meningitis was suspected. He was given appropriate doses of ceftriaxone and vancomycin starting at 9 a.m. On arrival to the medical floor at noon, you realize no cerebrospinal fluid (CSF) was obtained for analysis. Appropriate actions include:

    1. Perform a lumbar puncture and administer dexamethasone.

    2. Continue antibiotics for a 7-day course, but do not obtain CSF because it may be sterilized and produce a false-negative result.

    3. Add ampicillin, obtain a CSF sample, and administer dexamethasone.

    4. Perform a lumbar puncture, add ampicillin, and continue all three antibiotics for 7 days.

47. A 23-year-old male patient with a history of successful renal transplant 3 years ago presents with lethargy and an oral temperature of 102.5°F. On exam, while supine, his hips and knees flex involuntarily as you flex his neck forward. His exam:

    1. Demonstrates Kernig sign and is concerning for meningitis.

    2. Demonstrates Kernig sign and is not concerning for meningitis.

    3. Demonstrates Brudzinski sign and is concerning for meningitis.

    4. Demonstrates Brudzinski sign and is not concerning for meningitis.

48. A 23-year-old male patient with a history of successful renal transplant 3 years ago presents with lethargy, an oral temperature 102.5°F, and positive Brudzinski and Kernig signs. The next step in confirming your suspected diagnosis is:

    1. Empiric antibiotics.

    2. Computed tomography scan of the head without contrast.

    3. Lumbar puncture.

    4. Notification to the Centers for Disease Control and Prevention.

49. A 23-year-old male patient with a history of successful renal transplant 3 years ago, presents with lethargy, an oral temperature 102.5°F, and positive Brudzinski and Kernig signs. His symptoms evolved over 2 days. A lumbar puncture is performed and cerebropinal fluid (CSF) analysis reveals 150 white blood cells per cubic millimeter, no red blood cells, and a CSF/serum glucose ratio of 0.4. How should the AGACNP interpret the CSF results?

    1. These findings are equivocal for bacterial meningitis and further workup is needed.

    2. Initiate ceftriaxone, vancomycin, ampicillin, and dexamethasone.

    3. Initiate ceftriaxone, vancomycin, and ampicillin.

    4. Initiate ceftriaxone, vancomycin, and dexamethasone.

50. A patient with meningeal signs and symptoms developing over several days and a new-onset seizure undergoes a lumbar puncture with the following results: 110 white blood cells per cubic millimeter, 125 red blood cells, and a normal cerebrospinal fluid glucose. What urgent intervention is required to prevent the high possibility of a devastating neurological outcome?

    1. Steroids.

    2. Acyclovir.

    3. Protamine.

    4. Neurosurgical consult.

51. A 60-year-old female patient with type 2 diabetes and coronary artery disease underwent uncomplicated coronary bypass grafting 7 days ago and was discharged on postoperative day 10. She developed purulent sternal drainage and reported only small amounts of dark urine. Her labs include white blood cell count of 18,000 cells/mL³ and serum creatinine 1.7 mg/dL. Her heart rate is 110 beats/min and blood pressure is 110/60 mmHg. You have determined she needs antibiotics. What strategy and timing is appropriate?

    1. If she has good home care support, discharge from the emergency department with a prescription of cephalexin and instructions to follow up with cardiac surgery within 2 to 3 days.

    2. Check a lactate and if less than 1.2 mg/dL, then ensure intravenous vancomycin is initiated within 8 hours.

    3. She is septic and should have a wound culture obtained and vancomycin, piperacillin/tazobactam, and metronidazole started within an hour of presenting to the emergency department.

    4. She has septic shock and needs vancomycin, nafcillin, and metronidazole started after initial fluid resuscitation has been completed.

52. A 40-year-old female patient with a history of intravenous drug abuse presents with a complaint of not feeling well and had a fever of 103°F. Given your suspicion for infective endocarditis, where would you look for Janeway lesions?

    1. Sclera.

    2. Palms of hands and soles of feet.

    3. Antecubital fossa.

    4. Lung parenchyma on chest computed tomography.

53. A 40-year-old female patient with a history of intravenous drug abuse presents with a complaint of not feeling well and had a fever of 103°F. She has Janeway lesions. If she has three blood cultures positive for methicillin-resistant *Staphylococcus aureus* (MRSA), what is her diagnosis?

    1. Infective endocarditis.

    2. Unable to make a diagnosis without a transthoracic echocardiogram.

    3. Unable to make a diagnosis without a transesophageal echocardiogram.

    4. Sepsis from MRSA bacteremia.

54. A 40-year-old female patient with a history of intravenous drug abuse, fever of 103°F, Janeway lesions, and methicillin-resistant *Staphylococcus aureus* bacteremia had a transthoracic echocardiogram that did not identify any valvular or valve annulus abnormalities. Appropriate next steps in treating this patient include:

    1. Obtain daily blood cultures and continue intravenous vancomycin for 2 weeks following the first negative culture.

    2. Continue vancomycin for a total of 10 days.

    3. Obtain a transesophageal echocardiogram.

    4. The initial diagnosis of infective endocarditis is incorrect and noncardiac sources of the bacteremia should be explored.

55. A patient with methicillin-susceptible *Staphylococcus aureus* (MSSA) mitral valve endocarditis was being appropriately treated with intravenous nafcillin. The most recent blood culture reports an extended spectrum β-lactamase-producing strain. What should you do?

    1. Continue current therapy.

    2. Increase the nafcillin to exceed the minimal inhibitory concentration.

    3. Change to a carbapenem.

    4. Change to a fourth-generation cephalosporin.

56. A patient admitted with septic shock was found to have an abdominal abscess abutting the appendix. After starting empiric antibiotics to cover common pathogens and conducting fluid resuscitation and hemodynamic stabilization, what further treatment is necessary?

    1. Discuss options for draining the abscess percutaneously versus with open surgery.

    2. Obtain a colonoscopy.

    3. Anticipate renal failure and arrange for hemodialysis.

    4. Trend lactate, erythrocyte sedimentation rate, and C-reactive protein and deescalate antibiotics when these values are trending down.

57. A 60-year-old patient with no significant past medical history was admitted with severe influenza infection and respiratory failure. Twelve hours after arriving to the intensive care unit his vent settings are assist/control, tidal volume 6 mL/kg, positive end-expiratory pressure (PEEP) 18, and fraction of inspired oxygen 90%. Arterial blood gas is pH 7.20, P_{CO_2} 55, and Pa_{O_2} 50. The most appropriate next step in managing this patient is:

    1. Continue increasing PEEP until the Pa_{O_2} is greater than 60.

    2. This patient is a candidate for extracorporeal membrane oxygenation (ECMO); consult cardiac surgery emergently.

    3. This patient is too old for ECMO, consider discussing palliative measures.

    4. Cool the patient to 91°F to reduce oxygen consumption.

58. A patient is admitted with severe influenza infection and has a single-lobe infiltrate on chest x-ray. Antiinfective agents should include:

    1. Oseltamivir and ampicillin/sulbactam.

    2. Combivir and amoxicillin/clavulanate.

    3. Oseltamivir only.

    4. Darunavir, vancomycin, and cefepime.

59. An 80-year-old female patient weighing 90 kg is admitted for septic shock of unknown source. She was given a 1500-mL bolus of lactated Ringer's (LR) after which her mean arterial pressure (MAP) increased from 50 to 58 mmHg. You next intervention should be to

    1. Give an additional 1000- to 1500-mL bolus of LR.

    2. Start norepinephrine infusion and titrate to a MAP of greater than 60 to 65.

    3. Start epinephrine infusion and titrate to a MAP of greater than 60 to 65.

    4. Start vasopressin infusion and titrate to a MAP of greater than 60 to 65.

60. After adequate fluid resuscitation of a patient in septic shock, what is the most appropriate medication to improve organ perfusion?

    1. Dopamine.

    2. Epinephrine.

    3. Norepinephrine.

    4. Milrinone.

61. Assuming adequate volume resuscitation and hypotension refractory to high doses of vasopressors, which of the following is true of steroids for septic shock?

    1. Prednisone 60 mg daily is recommended to improve blood pressure.

    2. Hydrocortisone 50 mg every 6 hours has been shown to reduce the risk of death.

    3. Hydrocortisone or methylprednisolone should be used only if a patient has an inadequate response to synthetic adrenocorticotropic hormone (cosyntropin).

    4. The immune suppressive effect of steroids in septic shock increases mortality.

62. A 55-year-old male patient with no significant past medical history presented to the emergency department with a cough, temperature of 101°F, and pleuritic chest pain. His chest x-ray demonstrated a left upper lobe infiltrate. He has a normal neurological exam, blood urea nitrogen 25, respiratory rate 20, blood pressure 138/65 mmHg, and oxygen saturation 96%. How should this case be managed?

    1. Discharge to home with a prescription for azithromycin.

    2. Send to a 23-hour observation unit and treat with a β-lactam plus a macrolide.

    3. Admit to medical floor and treat with a respiratory fluoroquinolone such as levofloxacin or moxifloxacin, and obtain blood and respiratory cultures.

    4. Admit to the intensive care unit, obtain blood and respiratory cultures, and treat with ceftriaxone and azithromycin.

63. In a patient with type 2 diabetes and end-stage renal failure on hemodialysis who is appropriate for outpatient management of community-acquired pneumonia, what antibiotic strategy is preferred?

    1. Cefepime and vancomycin.

    2. Sulfamethoxazole/trimethoprim.

    3. A β-lactam, a fluoroquinolone, and oseltamivir.

    4. Moxifloxacin monotherapy.

64. A 70-year-old male patient with a history of a methicillin-resistant *Staphylococcus aureus* skin and soft tissue abscess of the leg 2 months ago and a penicillin allergy is admitted with sepsis and community-acquired pneumonia. What is the most appropriate initial antimicrobial regimen?

    1. Linezolid, cefepime, and azithromycin.

    2. Aztreonam, azithromycin, and vancomycin.

    3. Azithromycin and linezolid.

    4. Piperacillin-tazobactam, vancomycin, and levofloxacin.

65. A patient with community-acquired pneumonia was admitted to a medical floor 6 days ago, has been treated with appropriate antibiotics, and has been afebrile for the past 72 hours. What should the AGACNP do with the antibiotics?

    1. Discontinue the antibiotics today.

    2. De-escalate to ampicillin/sulbactam and discontinue after a total of 10 days of therapy.

    3. Stop the antibiotics after 10 days.

    4. Stop the antibiotics after 14 days.

66. A 51-year-old female patient with a history of methicillin-resistant *Staphylococcus aureus* (MRSA) bacteremia and endocarditis was admitted 3 days ago with an ischemic stroke. She is not intubated but has developed hypoxia and is requiring 6 L of oxygen to maintain an oxygen saturation of 92%. A chest x-ray revealed a right lower lobe infiltrate and her temperature is 100.9°F, but other vital signs are normal. She is already on vancomycin for endocarditis. Should you adjust her antibiotic regimen?

    1. No, her blood cultures grew a strain of MRSA that was susceptible to vancomycin.

    2. Yes, add piperacillin-tazobactam.

    3. Yes, stop vancomycin, add linezolid and amoxicillin-clavulanate.

    4. Yes, add both intravenous (IV) and inhaled tobramycin and IV cefepime.

67. A 46-year-old female patient with a history of uncontrolled diabetes has been an inpatient for the past 7 days because of poorly healing foot ulcers. She was transferred to the intensive care unit with septic shock. She was found to be hypoxic and had a left lower lobe pneumonia. What antibiotics should be started?

    1. Piperacillin-tazobactam, levofloxacin, and vancomycin.

    2. Cefepime and meropenem.

    3. Doxycycline and levofloxacin.

    4. Linezolid, cefepime, and piperacillin-tazobactam.

68. A 28-year-old male patient is admitted to the intensive care unit with ventilator-associated pneumonia and has been on linezolid, cefepime, and ciprofloxacin for 4 days. He has shown clinical improvement with decreasing oxygen requirements on the ventilator and he has been weaned off norepinephrine. His respiratory culture grew *Pseudomonas aeruginosa,* which was susceptible to ciprofloxacin. What should you do with his antibiotics?

    1. Continue all three for a total of 7 days.

    2. Continue all three for a total of 14 days.

    3. Stop linezolid and cefepime now and continue ciprofloxacin until day 7.

    4. Stop linezolid and cefepime now and continue ciprofloxacin until day 14.

69. In a patient with sepsis-induced severe acute respiratory distress syndrome, which strategy is *not* recommended to increase oxygenation?

    1. Prone positioning.

    2. Increase positive end-expiratory pressure.

    3. High-frequency oscillatory ventilation.

    4. Neuromuscular blockade.

70. Which upper glucose target in septic patients results in the best outcomes?

    1. Less than 110.

    2. Less than 140.

    3. Less than 180.

    4. Less than 200.

71. A patient with septic shock and acute respiratory distress syndrome has the following arterial blood gas values: pH 7.18, P_{CO_2} 45, P_{aO_2} 65, bicarbonate 12, and lactate 6. What is the most appropriate way to address this severe acidosis?

    1. Increase respiratory rate.

    2. Administer sodium bicarbonate 50 mEq intravenous push.

    3. Initiate sodium bicarbonate infusion.

    4. Give a bolus of lactated Ringer's.

72. A 50-year-old male patient was admitted for pneumonia and treated with levofloxacin for the past 5 days. His white blood count is 25,000, he has a fever of 101°F, and he recently developed diarrhea. What is the most appropriate initial treatment?

    1. Vancomycin 500 mg four times per day.

    2. Amoxicillin 250 mg every 8 hours.

    3. Metronidazole 500 mg three times per day.

    4. Fecal microbiota transplantation.

73. A 50-year-old male patient was admitted for pneumonia and treated with levofloxacin for 5 days. His white blood count is 27,000, he has a fever of 101.5°F, and he has developed an ileus and hypotension despite 2 days of treatment with oral vancomycin. What is the most appropriate modification to the current regimen?

    1. Add fidaxomicin 200 mg twice per day.

    2. Stop vancomycin and add fidaxomicin 200 mg twice per day.

    3. Add rectal vancomycin and intravenous metronidazole.

    4. Consider a fecal microbiota transplant.

74. A 25-year-old male patient is admitted to the intensive care unit after a motor vehicle collision resulting in a severe traumatic brain injury causing elevated intracranial pressure. He is on a ventilator and minimally responsive. On the second day of hospitalization, he has increasing vasopressor requirements and hourly urine output of 400 mL. To address this problem, you would order:

    1. Fluid restriction.

    2. Serum sodium and urine specific gravity.

    3. 24-hour urine protein and creatinine.

    4. STAT noncontrast head computed tomography.

75. A 25-year-old male patient is admitted to the intensive care unit after a motor vehicle collision resulting in a severe traumatic brain injury causing elevated intracranial pressure. He is on a ventilator and minimally responsive. On the second day of hospitalization, he has increasing vasopressor requirements and hourly urine output of 400 mL. His serum sodium increased from 146 to 155 mEq/L in the past 6 hours and urine specific gravity is 1.001. To address this problem, you would:

    1. Order 2 mcg desmopressin (DDAVP) intravenous (IV) and 1 L 0.9% normal saline.

    2. Increase maintenance fluids from 75 to 150 mL/hr and repeat serum sodium and specific gravity in 6 hours.

    3. Order 2 mcg DDAVP IV and fluid restriction.

    4. Calculate the free water deficit and order free water via nasogastric tube.

76. A 68-year-old 70-kg male patient with a history of tobacco abuse is admitted with dyspnea. A chest x-ray reveals a pulmonary mass, flattened bilateral diaphragm, and no pulmonary edema. He is alert and breathing comfortably after being started on 4 L O_2 via nasal cannula. His initial sodium is 128 mEq/L. Based on your knowledge of the probable diagnosis of syndrome of inappropriate antidiuretic hormone, how would you correct his sodium?

    1. Start 3% normal saline at 75 mL/hr.

    2. Start 0.9% normal saline at 1000 mL/hr.

    3. Institute a fluid restriction.

    4. Order 40 mg of furosemide and repeat serum sodium in 8 hours.

77. A 55-year-old female patient with history of type 2 diabetes and diverticulitis is admitted to the intensive care unit following laparotomy for colectomy. She remains intubated and requires norepinephrine at 0.06 mcg/kg/min to maintain a mean arterial pressure greater than 65 despite adequate intraoperative fluid resuscitation. Her blood glucose is 220 mg/dL. What will your initial glucose management strategy entail?

    1. Starting a regular insulin infusion with a target glucose less than 120 mg/dL.

    2. Starting regular insulin subcutaneously (SQ) on a sliding scale with a target glucose of 140 to 180 mg/dL.

    3. Starting regular insulin SQ on a sliding scale with a target glucose less than 120 mg/dL.

    4. Starting a regular insulin infusion with a target glucose of 140 to 180 mg/dL.

78. A 55-year-old female patient with history of type 2 diabetes and diverticulitis is admitted to the intensive care unit following laparotomy for colectomy. She was intubated and on norepinephrine for 3 days, but she is now extubated, weaned off the norepinephrine, and transferred to a medical-surgical unit. She is tolerating oral nutrition with a carbohydrate-controlled diet and is still on insulin infusion at 0.5 units/hr with a 24-hour glucose range of 150 to 180 mg/dL. Her home regimen involves metformin 1000 mg by mouth twice a day and a carbohydrate-controlled diet. Hemoglobin A1c is 7.8%. The most appropriate next step in the management of this patient's diabetes is to:

    1. Restart home metformin and monitor blood glucose before eating and every night at bedtime.

    2. Continue the insulin infusion for an additional 24 hours.

    3. Restart and increase the metformin to 2000 mg twice a day.

    4. Start insulin glargine, 12 units daily and a regular insulin sliding scale.

79. An 85-year-old female patient is admitted to a medical-surgical unit with a urinary tract infection and confusion. She is tolerating a regular diet and has no history of diabetes. The glucose on her initial chemistry panel is 230 mg/dL and her hemoglobin A1c is 10%. The most appropriate management of this patient's glucose is to:

    1. Start an insulin infusion and follow her serum glucose every hour.

    2. Initiate a subcutaneous basal, prandial correction regimen.

    3. Start metformin 1500 mg twice a day.

    4. Instruct the patient to follow up with her primary care provider 2 weeks after discharge.

80. An 85-year-old female patient is admitted to a medical-surgical unit with a urinary tract infection and confusion. She is tolerating a regular diet and has no history of diabetes. The glucose on her initial chemistry panel is 230 mg/dL and her hemoglobin A1c is 10%. Her glucose was 140 mg/dL with glargine and lispro. When planning the discharge for this patient, you learn that she plans to return home, but she is confused about insulin administration. What is the most appropriate next step based on the confusion about insulin administration?

    1. Transition to an oral agent and confirm that follow-up with a primary care provider is available.

    2. Discharge with prescriptions for glargine, lispro, and insulin syringes.

    3. Discharge with prescriptions for glargine and lispro insulin pens.

    4. Refer the patient to her home county's adult protective services.

81. In a patient with fatigue and weight loss, what would confirm a tentative diagnosis of primary adrenal insufficiency?

    1. 2 p.m. serum cortisol 180 nmol/L.

    2. 8 a.m. serum cortisol 150 nmol/L.

    3. 24-hour urinary free cortisol 8 mcg/24 hr.

    4. Corticotropin test with a peak cortisol greater than 550 nmol/L.

82. A patient with recent chronic obstructive pulmonary disease exacerbation presents to the emergency department because of lethargy. She recently completed a month-long course of prednisone 50 mg daily. Her blood pressure is 85/40 mmHg. What is her most likely diagnosis?

    1. Septic shock.

    2. Myxedema crisis.

    3. Thyroid storm.

    4. Adrenal insufficiency.

83. A 45-year-old male patient is admitted to the intensive care unit after resection of a pituitary adenoma. He develops vomiting, abdominal pain, myalgia, joint pains, and severe hypotension. This patient may have developed:

    1. Adrenal insufficiency.

    2. Diabetes insipidus.

    3. Abdominal compartment syndrome.

    4. Colonic ileus.

84. A 20-year-old college student with no past medical history is brought into the emergency department by friends after his mental status became altered. He has Kussmaul respirations, is confused, drowsy, and recently vomited. Which tests are required to confirm the most likely diagnosis?

    1. Serum glucose, bicarbonate, pH, and ketones.

    2. Serum sodium, chloride, and urinalysis.

    3. Arterial blood gas.

    4. Cerebrospinal fluid protein, glucose, and cell count.

85. A 20-year-old college student with no past medical history is brought into the emergency department by friends after his mental status became altered. He has Kussmaul respirations, is confused, drowsy, and recently vomited. His glucose is 380 mg/dL, bicarbonate 14 mEq/L, pH 7.27, and he has ketonuria. Other than tachypnea, vital signs are normal. In a healthy young adult, what additional test should be obtained to avoid the commonly fatal complication of this disease process?

    1. Lactate.

    2. Potassium.

    3. Arterial P_{CO_2}.

    4. Platelet count.

86. A 20-year-old college student with no past medical history is brought into the emergency department by friends after his mental status became altered. He has Kussmaul respirations, is confused, drowsy, and recently vomited. His glucose is 380 mg/dL, bicarbonate 14 mEq/L, pH 7.27, and he has ketonuria. Other than tachypnea, vital signs are normal. What are essential components of the initial therapy?

    1. Intravenous (IV) fluid, IV insulin infusion, and potassium replacement.

    2. Immediate intubation, IV insulin infusion, and IV fluids.

    3. Aggressive subcutaneous sliding scale regular insulin, and IV fluids.

    4. IV fluids, IV bicarbonate replacement, and IV insulin infusion.

87. A 60-year-old female patient with an established diagnosis of chronic autoimmune thyroiditis is in your office for routine follow-up of her thyroid labs, which are as follows: thyroid-stimulating hormone 7.0 mU/L (reference range 0.5–5.0 mU/L) and free T4 0.5 mU/L (0.7–1.4 mU/L). She is on levothyroxine 75 mcg by mouth daily for the past 2 months. What would you do with her levothyroxine dose?

    1. Keep the dose at 75 mcg daily.

    2. Decrease the dose to 50 mcg daily.

    3. Increase the dose to 100 mcg daily.

    4. Defer this decision for now, repeat the labs, and schedule a follow-up visit in 2 weeks.

88. A 55- year-old female patient with history of hypothyroidism and hyperlipidemia is admitted to a neuro floor following acute ischemic stroke. Her thyroid labs are as follows: thyroid-stimulating hormone 9.0 mU/L (reference range 0.5–5.0 mU/L) and free T4 0.3 mU/L

(reference range 0.7–1.4 mU/L). A review of her medical records reveals she is on levothyroxine 125 mcg by mouth (PO) daily and that her primary care provider adjusted the dose upward from 100 mcg PO daily 2 weeks before admission. What would you do with her levothyroxine dose?

    1. Keep it at 125 mcg daily.

    2. Decrease it to 100 mcg daily.

    3. Increase it to 150 mcg daily.

    4. Discontinue the levothyroxine.

89. A 70-year-old male patient with idiopathic hypothyroidism is admitted to a medical-surgical unit with community-acquired pneumonia, hypoxia requiring 3 L O_2 per nasal cannula, and several months of lethargy. His thyroid labs were obtained and are as follows: thyroid-stimulating hormone 15.0 mU/L (reference range 0.5–5.0 mU/L) and free T4 0.2 mU/L (reference range 0.7–1.4 mU/L). He reports over the past 6 months his primary care provider has increased his levothyroxine four times to a current dose of 250 mcg by mouth (PO) daily with the last dose adjustment 6 weeks ago. He denies medical nonadherence, and his spouse confirmed he takes it every morning with breakfast. Which of the following will properly address his abnormal lab values?

    1. Increase the levothyroxine dose to 275 mcg PO daily.

    2. Prescribe Synthroid 250 mcg PO daily, "dispense as written."

    3. Change the time of day that the current dose is taken.

    4. Place a referral for radioactive thyroid ablation.

90. A 58-year-old male patient is admitted to a cardiac unit following non-ST elevation myocardial infarction. He had cardiogenic shock and has been weaned off pressor and inotropic support. During his hospitalization, thyroid function tests were obtained: thyroid-stimulating hormone 6.5 mU/L (reference range 0.5–5.0 mU/L), free T3 1.1 mU/L (reference range 1.7–3.7 mU/L), and free T4 0.6 mU/L (reference range 0.7–1.4 mU/L). How will you address these thyroid function tests?

    1. Initiate levothyroxine 1.7 mcg/kg ideal body weight by mouth (PO) daily.

    2. Initiate levothyroxine 25 mcg PO daily.

    3. Initiate levothyroxine 50 mcg intravenously once, followed by 25 mcg PO daily.

    4. Instruct the patient to follow up with his primary care provider to have his thyroid function rechecked in about 1 month.

91. A 50-year-old male patient with type 2 diabetes says 3 days ago, he was diagnosed with community-acquired pneumonia and presents to the emergency department with a chief complaint of "not feeling well." He has a temperature of 96.5°F, Heart rate 120 beats/min, and blood pressure 90/50 mmHg. Labs include white blood cell count 14,000/mcL, plasma glucose 650 mg/dL, and a urinalysis was negative for infection or ketones. What is the diagnosis?

    1. Diabetic ketoacidosis.
    2. Hyperglycemic hyperosmolar state.
    3. Unable to determine without a serum β-hydroxybutyrate.
    4. Hypoxic osmotic nonketosis.

92. A 55-year-old woman with a history of hypertension presented with sudden onset of severe headache that started 1 hour ago; she also has nausea. She has no history of recent trauma. On exam, there was neck rigidity. Head computed tomography showed a hyperdense lesion in sulci and interhemispheric fissure. Which of the following is *not* a complication to this condition?

    1. Hydrocephalus.
    2. Alzheimer dementia.
    3. Seizure.
    4. Syndrome of inappropriate antidiuretic hormone.

93. A 32-year-old male patient arrives via ambulance to the emergency department after being in a motor vehicle accident. He is unconscious but his pupils are reactive; his Glasgow Coma Scale is 6. Head computed tomography showed multiple punctate hemorrhages in different areas of the brain and a foggy appearance in gray–white matter. What is the most likely diagnosis in this patient?

    1. Epidural hematoma.
    2. Subdural hematoma.
    3. Subarachnoid hemorrhage.
    4. Diffuse axonal injury.

94. A 25-year-old male patient visited his nurse practitioner for follow-up. He has a history of epilepsy. He is now on lamotrigine after sodium valproate failed to control his seizures, but he still has a seizure episode every week, so he decides to add sodium valproate to his regime. Which of the following is an increased risk in this patient?

    1. Myocardial infarction.
    2. Addiction.
    3. Pancreatitis.
    4. Stevens–Johnson syndrome.

95. A 40-year-old male alcoholic is brought to the emergency department with an ataxic gait and decreased level of consciousness. On exam, he was confused and disoriented with slurred speech, but his pupils are reactive to light. Which of the following will be found on further exam of this patient?

    1. Pinpoint pupils.
    2. Nystagmus.
    3. Elevated blood pressure.
    4. Fever.

96. A 40-year-old female patient who was diagnosed with polycystic kidney disease 1 year ago visits her nurse practitioner for routine follow-up. Her brother died 2 years ago from hemorrhagic stroke. If the patient underwent computed tomography angiography, what is she at risk for having?

    1. Posterior communication artery aneurysm.
    2. Chronic subdural hematoma.
    3. Berry aneurysm.
    4. Hydrocephalus.

97. A 50-year-old homeless man presented with headache that started 2 days ago associated with projectile vomiting and photophobia. He has no history of any chronic disease. On exam, he has a stiff neck. Brain computed tomography was normal and lumbar puncture showed high opening cerebrospinal fluid pressure with low glucose, high protein, and leukocytosis. Which of the following is the most likely organism causing the patients symptoms?

    1. *Escherichia coli.*
    2. *Streptococcus pneumoniae.*
    3. *Proteus mirabilis.*
    4. *Staphylococcus aureus.*

98. A 50-year-old man complains of urinary incontinence that began this morning. He also has severe back pain for the past 2 days. On exam, there was a significant weakness in the patient's right lower limb associated with hyporeflexia. Which of the following symptoms does the nurse practitioner expect to find in this patient?

    1. Scrotal swelling.
    2. Nystagmus.
    3. Positive Babinski.
    4. Loss of bowel control.

99. A 55-year-old man presented to the emergency department with sudden severe back pain that started 1 day ago. He also had a history of urinary and fecal incontinence. On exam, he had bilateral lower limb weakness and hyperreflexia with a positive Babinski. Which of the following is the site of lesion in this patient?

    1. Cervical spinal cord.

    2. Conus medullaris.

    3. Cauda equina.

    4. Lumbar spinal cord.

100. A 45-year-old male patient is evaluated for chronic headache that has been going on for more than 3 months. When he leans forward, the headache is worse. Also, he is having nausea and blurred vision. There is no history of trauma or neurological deficit. On exam, he appears confused, his blood pressure is 155/95 mmHg, and his pulse is 55 beats/min. Which of the following is the most likely diagnosis?

    1. Increase intracranial pressure.

    2. Ischemic stroke.

    3. Pontine hemorrhage.

    4. Chronic sinusitis.

101. A middle-aged man complains of headaches that started 1 month ago after sustaining a fall down a flight of stairs. He denies losing consciousness, nausea, vomiting, or neurological deficits. Head computed tomography showed 2-cm subdural hematoma. Which of the following is the best treatment option for this patient?

    1. Observation.

    2. Ventriculoperitoneal shunt.

    3. Burr hole drain.

    4. Craniotomy.

102. A 65-year-old woman, with a history of diabetes and hypertension presents to the emergency department with right arm weakness that started 1 hour ago. Also, she has a history of dysarthria. On exam, her strength in the right arm is 1/5 with right facial paralysis, whereas the strength in the right leg is 4/5. Head computed tomography shows no intracerebral hemorrhage. What is a contraindication for thrombolytic therapy?

    1. Surgery in the past 6 months.

    2. Platelet count is 110,000/mm³.

    3. Blood pressure 220/130 mmHg.

    4. Patient with a history of coffee ground emesis 6 months ago.

103. A 30-year-old man presents to the emergency department after a motor vehicle accident. The patient opens his eyes when his name is called, but he could not localize a pain stimulus or withdraw his arm. His speech is also just jumbled, incoherent words. What is the Glasgow Coma Scale for this patient?

    1. 10.

    2. 7.

    3. 12.

    4. 8.

104. A 30-year-old homeless man and drug abuser presents to the emergency department with a fever that started 3 days ago. He also complains of low back pain that radiates to his left leg. He also reports new-onset fecal incontinence. On exam, he appears acutely ill, his temperature is 102.9°F, muscle strength was 1/5 in his left leg and 3/5 in the right with sensory loss in both limbs with tenderness in the lower part of the back. Which of the following is the best treatment for this patient?

    1. Epidural injection.

    2. Spinal surgery compression with antibiotics.

    3. High-dose prednisone.

    4. Muscle relaxant with physiotherapy.

105. A 22-year-old man presented to the emergency department after a motorcycle accident. He was conscious and oriented with a Glasgow Coma Scale of 15 but he had clear fluid draining from his nose. Head computed tomography showed a depressed skull base fracture. What is the most appropriate next step?

    1. Observation.

    2. Repair dura immediately.

    3. Prescribe antibiotics.

    4. Elevate his head 60 degrees.

106. A 35-year-old male alcoholic was found in the street. He was confused and had an ataxic gait, so he was taken to the emergency department. On exam, he was confused and disoriented with slurred speech, his pupils are dilated and reactive to light. What is the next step the nurse practitioner should take?

    1. Order a head computed tomography.

    2. Give thiamine.

    3. Start empiric antibiotics.

    4. Give naloxone.

107. A 34-year-old man presented to the emergency department after a motorcycle accident. He was conscious and oriented, but his skull x-ray showed a skull fracture. Half an hour later he lost consciousness and his right pupil became dilated, but the left pupil is normal. What will the head computed tomography show?

    1. A hyperdense lesion in the interhemispheric fissure.

    2. Hyperdense biconcave lesion between dura and skull.

    3. An intraventricular hyperdense lesion.

    4. An intracerebral hyperdense lesion.

108. A 65-year-old woman, with diabetes and hypertension presented to her nurse practitioner with right arm weakness that started 1 hour ago. Also, she has a history of dysarthria. She used to smoke 1 pack for 30 years and she has a history of hyperlipidemia on atorvastatin. On exam, her blood pressure is 160/90 mmHg, strength in the right arm is 1/5 with right facial paralysis, whereas strength in the right leg is 4/5. Head computed tomography showed no intracerebral hemorrhage. Which of the following is the strongest risk factor for the patient's condition?

    1. Hypertension.

    2. Hyperlipidemia.

    3. Smoking.

    4. Alcohol intake.

109. The patient is a 58-year-old male patient who is being managed for emboli prophylaxis because of his diagnosis of atrial fibrillation. He is on warfarin 2 mg by mouth (PO) every Monday, Wednesday, and Friday and 4 mg PO on Tuesday, Thursday, Saturday, and Sunday. Today his prothrombin time is 37 seconds and his international normalized ratio (INR) is 2.9. The Adult-Gerontology Acute Care Nurse Practitioner knows that the appropriate action is to

    1. Make no change to dose but reevaluate in 3 to 5 days.

    2. Continue his current dose and recheck INR in 2 to 4 weeks.

    3. Increase his dose to 4 mg daily.

    4. Decrease his dose to 2 mg daily.

110. The patient presents for a routine wellness exam, and the review of systems is significant only for a markedly decreased capacity for intake and a vague sense of nausea after eating. The patient denies any other symptoms; the remainder of the gastrointestinal review of systems is negative. His medical history is significant for complicated peptic ulcer disease that finally required resection

for a perforated ulcer. The Adult-Gerontology Acute Care Nurse Practitioner advises the patient that:

    1. He will need an endoscopy to evaluate the problem.

    2. He will need lifelong PPI medication.

    3. Chronic gastroparesis is a known complication of ulcer surgery.

    4. He needs to be referred to a surgeon for further evaluation.

111. A 60-year-old man presents to his nurse practitioner with complaints of weakness and fatigue. He is a heavy smoker and was recently diagnosed with small cell carcinoma. On exam, his vital signs are stable. There is an obvious weakness in his proximal muscles with loss of deep tendon reflexes. His chemistry test was within normal. Which of the following is the next step of management?

    1. Atropine.

    2. Edrophonium.

    3. Plasmapheresis.

    4. Levothyroxine.

112. A 70-year-old man with a history of diabetes presented to the emergency department with right arm weakness that started 1 hour ago. He has a history of dysarthria. On exam, his blood pressure is 160/90 mmHg, and strength in the right arm is 1/5 with right facial paralysis, whereas strength in the right leg is 4/5. Head computed tomography showed no intracerebral hemorrhage. Which of the following is a contraindication for thrombolysis?

    1. Ischemic stroke.

    2. Thrombolysis was started within 3 hours of presentation.

    3. The symptom was not relieved before the start of treatment.

    4. Seizure at the onset of a stroke.

113. A 30-year-old homeless man and drug abuser presents with a fever that started 3 days ago. It is associated with low back pain that radiates to his lower limbs. Also, he has fecal incontinence. On exam, he appears ill, his temperature is 102.9°F, muscle strength of the left leg was 1/5 and 3/5 in the right leg with sensory loss in both limbs with tenderness in the lower part of the back. Which of the following is the next step of management?

    1. Blood culture.

    2. Lumbar puncture.

    3. Spinal magnetic resonance imaging.

    4. Head computed tomography.

114. A 30-year-old obese female patient with a 10 pack/year smoking history presents to her nurse practitioner with a chronic headache that has been present for the past 3 months. The headache is worse at night and wakes her up. She also has nausea associated with the headache. There is no history of trauma or other neurological deficits. Her head computed tomography was normal and lumbar puncture showed high opening pressure with normal cerebrospinal fluid analysis. Which of the following is a risk factor for this patient's condition?

    1. Diabetes mellitus.

    2. Hypertension.

    3. Obesity.

    4. Smoking.

115. A 26-year-old man presented to the emergency department after being stabbed in his back and hitting his spine. He was conscious and oriented with right-sided paralysis. On exam, his blood pressure is 120/80 mmHg. The strength on his right side was 1/5. Also, he lost the sensation to heat in the left arm. What is the diagnosis in this patient?

    1. Anterior cord syndrome.

    2. Posterior cord syndrome.

    3. Brown–Sequard syndrome.

    4. Cauda equine syndrome.

116. A 34-year-old female patient presented with fever and productive cough that started 2 days ago. She has a history of myasthenia gravis and is on pyridostigmine. On exam, she appeared tired and in distress, her pulse was 150 beats/min and her respiratory rate was 30 breaths/min with shallow breathing and subcostal muscle retractions. She was intubated and admitted to the intensive care unit. Which of the following is the next step of management?

    1. Atropine.

    2. Physiotherapy.

    3. Plasmapheresis.

    4. Bronchoscopy.

117. A 30-year-old male patient was admitted to the hospital department after a motorcycle accident; He was not wearing a helmet. At the time of admission, he was conscious but had a headache. One hour later, he lost consciousness and his right pupil was dilated but the left pupil was normal. Which of the following is the mechanism behind the patient's condition?

    1. Rupture of the middle meningeal artery.

    2. Rupture of berry aneurysm.

    3. Sinus venous thrombosis.

    4. Rupture of intracranial vein.

Multisystem Answers & Rationales 11

1. Answer: 2

Rationale: Pain is an early symptom of compartment syndrome, whereas pulselessness, paralysis, and edema are late signs.

2. Answer: 3

Rationale: Obtain quantitative pressures in all four compartments and consult surgery for a fasciotomy if tissue perfusion pressure (i.e., diastolic blood pressure minus compartment pressure) is less than 30 mmHg. All four compartments in the lower leg should have pressures checked. Historically, a pressure greater than 30 mmHg has been used, but other studies have suggested the use of tissue perfusion pressure, or delta pressure, to account for the variability of the blood pressure and thus tissue perfusion as an indication for surgical decompression.

3. Answer: 1

Rationale: Assess for pain with passive range of motion of the toes and ankle. Pain with passive range of motion through the affected compartment points toward a diagnosis of compartment syndrome.

4. Answer: 2

Rationale: Decompress intraluminal components via nasogastric and/or rectal tubes. Although opening the abdominal compartment remains the definitive management of abdominal compartment syndrome, less invasive means of reducing intraabdominal volume may reduce pressure and avoid surgery.

5. Answer: 4

Rationale: Central venous pressure is typically reduced in severe abdominal compartment syndrome because of decreased venous return from the inferior vena cava.

6. Answer: 1

Rationale: Patients with pancreatitis can develop abdominal compartment syndrome caused by peripancreatic inflammation, visceral edema secondary to resuscitation, and ileus, thus checking abdominal pressures could explain hypotension and renal failure.

7. Answer: 1

Rationale: Before decompression transpulmonary pressure from a distended abdomen will often result in high pressures. After decompression, tidal volume and positive end-expiratory pressure should be carefully reduced to avoid overexpansion of the lungs.

8. Answer: 3

Rationale: Patients with these symptoms after a tibial fracture have greater than 90% likelihood of having compartment syndrome. Loss of pulses is a very late finding, and the presence of distal pulses should not be taken as a reassuring finding.

9. Answer: 4

Rationale: The diagnosis of compartment syndrome requires a high degree of clinical suspicion and rapid measurement of compartment pressures. Diagnosis of compartment syndrome must occur rapidly and typically includes both clinical exam findings and measurement of intramuscular pressures as neither is completely diagnostic. Pressures near a fracture or deeper in the muscle are typically higher, and myonecrosis occurs in approximately 2 hours.

10. Answer: 4

Rationale: A clue to this scenario is a farm worker, who potentially has exposure to large amounts of organophosphate insecticides. Signs of organophosphate toxidrome include diaphoresis, urination, miosis, bronchorrhea, emesis, lacrimation, lethargy, and salivation.

11. Answer: 3

Rationale: Organophosphate toxicity causes excessive acetylcholine at the muscarinic receptors and atropine competitively inhibits acetylcholine. Dosing starts at 1 to 3 mg for adults, with doubling of the dose every 5 minutes until airway secretions are controlled.

12. Answer: 3

Rationale: The antidote *N*-acetylcysteine (NAC) should be administered as soon as possible, preferably within 8 hours of ingestion to reduce the risk of liver injury from the highly cytotoxic metabolite of acetaminophen, *N*-acetyl-*p*-benzoquinone imine. Charcoal may be useful within 2 hours but should not influence the decision to use NAC.

13. Answer: 4

Rationale: Patients who have consumed greater than 6 g/day for more than 48 hours or who are symptomatic with right upper quadrant pain, jaundice, or vomiting should receive the antidote *N*-acetylcysteine.

14. Answer: 1

Rationale: Tricyclic antidepressant overdose leads to anticholinergic symptoms such as dry mucosal membranes; urinary retention; and hot, dry skin within the first 2 hours. Later, the sodium channel blockade leads to prolonged QRS and QT, seizures, and hypotension.

15. Answer: 4

Rationale: Bicarbonate should be used in patients with evidence of sodium channel blockade such as prolonged QRS. Benzodiazepines should be used for seizures.

16. Answer: 4

Rationale: Cyanide is a chemical asphyxiant that is used in some industrial settings. Venous blood can become arterialized as the cyanide prevents oxygen extraction at the tissue level. Treatment cannot wait for further testing and includes the use of a three-part antidote kit.

17. Answer: 2

Rationale: The opioid toxidrome classically includes central nervous system depression, respiratory depression, and miosis. Bradycardia is also associated with opioid overdose and can occur as a result of respiratory depression. Patients admitted to the hospital also can have illicit drug use from items stowed in their personnel effects or delivered by visitors.

18. Answer: 4

Rationale: Serotonin syndrome can occur after exposure to serotonergic medications such as selective serotonin reuptake inhibitors, metoclopramide, selective norepinephrine reuptake inhibitors, tricyclic antidepressants, ondansetron and recreational drugs like cocaine and ecstasy (MDMA).

19. Answer: 1

Rationale: Treatment of serotonin syndrome is mostly supportive and involves rehydration with crystalloids and stopping the offending medications. In cases with very high fevers (i.e., 106°F) and hypotension, therapy may include vasopressors, intubation and paralysis, and cyproheptadine if other therapy has failed. The case described does not meet these thresholds for escalation.

20. Answer: 2

Rationale: Controlling the source of hemorrhage and restoration of the oxygen-carrying capacity limit the depth and duration of the shock state by restoring oxygen delivery at the cellular level.

21. Answer: 3

Rationale: This patient has hemorrhagic shock from penetrating trauma. Evidence suggests that a fluid-limited strategy reduces hemodilution and coagulopathy and blood products, in ratios to approximate whole blood, should be given.

22. Answer: 3

Rationale: Blood products contain the anticoagulant, citrate, which accumulates when many transfusions are given and can cause a life-threatening hypocalcemia and coagulopathy, thus empiric dosing of calcium chloride is necessary.

23. Answer: 2

Rationale: Patient with a Glasgow Coma Scale less than or equal to 8 is categorized as a severe traumatic brain injury and has a higher blood pressure target to maintain brain perfusion and avoid secondary injury.

24. Answer: 4

Rationale: Early surgery or embolization stops blood loss; the other options are incorrect.

25. Answer: 3

Rationale: The American Association of Neurological Surgeons and the Congress of Neurological Surgeons' Guidelines for the Management of Acute Cervical Spine and Spinal Cord Injuries recommend a mean arterial pressure goal of 85 to 90 mmHg. Steroids have not been shown to improve outcomes in traumatic spine injuries.

26. Answer: 2

Rationale: Norepinephrine has the most favorable profile to influence these vital signs. Phenylephrine can cause a reflex bradycardia and isoproterenol will not increase the mean arterial pressure to the goal of 85 mmHg.

27. Answer: 3

Rationale: Neurogenic shock results in loss of sympathetic tone and is characterized by warm dry skin, bradycardia, and hypotension caused by an inability to redirect blood from the peripheral circulation. There is no evidence for septic or hemorrhagic shock. Spinal shock has nothing to do with hemodynamics.

28. Answer: 2

Rationale: According to the Canadian C-Spine Rules, patients greater than 65 years of age or those with dangerous mechanisms such as high-speed motor vehicle crash, struck bicycle, and falls from greater than 3 feet require imaging, and a computed tomography is the most appropriate modality.

29. Answer: 1

Rationale: Administer blood via a warming device, and use a warming blanket to normalize body temperature. Hypothermia is common among trauma patients and associated with higher mortality.

30. Answer: 1

Rationale: Early (before 3 hours) administration of tranexamic acid reduces hemorrhage-induced mortality.

31. Answer: 3

Rationale: The urgent administration of blood products with a crystalloid-restrictive strategy is recommended in the newest trauma guidelines.

32. Answer: 2

Rationale: The "lethal triad" consists of hypothermia, acidosis, and coagulopathy; these are caused by severe bleeding and form a positive feedback cycle that perpetuates worsening of the triad and bleeding.

33. Answer: 3

Rationale: The newest Advanced Trauma Life Support guidelines suggest a target blood pressure of greater than 100 mmHg among 50- to 69-year-olds and greater than 110 among 15- to 49-year-olds and 70-year-olds.

34. Answer: 2

Rationale: Consider the cerebral perfusion pressure (CPP), which is calculated by subtracting intracranial pressure from mean arterial pressure. The CPP should be greater than 60.

35. Answer: 3

Rationale: The Parkland formula (mass in kg × percentage of total body surface area burned × 4) suggests 6 L for this patient. Actual volume can vary depending on the urine volume.

36. Answer: 3

Rationale: Most burn injuries do not need to be specifically addressed within the first hour; however, airway, breathing, and circulation remain emergent concerns to address. People who sustain burns in confined spaces are presumed to have carbon monoxide poisoning.

37. Answer: 3

Rationale: Exploration of the supraaortic and intracranial arteries should occur if patients with basilar skull fractures,

LeFort II or III type facial fractures, cervical spine fracture, or focal neurological deficit are not explained by brain imaging.

38. Answer: 4

Rationale: An appropriate $Paco_2$ target for a patient with acute brain herniation syndrome is 30 to 35 to induce mild cerebral arterial vasoconstriction; thus decrease the volume of blood within the skull and reduce intracranial pressure until further treatments can be initiated. Inducing hypoventilation can worsen intracranial pressure.

39. Answer: 4

Rationale: Patients with cool skin and tachycardia should be presumed to have early hemorrhagic shock. Femur fractures can result in massive internal blood loss and an initial normal hemoglobin/hematocrit is unreliable for excluding hemorrhagic shock.

40. Answer: 2

Rationale: Guidelines recommend intramuscular epinephrine as soon as anaphylactic shock is suspected.

41. Answer: 1

Rationale: The patient's oxygenation status needs to be evaluated immediately. If supplemental oxygen were an answer choice, that would be the first action. At this point, the patient does not need to be electively intubated. A chest x-ray does need to be done, but the arterial blood gas should be done first. The patient needs to be stabilized before transferring to another unit.

42. Answer: 3

Rationale: This patient is hypoxic with impending respiratory collapse and is likely to require intubation if the initial dose of epinephrine does not rapidly reverse her anaphylaxis.

43. Answer: 2

Rationale: Glucagon can bypass the β-receptor in patients on a beta-blocker, providing direct inotropic and chronotropic effects, restoring hemodynamic stability.

44. Answer: 2

Rationale: This patient's sequential organ failure assessment score is greater than 2 and she should be treated for sepsis. The Surviving Sepsis Campaign's 2016 guidelines recommend an urgent 30-mL/kg bolus for all septic patients followed by cultures and antibiotics.

45. Answer: 3

Rationale: Removing implanted devices, particularly those in contact with infected tissue and have likely been colonized, can aid with clearance of infection.

46. Answer: 1

Rationale: Cerebrospinal fluid is unlikely to sterilize for 6 hours following initiation of antibiotics. Dexamethasone reduces mortality and other unfavorable outcomes in acute bacterial meningitis, particularly those caused by *Streptococcus pneumoniae,* which is a common pathogen among middle-aged adults in which symptoms evolve over hours.

47. Answer: 3

Rationale: Reflexive flexion of the hips and knees while the examiner flexes the patient's neck is a Brudzinski sign, which is concerning for meningitis.

48. Answer: 2

Rationale: Patients with an abnormal neurological exam should have a head computed tomography performed before performing a lumbar puncture to rule out a mass-occupying lesion and avoid downward herniation as the cerebrospinal fluid is drained.

49. Answer: 3

Rationale: Initial empiric meningitis coverage includes a third-generation cephalosporin and vancomycin. Immunosuppressed patients and the elderly also require ampicillin because of their increased risk of *Listeria monocytogenes.* Dexamethasone is not necessary because his symptoms evolved over days making *Streptococcus pneumoniae* less likely.

50. Answer: 2

Rationale: Herpes encephalitis results in rapid destruction of the temporal lobe, which can cause seizures, leads to both high red and white cells in the cerebrospinal fluid (CSF), and should be treated with urgent empiric acyclovir until it can be ruled out with polymerase chain reaction testing on the CSF.

51. Answer: 3

Rationale: She is septic and should have a wound culture obtained and vancomycin, piperacillin/tazobactam, and metronidazole started within an hour of presenting to the emergency department. This patient has a source of infection and new-onset organ failure and meets the criteria for sepsis. She does not have shock. Broad antibiotic coverage against methicillin-resistant gram-positive, gram-negative, and anaerobic organisms is necessary.

52. Answer: 2

Rationale: Janeway lesions are characteristic of infective endocarditis and are erythematous or hemorrhagic spots less than a few millimeters found on the palms and soles.

53. Answer: 1

Rationale: This patient meets the Duke criteria for infective endocarditis with one major criterion (two or more blood cultures positive for a typical organism), and three or more minor criteria (fever greater than 100.4°F, vascular phenomenon [Janeway lesions], and a predisposing condition [intravenous drug abuse]).

54. Answer: 3

Rationale: The diagnosis of infective endocarditis stands; transthoracic echocardiograms can produce false negatives and transesophageal echocardiograms are more sensitive. In this scenario, the clinical suspicion is very high.

55. Answer: 3

Rationale: Use of β-lactams, such as penicillins and cephalosporins, are unlikely to be effective when the bacteria are producing β-lactamase.

56. Answer: 1

Rationale: Source control is an important step in treating sepsis because infections are unlikely to clear in the setting of an undrained abscess. The least invasive method of source control is recommended in the Surviving Sepsis Campaign's guidelines; however, organ injury, fistula formation, and other considerations may impact the appropriate method to drain an abscess.

57. Answer: 2

Rationale: This patient does not have contraindications to extracorporeal membrane oxygenation, which could be a life-saving measure for this patient.

58. Answer: 1

Rationale: Oseltamivir plus ampicillin/sulbactam, amoxicillin/clavulanate, third-generation cephalosporins, and respiratory quinolones that show an antibacterial activity to *Staphylococcus aureus, Streptococcus pneumoniae, S. pyogenes,* and *Moraxella catarrhalis* are recommended in patients with concurrent pneumonia and severe influenza.

59. Answer: 1

Rationale: The recommended initial bolus for septic shock is 30 mL/kg, which is 2700 mL. This should be completed before initiating vasopressors.

60. Answer: 3

Rationale: In the absence of ventricular dysfunction or other mitigating factors, norepinephrine is the vasopressor recommended by the Surviving Sepsis Campaign's sepsis guidelines.

61. Answer: 2

Rationale: The Society of Critical Care Medicine and European Society of Intensive Care Medicine's 2017 guidelines on addressing corticosteroid deficiency cite numerous studies and recommend hydrocortisone dosed at less than 400 mg/day for greater than 3 days in this circumstance. The Surviving Sepsis Guidelines suggest hydrocortisone 200 mg/day if hypotension is refractory to fluids and vasopressors.

62. Answer: 1

Rationale: Severity scores such as the CURB-65 (confusion, uremia, respiratory rate, low blood pressure, age 65 years or greater) should be used to determine severity of illness. In this case, the patient does not meet any of the criteria for admission and can be managed as an outpatient. Treatment with a macrolide is preferred, alternatively doxycycline.

63. Answer: 4

Rationale: Patient with community-acquired pneumonia who are appropriate for outpatient therapy and have comorbidities such as chronic heart, lung, liver, or renal disease; diabetes mellitus; alcoholism; malignancies; asplenia; immunosuppressing conditions; or use of immunosuppressing drugs should be treated with a respiratory fluoroquinolone or a β-lactam plus a macrolide.

64. Answer: 2

Rationale: Patients with community-acquired pneumonia admitted to the intensive care unit generally need a β-lactam plus either azithromycin or a fluoroquinolone. In this case of penicillin allergy, aztreonam is substituted for the β-lactam and given the history of methicillin-resistant *Staphylococcus aureus*, either vancomycin or linezolid should be added.

65. Answer: 1

Rationale: Duration of treatment for community-acquired pneumonia should typically be 5 days. Treatment could be longer if the initial therapy did not provide adequate coverage or if the patient's fever has continued.

66. Answer: 2

Rationale: Treatment for hospital-acquired pneumonia for patients with high risk of multidrug-resistant organism (in this case, exposure to intravenous antibiotics), treatment should include an antipseudomonal β-lactam plus vancomycin or linezolid. In this complicated case, changing the vancomycin to linezolid would provide inadequate coverage for the bacteremia because linezolid is not bactericidal. If there is concern for inadequately treated endocarditis, vancomycin

should be replaced. It would be reasonable to consider an infectious disease consult.

67. Answer: 1

Rationale: Patients with a high risk of death from hospital-acquired pneumonia (i.e., septic shock) with risk factors for pseudomonas should have double pseudomonal coverage, but not two β-lactams. This patient is also at risk for methicillin-resistant *Staphylococcus aureus* and needs vancomycin or linezolid.

68. Answer: 3

Rationale: The Infectious Diseases Society of America/American Thoracic Society guidelines for hospital-acquired and ventilator-associated pneumonias recommend a 7-day course and de-escalation based on susceptibilities, assuming clinical improvement.

69. Answer: 3

Rationale: High-frequency oscillatory ventilation has theoretical advantages in acute respiratory distress syndrome but has been shown to worsen mortality.

70. Answer: 3

Rationale: The Surviving Sepsis Campaign guidelines recommend keeping arterial blood glucose less than 180. Lower targets result in more hypoglycemia.

71. Answer: 4

Rationale: The goal is to improve tissue perfusion and oxygenation, and giving the fluids is the best of these options. Bicarbonate is not indicated unless pH is less than 7.15 and is associated with increased Pco_2, and lactate and can result in intracellular acidosis even though blood pH increases after administration.

72. Answer: 1

Rationale: This case of *Clostridium difficile* is categorized as severe because white blood cells are greater than 15,000 or a serum creatinine is greater than 1.5 mg/dL. An initial episode of severe *C. difficile* should be treated with enteral vancomycin or fidaxomicin.

73. Answer: 3

Rationale: The addition of hypotension or ileus to the scenario recategorizes it as fulminant *Clostridium difficile* infection. When ileus is present the addition of vancomycin via retention enema aids in delivering the drug to the site of infection.

74. Answer: 2

Rationale: This scenario suggests a diagnosis of diabetes insipidus, for which serum sodium and urine specific gravity will aid in the diagnosis.

75. Answer: 1

Rationale: This patient has central diabetes insipidus from pituitary compression; treatment involves urgent administration of desmopressin and fluids to attenuate the hypernatremia.

76. Answer: 3

Rationale: Syndrome of inappropriate antidiuretic hormone is commonly caused by pulmonary disease and malignancy, and first-line treatment is a fluid restriction in the absence of symptoms such as seizure, mental status change, or falls.

77. Answer: 4

Rationale: The preferred insulin route in the intensive care unit setting is intravenous infusion with a target of 140 to 180 mg/dL to avoid hypoglycemic complications. Vasoconstriction and edema of subcutaneous tissue can alter absorption.

78. Answer: 1

Rationale: This patient had adequate control and can be safely transitioned back to her home regimen in the absence of other contraindications.

79. Answer: 2

Rationale: Hospitalized patients with new hyperglycemia should be managed with a basal, prandial correction regimen.

80. Answer: 1

Rationale: If you are unable to ensure that the patient comprehends her insulin administration regimen, this is not safe, despite it being the preferred initial treatment. Therefore, the next most reasonable option is an oral agent with follow-up.

81. Answer: 2

Rationale: A cortisol level should be checked at 8 a.m., and a level less than 165 is consistent with adrenal insufficiency. Urinary cortisol is not helpful in diagnosis, and the cortisol level after a corticotropin test less than 500 is diagnostic of adrenal insufficiency.

82. Answer: 4

Rationale: Abrupt cessation of steroids after greater than 2 to 3 weeks can result in adrenal insufficiency. Signs of adrenal insufficiency include hypotension and fatigue.

83. Answer: 1

Rationale: Vomiting, abdominal pain, myalgia, joint pains, and severe hypotension are hallmark features of adrenal insufficiency. Additionally, recent surgical manipulation of the pituitary is the likely etiology of low corticotropin secretion leading to adrenal insufficiency.

84. Answer: 1

Rationale: Kussmaul respirations, confusion, drowsiness, and vomiting are suggestive of diabetic ketoacidosis (DKA). Diagnostic criteria for DKA are serum glucose greater than 200 to 300 mg/dL, bicarbonate less than 15 to 18 mEq/L, pH less than 7.3, and ketones present in the blood or urine.

85. Answer: 2

Rationale: Mortality is most common in diabetic ketoacidosis from the precipitating illness (e.g., myocardial infarct or sepsis), but in the absence of a precipitating illness, hypokalemia can be fatal.

86. Answer: 1

Rationale: Urgent initial therapy consists of intravenous fluids, insulin, and potassium and close monitoring of blood glucose and potassium levels to avoid hypoglycemia and hypokalemia.

87. Answer: 3

Rationale: High thyroid-stimulating hormone and low free T4 are consistent with undertreated hypothyroidism.

88. Answer: 1

Rationale: Although these labs would generally indicate undertreated hypothyroidism, thyroxine (T4) has a serum half-life of 1 week and dose adjustments are typically only made no more frequently than every 4 to 6 weeks.

89. Answer: 3

Rationale: Levothyroxine absorption is altered when coadministered with food, supplements, and some medications and should be taken on an empty stomach, 1 hour before or 4 hours after a meal.

90. Answer: 4

Rationale: During critical illness, the normal negative feedback loop is altered, resulting in nonthyroidal illness syndrome or euthyroid sick syndrome, especially in patients with cardiac illness. There is scant evidence to support starting thyroid replacement in the acute setting.

91. Answer: 2

Rationale: Absence of ketones rules out diabetic ketoacidosis and glucose greater than 600 mg/dL, hypovolemia, and hypothermia point to a hyperglycemic hyperosmolar state (synonymous with and formerly referred to as hyperglycemic hyperosmolar nonketotic coma [HONK] and hyperosmolar hyperglycemic nonketotic syndrome [HHNS]).

92. Answer: 2

Rationale: This patient presented with a sudden severe headache, which is a typical presentation of subarachnoid hemorrhage (SAH). SAH appears on head computed tomography as a hyperdense lesion in the interhemispheric fissure. There are many complications for SAH including hydrocephalus, seizure, and electrolyte abnormalities caused by syndrome of inappropriate antidiuretic hormone secretion or diabetes insipidus.

93. Answer: 4

Rationale: Diffuse axonal injury happens with a sudden acceleration–deceleration event and has high morbidity and mortality. It mainly affects the brain at the level of the gray–white matter junction. The diffuse axonal injury appears in head computed tomography with multiple punctate hemorrhages with blurring white–gray matter interference.

94. Answer: 4

Rationale: In the treatment of epilepsy, monotherapy is preferred, and the first line of management is sodium valproate, but if the patient still has seizures, he should be switched to lamotrigine. If the seizure is still uncontrolled, you can use both drugs together, but the practitioner should use caution because the risk of Stevens–Johnson syndrome is increased in this patient.

95. Answer: 2

Rationale: Patients with Wernicke encephalopathy will have an ataxic gait, slurred speech, confusion, dilation of pupils, and nystagmus. All these signs raise suspicion for Wernicke encephalopathy, which happens in alcoholics. The treatment of this condition is thiamine, which can reverse Wernicke encephalopathy and prevent it.

96. Answer: 3

Rationale: Any patient diagnosed with polycystic kidney disease with a family history of hemorrhagic stroke or intracranial aneurysm is at risk of developing a berry aneurysm.

97. Answer: 2

Rationale: This patient has symptoms of meningitis. Also, the characteristics of cerebrospinal fluid findings in bacterial meningitis were found in this patient, including high protein, increased polymorphonuclear leukocytes, and low glucose. The most common organism in bacterial meningitis is *Streptococcus pneumoniae.*

98. Answer: 4

Rationale: This patient has the symptoms of cauda equine syndrome, which can happen as a result of trauma and leads to the rupture of the disc or caused by inflammatory conditions. This is an emergent situation that needs rapid intervention to release the compression before ischemia happens.

99. Answer: 2

Rationale: This patient has the symptoms of conus medullaris syndrome, which can present with symmetrical motor weakness, early bladder and bowel dysfunction with hyperreflexia, and sudden back pain. Conus medullaris syndrome is an emergency that needs urgent surgical decompression.

100. Answer: 1

Rationale: The patient has symptoms of increased intracranial pressure, which includes headache, nausea, papilledema, and high opening cerebrospinal fluid pressure. There are many causes that lead to increased intracranial pressure including space-occupying lesions, intracerebral hemorrhage, and idiopathic causes.

101. Answer: 3

Rationale: Symptomatic subdural hematomas or any chronic hematoma larger than 1 cm needs surgical drainage. A simple burr hole is effective in this condition. A craniotomy can be the choice only if the burr hole has failed because the blood is congealed too much. Ventriculoperitoneal shunt is also used in the treatment of subdural hematoma.

102. Answer: 3

Rationale: The patient presents with symptoms of acute ischemic stroke. The head computed tomography showed no intracerebral hemorrhage so the next step of management is alteplase, which is a thrombolytic therapy that can be used for ischemic stroke within 3 hours from symptom initiation. There are several contraindications for thrombolytic therapy including previous hemorrhagic stroke, blood pressure greater than 180 mmHg, and previous surgery or gastrointestinal bleeding within 3 months.

103. Answer: 1

Rationale: The Glasgow Coma Scale is a measure of the best response of a patient for each group. The groups include motor scores that range from 1 to 6, a verbal category that ranges from 1 to 5, and an eye category that ranges from 1 to 4. When you add the totals together they range should be between 3 and 15.

104. Answer: 2

Rationale: This patient has signs of spinal cord compression, with several possible causes. He also had rapid deterioration with fever, which suggests spinal epidural abscess. An epidural abscess is considered an emergency and needs urgent magnetic resonance imaging to diagnose it. The treatment regime usually includes surgical compression with antibiotics.

105. Answer: 2

Rationale: This patient had cerebrospinal fluid leaking from his nose, which happens if there is a fracture in the area of the paranasal sinus, the mastoid air cell, or the middle ear. With evidence of depressed fracture surgery, intervention to repair dura is needed immediately to prevent other sequels like meningitis.

106. Answer: 2

Rationale: This patient has an ataxic gain, slurred speech, confusion, and dilation of pupils. All of these signs raise suspicion for Wernicke encephalopathy, which happens in alcoholics and people who are malnourished. The treatment of this condition is thiamine, which can reverse Wernicke encephalopathy and prevent it.

107. Answer: 2

Rationale: Epidural hematomas are characterized by a lucid interval at presentation, but the patient will then suddenly deteriorate. An epidural hematoma is a result of rupture of the middle meningeal artery. The first step to diagnosis an epidural hematoma is a head computed tomography (CT), and then the patient needs to have a craniotomy to evacuate the hematoma. An epidural hematoma appears in a head CT as a hyperdense biconcave lesion between dura and skull.

108. Answer: 1

Rationale: The patient presented with symptoms of acute ischemic stroke, and head computed tomography showed no intracerebral involvement. There are many risk factors for ischemic strokes including hypertension, diabetes, hyperlipidemia, and smoking, but the major risk factor and the most important one is hypertension.

109. Answer: 2

Rationale: The dose does not need to be changed at this point. Ongoing monitoring is the only thing required.

110. Answer: 3

Rationale: Chronic gastroparesis is a known complication of ulcer surgery. The patient should eat small, frequent meals.

111. Answer: 3

Rationale: The patient has a history of small cell carcinoma and presented with proximal muscle weakness, suggesting this patient has Lambert–Eaton myasthenic syndrome, which is a paraneoplastic syndrome. In this syndrome, the body develops an antibody against presynaptic calcium channel blockers. The treatment of this disease includes plasmapheresis and immunosuppression drugs.

112. Answer: 4

Rationale: The patient presented with symptoms of acute ischemic stroke and head computed tomography showed no intracerebral hemorrhage. The next step of management is alteplase, which is thrombolytic therapy that can be used for ischemic stroke within 3 hours from symptom initiation. There are several contraindications for thrombolytic therapy including previous hemorrhagic stroke, blood pressure greater than 180 mmHg, and previous surgery or gastrointestinal bleeding within 3 months.

113. Answer: 3

Rationale: This patient has signs of spinal cord compression. There are several causes that can lead to this, but he also had rapid deterioration with fever, which suggests spinal epidural abscess. Epidural abscess is considered an emergent case and needs urgent magnetic resonance imaging to diagnose it. The treatment regime usually includes surgical compression with antibiotics.

114. Answer: 3

Rationale: The patient has symptoms of increased intracranial pressure, which includes headache, nausea, papilledema, and high opening cerebrospinal fluid pressure. On the other hand, there is no abnormality in the investigation and no neurological deficit. All this suggests idiopathic intracranial hypertension or pseudotumor cerebri. Obesity and hypervitaminosis A are risk factors that can lead to pseudotumor cerebri. The first line of management includes acetazolamide or furosemide. Weight loss can reduce the symptoms in obese patients.

115. Answer: 3

Rationale: This patient presented with typical symptoms of Brown–Sequard syndrome, which includes loss of motor and proprioception ipsilaterally, and loss of thermoception in the contralateral side. The primary mechanism for this syndrome is stabbing or a gunshot injury.

116. Answer: 3

Rationale: This patient presented with signs and symptoms of myasthenia crisis, which can happen because of respiratory tract infection. It is a life-threatening condition. The management of myasthenia gravis includes intubating the patient then starting plasmapheresis or intravenous immunoglobulin with steroids.

117. Answer: 1

Rationale: An epidural hematoma is characterized by a lucid interval. At presentation the patient appears conscious with a good general condition and then the patient's condition will suddenly deteriorate. An epidural hematoma is the result of the rupture of the middle meningeal artery, whereas subdural hematoma mainly happens from the rupture of the intracranial vein and rupture of an aneurysm that can cause an intracerebral hemorrhage.

12

Psychosocial/Cognitive/Behavioral Health

1. The patient is a 27-year-old woman who presents to your health care facility with a history of depressed mood that has worsened during the past few weeks. She gained 8 kg in the past 2 months; she reports that she is eating when she is not sleeping. She is very stressed and worried about her job. She has passive thoughts of harming herself but no definite plan. Her medical history includes anxiety, and she takes 0.5 mg of alprazolam three times daily. Which medication is the best to treat this patient?

   1. Paroxetine.

   2. Fluoxetine.

   3. Imipramine.

   4. Mirtazapine.

2. The patient is a 43-year-old Hispanic man who is getting ready to be discharged from your health care facility after a myocardial infarction. He has a 23-year history of cigarette smoking and smokes 1 pack/day. He has tried to quit several times, but he was unsuccessful. He tried 2-mg nicotine gum, and to save money, he chewed only 6 pieces daily. He has a history of depression along with his cardiac problems. Which medication is the best for this patient?

   1. Nicotine 4-mg gum.

   2. Varenicline 0.5 mg once daily.

   3. Bupropion SR 150 mg twice daily.

   4. Nicotine patch 21 mg/day.

3. The patient is a 53-year-old African American woman (weight 95 kg, height 73 inches) who comes to your clinic for management of her type 2 diabetes, mild congestive heart disease, neuropathy, and recurrent major depression. Her medications are metformin 1000 mg twice daily, carvedilol 12.5 mg twice daily, citalopram 40 mg daily, and ramipril 10 mg daily. She still has depressive symptoms and wants to change her medication. What is the best action for her?

   1. Duloxetine.

   2. Desipramine.

   3. Sertraline.

   4. Bupropion.

4. The patient is a 58-year-old Asian man with a 25-year history of alcoholic dependence. He drinks 1 cup of vodka every day. He has tried to quit several times without success. His laboratory tests reveal aspartate aminotransferase 135 international units/L, alanine aminotransferase 75 international units/L, albumin 4 g/dL, total bilirubin 0.3 mg/dL, prothrombin time 0.8 seconds, platelet count 350,000/mm^3, and creatinine clearance 35 mL/min. After detoxification, which maintenance treatment is most appropriate?

   1. Chlordiazepoxide.

   2. Disulfiram.

   3. Naltrexone.

   4. Acamprosate.

5. The patient is a 35-year-old white woman admitted to the emergency department with agitation, diaphoresis, and fever (103.5°F). Also, her eyelid has been twitching for 2 hours. She reports cold symptoms for the past 3 days, and she took dextromethorphan and pseudoephedrine. Her medical history includes depression, hypertension, and osteoarthritis. She currently takes sertraline 100 mg daily, glipizide 5 mg daily, diltiazem XR 240 mg daily, calcium 500 mg daily, and acetaminophen 650 mg every 6 hours. Which combination of medications is most likely contributing to her symptoms?

   1. Dextromethorphan and paroxetine.

   2. Paroxetine and acetaminophen.

   3. Paroxetine and glipizide.

   4. Dextromethorphan and pseudoephedrine.

6. The patient is a 23-year-old Asian woman with a 2-year history of heroin addiction. She has successfully been maintained on methadone 40 mg daily for 1 year. Now, she does not want to go to a daily opioid treatment program to get her methadone dose. Which treatment regimen could be changed and is appropriate for her?

    1. Initiate naltrexone.

    2. Administer naltrexone/buprenorphine.

    3. Change to buprenorphine × 2 days, then administer naltrexone/buprenorphine.

    4. Taper to methadone 30 mg, then change to buprenorphine.

7. A 29-year-old woman presents to the psychiatric clinic complaining of losing interest in her job and she wants to be alone. She has a 6-year history of type I bipolar disorder and takes lithium 300 mg twice daily. She states that she takes her medicine every day just as prescribed. Her lithium level today is 1.0 mEq/L. She has been without manic disorders for the past 5 years. Which medication is the best for her acute depression symptoms?

    1. Venlafaxine.

    2. Quetiapine.

    3. Aripiprazole.

    4. Lamotrigine.

8. A 29-year-old woman presents to the psychiatric clinic complaining of losing interest in her job and wants to be alone all the time. She has a 6-year of history of type I bipolar disorder and takes lithium 300 mg twice daily. She states that she takes her medicine every day just as prescribed. Her lithium level today is 1.0 mEq/L. She has been without manic disorders for the past 5 years. Which therapy would be the best for the maintenance depression symptoms?

    1. Venlafaxine.

    2. Sertraline.

    3. Aripiprazole.

    4. Lamotrigine.

9. The patient is a 67-year-old white man who has a difficulty going to sleep. Once he falls to sleep, he rests comfortably throughout the night. The physical examination reveals no contributing factors. The patient has a history of myocardial infarction 2 years ago, mild congestive heart failure, and hypertension. He has tried diphenhydramine, but he complained of hangover symptoms. Which medication has the least hangover effect and would be appropriate for his insomnia symptoms?

    1. Ramelteon.

    2. Suvorexant.

    3. Zolpidem.

    4. Eszopiclone.

10. The patient is a 48-year-old woman who comes to the clinic with symptoms of generalized anxiety disorder. Her medical history includes hypertension, breast cancer, osteoporosis, vasomotor symptoms, and newly diagnosed type 2 diabetes mellitus. She currently takes lorazepam, alendronate, calcium supplement, ramipril, tamoxifen, metformin, and vitamin D supplements. The nurse practitioner recommends tapering off lorazepam. Which medication is the best for controlling her anxiety symptoms?

    1. Pregabalin.

    2. Venlafaxine.

    3. Fluoxetine.

    4. Bupropion.

11. The patient is a 27-year-old white man who presented to the emergency department with trembling, sweating, chest pain, and shortness of breath. His physical examination does not note any cardiac problems; the nurse practitioner diagnosed him with panic disorder. Which therapy is the best for his acute symptoms?

    1. Sertraline.

    2. Buspirone.

    3. Bupropion.

    4. Chlordiazepoxide.

12. The patient is a 27-year-old white man who presented to the emergency department with trembling, sweating, chest pain, and shortness of breath. His physical examination rules out any cardiac problems; the nurse practitioner diagnosed him with panic disorder. He takes alprazolam to treat his acute symptoms. Which action would be the best for long-term management of his panic disorders?

    1. Initiate cognitive behavioral therapy (CBT) and buspirone.

    2. Initiate CBT and bupropion.

    3. Initiate CBT and hydroxyzine.

    4. Initiate CBT and escitalopram.

13. The patient is a 37-year-old American African man who presents to the psychiatry clinic for follow-up. His medical history includes type I bipolar disorder, and reports that he has had about an 8-kg weight gain over the past 2 months. He takes lithium 450 mg twice daily for the past 8 months, olanzapine 10 mg once daily, and a multivitamin supplement. The laboratory tests reveal the lithium concentration is 0.8 mEq/L, sodium is 135 mEq/L, potassium is 4.5 mEq/L, serum creatinine is 0.9 mg/mL, glucose is 120 mg/dL, and thyroid-stimulating hormone is 26 units/mL. Which most likely accounts for the objective finding?

    1. Olanzapine.

    2. Multivitamin supplements.

    3. Hypothyroidism.

    4. Lithium concentration.

14. The patient is a 37-year-old American African man who presents to the psychiatry clinic for follow-up. His history includes type I bipolar disorder, and reports that he has had about an 8-kg weight gain over the past 2 months. He takes lithium 450 mg twice daily for the past 8 months, olanzapine 10 mg once daily, and a multivitamin supplement. The laboratory tests reveal the lithium concentration is 0.8 mEq/L, sodium is 135 mEq/L, potassium is 4.5 mEq/L, serum creatinine is 0.9 mg/mL, glucose is 120 mg/dL, and thyroid-stimulating hormone is 26 units/mL. From the objective finding, which medication is considered the best for this patient?

    1. Levothyroxine.

    2. Insulin glargine.

    3. Propranolol.

    4. Propylthiouracil.

15. A 27-year-old Hispanic woman (weight 93 kg, height 73 inches) presents to your health care facility for a checkup. The patient has a 3-year history of type I bipolar disorder and hypertension. She currently takes lithium 450 mg twice daily and ramipril 10 mg twice daily. Her lithium concentration has been evaluated, and it is 1.2 mEq/L. Her laboratory tests show sodium 147 mEq/L, potassium 4.7 mEq/L, and serum creatinine 1.0 mg/mL. Which condition could cause a drug interaction and increase the lithium concentration?

    1. Theophylline.

    2. Ramipril.

    3. Pregnancy.

    4. Amiloride.

16. A 37-year-old Asian man with a history of rapid-cycling bipolar disorder, hypertension, and dyslipidemia presents to your psychiatric clinic. He has been taking lithium 450 mg twice daily for the past 3 years, then his lithium was changed to divalproex sodium 500 mg daily. He also takes lisinopril 20 mg daily, multivitamin supplements, and pitavastatin 4 mg daily. He complains of abdominal pain, nausea, vomiting, and rebound tenderness. The laboratory tests reveal sodium 135 mEq/L, potassium 4 mEq/L, chloride 95 mEq/L, glucose 90 mg/dL, serum creatinine 0.9 mg/mL, aspartate aminotransferase 26 international units/L, alanine aminotransferase 20 international units/L, amylase 460 international units/L, and lipase 380 international units/L. Which medication is most likely responsible for his laboratory finding?

    1. Lisinopril.

    2. Divalproex sodium.

    3. Multivitamin supplements.

    4. Pitavastatin.

17. A 47-year-old Asian woman with a history of rapid-cycling bipolar disorder, hypertension, and dyslipidemia presents to your psychiatric clinic. She has been taking lithium 450 mg twice daily for the past 3 years, but there is a recurrence of her mania symptoms. Which medication is the best for this presentation?

    1. Divalproex sodium.

    2. Lamotrigine.

    3. Sertraline.

    4. Alprazolam.

18. The patient is a 37-year-old African American woman who has a 5-year history of schizophrenia. She was diagnosed with type 2 diabetes, obesity, and dyslipidemia in the past 6 months. She takes risperidone, metformin, atorvastatin, and insulin glargine. She complained of galactorrhea, which was induced by risperidone. Which medication is most appropriate for this patient?

    1. Olanzapine.

    2. Paliperidone.

    3. Ziprasidone.

    4. Clozapine.

19. The patient is a 47-year-old woman with a 17-year history of schizophrenia. She has been taking haloperidol, but this was recently changed to aripiprazole. Today, she comes to the psychiatric clinic with anxiety and agitation. She feels "uncomfortable in her skin." She reports that she regularly drinks alcohol. Which medication is most appropriate to relieve her symptoms?

    1. Propranolol.

    2. Alprazolam.

    3. Benztropine.

    4. Dantrolene.

20. The patient is a 63-year-old white woman with a 25-year history of schizophrenia who is admitted to the emergency department with involuntary chewing motions and abnormal blinking for the past 6 months. The patient was on haloperidol 5 mg twice daily, but the dose was decreased to 2.5 mg twice daily. The symptoms started to decrease, but the patient still is uncomfortable and she wants to change her antipsychotic medication. Which medication is the best for her?

    1. Risperidone.

    2. Clozapine.

    3. Thioridazine.

    4. Aripiprazole.

21. A 20-year-old white woman comes with her parents to your psychiatric clinic. The parents are concerned about her isolative behavior. She reports that she hears voices that told her that she is not a good person and she should jump off a bridge. She denies any alcohol or drug abuse. She is diagnosed with schizophrenia and is prescribed haloperidol. After she took the haloperidol, she had neck stiffness and an oculogyric crisis. Which medication is most appropriate for her symptoms?

    1. Propranolol.

    2. Benztropine.

    3. Dantrolene.

    4. Quetiapine.

22. A 20-year-old white woman comes with her parents to your psychiatric clinic. The parents are concerned about her isolative behavior. She reports that she hears voices that told her that she is not good person and she should jump off a bridge. She denies any alcohol or drug abuse. She is diagnosed with schizophrenia and is prescribed haloperidol. After she took the haloperidol dose, she had neck stiffness and an oculogyric crisis. She was treated with benztropine and changed her haloperidol to risperidone. She said that she forgets to take her vitamin every day. Which statement is the most correct regarding risperidone?

    1. Risperidone is effective for decreasing the patient's positive symptoms.

    2. Risperidone has the minimal risk of causing extrapyramidal symptoms.

    3. Risperidone is available in a long-acting injection to increase adherence.

    4. Risperidone can be dosed once daily after titration to target dose.

23. A 20-year-old white woman comes with her parents to your psychiatric clinic. The parents are concerned about her isolative behavior. She reports that she hears voices that told her that she is not good person and she should jump off a bridge. She denies any alcohol or drug abuse. She is diagnosed with schizophrenia and is prescribed haloperidol. After she took the haloperidol dose, she had neck stiffness and an oculogyric crisis. She was treated with benztropine and her haloperidol was changed to risperidone. She said that she forgets to take her vitamin every day. One year later, she is no longer responding to risperidone. The nurse practitioner needs to change her medication prescription. Which drug is the best for her?

    1. Quetiapine.

    2. Olanzapine.

    3. Thioridazine.

    4. Fluphenazine.

24. The patient is a 37-year-old Hispanic man with hypertension, type 2 diabetes, and chronic pain. He presents to the psychiatric unit for assessment of his depressive symptoms. He reports general sadness; feelings of hopelessness, worthlessness, and guilt; weight loss (6 kg); and poor concentration. He denies any suicidal ideas; he denies any alcohol or drug abuse. Also, he reports that he lost interest in his hobbies and has become more isolated. His medications are metformin, captopril, and hydrocodone/acetaminophen. Which selective serotonin reuptake inhibitors could interact with his medications?

    1. Paroxetine.

    2. Fluvoxamine.

    3. Sertraline.

    4. Citalopram.

25. The patient is a 37-year-old Hispanic man with hypertension, diabetes type 2, and chronic pain. He presents to the psychiatric unit for assessment of his depressive symptoms. He reports general sadness, feeling hopelessness, worthlessness, guilty, and weight loss (6 kg) and poor concentration. He denies any suicidal ideas; he denies any alcohol or drug abuse. Also, he reports that he lost interest in his hobbies and has become more isolated. His medications are metformin, captopril, and hydrocodone/acetaminophen. You evaluate his blood pressure, and it is elevated to 155/100 mmHg. Which medication is the best for this patient?

    1. Venlafaxine.

    2. Bupropion.

    3. Mirtazapine.

    4. Fluoxetine.

26. The patient is a 47-year-old African American woman who presents to your psychiatric unit to evaluate her depressive symptoms. She reports feeling sadness, hopelessness and worthlessness, loss of interest to go outside, and a weight loss of 8 kg over the past 6 weeks. The nurse practitioner prescribes citalopram 20 mg daily. After 4 weeks, she starts to gain some weight, but she still has sadness and anhedonia. What is the best action to optimize her medication?

    1. Change to another selective serotonin reuptake inhibitor.

    2. Continue at her current dose.

    3. Increase her dose to 40 mg daily.

    4. Add bupropion 150 mg twice daily.

27. The patient is a 47-year-old African American woman who presents to your psychiatric unit to evaluate her depressive symptoms. She has feelings of sadness, hopelessness and worthlessness, loss of interest to go outside, and a weight loss of 8 kg over the past 6 weeks. The nurse practitioner prescribes citalopram 20 mg daily. After 4 weeks, she starts to gain some weight, but she still has sad feelings and anhedonia. The nurse practitioner recommends increasing her citalopram dose. After 6 months, she presents to the unit complaining of anorgasmia; however, her depressive symptoms have resolved. Which action would be appropriate for her case?

    1. Stopping citalopram.

    2. Changing to another selective serotonin reuptake inhibitor.

    3. Add bupropion to citalopram.

    4. Add mirtazapine to citalopram.

28. A 33-year-old white man presents to the health care facility with a 6-week history of anhedonia and loss of concentration. The nurse practitioner evaluates his depressive symptoms with a psychometric assessment. Which instrument is the best to assess this patient's symptoms by the physician?

    1. Beck Depression Inventory.

    2. Patient Health Questionnaire-9.

    3. Quick Inventory of Depressive Symptoms Self-Rated.

    4. Hamilton Rating Scale for Depression.

29. The patient is a 24-year-old man with a 7-month history of major depressive disorders. He is treated with sertraline 100 mg daily and is responsive to this treatment. He denies any suicidal or harmful ideas. Which patient rating scale is the best to manage his symptoms?

    1. Patient Health Questionnaire-9.

    2. Hamilton Rating Scale for Depression.

    3. Clinical Global Impressions.

    4. Montgomery–Äsberg Depression Rating Scale.

30. The patient is a 36-year-old Asian man who presents to your unit with his wife. The patient is hyperverbal and has not slept in the past 48 hours. He has been hospitalized in the past 2 months with depressive symptoms and suicidal ideas. He has a history of being hospitalized more than four times over the past year. His wife reports that he is not adherent with his prescribed medication. He has a history of alcoholic cirrhosis. Which statement is the most appropriate for managing his symptoms?

    1. Lithium is effective for his manic phase and prevents future episodes.

    2. Divalproex should be tried because it is good for maintenance treatment.

    3. Carbamazepine should be tried because it is effective for maintenance treatment.

    4. Lamotrigine should be tried because it is good for maintenance treatment.

31. The patient is a 36-year-old Asian man who presents to your unit with his wife. The patient is hyperverbal and has not slept for the past 48 hours. He has been hospitalized in the past 2 months with depressive symptoms and suicidal ideas. He has a history of being hospitalized more than four times over the past year. His wife reports that he is not adherent with his prescribed medication. He has a history of alcoholic cirrhosis. The nurse practitioner prescribed lithium 450 mg twice daily for him. Which adverse effect requires immediate evaluation for this patient?

    1. Hypothyroidism.

    2. Abdominal bloating and gas.

    3. Coarse tremors.

    4. Weight gain.

32. A 43-year-old Hispanic man presents to the clinic with a history of type I bipolar disorder, osteopenia, and gastroesophageal reflux disease for consultation. His medications include lamotrigine, calcium supplements, and ranitidine. Which statement is incorrect regarding lamotrigine?

    1. Rash occurs within the first 2 to 8 weeks of therapy.

    2. Lamotrigine is approved for acute therapy.

    3. Lamotrigine has been associated with aseptic meningitis.

    4. Lamotrigine dose should be halved in the presence of divalproex.

33. A 49-year-old Asian woman presents to the psychiatry unit with a history of rapid speech, insomnia lasting more than 48 hours, poor attention, and flight of ideas. The patient has had a history of hospitalization three times for mania. She also reports intermittent depression, but she denies any suicidal ideation. She takes lithium 450 mg twice daily, but she reports that she forgets to take it several days a week. Which statement is the best for bipolar disorders?

    1. Type I bipolar disorder is often misdiagnosed as major depression.

    2. Type II bipolar disorder is often misdiagnosed as major depression.

    3. Rapid cycling is at least four episodes of mania in 2 years.

    4. Rapid cycling is at least four episodes of depression in 2 years.

34. A 52-year-old white man (weight 73 kg, height 75 inches) with a 7-year history of bipolar disorder comes to your unit complaining of neck stiffness, muscle pain, confusion, and headache. His medication list includes lamotrigine, and lisinopril and hydrochlorothiazide for hypertension. He is afebrile. The laboratory test reveals the white blood cell count is 6000 cells/mL. Which statement is the most correct for this presentation?

    1. Lamotrigine is associated with development of meningitis.

    2. The patient should be treated with ceftriaxone and vancomycin.

    3. The patient should be treated with ceftriaxone only.

    4. The patient should be treated with vancomycin only.

35. The patient is a 43-year-old male Iraq war veteran who comes to the health care facility complaining of nightmares and having flashbacks to his deployment in Iraq. Also, he has been on sertraline for the past 2.5 weeks for depression. He feels that his sad mood and poor concentration are better, but his nightmares are worse. Which therapy is the best for his case?

    1. Change sertraline to paroxetine.

    2. Add buspirone to his therapy.

    3. Add quetiapine to his therapy.

    4. Continue on his current regimen with cognitive behavioral therapy.

36. The patient is a 43-year-old male Iraq war veteran who comes to the health care facility complaining of nightmares and having flashbacks to his deployment in Iraq. Also, he has been on sertraline for the past 2.5 weeks for depression. He feels that his sad mood and poor concentration are better, but his nightmares are worse. After 2 months, his nightmares start to disappear, but he feels very irritable and he becomes very aggressive toward others. Which adjunctive medication should be added for his case?

    1. Lithium.

    2. Alprazolam.

    3. Buspirone.

    4. Divalproex.

37. The patient is a 43-year-old male Iraq war veteran who comes to the health care facility complaining of nightmares and having flashbacks to his deployment in Iraq. Also, he has been on sertraline for the past 2.5 weeks for depression. He feels that his sad mood and poor concentration are better, but his nightmares are worse. After 2 months, his nightmares start to disappear, but he feels very irritable and he becomes very aggressive toward others. The nurse practitioner recommends divalproex sodium for him. After 8 months, he becomes tolerant to his medication. He read about buspirone and he wants to know if this medication is appropriate for him or not. Which statement is correct regarding buspirone for him?

    1. Buspirone can treat the nightmares.

    2. Buspirone can treat the irritability and aggression.

    3. Buspirone has little dependence potential.

    4. Buspirone dosed with one tablet daily.

38. A 33-year-old white woman presents to your clinic with her boyfriend. She has a history of obsessive-compulsive disorders (OCD) and takes lorazepam, but this is not helping her OCD. Which medication is the best for her?

    1. Amitriptyline.

    2. Desipramine.

    3. Clomipramine.

    4. Nortriptyline.

39. The patient is a 33-year-old African American woman who presents to your clinic with noticeable dark circles under her eyes. She complains of difficulties sleeping. It takes her 20 minutes to fall asleep, but she wakes up after 3 hours and cannot return to sleep. She tried diphenhydramine, but she wakes up with hangover symptoms. Her medical history includes hypothyroidism, hypertension, occasional neck pain, and depression. Her medications are levothyroxine 112 mcg at bedtime, ramipril 20 mg daily and hydrochlorothiazide 25 mg in the morning, ketoprofen 50 mg as needed for pain, and paroxetine 20 mg daily at morning. Which medication is most likely contributing to her insomnia?

    1. Ketoprofen.

    2. Paroxetine.

    3. Levothyroxine.

    4. Ramipril.

1. Answer: 2

Rationale: The patient presents with signs and symptoms of major depressive disorder. Selective serotonin receptor inhibitors are considered a first-line agent in treatment for this patient. The patient gained 8 kg in the past 2 months; therefore paroxetine (answer 1) is not recommended for her case because it leads to increased appetite and causes somnolence. Fluoxetine (answer 2) is the best medication for this patient because it does not affect weight or appetite. In addition, fluoxetine could concomitantly relieve her symptoms of anxiety. Imipramine is a tricyclic antidepressant agent (TCA) that has a warning that patients with passive suicidal ideas should not receive TCAs (answer 3). Mirtazapine (answer 4), like paroxetine, could increase appetite and lead to weight gain.

2. Answer: 3

Rationale: The patient's previous attempt to quit smoking with nicotine gum was probably unsuccessful because the gum strength (2 mg) and the frequency of use (fewer than 9 pieces a day) were too low to manage his nicotine craving; therefore his previous use of nicotine gum is not a true treatment failure. Varenicline (answer 2) is not contraindicated because of the cardiac problems, but it is contraindicated because the patient has a depression history. Bupropion (answer 3) is a better fit because of its appropriateness for depressive disorders. Nicotine gum (answer 1) or patch (answer 4) are appropriate and can be added when bupropion fails as monotherapy to treat his nicotine craving.

3. Answer: 1

Rationale: This patient still has depressive symptoms and diabetic neuropathy; therefore duloxetine (answer 1) is the best choice for this patient. Although desipramine (answer 2) could be used for treating her neuropathy, it is not a good choice because of her heart disease. Sertraline (answer 3) would be a better choice for her depression, but it does not help diabetic neuropathy. However, bupropion can lead to weight loss, but data are not strong for treatment of neuropathy (answer 4).

4. Answer: 4

Rationale: This patient has alcoholic hepatitis, as indicated by his elevated liver enzymes; thus it could improve with abstinence. His liver function is normal, as evidenced by his albumin, prothrombin time. and platelet count. Chlordiazepoxide (answer 1) has an important role in acute alcohol detoxification, but there are limited data about its role for the maintenance treatment. Disulfiram (answer 2) requires a strong recommendation from the patient to abstain. Moreover, it should be used with caution for patients with active liver disease. Naltrexone (answer 3) should be used with caution for patients with acute liver disease. Acamprosate (answer 4) is the most appropriate medication for this patient. In addition, the dose of Acamprosate should be reduced for patients with a creatinine clearance between 50 and 30 mL/min.

5. Answer: 1

Rationale: The patient presents to the emergency department with signs and symptoms of serotonin syndrome (myoclonus, agitation, and diaphoresis). The medications most likely contributing to her symptoms are dextromethorphan and paroxetine because both agents have serotonergic activity. Moreover, paroxetine inhibits CYP2D6, which is responsible for metabolism of dextromethorphan, so it could increase the serotonergic activity (answer 1). Thus none of the other choices leads to serotonergic activity, so answers 2, 3, and 4 are incorrect.

6. Answer: 4

Rationale: Initiation of naltrexone as monotherapy is inappropriate because it could precipitate withdrawal symptoms of methadone (answer 1). Patients who take long-acting opioids such as methadone should be changed to buprenorphine first before being advanced to buprenorphine/naltrexone (answer 2). Initiation of buprenorphine with a higher dose of methadone could precipitate the withdrawal symptoms because of higher binding affinity of buprenorphine for the mu receptor with less activity and the added antagonism at the kappa receptor (answer 3). Therefore patients who take long-acting opioid should be tapered, to avoid withdrawal symptoms, before changing to buprenorphine (answer 4).

7. Answer: 2

Rationale: This patient has a history of type I bipolar disorder. She has been on lithium for 6 years, with an acceptable therapeutic range, which is long enough to derive any antidepressant effects. Venlafaxine (answer 1) is a serotonin and norepinephrine reuptake inhibitor that could lead to mania. Moreover, the effect of antidepressants for treatment of depression disorders associated with bipolar disorders is still questionable. Quetiapine (answer 2) has a Food and Drug Administration indication for the treatment of depression symptoms associated with bipolar disorders because of its rapid onset of action. Aripiprazole (answer 3) is inappropriate for treatment of depression symptoms associated with bipolar disorders because it is not effective and there is not enough data to support its effectiveness. Lamotrigine (answer 4) is appropriate for maintenance treatment because of its slow onset and it requires a slow titration to reach therapeutic doses.

8. Answer: 4

Rationale: The patient has depressive symptoms associated with bipolar disorders and is treated with quetiapine for her acute symptoms because of its rapid onset. Venlafaxine (answer 1) is a serotonin and norepinephrine reuptake inhibitor and sertraline (answer 2) is a selective serotonin reuptake inhibitor. These are inappropriate for the treatment of depression symptoms associated with bipolar disorders because their affect is still questionable and there is not enough data for their effectiveness. In addition, they could cause mania. Aripiprazole (answer 3) is inappropriate for treatment of depression symptoms associated with bipolar disorder because of lack of effectiveness. Lamotrigine (answer 4) is indicated for maintenance treatment because of its slow onset, and it requires a slow titration to reach therapeutic doses.

9. Answer: 1

Rationale: The patient has difficulty with sleep and he would benefit from a medication that could decrease sleep latency and does not prolong sleep. Ramelteon (answer 1) is the best agent for his symptoms because its melatonin analog may help older patients who have difficulty with circadian rhythm. Moreover, ramelteon is indicated for treatment of chronic insomnia. Suvorexant (answer 2) could treat sleep maintenance but causes hangover symptoms. Zolpidem (answer 3) received recent labeling changes for reduced doses and has a reduced metabolism in older patients. Eszopiclone (answer 4) could decrease the time it takes to fall sleep, but its long half-life could lead to hangover symptoms.

10. Answer: 2

The patient presents with generalized anxiety disorder (GAD), which could be treated with selective serotonin reuptake inhibitors as a first-line agent. Pregabalin could be appropriate as a second-line or third-line agent, but the clinical data are not strong (answer 1). Venlafaxine (answer 2) is a serotonin and norepinephrine reuptake inhibitor with proven efficacy against GAD and vasomotor symptoms. Although fluoxetine (answer 3) has a proven efficacy for treating patients with GAD symptoms, it is a CYP2D6 inhibitor, which could affect tamoxifen metabolism. Bupropion (answer 4) is a CYP2D6 inhibitor, which could affect tamoxifen efficacy. Moreover, bupropion is ineffective against most anxiety symptoms.

11. Answer: 4

Rationale: This patient comes in with panic disorder, which could be treated with selective serotonin reuptake inhibitors, but they take time to achieve full efficacy. Thus sertraline (answer 1) would not be helpful for treatment of his acute symptoms. Buspirone (answer 2) and bupropion (answer 3) are not effective for panic attacks. Using benzodiazepines would be appropriate to treat the acute symptoms of panic disorders because of their rapid onset (answer 4).

12. Answer: 4

Rationale: The patient has panic disorder and is treated with benzodiazepine to manage his acute symptoms. Initiating cognitive and behavioral therapy would be recommended because of its effectiveness, but buspirone (answer 1) and bupropion (answer 2) are not effective against generalized anxiety disorders (GADs); therefore these answers are incorrect. Hydroxyzine is an antihistaminic agent that is inappropriate in the treatment of GAD. In addition, it could cause hangover symptoms (answer 3). Initiating selective serotonin reuptake inhibitors would be appropriate because they are the first-line agents for preventing panic disorders (answer 4).

13. Answer: 3

Rationale: From the objective findings, this patient has an elevated thyroid-stimulating hormone (TSH). The patient takes olanzapine tablets, which leads to metabolic syndrome with glucose intolerance and obesity, but it does not cause elevation in TSH (answer 1). Multivitamin supplement could not cause a TSH elevation (answer 2). Lithium could induce a TSH elevation, which is not dose dependent, within the first 2 months of treatment (answer 3). The acceptable lithium therapeutic maintenance range is between 0.6 and 1.0 mEq/L); thus his lithium concentration is in the normal range (answer 4).

14. Answer: 1

Rationale: This patient presents with a thyroid-stimulating hormone elevation caused by lithium-induced hypothyroidism; thus levothyroxine treatment is the best treatment for hypothyroidism (answer 1). Olanzapine could lead to metabolic disorders such as hyperglycemia and obesity, but this patient is not complaining of a glucose elevation (answer 2). Propranolol (answer 3) could be used for treatment of an acute symptomatic disorder related to hyperthyroidism. Propylthiouracil (answer 4) is appropriate for treatment of hyperthyroidism, nor hypothyroidism.

15. Answer: 1

Rationale: The patient presents with an elevation in lithium concentration; the acceptable normal therapeutic range at maintenance state is between 0.6 and 1.0 mEq/L. Theophylline (answer 1) could decrease the lithium concentration. Ramipril (answer 2) could increase the lithium concentration; therefore it should be avoided or the dose reduced. Pregnancy (answer 3) could increase the glomerular filtration rate, which leads to a decrease in lithium concentration. Amiloride (answer 4) has little effect on lithium.

16. Answer: 2

Rationale: From the laboratory findings, this patient presents with an elevation in the pancreatic enzymes, which means acute pancreatitis. Although the incidence of acute pancreatitis is rare, divalproex sodium could cause this condition. Furthermore, this condition must be managed by discontinuing divalproex sodium because it is a reversible condition. Thus, answer 2 is correct. There are no reports that other medications such as lisinopril, pitavastatin, and multivitamins cause acute pancreatitis, so answers 1, 3, and 4 are incorrect.

17. Answer: 1

Rationale: This patient complains of recurrence of mania symptoms and lithium intolerance. Divalproex sodium (answer 1) is the best choice for this condition because it is as effective as lithium in acute and prophylactic management. Moreover, it is good in rapid cyclers. Lamotrigine is the best at a maintenance state because it needs a gradual titration to reach the therapeutic concentration, and it does not cause side effects such as a rash or Stevens–Johnson syndrome (answer 2). Selective serotonin reuptake inhibitors are not appropriate for treatment of type I bipolar disorders because there is a potential for switching to the manic phase (answer 3). Alprazolam is a benzodiazepine and could only be used in acute agitation. It is not helpful for the core symptoms (answer 4).

18. Answer: 3

Rationale: This patient has metabolic syndrome (weight gain, diabetes, and dyslipidemia) caused by taking risperidone. Olanzapine (answer 1) is associated with a high incidence of metabolic syndrome. Paliperidone (answer 2) could metabolize to risperidone, which has a similar pharmacological profile. It also could induce galactorrhea as risperidone. Ziprasidone (answer 3) has a low incidence of metabolic syndrome; therefore it is the best choice for this patient. Clozapine (answer 4) like olanzapine has a high incidence of metabolic syndrome.

19. Answer: 1

Rationale: The patient has anxiety, agitation, and feels uncomfortable in her skin. These symptoms resemble akathisia; therefore the best treatment for this case is a lipophilic beta-blocker such as propranolol (answer 1). Benzodiazepines (answer 2) might be efficacious for akathisia, but the patient has a history of alcohol abuse. Benztropine (answer 3) is an anticholinergic agent that is effective against dystonia and parkinsonism symptoms but not akathisia. Dantrolene (answer 4) is more effective against neuroleptic malignant syndrome.

20. Answer: 2

Rationale: The patient has involuntary facial muscles, which is called tardive dyskinesia. Risperidone has fewer extrapyramidal side effects (EPSs), but it is not the best treatment for tardive dyskinesia (answer 1). Clozapine (answer 2) is the best choice because of its low-to-nonexistent incidence of tardive dyskinesia. Thioridazine (answer 3) is a first-generation antipsychotic agent associated with the development tardive dyskinesia. Aripiprazole (answer 4) has fewer EPSs, but it is associated with akathisia and tardive dyskinesia.

21. Answer: 2

Rationale: The patient presents with schizophrenic symptoms and takes haloperidol, which is related to the extrapyramidal side effects (EPSs). She complains of neck stiffness and oculogyric crisis; therefore propranolol is inappropriate for her (answer 1). Benztropine (answer 2) is an anticholinergic agent that could reverse her EPSs and relieve her neck stiffness. Dantrolene (answer 3) is a muscle relaxant that is appropriate for management of neuroleptic malignant syndrome. Although quetiapine has fewer EPSs, it could not manage these acute symptoms at this time (answer 4).

22. Answer: 3

Rationale: Risperidone is effective for decreasing both negative and positive symptoms (answer 1). Although risperidone has a fewer extrapyramidal side effects (EPSs) than haloperidol, its EPSs are dose-related for doses greater than 6 mg daily (answer 2). This patient reports that she forgets to take her vitamin so she may have an adherence problem; thus the long-acting injection for risperidone is the best for her presentation (answer 3). Oral doses (answer 4) are not appropriate for her case.

23. Answer: 1

Rationale: This patient has a history with dystonia. Quetiapine (answer 1) has minimal extrapyramidal side effects (EPSs) compared with risperidone and haloperidol. Olanzapine (answer 2) would not be the best choice because it has a high risk for metabolic syndromes in youth. Thioridazine (answer 3) and fluphenazine (answer 4) are inappropriate because they are first-generation agents, which have the highest risk for EPSs.

24. Answer: 1

Rationale: Paroxetine is a CYP2D6 inhibitor that interacts with the metabolism of hydrocodone (answer 1). Fluvoxamine (answer 2) is a CYP1A2 inhibitor that can interact with metformin or opiates. Sertraline (answer 3) could affect the metabolite of hydrocodone because sertraline is a CYP3A4 inhibitor, but it is less effective than paroxetine. Citalopram (answer 4) can interact with his current medications.

25. Answer: 3

Rationale: This patient has increased blood pressure and is taking a high dose of venlafaxine. This could worsen his blood pressure (answer 1). Bupropion (answer 2) could decrease his appetite and this patient already has weight loss. Mirtazapine (answer 3) is the best medication for this patient because it could improve his appetite and increase his weight. In addition, mirtazapine does not have any interactions with his current medications. Fluoxetine (answer 4) would not improve his appetite; therefore it would not the best medication for his case.

26. Answer: 3

Rationale: This patient experienced partial relief with citalopram 20 mg daily; therefore changing to another selective serotonin reuptake inhibitor could be an option after citalopram is maxed out (answer 1 is incorrect). The patient has taken citalopram for 4 weeks, and possibly at a subtherapeutic dose; thus answer 2 is incorrect and answer 3 is correct. Adding bupropion would be appropriate after reaching the maximum tolerated dose of citalopram for 6 to 8 weeks (answer 4 is incorrect).

27. Answer: 3

Rationale: Although this patient experienced resolution of depressive symptoms, she still needs her therapeutic dose of citalopram (answer 1). However, changing to another selective serotonin reuptake inhibitor (SSRI) could be inappropriate because all SSRIs can cause anorgasmia (answer 2). Adding bupropion to her therapy would be the best choice for her case because bupropion could treat her anorgasmia and may enhance her mood (answer 3). Adding mirtazapine to her therapy would be inappropriate because it will not treat her anorgasmia (answer 4).

28. Answer: 4

Rationale: This patient has depressive symptoms, which should be assessed by using clinical rating scales. These instruments are used to identify depression and assess its severity. The Beck Depression Inventory (answer 1) is a patient rating scale and not a clinical rating scale. The Patient Health Questionnare-9 (answer 2) is a patient rating scale that is based on the diagnostic criteria for major depression (Diagnostic and Statistical Manual of Mental Disorders, 5th edition). Moreover, the Patient Health Questionnare-9 can be used to monitor treatment response. The Quick Inventory of Depressive Symptoms Self-Rated (answer 3) is a patient rating scale and not a clinical rating scale. The Hamilton Rating Scale for Depression (answer 4) is the best choice because it is a clinical rating scale, which is often used to show efficacy in clinical trials for the antidepressants approved by the Food and Drug Administration.

29. Answer: 1

Rationale: This patient has a history of major depressive disorder (MDD) and needs a patient scale rating to assess his symptoms. Patient Health Questionnare-9 (answer 1) is a patient rating scale, which is based on the diagnostic criteria for major depression (Diagnostic and Statistical Manual of Mental Disorders, 5th edition). Also, it is easily administered and assessed, and it could be used to monitor treatment response. The Hamilton Rating Scale for Depression (answer 2) is a clinical rating scale, not a patient rating scale. Clinical Global Impressions (answer 3) is a clinical rating scale used to evaluate the severity and improvement of the patient overall. The Montgomery–Äsberg Depression Rating Scale (answer 4) is a clinical rating scale used for evaluation of depressive symptoms.

30. Answer: 1

Rationale: This patient presents to the unit with type I bipolar disorder; therefore lithium is the best therapy for his symptoms and to control his manic phase. Lithium is considered a first-line treatment therapy for bipolar disorder type I (answer 1). Divalproex is the best therapy for rapid cycling, but the patient has liver disease, so divalproex is contraindicated (answer 2). Carbamazepine should be tried as the second or third line of treatment (answer 3). Lamotrigine is effective for maintenance, but it is not effective for the manic phase (answer 4).

31. Answer: 3

Rationale: Lithium has many adverse drug effects such as hypothyroidism (answer 1), gastrointestinal disturbance (answer 2), and weight gain (answer 4). All these adverse effects require lifestyle modifications, but coarse tremors (answer 3) are associated with lithium toxicity and require immediate evaluation.

32. Answer: 2

Rationale: Lamotrigine has a delayed risk of rash, which appears within the first 2 to 8 weeks after initiation of therapy; therefore it should be titrated gradually to avoid a Stevens–Johnson type of rash (answer 1). Lamotrigine is approved for maintenance therapy, and appears particularly effective for prevention of future depressive disorders. It has fewer side effects for prevention of the manic phase (answer 2). Lamotrigine is associated with development of aseptic meningitis within 1 to 42 days, which requires hospitalization (answer 3). The lamotrigine dosage should be decreased to half in the presence of divalproex because divalproex is an enzyme inhibitor that leads to accumulation of lamotrigine (answer 4).

33. Answer: 2

Rationale: There are two types of bipolar disorders. Type I bipolar disorder is marked by one or more manic mixed episodes with major depressive disorders (MDDs), so it is easy to differentiate it from MDDs (answer 1 is incorrect). Bipolar disorder type II is marked by one or more MDDs mixed with at least one hypomania episode; therefore it is often misdiagnosed as an MDD (answer 2 is correct). Rapid cycling is at least four episodes of mania or depression in 1 year, so answers 3 and 4 are incorrect.

34. Answer: 1

Rationale: This patient presents with signs and symptoms of meningitis, but his temperature and white blood cell count are in the normal range, so this patient does not have an infection. This means that answers 2, 3, and 4 are incorrect because antibiotic therapies are inappropriate for his presentation. Lamotrigine is associated with development of aseptic meningitis, which often occurs within 1 to 42 days of therapy initiation, so answer 1 is correct.

35. Answer: 4

Rationale: The patient presents with a history of posttraumatic stress disorder (PTSD) and major depressive disorder (MDD). Physiotherapy is the cornerstone for this case, not only the pharmacotherapy. Changing to another selective serotonin reuptake inhibitor (SSRI) would be inappropriate because this patient experienced an improvement in his depressive disorders, so there is no reason to change it to paroxetine (answer 1). Adding buspirone as adjunctive is not indicated at this time because sertraline does not reach the maximal therapeutic effect (answer 2). Adding quetiapine (answer 3) is not indicated for treatment of PTSD. Continuing with sertraline and cognitive behavioral therapy is the best choice because SSRIs are first-line PTSD treatment (answer 4).

36. Answer: 4

Rationale: The patient has agitation, so another medication needs to be added. Lithium (answer 1) may control the mood liability, but it needs close monitoring. A Benzodiazepine (answer 2) could be used for a short time; however, it is not being used to target the aggressive symptoms. Buspirone (answer 3) does not have any effect on posttraumatic stress disorder (PTSD). Divalproex (answer 4) is often used to treat the aggressive and irritability symptoms for patients with PTSD.

37. Answer: 3

Rationale: Buspirone is ineffective against nightmares or aggression and irritability, so answers 1 and 2 are incorrect. Buspirone does not have much dependence potential (answer 3 is correct). Buspirone should be dosed three times daily (answer 4 is incorrect).

38. Answer: 3

Rationale: Clomipramine is the most serotonergic drug of the choices provided and is highly effective against obsessive-compulsive disorder (answer 3 is correct, and answers 1, 2, and 4 are incorrect).

39. Answer: 3

Rationale: This patient has insomnia, and one of the drug choices can increase her insomnia symptoms. Ketoprofen (answer 1) does not have any association with her insomnia symptoms. Paroxetine (answer 2) may lead to insomnia in certain patients, but this patient takes her medication in the morning, so she has a low risk for this. Levothyroxine (answer 3) can contribute to insomnia. Moreover, this patient takes her medication at bedtime. Ramipril (answer 4) does not cause insomnia.

13

Advocacy and Moral Agency

1. Angie is a 19-year-old patient recently been diagnosed with leukemia. She is to undergo her first chemotherapy session. Her prechemotherapy vital signs are blood pressure 120/80 mmHg, respiratory rate 18 beats/min, pulse rate 65 breaths/min, and temperature 36.8°C. As Jehovah's Witnesses, Angie's parents refused blood transfusion, but Angie gave her consent for it. Whose decision will you follow?

   1. The physician's decision.

   2. The parent's decision.

   3. Angie's decision.

   4. Your own personal decision.

2. A nurse in another department approached you. She said that your patient, Angie, is her friend and asked how she was doing with her first chemotherapy. What should you do?

   1. Provide information because all tests came out normal.

   2. Refuse to talk about the patient.

   3. Tell the nurse to ask the nurse assigned.

   4. Inform the nurse that you will provide her a copy of Angie's tests.

3. A patient with cancer is being discharged from the hospital and she suddenly burst into tears saying that she is afraid to die. To offer comfort, what should you consider?

   1. If her family is aware of her mental state.

   2. Patient's cultural background.

   3. Patient's vital signs.

   4. The patient's relationship status.

4. A nurse practitioner is also an advocate for the patients. Which of these statements is considered the *best* action for an advocate?

   1. Document clinical changes every hour.

   2. Assess patient and wait for a physician to provide any medication.

   3. Allow registered nurses and their supervisors to solve any form of conflict.

   4. Assess the patient's perspective and explain when necessary.

5. A patient went to the nurse's station and asked if he could go to the pantry to get something to eat. Hospital policy does not permit patients going into the pantry, so you politely refused the patient's request. The patient started verbally abusing you. What do you do?

   1. Inform the patient that you will get what he wants from the pantry and deliver it to his room.

   2. Ask the patient to lower his voice so other patients will not be disturbed.

   3. Have the registered nurse assist and bring the patient to the cafeteria.

   4. Calmly and firmly, escort the patient back to his room.

6. A patient was prescribed haloperidol (Haldol) and is taking 2 mg by mouth twice a day. Which menu would you choose for the patient?

   1. 3 ounces of baked chicken with steamed rice, green beans, a slice of bread, banana, and milk.

   2. Double cheeseburger, large-sized french fries, three chocolate chip cookies, one banana, and milk.

   3. 3 ounces of baked fish, one piece of bread, ice cream, pineapple juice.

   4. 3 ounces of roast beef with mashed potatoes, dressed salad, 1 dill pickle, baked apple pie, and milk.

7. After surgery, a patient is informed that he has terminal cancer. The patient starts to yell at the hospital staff saying, "I can't get enough sleep because you keep coming here! I'm so tired of all of you!" What stage of grief is the patient in?

    1. Denial.

    2. Depression.

    3. Anger.

    4. Acceptance.

8. In the United States, the Patient Self-Determination Act protects patients in terms of their rights to what? Select *all* that apply.

    1. Informed fully about treatments including the benefits, risk, and even the alternatives so they are knowledgeable enough to provide an informed decision whether they want the treatment or not.

    2. To be able to make decisions about whom their health care provider will be without coercion or undue influence, which includes influence from health care providers.

    3. Make decisions about health care and have those decisions communicated and protected to others when the decision maker is no longer competent to do so.

    4. Privacy and confidentiality when it comes to their medical records and will only be shared to others such as family members when the patient formally approves it.

9. As an advocate for the patient, the nurse practitioner needs to make sure that "safe and effective care" is provided in conformity with the:

    1. American Nursing Association.

    2. National Council for Licensure Examinations.

    3. Nurse Practice Act.

    4. State Board of Licensure.

10. You notice that a physician has prescribed a medicine that is three times the recommended dose. What is your initial action?

    1. Write another order without discontinuing the old order.

    2. Contact the physician immediately and clarify.

    3. Do not give the medication.

    4. Lower the dose to its ideal one without consultation.

11. A patient's family asks you what "palliative care" means. What is your response?

    1. Palliative care means that the patient and the patient's family will take a more passive role and the physician will focus on the physiological needs of the patient. The location of death will most likely occur in the hospital setting.

    2. Palliative care is provided to those who have less than 6 months to live.

    3. Palliative care aims to relieve or reduce the symptoms of the disease of the patient.

    4. The goal of palliative care is to affect a cure for a serious disease or illness.

12. A retired nurse practitioner (NP) stops to help in an emergency along the road. When the injured party files suit, the retired NP would be covered by:

    1. The Good Samaritan Law.

    2. The National Care Act.

    3. Automobile insurance.

    4. Medicare.

13. In the hospital setting, which two people (choose two answers) have the responsibility of obtaining informed consent?

    1. The nurse manager.

    2. The nurse.

    3. The nurse practitioner.

    4. The physician.

14. When signing a form as a witness, your signature shows that the patient:

    1. Was not medicated with narcotics and was in fact, awake and alert.

    2. Was fully informed and is aware of all consequences.

    3. Was able to freely sign without any pressure.

    4. None of these.

15. You are showing the patient how to use his crutches at home and instructing his wife on how to change his bandages. You are primarily acting as a:

    1. Patient advocate.

    2. Manager of care.

    3. Decision-maker.

    4. Teacher.

16. Liza, a registered nurse, came to work late and looks unkempt. Julie, a nurse practitioner, approaches Liza when she notices her zigzagging through the hallway. Liza's breath reeks of mints and rum and Julie believes Liza is intoxicated. What is the best initial nursing action for Julie to take?

    1. Call the supervisor and report Liza immediately.

    2. Confront Liza about her movements and that you believe her to be intoxicated. You also relieve her of her nursing duties immediately.

    3. Just ignore the situation.

    4. Give Liza a lecture about substance abuse and send her off with a warning.

17. Joel is admitted with a diagnosis of schizophrenia. He refuses to take his medication and states, "I believe I don't need those medications. They make me sleepy and drowsy. I insist that you explain their use and side effects." The nurse practitioner should understand that:

    1. The patient needs to be referred to a psychiatrist to change his mind.

    2. The patient has a right to know about the prescribed medications.

    3. Educating patients about their medications is an optional responsibility of a nurse practitioner.

    4. Patients with schizophrenia are at a higher risk of psychosocial complications when they know about their medication side effects. It is better not to let them know.

18. A patient tells the nurse practitioner (NP) on duty, "I have something very important to tell you if you promise that you will not tell anyone." The best response by the NP is:

    1. "I am obligated to document and report any important information."

    2. "I won't make such a promise."

    3. "That depends on what you will be telling me."

    4. "I must report everything to the treatment team."

19. A patient asked the nurse practitioner (NP) to call the police and states, "I need to report that I am being abused by a nurse." What should the NP do first?

    1. Make sure the patient is not delirious.

    2. Report of the patient's complaint to the police.

    3. Obtain as much detail as possible about the patient's claim of abuse.

    4. Document the statement on the patient's chart with a report to the manager.

20. A 22-year-old woman is scheduled to have surgery today. Her vital signs are blood pressure 110/80 mmHg, respiratory rate 15 breaths/min, pulse rate 80 beats/min, and temperature 36.8°C. Based on her vital signs, she was premedicated for the surgery. While the nurse practitioner (NP) reviews her chart, she discovers that the consent form was not signed. The NP's actions would be based on the understanding that:

    1. Because the patient came to the hospital, consent is implied even if the consent for the surgery has not been signed.

    2. All invasive procedures require a consent form.

    3. The NP should have him sign a consent form immediately.

    4. The NP should have the next of kin sign the necessary consent form.

21. Your patient's father is a physician, but not the physician of record. He casually enters the nursing station and asks for his daughter's chart. What is the best action for the nurse practitioner (NP) to take?

    1. Give him the chart as requested.

    2. Do not to allow him to read the chart.

    3. The NP will have to ask the attending surgeon if it is permissible for him to read the chart.

    4. The NP will have to ask the patient if she wants him to read her chart.

22. The patient has advanced directives on her chart. What guideline should the nurse practitioner (NP) keep in mind?

    1. In health care, the power of attorney is invoked only when the patient has a terminal condition or is in a vegetative state.

    2. When a patient is already incapacitated, a living will allows an appointed person to make health care decisions on his or her behalf.

    3. The living will is invoked only when a patient has a terminal condition or is a vegetative state.

    4. No change is allowed by the patient once he or she is admitted to the hospital.

23. John is a 28-year-old male patient admitted with persistent diarrhea and rapid weight loss. Lab values show the following: red blood cell count is 5 million cells/μL, platelet count is 80,000 μL, and CD4 is 150 cells/mm^3. What is the nurse practitioner's initial working diagnosis?

    1. John has AIDS.

    2. John has HIV.

    3. John has hepatitis B.

    4. John has hepatitis C.

24. You are teaching John, who was recently diagnosed with AIDS, about multidrug therapy. Which of the following will best explain the rationale for John to use more than one antiretroviral medication to treat AIDS?

    1. "This is to make sure that the virus does not develop any resistance to the medications."

    2. "You will not experience any side effects when you take a combination of medications."

    3. "While taking this medication, you will not be able to transmit the disease."

    4. "This combination of medications will completely eliminate the AIDS virus from your body."

25. The nurse practitioner gave John, a 28-year-old patient with HIV/AIDS, his first medication. While recapping the needle, she accidentally stuck herself. What should be her initial action?

    1. Provide consent for testing.

    2. Notify the supervisor.

    3. Start postexposure prophylaxis.

    4. Document the exposure.

26. You overheard another nurse practitioner (NP) say that John was "a nasty old man because he has HIV." What ethical dilemma is the NP exhibiting?

    1. Gender bias and ageism.

    2. Code of ethics violation.

    3. Beneficence.

    4. Justice.

27. Which statement by John shows that he requires further education when discussing AIDS and its prevention and transmission?

    1. "I should always wear a condom during sexual activity."

    2. "AIDS can be transmitted through sharing of utensils."

3. "Sharing needles with others is one mean of transmitting the disease."

4. "There's a big possibility that I have transmitted the disease to my wife."

28. You are preparing John, a 28-year-old patient with HIV/AIDS, for discharge to home. Which of the following instructions is best for you to include in the instructions?

    1. Never share eating utensils with your family members.

    2. Do not spend too much time in public places.

    3. Avoid sharing razors and toothbrushes with others.

    4. Do not eat from the same serving dishes that are shared by others.

29. John thinks he might have transmitted HIV/AIDS to his wife. What would be the best response?

    1. Yes, you did.

    2. It is sexually transmitted, which means there is a big possibility that you transmitted it to your partner.

    3. It is better for her to come and be tested.

    4. The disease is not always transmitted. Just pray that she was not affected.

30. Lucy is an 85-year-old female patient who was diagnosed with stage 4 colon cancer. She is starting to grieve. What does the nurse practitioner (NP) need to keep in mind about the grief process?

    1. The stages of grief do not have to be in order. Grief may occur, recur, or even be skipped.

    2. Lucy wants to be left alone.

    3. Coping mechanisms in the past should be discarded during the current grieving.

    4. The person's loss has nothing to do with the grieving process.

31. When caring for a terminally ill patient, it is important for the nurse to maintain the patient's dignity. This can be facilitated by:

    1. Making firm decisions on behalf of patient.

    2. Making sure to put the patient in a private room.

    3. Not putting any emphasis on patient's appearance to decrease anxiety.

    4. Spending time to let the patient share his or her experiences and life stories.

32. The patient's family was just sitting at her bedside in the hospital during the final stages of her terminal cancer. What can the nurse practitioner do to help the family during this difficult time?

    1. Find simple activities for the family to do together, which will be aimed at taking care of the patient.

    2. Lie about the patient's real condition so the family will not lose hope.

    3. Do not allow the family to do any spiritual practices because this is not allowed in the hospital.

    4. Limit visitors so the patient can be left alone.

33. When a patient refuses standard treatment and is suddenly researching experimental and questionable therapies, which stage of dying is the patient exhibiting?

    1. Denial.

    2. Anger.

    3. Bargaining.

    4. Depression.

34. All of the following are crucial needs of the dying patient *except*:

    1. The preservation of one's dignity and self-worth.

    2. Pain control.

    3. Love and belongingness.

    4. The freedom from decision-making.

35. Lucy, an 85-year-old female patient who was diagnosed with stage 4 colon cancer, has already refused treatment. What law states that the patient has the right to refuse treatment?

    1. The Nursing Care Act.

    2. Common law.

    3. Civil law.

    4. Statutory law.

36. When a loved one dies, bereavement happens. How can bereavement be defined?

    1. The social and outward expression of one's loss.

    2. Delaying and denying the awareness of the reality of the loss.

3. A person's emotional response to loss.

4. The outward expression and inner feeling of the one left behind.

37. A patient who just died had a "Do Not Resuscitate" order. Once no pulse or respiration is verified, what is the next action?

    1. Vital organs should be retrieved by the transplant team.

    2. If the deceased is not an organ donor, remove all tubes and equipment and prepare the body by cleansing and positioning it properly.

    3. Have family members say their goodbyes.

    4. Have the body removed by the funeral home immediately.

38. The nurse practitioner has shared to the other members of the health team the patient's values, preferences, and expressed needs. Under Quality and Safety in the Education of Nurses, this falls under what competency?

    1. Quality improvement.

    2. Patient-centered care.

    3. Evidence-based practice.

    4. Safety.

39. Lucy, who is terminally ill, has agreed to hospice care. Which statement by Lucy's husband shows that he needs further education by the nurse practitioner?

    1. "You will help to keep my spouse as comfortable as possible while under your care."

    2. "You will help my spouse get cured so we can get back to our normal life."

    3. "The main reason we brought her here is to make the end of my spouse's life as comfortable as possible."

    4. "Your team will provide me with support during this difficult time."

Advocacy and Moral Agency Answers & Rationales 13

1. Answer: 3

Rationale: Angie's decision is followed based on the autonomy principle, which refers to the right of individuals to make decisions for themselves.

2. Answer: 2

Rationale: Providing any information about a patient's condition to an uninvolved person is a violation of the patient's right to privacy and confidentiality.

3. Answer: 2

Rationale: Before comforting a patient, you should consider his or her cultural background. Therapeutic touch may be considered normal, and even recommended in this situation, but in other cultures and religions, it can be a violation to privacy.

4. Answer: 4

Rationale: It is important to know and understand the patient's perspective. When you do, it is easier to defend the patient's point of view. This is a way to advocate for your patients.

5. Answer: 4

Rationale: Patient's need clear and direct instructions and limitations. Abusive behavior should not be reinforced.

6. Answer: 1

Rationale: Haldol is an antipsychotic drug and does not have meal restrictions; therefore you are looking for the most balanced diet. Most balanced are answers 1 and 4. In 4, the dill pickle is very high in sodium, which leaves answer 1 as the most balanced.

7. Answer: 3

Rationale: There are five Kübler-Ross stages of dying. The patient is exhibiting the stage of anger when the individual resists the loss and may strike out at everyone and everything, in this case, the hospital staff.

8. Answers: 2 and 3

Rationale: The Patient Self-Determination Act gives Americans the right to make health care decisions and have these decisions protected and communicated to others when the patient is not competent to do so. Included are rejections of future care and treatments that are reflected in advance directives. The act also provides the patient to be free of any coercion and undue influence of others, which includes influence from health care providers.

9. Answer: 3

Rationale: In the Nurse Practice Act, as a nurse practitioner, you are still an advocate for the patient and need to make sure you provide "safe and effective care" for the patient.

10. Answer: 2

Rationale: Contact the physician immediately and clarify the order. Never change an order without clarifying it with the physician who prescribed it.

11. Answer: 3

Rationale: The main goal of palliative care is the relief, prevention, reduction, or soothing of symptoms of disease. Hospice care is the care that occurs for those who have less than 6 months to live.

12. Answer: 1

Rationale: Good Samaritan laws grant immunity from suit if there is no gross negligence.

13. Answers: 3 and 4

Rationale: The nurse practitioner and physician are responsible for obtaining an informed consent. The nurse can witness that the signature was obtained by the patient.

14. Answer: 4

Rationale: When a nurse practitioner signs as a witness to an informed consent, he or she is only witnessing what is being done.

15. Answer: 1

Rationale: Showing the patient and his wife how to take care of him at home makes you a patient advocate in this scenario.

16. Answer: 2

Rationale: Calling the supervisor is only a secondary measure after confronting the nurse practitioner and removing her from possible patient harm. Patient safety should always be the priority. Ignoring the situation is unethical. In her current condition, a lecture is probably futile.

17. Answer: 2

Rationale: Patients have a right to informed consent, which includes information about medications, treatments, and even diagnostic studies.

18. Answer: 2

Rationale: Secrets are highly inappropriate in therapeutic relationships. Some secrets may be related to risk for harm to self or others. The nurse must honor and help the patient to understand rights, limitations, and boundaries regarding his or her confidentiality.

19. Answer: 3

Rationale: It is your duty as nurse practitioner to obtain more details of the patient's claim of abuse. You are to gather all the information you can find about the incident before reporting or documenting it.

20. Answer: 2

Rationale: We cannot legally assume that the patient consents to a procedure for which he has not given consent to. This will not be legally defensible. It is known that all invasive procedures require informed consent. Other facts that are to be considered include the patient is an adult and the surgery was scheduled, which means it is not an emergency. Because the patient was already premedicated, she is not in the position to make or sign an informed consent anymore. The surgeon needs to be informed right away.

21. Answer: 2

Rationale: It is the nurse's duty to maintain the patient's right of confidentiality. He is not the patient's physician and does not have a medical need to see her chart. The father should not be allowed to read the chart without written permission from the patient, who is past the age of majority. The attending surgeon cannot give him permission to review the chart either; only the patient can give permission. The patient must provide written permission for unauthorized persons to review her chart. Because this patient just had surgery and is not alert enough to give written legal permission, the father is not allowed to see the chart.

22. Answer: 3

Rationale: A living will directs the patient's health care in the event of a terminal illness. The patient has the right to change an advance directive at any time.

23. Answer: 2

Rationale: The normal CD4 rate is 500 to 1600 cells/mm^3; 200 to 500 cells/mm^3 would mean the patient has HIV. Less than 200 cells/mm^3 would mean that John now has AIDS. Low platelet count also may be caused by the presence of AIDS.

24. Answer: 1

Rationale: The medications will not kill or even cure the virus. The main purpose of encouraging antiretroviral medications is to prevent the virus from becoming resistant to the medications.

25. Answer: 2

Rationale: The nurse practitioner should be informed right away. Testing will not show any positive result because it takes 4 to 6 weeks before the virus is detected.

26. Answer: 1

Rationale: When the nurse describes the patient as a "nasty old man," this is gender bias and ageism. It is also stereotyping. The statement is also a negative connotation to the patient.

27. Answer: 2

Rationale: HIV/AIDS is sexually transmitted through blood. This means that it is not transmitted via saliva by sharing the use of utensils.

28. Answer: 3

Rationale: It is possible for razors to have blood on them during cuts and toothbrushes during hard brushing. Because AIDS may also be transmitted through blood, it is safer to not share those kinds of articles with others.

29. Answer: 3

Rationale: Because HIV/AIDS is sexually transmitted and it takes 4 to 6 weeks before it shows up on the tests, there is a possibility that John's wife may be affected. As practitioners, we are *never* to assume. We always advise patients to get the necessary lab tests done for confirmation.

30. Answer: 1

Rationale: Reaction to grief varies greatly; the stages are not always followed. Every grieving process may be different.

31. Answer: 4

Rationale: Spending time to let patients share their life experiences and life stories enables the nurse practitioner (NP) to know patients better. In knowing the patient's better, the attending NP will understand more about how to approach the situation for better patient care.

32. Answer: 1

Rationale: Let the families do simple things like combing the patient's hair or feeding the patient. This will encourage the bond between patient and family members. You cannot assume that the patient wants to be left alone.

33. Answer: 3

Rationale: When the patient decides to forego standard therapies and starts searching for alternative, nonproven treatments, he or she is exhibiting bargaining behavior.

34. Answer: 4

Rationale: The freedom of decision is not a crucial need compared with the other choices.

35. Answer: 2

Rationale: Common law states that all competent adults can consent to and refuse medical treatment.

36. Answer: 4

Rationale: Bereavement refers not only to the emotional state but also to the outer reaction of the survivor.

37. Answer: 2

Rationale: Before the family can view and say their goodbyes to the deceased, the room and the body must be cleaned and prepared. This includes removing all equipment that is attached to the patient. Removing the dirty linens is also part of the protocol. Preparing the patient would mean bathing him or her and positioning the body on the bed properly.

38. Answer: 2

Rationale: The action shows patient-centered care. This happens when the patient's desires and needs are the driving force on which his health care plan and actions are based.

39. Answer: 2

Rationale: When in hospice care, the goal of the institution is to make the patient and family as comfortable as possible during the end-of-life stage. Hospice care is not a cure.

14

Caring Practices

1. Mariel is a 72-year-old female patient admitted for stroke. She can hardly move the left side of her body. Her vital signs on assessment are blood pressure 180/100 mmHg, respiratory rate 20 breaths/min, heart rate 80 beats/min, and temperature 36.9°C. As a nurse practitioner, your care must be patient focused. A patient-focused goal setting means:

   1. Keeping it short and simple.

   2. It should be controlled by the physician.

   3. Focusing on short-term goals rather than long-term goals.

   4. Keeping it measurable, attainable, and reasonable.

2. Mariel has insurance with Medicare. The nurse practitioner's services to meet the coverage requirement of Medicare must be:

   1. In accordance with state restrictions and supervision requirements.

   2. Under direct supervision.

   3. Through physician-directed clinic or hospital only.

   4. Only provided in a rural health clinic or federally qualified health center.

3. Mariel was given an angiotensin-converting enzyme (ACE) inhibitor during admission. An ACE inhibitor is contraindicated for:

   1. Diabetes mellitus.

   2. Renal failure.

   3. Heart failure.

   4. Hypertension.

4. While you were visiting Mariel, she had an episode of epistaxis. She was swallowing and bleeding from both posterior nares. What is your best action to control the bleeding?

   1. Apply topical vasoconstrictor and pack the nares.

   2. Let patient tilt her head up and pinch her nose.

   3. Allow the patient to lean forward and apply heat pack on the nose.

   4. Put ice pack on the back of the patient's neck.

5. The bleeding has stopped after 30 minutes. Which of the following blood tests would you order for the patient as a follow-up?

   1. Coagulation panel.

   2. No blood test is necessary.

   3. Complete blood count.

   4. Hematocrit and hemoglobin.

6. Mariel was found to have a galloping rhythm. Through auscultation, the nurse practitioner has detected S3 occurring after S2 while the patient was lying on her left side. This is an indication of:

   1. Mitral stenosis.

   2. Heart failure.

   3. Aortic stenosis.

   4. Myocarditis.

7. In relation to heart problems, when a patient is ordered to wear a Holter monitor, what does the patient need to keep in mind?

   1. To turn the monitor before going to bed.

   2. To write daily activities and keep an activity journal.

   3. Limit activities.

   4. Stop all medications.

8. A patient was admitted for an ischemic stroke. The patient received unfractionated heparin. The patient's baseline platelet count was 119,000 mm³. The patient's platelet count suddenly decreased to 40,000 mm³ after 5 days of treatment. This is suggesting that the patient may have heparin-induced thrombocytopenia. What is this patient at risk for?

   1. Infection.

   2. Shock.

   3. Hemorrhage.

   4. Vessel occlusion and thrombosis.

9. Jared is a 20-year-old male patient who was in a motorcycle accident. He has multiple long bone fractures and suspected spinal injuries. During assessment, which of the following is not an internal bleeding warning sign?

   1. Board-like abdomen.

   2. Hematomas.

   3. Vomiting of bile.

   4. Deformed extremities.

10. Jared is at risk for fat emboli. To help determine fat emboli, what are the signs and symptoms to watch for?

    1. Bradycardia, bradypnea, high fever of more than 100.4°F, decreased pulse rate.

    2. Bradycardia, bradypnea, low body temperature, increased pulse rate.

    3. Tachycardia, high fever of more than 100.4°F, jaundice.

    4. Tachycardia, high fever of more than 100.4°F, eczema.

11. Jared was suspected of having spinal cord injury. Forty-eight hours ago, he had a flushed face and neck, severe headache, and diaphoresis. The nurse practitioner assessed him further. His vital signs are blood pressure 200/110 mmHg, respiratory rate 20 breaths/min, heart rate 50 beats/min, and temperature 98.6°F. What do these signs indicate?

    1. Pulmonary embolism.

    2. Malignant hypertension.

    3. Spinal shock.

    4. Autonomic dysreflexia.

12. One of the nurse practitioner's patients has ketoacidosis. She worries that the patient may develop further acidosis. The latest arterial blood gas shows a pH of 7.0. What treatment may correct this imbalance?

    1. Fluids and potassium replacement.

    2. Fluids and insulin.

    3. Oxygenation and insulin.

    4. Fluids and arterial blood gases every 4 hours.

13. A nurse practitioner is tasked to teach new nurses about the neurological system. How is the purpose of the cerebrospinal fluid best described?

    1. It acts as a cushion for the brain and the spinal cord.

    2. It transports fluid to the ventricles.

    3. It helps develop neurotransmitters.

    4. It helps in maintaining cerebral perfusion pressures.

14. Which of the following is the leading cause of acute tubular necrosis?

    1. Shock.

    2. Gastrointestinal bleeding.

    3. Hypertension.

    4. Sepsis.

15. Your 78-year-old patient with diabetes was diagnosed with acute tubular necrosis. Which would likely indicate that the patient is in the initial phase?

    1. Blood pressure of more than 180/100 mmHg.

    2. Urine output of less than 400 mL/day.

    3. Creatine level of 1.1 mg/dL.

    4. Abdominal pain and nausea.

16. The patient has pancreatitis. Which medication is effective in decreasing the vagal stimulation, ampullary spasm, and pancreatic secretion?

    1. Anticholinergics.

    2. Opioid analgesics.

    3. Antispasmodic.

    4. Antiemetics.

17. A 62-year-old male patient is admitted to the intensive care unit for hepatic failure. Which of his previous conditions does not predispose him to hepatic failure?

    1. Pancreatitis.

    2. Acetaminophen overdose.

    3. Viral hepatitis.

    4. Biliary atresia.

18. Which of the following conditions causes significant complications in intermittent hemodialysis?

    1. Cerebral edema.

    2. Arrhythmias.

    3. Hypertension.

    4. Hypotension.

19. Which lab value in a patient with end-stage renal disease needs to be monitored for a potential sign of bleeding?

    1. Hemoglobin.

    2. Platelet.

    3. Hematocrit.

    4. Prothrombin time.

20. The patient who just returned from abdominal surgery is forcefully coughing without abdomen protection. The nurse practitioner is teaching the patient to put a pillow on his abdomen when coughing. This action is to avoid what postoperative complication?

    1. Tension pneumothorax.

    2. Paralytic ileus.

    3. Dehiscence.

    4. Atelectasis.

21. A 43-year-old male patient arrived in the emergency department and has symptoms of acute renal failure. What is the most accurate measure of renal function?

    1. Creatinine.

    2. Urine output.

    3. Glomerular filtration rate.

    4. Urea.

22. As the nurse practitioner was assessing a patient for pressure ulcers, he noticed a 1×0.5–inch, red shallow crater on the patient's heel. This crater is surrounded by bright pink skin and has a small amount of white drainage. How would this be documented?

    1. Stage 1 pressure ulcer, blanchable.

    2. Stage 2 partial-thickness wound.

    3. Stage 3 full-thickness wound.

    4. No stageable wound.

23. Because of coronary syndrome, a patient suffers a myocardial infarction. The physician ordered bivalirudin in preparation for the patient undergoing percutaneous coronary intervention. For a patient receiving bivalirudin, what is the most important symptom to watch out for?

    1. Bradycardia.

    2. Bleeding.

    3. Hypotension.

    4. All of the above.

24. A father of two had a motor vehicular accident. His blood pressure is 70/40 mmHg. This patient has a do not resuscitate order in his chart. After a few hours, he went into cardiac arrest. One of his daughters wants the health personnel to do everything to save him. What is the appropriate action in this scenario?

    1. Do not resuscitate.

    2. Follow the daughter's orders.

    3. Contact the ethics committee of the hospital.

    4. Ask the registered nurse to resuscitate.

25. As a nurse practitioner, you need to be aware of the hospital or health care center visitation policy. What is the best action to make when a family member of a critically ill patient wants to stay for the night, which is contrary to visiting policy?

    1. Allow the entire family to stay in the room.

    2. Suggest that they stay in a motel near the hospital instead.

    3. Allow one or two family members to stay, then evaluate the patient's response.

    4. Stick to the policy and educate the family about it.

26. A 14-year-old patient's mother called and asked about her son's plan of care and several other questions about his condition. What would be the appropriate response from the nurse practitioner?

    1. "Sure. One moment please."

    2. "I'll put you through to the patient's room and you may ask him yourself."

    3. "I'm sorry. I cannot give you any information about the patient."

    4. "Let me verify a few things first. What is the patient's birth date? Can you provide his middle name please?"

27. The nurse practitioner is assessing a 30-year-old male patient who is suspected for rheumatic fever. Which of the following would confirm this diagnosis?

    1. Petechial rashes all over the body and a fewer of over 101°F.

    2. A positive x-ray with white masses.

    3. Productive cough with yellow sputum and a sore throat that has lasted for 3 weeks.

    4. A positive antistreptolysin O titer.

28. A patient with ruled-out cerebrovascular accident is to undergo magnetic resonance imaging (MRI). What would be a contraindication for the MRI?

    1. History of heart attack.

    2. Implanted pacemaker.

    3. Allergy to poison ivy.

    4. History of anxiety.

29. What type of anxiety disorder is guided exposure therapy used for?

    1. Posttraumatic stress disorder.

    2. Panic disorder.

    3. Specific phobias.

    4. Generalized anxiety disorder.

30. The nurse practitioner is teaching the patient with iron-deficiency anemia about nutrition. Which meal is recommended for the patient?

    1. Hamburger, green salad, green beans, and chocolate cake.

    2. Pork chop, applesauce, cornbread, and apple pie.

    3. Chicken salad sandwich, potato salad, and ice cream.

    4. Egg salad on wheat bread, carrot sticks, lettuce salad, and raisin oatmeal cookies.

31. While transporting a patient with methicillin-resistant *Streptococcus aureus* (MRSA) for surgery, precautions for infection control in the operating room were done. Which action by the nurse practitioner shows that she is taking precautions?

    1. Placing a surgical mask on the patient when outside of the room.

    2. Placing a sign on the patient's chart to alert the staff in the operating room.

    3. Wearing a mask and gloves when transporting the patient to the operating room.

    4. Placing the patient's chart in a bag before transporting the patient.

32. A cancer patient who is undergoing chemotherapy has a platelet count of 20,000/mL. What does the nurse practitioner need to teach the patient?

    1. Sleep at least 13 hours a day.

    2. Take aspirin for headaches.

    3. Avoid anyone with a cold or flu.

    4. Avoid participating in activities that could cause injury.

33. Which of the following is not a nurse practitioner intervention for a patient with tonic-clonic seizures?

    1. Restraining a patient during a seizure.

    2. Clear the area of hard objects.

    3. Turn the patient's head or turn him on his side.

    4. Assist the patient to a lying position and loosen any tight clothing.

34. The nurse practitioner is checking for an adverse effect to the contrast medium after a patient has undergone a computerized tomography (CT) scan. Which of the following is *not* an adverse reaction to the contrast medium?

    1. Restlessness.

    2. Facial flushing.

    3. Urticaria.

    4. Bradycardia.

35. Which of the following is the most common cause for cardiogenic shock?

    1. Hypertensive crisis.

    2. Stroke.

    3. Myocardial infarction.

    4. Acute pulmonary emboli.

36. Which of the following is *not* an indication for heparin?

    1. Ischemic stroke.

    2. Cerebral thrombosis.

    3. Embolism prophylaxis.

    4. New-onset atrial fibrillation.

37. Which precaution should the nurse practitioner follow when administering phenytoin to a patient?

    1. Give fosphenytoin instead because not everyone reacts well to phenytoin.

    2. Phenytoin should only be given as a pill.

    3. Mixing phenytoin with dextrose solution should be avoided.

    4. Mixing phenytoin with dextrose solution should always be done when given in an intravenous form.

38. A 21-year-old male patient has a body mass index of 33. He is admitted because of difficulty in breathing and recurrent chest pains. The assessment shows that both parents of the patient have suffered from myocardial infarction before they turned 50 years old. What would be the first step to prevent the patient from developing myocardial infarction?

    1. Teach the patient the right food for his body and instruct him to avoid fatty and high-calorie foods.

    2. Encourage the patient to have a regular exercise program.

    3. Assess the patient's level of interest in weight loss programs.

    4. Educate the patient about obesity and its risks.

39. The nurse practitioner is taking care of a 55-year-old patient with acute lymphocytic leukemia. The patient's white blood cell count is 6000 cells/mcL. What would be done to prevent the patient from developing an infection?

    1. Take vital signs every 2 hours.

    2. Insert a Foley catheter.

    3. Frequently check patient's mouth and give saline solution rinses.

    4. When the patient's white blood cells drop, immediately start the patient on antibiotic therapy.

40. A patient is admitted to the coronary care unit with a blood pressure of 90/60 mmHg, a heart rate of 125 beats/min, and complaints of chest pain rating it 8 of 10. The patient already took a 0.04-mg tablet of nitroglycerin 5 minutes ago. What would be the nurse practitioner's next intervention?

    1. Obtain a STAT electrocardiogram.

    2. Administer another dose of 0.04 mg tablet of nitroglycerin.

    3. Take the patient's blood pressure and put on the monitor.

    4. Administer a dose of morphine 2 mg intravenously and assess pain in 10 minutes.

41. The nurse practitioner is assisting a physician during an abdominal paracentesis. What is the maximum amount of fluid that may be aspirated?

    1. 2000 to 2500 mL.

    2. 1000 to 1500 mL.

    3. 2500 to 3000 mL.

    4. 1500 to 2000 mL.

42. A patient has acute respiratory acidosis. He has a pH of 7.25 and a $Paco_2$ of 55. As a nurse practitioner, you know that the underlying cause of acute respiratory acidosis is what?

    1. There is no underlying cause.

    2. The lungs are ventilating insufficiently.

    3. The aldosterone level is elevated.

    4. There is an underlying gastric disorder.

43. What would be the nurse practitioner's first step in treating a patient with acute respiratory distress syndrome?

    1. Prevent respiratory and metabolic complications.

    2. Provide adequate nutrition.

    3. Maintain oxygenation.

    4. Maintain fluid and electrolyte balance.

44. The nurse practitioner is assessing a 48-year-old patient in the intensive care unit. She has been experiencing severe vomiting and diarrhea for the past for 4 days. What signs and symptoms would show that it has progressed to complications of shock related to hypovolemia?

    1. Blood pressure 98/48 mmHg, heart rate 120 beats/min, cold feet and hands.

    2. Mental status changes, acute abdominal pain, and normal vital signs.

    3. Mental status change, blood pressure 130/80 mmHg; temperature of 99.4°F.

    4. Blood pressure 150/80 mmHg, heart rate 120 beats/min, afebrile.

45. A 55-year-old woman has been admitted with a diagnosis of sepsis. What would be the first signs and symptoms if the patient is having gastrointestinal bleeding?

    1. Bloody feces.

    2. Weight loss and anorexia.

    3. Fatigue and weakness.

    4. Abdominal pain and discomfort.

46. As a nurse practitioner, you are managing the care of multiple patients. Which patient would be at greatest risk for septic shock?

    1. A 38-year-old woman who is 2 days' post appendectomy.

    2. A 54-year-old woman who is diagnosed with pneumonia.

    3. An 80-year-old woman with stage 4 pressure ulcer on her coccyx, insulin dependent, with a long-term Foley catheter.

    4. An 85-year-old woman who had bypass surgery 2 weeks ago.

47. In assessing the gag reflex, which cranial nerve would be tested?

    1. Trochlear.

    2. Trigeminal.

    3. Vagus.

    4. Glossopharyngeal.

48. Victoria has been admitted three times in the past 14 months because of exacerbated congestive heart failure. What should the nurse practitioner do to lower the likelihood of readmission?

    1. Advise the patient to increase the number of doctor visits.

    2. Properly educate the patient about the condition and how to manage it properly. Follow up with the patient within 1 week.

    3. Let patient increase diuretic dose on discharge.

    4. Let patient stay in the hospital for an additional 72 hours to monitor condition.

49. Victoria was admitted to the intensive care unit again with the exacerbation of congestive heart failure. Her oxygen saturation is 90% on 2 L oxygen. She is breathing rapidly with a heart rate of 145 beats/min. Victoria has been taking beta-blockers for her heart failure at home. Which drug would be best to give the patient to increase her heart's contractility?

    1. Primacor.

    2. Dopamine.

    3. Digoxin.

    4. Nitroglycerin.

50. The nurse practitioner is assessing a patient with worsening congestive heart failure. Which part of the heart would be involved in such a condition?

    1. Mitral valve.

    2. Left ventricle.

    3. Right ventricle.

    4. Aorta.

51. A patient is ordered for tube feeding. The nurse practitioner knows that the best position of the patient when feeding is finished is:

    1. High-Fowler's.

    2. Left side with head of the bed elevated.

    3. Semi-Fowler's.

    4. Right side with head of the bed elevated.

52. The nurse is providing a patient with type 1 diabetes exercise guidelines. Which of the following are most appropriate? *Select all that apply.*

    (1) Eat more complex carbohydrate before exercising.

    (2) Do not administer insulin immediately before and after exercise.

    (3) Leave an energy drink with electrolytes in your locker in case you need it.

    (4) Inform your gym that you have type 1 diabetes.

    (5) Eat a simple carbohydrates snack before you exercise.

        1. 1, 2, 3, 5.

        2. 2, 4, 5.

        3. 1, 4, 5.

        4. 1, 2, 3, 4, 5.

53. The nurse practitioner is screening patients for colon cancer. Which of the following are considered risk factors for colorectal cancer? *Select all that apply.*

    (1) 55 years of age and above.

    (2) Diet high in beef.

    (3) Gluten-free diet.

    (4) Type 2 diabetes.

    (5) History of inflammatory bowel syndrome.

        1. 1 and 4 only.

        2. 1, 4, 5.

        3. 1, 2, 3, 4, 5.

        4. 1, 2, 4, 5.

54. Which of the following opportunistic infections adversely affect HIV/AIDS patients? *Select all that apply.*

    (1) Blindness.

    (2) Kaposi sarcoma.

    (3) Tuberculosis.

    (4) *Toxoplasma gondii.*

    (5) Peripheral neuropathy.

        1. 2, 3, 4.

        2. 1, 3, 4, 5.

        3. 1, 2, 4, 5.

        4. 1, 2, 3, 4, 5.

55. What is the goal of performance improvement activities?

    1. To improve policies.

    2. To stay in budget.

    3. To improve process.

    4. To increase efficiency.

56. Which of the following smoking cessation medication needs close monitoring because of its potentially lethal side effects?

    1. Varenicline (Chantix).

    2. Nicotine nasal spray.

    3. Nicotine inhaler.

    4. Bupropion (Zyban).

57. Kathleen, a 35-year-old female patient, is complaining of lower back pain. She is suspected of having herniated nucleus pulposus. Vertebral herniation may likely be found in which areas?

    1. L1-L2, L4-L5.

    2. L2-L3, L3-L4.

    3. L4-L5, L5-S1.

    4. S1-S2, S2-S3.

58. The nurse practitioner is assessing a patient with multiple myeloma. Which of the following signs shows that the patient is experiencing hypercalcemia?

    1. Twitching of hands.

    2. Decreased motility of the gastrointestinal tract.

    3. Diarrhea.

    4. Hyperactive deep tendon reflexes.

59. Your patient is suspected of having von Willebrand disease. Which of the statements is incorrect about its characteristics?

    1. The deficiency is only moderate.

    2. The von Willebrand factor allows adhesion of platelets to a glycoprotein Ib-IX.

    3. The von Willebrand factor functions independent of factor VIII.

    4. It is a qualitative platelet defect.

60. The nurse practitioner is assessing a patient who is suspected of severe anemia. Along with the lab work and vital signs, what physical assessment is another indication of severe anemia?

    1. Pedal edema.

    2. Bluish color on the abdomen.

    3. Abnormalities on the patient's nails.

    4. Wrist and arm jerk when blood pressure cuff is applied.

61. Which of the following diagnoses decreases the metabolic rate?

    1. Cardiac failure.

    2. Hypothyroidism.

    3. Chronic obstructive pulmonary disease.

    4. Cancer.

62. What condition is malnutrition, ill health, and wasting associated with as a result of a chronic disease?

    1. Surgical asepsis.

    2. Venous stasis.

    3. Cachexia.

    4. Catabolism.

63. Which of the following patients is more likely at risk for Osgood–Schlatter disease?

    1. Ryan, a 16-year-old athlete, who is physically active and is the captain of their soccer team.

    2. Khloe is a 23-year-old pregnant woman who is in her first trimester.

    3. A 45-year-old man, Mario, who has been exposed to asbestos at work.

    4. Janet is a 68-year-old woman admitted for hip fracture.

64. Your patient has fever, occult, night sweats, hematuria, tenderness of the spleen, and Osler nodes. What disorder would you suspect the patient is experiencing?

    1. AIDS/HIV.

    2. Tuberculosis.

    3. Pericarditis.

    4. Endocarditis.

65. The nurse practitioner is caring for a patient with septic shock. Which of the following should be administered first?

    1. Start antibiotic therapy to treat underlying infection.

    2. Administer corticosteroids to reduce inflammation.

    3. Intravenous fluids to increase intravascular volume.

    4. Vasopressors to increase patient's blood pressure.

66. As the nurse practitioner for a patient on a ventilator with an endotracheal tube, what assessment data would indicate that the tube has migrated too far down the trachea?

    1. Decreased breath sounds on the left side of the chest.

    2. Increased breath sounds on the left side of the chest.

    3. Low pressure alarm sound.

    4. High pressure alarm sound.

67. When the nurse practitioner is assessing a patient with osteoarthritis, which characteristic is a symptom of this condition?

    1. Waddling gait.

    2. Joint crepitus.

    3. Decreased grip strength.

    4. Bilateral joint swelling.

68. A patient was brought to the emergency department complaining of watery stool for the past 3 days. On assessment, the patient's blood pressure is 100/60 mmHg, pulse rate is 108 beats/min, and there are dry mucous membranes. Which fluid would the nurse practitioner use for the patient's intravenous therapy?

    1. Hypotonic crystalloid.

    2. Hypertonic crystalloid.

    3. Colloid solution.

    4. Isotonic crystalloid.

69. The nurse practitioner is caring for a patient with end-stage chronic obstructive pulmonary disease. Which of the following is an indication that the patient has developed cor pulmonale?

    1. Venous stasis ulcers.

    2. Hepatomegaly.

    3. Night sweats.

    4. Hypocapnia.

70. The patient is observed by the nurse practitioner to have a pulsating abdominal mass. What would be the appropriate next step?

    1. Measure the abdominal circumference.

    2. Assess femoral pulses.

    3. Make an order for a bladder scan.

    4. Ask patient to perform the Valsalva maneuver.

71. The nurse practitioner is taking care of a patient who is diagnosed with Crohn disease and currently has a colostomy. When assessing the stoma, what condition indicates that the stoma has retracted?

    1. Narrowed and flattened.

    2. Dry and reddish-purple.

    3. Pinkish-red and moist.

    4. Concave and bowl-shaped.

72. The nurse practitioner is preparing a pneumococcal vaccine for a 65-year-old patient with chronic bronchitis. The patient said that she already had that vaccine 5 years before. What is the nurse practitioner's most appropriate response?

    1. "You were only 60 then, a repeat vaccination is recommended."

    2. "Just like the flu shot, you need this vaccine annually."

    3. "I can give you a flu shot instead of a pneumococcal vaccination."

    4. "This vaccine is given yearly to anyone with lung disease."

73. A patient is diagnosed with Wolff-Parkinson-White syndrome. He is undergoing catheter ablation procedure. What would be the priority care after the procedure?

    1. Monitor insertion site and distal pulses.

    2. Auscultate apical pulse for a full minute every hour.

    3. Assist the patient to the bathroom to void.

    4. Assess level of consciousness every 30 minutes.

74. A patient who is diagnosed with type 2 diabetes is admitted because of pneumonia. The patient is now receiving insulin for glucose control because his oral antidiabetic has been discontinued. What is the rationale for the change of medication?

    1. An illness like pneumonia will cause increased insulin resistance.

    2. Infection has compromised beta-cell function so the patient will start needing insulin.

    3. Insulin will help prevent hypoglycemia during the illness.

    4. Stress-related states such as infections increase risk of hyperglycemia.

75. As the nurse practitioner caring for a patient with a pneumothorax, which of the following needs to be included in your plan of care?

    1. Empty the drainage chamber every shift and record the amount of drainage collected.

    2. Daily dressing change for the insertion site using aseptic technique.

    3. Encourage the patient to regularly cough and do deep breathing.

    4. Massage the tube every 2 hours vigorously to promote drainage.

76. Which of the following lab value alteration is likely a result of corticosteroid treatment for a patient with type 1 diabetes and recently diagnosed with pneumonitis?

    1. Albumin 3.5 g/dL (0.05 mmol/L).

    2. Potassium 5.1 mEq/L (5.1 mmol/L).

    3. Sodium 138 mEq/L (138 mmol/L).

    4. Glucose 200 mg/dL (11.1 mmol/L).

77. A patient is to receive total parenteral nutrition and lipids during acute exacerbation of inflammatory bowel disease. Which of the following is the priority when caring for the patient?

    1. Every 72 hours, change the administration set.

    2. Every shift, monitor the urine's specific gravity.

    3. Monitor the patient's blood glucose per protocol.

    4. Infuse the solution in a large peripheral vein.

78. A patient with a platelet count of 40,000 mcL (40×10^9/L) is to be discharged. What is the most important discharge teaching by the nurse practitioner?

    1. "Take your aspirin with meals every day."

    2. "Take multivitamins every day."

    3. "When you shave, use a straight edge razor."

    4. "Floss gently and use a soft-bristled toothbrush."

Caring Practices Answers & Rationales   **14**

1. Answer: 4

Rationale: A goal, even in health care, needs to be SMART.

S-Specific

M-Measurable

A-Attainable

R-Relevant/realistic/reasonable

T-Timely

2. Answer: 1

Rationale: The nurse practitioner may bill Medicare for one's services in accordance with his or her current state restrictions and supervision requirement. One state may differ from another.

3. Answer: 2

Rationale: Angiotensin-converting enzyme inhibitors are contraindicated for patients with kidney failure. Because of the inhibition of angiotensin, this may cause azotemia resulting from preferential efferent arteriolar vasodilation in the renal glomerulus.

4. Answer: 1

Rationale: Applying a topical vasoconstrictor and pack is done to slow down the bleeding. This is the best action to take. Letting patient tilt head was an old practice and is not advisable. Heat causes vasodilation and will trigger more bleeding. Putting ice pack on the back of the neck has very little effect in terms of slowing down the bleeding.

5. Answer: 4

Rationale: You may order hematocrit and hemoglobin count to determine the patient's blood loss. Posterior bleeding of the nares is dangerous and may result in significant blood loss.

6. Answer: 2

Rationale: A galloping rhythm in elder adults may indicate heart failure or left ventricular failure. In children and young adults, a gallop may be normal.

7. Answer: 2

Rationale: The patient needs to keep track of his activities so the Holter monitor can help determine whether a specific activity is a trigger for any abnormality. The patient needs to continue taking his medications and continue with his normal, daily activities. He needs to keep the monitor on before going to bed because during sleep is when some abnormalities happen.

8. Answer: 4

Rationale: The patient is at risk for vessel occlusion and thrombosis rather than hemorrhage because of heparin-induced thrombocytopenia. A platelet count below 50,000 mm^3 indicates that it is type II, which is an autoimmune reaction to heparin.

9. Answer: 3

Rationale: Vomiting of blood is a warning sign for internal bleeding, not vomiting of bile. Board-like abdomen may indicate that there is blood spill in the peritoneal cavity.

10. Answer: 3

Rationale: Some signs and symptoms of fat emboli include tachycardia (heart rate greater than 110 beats/min), pyrexia (temperature greater than 100.4°F), retinal changes of fat or petechiae, renal dysfunction, jaundice, and sudden thrombocytopenia.

11. Answer: 4

Rationale: Autonomic dysreflexia is caused by T6 or above spinal cord injury. This causes imbalance reflex sympathetic discharge and can lead to life-threatening hypertension. All caregivers need to be aware of its signs and symptoms.

12. Answer: 2

Rationale: The treatment may be to turn around the additional complication of the patient's acidosis level with fluids and insulin. Potassium is used to treat hypokalemia. Drawing arterial blood gas is a diagnostic tool and is not used for treatment.

13. Answer: 1

Rationale: The cerebrospinal fluid cushions the brain and the spinal cord. It is the shock absorber that helps protect the brain from injury.

14. Answer: 4

Rationale: Sepsis is the leading cause of tubular necrosis. This is precipitated by a hypotensive event. Tubular necrosis is a severe form of renal failure that usually develops in patients who are critically ill.

15. Answer: 2

Rationale: One indicator that the patient is in the initial phase of acute tubular necrosis is oliguria or urine output less than 400 mL/day. Abdominal pain, the creatinine level, and blood pressure measurement are not indications of the initial phase of a patient with acute tubular necrosis (ATN).

16. Answer: 1

Rationale: Anticholinergics like atropine and propantheline are medications that are effective in decreasing vagal stimulation, ampullary spasm, and pancreatic secretion.

17. Answer: 1

Rationale: The other three choices are conditions that can prelude liver failure. Pancreatitis does not predispose a patient to hepatic failure.

18. Answer: 4

Rationale: In an intensive care unit setting, the nurse practitioner should watch for hypotension. Hemodialysis can cause hemodynamic instability with critically ill patients, which is quickly seen in the patient's blood pressure.

19. Answer: 2

Rationale: The lab value related to bleeding that needs to be monitored is the platelet level of the patient. Patients with end-stage renal disease are at risk for bleeding because they are at risk for platelet dysfunction.

20. Answer: 3

Rationale: Wound dehiscence may occur postoperatively when the wound edges separate, and it can lead to evisceration. The nurse practitioner was right in teaching the patient to use an abdominal pillow when he coughs to prevent such a complication.

21. Answer: 3

Rationale: Glomerular filtration rate (GFR) is the most accurate measure to determine acute renal failure. GFR estimates how much blood passes through the glomeruli each minute.

22. Answer: 2

Rationale: The crater on the patient's heel is a stage 2 partial-thickness partial ulcer. Two skin layers are involved, the epidermis and the dermis. The shallow crater broke through the first layer.

23. Answer: 4

Rationale: It is important to watch out for bradycardia, bleeding, and hypotension when a patient is taking bivalirudin. It is a direct thrombin inhibitor used to prevent blood clots.

24. Answer: 1

Rationale: The only appropriate action would be not to resuscitate. A do not resuscitate order means no attempt to resuscitate should be done when the patient suffers an arrest.

25. Answer: 3

Rationale: The best action would be to allow one or two family members to stay the night as they wish. Once done, evaluate the patient's response. The presence of a support person may be therapeutic for the patient.

26. Answer: 3

Rationale: According to the Health Insurance Portability and Accountability Act, a health practitioner is not allowed to give any information about the patient to anyone who is not directly involved in the patient's care. Sharing of information is not allowed without the patient's consent.

27. Answer: 4

Rationale: A positive antistreptolysin O titer is the diagnostic test to confirm acute rheumatic fever.

28. Answer: 2

Rationale: The presence of a pacemaker would be contraindicated for someone who is to undergo magnetic resonance imaging. Any metal embedded in the body is contraindicated, even metal fragments.

29. Answer: 3

Rationale: Guided exposure therapy is used for patients with specific phobias. The therapy includes relaxation and imagery techniques. Patients are also educated more about their conditions.

30. Answer: 4

Rationale: A diet that includes eggs, wheat bread, carrots, raisins, and other leafy vegetables are ideal for someone with iron-deficiency anemia.

31. Answer: 1

Rationale: Placing a mask on the patient before entering the operating room is a precautious action for infection control. When a patient has an infection that requires isolation, the patient must wear a surgical mask when outside of his or her room.

32. Answer: 4

Rationale: The nurse practitioner needs to educate the patient about the risk of bleeding. Activities that can potentially cause injury need to be avoided. Aspirin can cause bleeding and should be discouraged.

33. Answer: 1

Rationale: Restraining the patient during the seizure is not a nurse practitioner (NP) intervention. For the clonic phase, the patient's entire body is rigid and in the tonic phase, there is uncontrollable jerking. The other choices are appropriate NP interventions.

34. Answer: 4

Rationale: All three choices are signs of adverse effects to the contrast medium except for bradycardia. The patient may be having allergic reactions to the material.

35. Answer: 3

Rationale: Myocardial infarction continues to be the most common cause of cardiogenic shock. Cardiogenic shock presents with low systolic blood pressure and clinical signs of hypoperfusion.

36. Answer: 1

Rationale: Anticoagulants are not suggested for patients with hemorrhagic stroke. Heparin may cause severe bleeding in the brain.

37. Answer: 3

Rationale: Phenytoin should not be administered with dextrose solution because it will precipitate and crystallize the solution.

38. Answer: 3

Rationale: The first step would be to assess the patient's interest in weight loss programs because the patient needs to be willing enough to commit to it.

39. Answer: 2

Rationale: Inserting a Foley catheter or any other noncritical device would put the patient at risk for infection. The nurse practitioner should monitor vital signs every 2 to 4 hours, check patient's mouth for ulcerations, and quickly give antibiotic therapy once the white blood cell count drops.

40. Answer: 2

Rationale: The nurse practitioner (NP) should give the patient another 0.04-mg tablet of nitroglycerin. Patients can take up to three sublingual nitroglycerin tablets within 15 minutes. Expect chest pain to elevate within 5 to 10 minutes. After giving the nitroglycerin, the NP can then take vital sign and obtain an electrocardiogram.

41. Answer: 4

Rationale: From 1500 to 2000 mL is the maximum amount of fluid that should be aspirated in one paracentesis. Aspirating more than 2000 mL may lead the patient into hypovolemic shock.

42. Answer: 2

Rationale: Insufficient ventilation of the lungs is the underlying cause of acute respiratory acidosis. The sudden collapse of the body's ventilation system may result from chronic obstructive pulmonary disease, drugs or toxins, and central nervous system disease.

43. Answer: 3

Rationale: The very first step is to maintain oxygenation. First, supplemental oxygenation is tried, and if this is not sufficient, then a mechanical ventilator will be used after intubation.

44. Answer: 1

Rationale: Signs and symptoms that suggest hypovolemic shock are low blood pressure, tachycardia, and cold extremities. Shock is a sign of a critical illness and needs to be treated quickly.

45. Answer: 1

Rationale: Bloody feces is the first indicator that the patient is having gastrointestinal bleeding. Melena, a black, tarry stool, is an indication of upper gastrointestinal disease that causes bleeding.

46. Answer: 3

Rationale: The patient in answer 3 is at high risk for septic shock because she is elderly, she has an open wound, her diabetes will delay wound healing, and an indwelling Foley catheter is another entrance for bacteria. The patient in answer 1 is young, with no comorbidities, and likely had a laproscopic procedure. The patient in answer 2 has no comorbidities and is relatively young. The patient in answer 4, although older, has no comorbidities.

47. Answer: 4

Rationale: The cranial nerve used for assessing the gag reflex is the glossopharyngeal nerve. The trochlear nerve is used to check one's ability to move their eyes, the trigeminal nerve assesses one's ability to swallow, and the vagus nerve identifies the symmetry arch of one's tongue.

48. Answer: 2

Rationale: The nurse practitioner needs to properly educate the patient about her condition and its management. Once she understands her condition, she more likely will take care of herself by assessing for warning signs calling the doctor when necessary.

49. Answer: 1

Rationale: The best drug to give Victoria would be Primacor. The dopamine will not work because she has been taking beta-blockers at home, so the needed receptors are already being used.

50. Answer: 2

Rationale: Heart failure is a condition that affects the ventricles. The left ventricular function would show deterioration because it will affect the left side before it affects the right side.

51. Answer: 4

Rationale: Once feeding is done, the best position for the patient is to be on his right side for digestion with an elevated bed head to prevent aspiration.

52. Answer: 2

Rationale: It is best for a type 1 diabetic to eat a simple carbohydrate snack before exercising. When you give insulin right before or right after exercising, the patient may bottom out.

53. Answer: 4

Rationale: A gluten-free diet does not put one at risk for colorectal cancer.

54. Answer: 1

Rationale: Kaposi sarcoma, tuberculosis, and *Toxoplasma gondii, Mycobacterium avium*, herpes simplex, and *Salmonella* are HIV/AIDS-associated opportunistic infections. Although some patients do experience blindness and peripheral neuropathy, these are because of nervous system impairment rather than an infection.

55. Answer: 3

Rationale: The main purpose of performance improvement activities is to improve the process. These activities will help identify flaws in the process. Then the current process can be changed and improved, which helps lower human error and possible harm to patients.

56. Answer: 1

Rationale: When a patient is taking varenicline, he needs to be closely monitored because it is one of the most potentially lethal drugs. It can cause seizures, myocardial infarction, psychosis, and many more complications. Safer medications to curb smoking would be the nicotine inhaler or nicotine nasal spray and bupropion (Zyban). The latter may cause dry mouth and insomnia but nothing lethal.

57. Answer: 3

Rationale: L4-L5 and L5-S1 are the most common areas for herniated discs because these areas bear most of the body's weight.

58. Answer: 2

Rationale: Decreased motility of the gastrointestinal tract is a sign of hypercalcemia. Patients who are diagnosed with multiple myeloma are at risk for hypercalcemia.

59. Answer: 3

Rationale: The von Willebrand disease is a hereditary disease of the von Willebrand factor. It functions together with factor VIII because the von Willebrand factor is needed to maintain normal plasma factor VIII levels.

60. Answer: 3

Rationale: Along with lab work and vital signs, pedal edema is an indicator, and it may be seen on the patient's nails. Nail abnormalities may include spoon shape, long-shaped striations, and clubbing. The patient may also have retinal hemorrhages.

61. Answer: 2

Rationale: Fewer calories are required in hypothyroidism because there is a decreased metabolic demand. Cardiac failure, chronic obstructive pulmonary disease, and cancer are conditions in which the metabolic demand is increased.

62. Answer: 3

Rationale: Malnutrition, ill health, and wasting are a result of chronic disease and are all associated with cachexia. Cachexia also may be caused by dehiscence or wound rupture. Surgical asepsis is a sterile technique, catabolism is the breakdown of tissue after crush injury or severe trauma, and venous stasis is a disorder related to the pooling of blood in a vein.

63. Answer: 1

Rationale: Osgood–Schlatter is a disease caused by overuse of the knee. This is characterized by an inflammation in the patellar tendon. Exposure to asbestos may lead to a condition called mesothelioma.

64. Answer: 4

Rationale: The signs and symptoms all lead to a diagnosis of endocarditis.

65. Answer: 3

Rationale: The nurse practitioner needs to address the circulation and perfusion first, so intravenous fluids should be started immediately. Vasopressors are administered if the patient will not respond to the fluids.

66. Answer: 1

Rationale: Once the endotracheal tube has been inserted too far, it goes to the right main stem bronchus. Air is then delivered to the right lung instead of the left. A low-pressure alarm is an indication of disconnection or leak in the circuit. A high pressure alarm can indicate an obstruction.

67. Answer: 2

Rationale: Crepitus or crepitation is described as the grinding, crackling, or popping sound that occurs during joint movement. It is also present when cartilage is lost. Decreased grip strength and bilateral joint swelling is usually seen in rheumatoid arthritis.

68. Answer: 4

Rationale: An isotonic crystalloid solution will expand the intravascular compartment. It will not affect other cells and tissues in other fluid compartments. This solution is used in this scenario because hypovolemia is corrected by expanding the intravascular compartment.

69. Answer: 2

Rationale: Cor pulmonale or right-sided heart failure is a result of chronic lung conditions like bronchitis or chronic obstructive pulmonary disease. Hepatomegaly/liver pulsatility is present if there is significant tricuspid regurgitation. It is just one sign that indicates cor pulmonale.

70. Answer: 2

Rationale: Abdominal aortic aneurysm may be present when one has pulsating mass. Assessing the pulses distal to the aneurysm will provide information regarding the degree of circulatory compromise. The Valsalva maneuver is done when hernia is suspected. A bladder scan is ordered when a distended bladder is suspected, which is present as a nonpulsating suprapubic enlargement.

71. Answer: 4

Rationale: A concave and bowl-shaped stoma means it has retracted. It is hard to take care of a retracted stoma. A healthy-looking stoma should be pinkish-red and moist.

72. Answer: 1

Rationale: Anyone who got their pneumococcal vaccine before they turned 65 is recommended to get it again. Patients who are 65 years old or older should receive both PCV13 and PCV23 vaccines.

73. Answer: 1

Rationale: The catheter may cause trauma to the vessels. The nurse practitioner (NP) needs to monitor for hematoma formation and interference of circulation distal to the insertion site. The other options are also NP care, but they are not a priority.

74. Answer: 4

Rationale: An infection will cause a stress response in the body. The stress response increases the epinephrine and hormone glucocorticoids, which suppresses the natural immune response. This will take more time for the body to fight infection.

75. Answer: 3

Rationale: Regular coughing and deep breathing will help re-expand a collapsed lung. The dressing change is protocol when the site is soiled. Massaging the tube vigorously will increase intrapulmonary pressure and can damage the lung.

76. Answer: 4

Rationale: Corticosteroids can cause a rise in blood sugar, even in nondiabetic patients. This triggers the liver to release additional glucose. Albumin, potassium, and sodium are not expected findings for the scenario given.

77. Answer: 3

Rationale: Blood glucose levels should be closely monitored since total parenteral nutrition (TPN) can cause hyperglycemia. Because of the hypertonicity of TPN solution, it must be administered via a central venous catheter. The set needs to be changed every 24 hours if the TPN contains lipids.

78. Answer: 4

Rationale: The normal range for platelets is 150,000 to 400,000 mcL (150–400 × 10^9/L). The patient has thrombocytopenia and should be cautious about bleeding. Using a soft-bristled toothbrush and flossing will prevent the gums from bleeding.

15

Collaborative Practice

1. Collaborative Practice in health care is widely used and has proven to be effective in reducing risk and errors in practice. This has also proven that effective communication is possible in a multidisciplinary setting. Which of the following best defines collaborative practice?

    1. Collaborative practice is when one member of the health care team learns from another member.

    2. Collaborative practice is when multiple health workers from different professional backgrounds work together with patients, families, caregivers, and communities to deliver the highest quality of care.

    3. Collaborative practice happens when one department of the health care industry benefits from another department, providing the highest quality of care.

    4. Collaborative practice is being able to work with other members of the health care team without conflicts. Teamwork is the main goal of this practice.

2. Ryan, a nurse practitioner, is acting as the coordinator of the interprofessional health care team. The team is caring for a patient who has recently experienced a stroke. The patient is having problems swallowing. Which of the following health care providers should be consulted?

    1. Occupational therapist.

    2. Registered dietitian.

    3. Respiratory therapist.

    4. Speech-language pathologist.

3. Nurse practitioner or advanced practice nurses are vital to the health care team. Which of the following is true about advanced practice nurses?

    1. They are considered experts in a specialty area.

    2. Can only prescribe medication in collaboration with a medical doctor.

    3. Focus primarily on health promotion interventions.

    4. Have a registered nurse doctorate-level degree.

4. Ryan, the nurse practitioner, is part of a multidisciplinary team. The team's goal is to meet the patient's needs at home. Who is responsible for the coordination of care that is to be provided?

    1. Physician.

    2. Registered nurse.

    3. Licensed practical nurse.

    4. Nurse practitioner.

5. Your patient who is home alone is struggling to take care of herself. She verbalized "What do I do? I need more help." What would be most important for you to do?

    1. Call another nurse and figure out how to help the patient.

    2. Call the physician and confirm you prescribed Xanax to calm the patient.

    3. Call a licensed practical nurse to help the patient with her activities of daily living.

    4. Call a social worker to discuss care options for the patient.

6. When a patient that you are caring for is at risk for falls because of impaired gait, who is the best person to collaborate with?

    1. Occupational therapist.

    2. Dietician.

    3. Psychiatrist.

    4. Physical therapist.

7. Your patient can benefit from the use of an adaptive device for cutting food. Which member of the multidisciplinary team would be best to collaborate with?

   1. Occupational therapist.

   2. Dietician.

   3. Psychiatrist.

   4. Physical therapist.

8. Jerome, a nurse practitioner, is working at a tertiary hospital. The nursing team in his department consists of himself, one registered nurse, two licensed practical nurses, and one nursing assistant. As the nurse practitioner, it is important for Jerome to have the knowledge of which responsibility may be done by whom. Which of the following patient assignments is appropriate for the nursing assistant?

   1. A colostomy patient requesting assistance with irrigation.

   2. A patient who was diagnosed with cerebral vascular accident just 3 days prior needs assistance to go to the bathroom.

   3. Medication for patient with cerebral palsy.

   4. Patient with sepsis who needs an intravenous push medication.

9. Janelle, a nurse practitioner, is the team leader of nursing care in a busy medical/surgical unit. Which of the following would need immediate intervention by Janelle?

   1. A nurse is talking with the patient's family with direct permission from the patient.

   2. A registered nurse who wears gloves with her gown before she enters the room of a patient who is diagnosed with localized herpes zoster.

   3. A licensed practical nurse who has gathered all the supplies necessary for sterile dressing change before going into the patient's room.

   4. The registered nurse who changes the linens on the bed while the patient with Ménière disease goes to the bathroom.

10. The nurse practitioner asked a nursing assistant to assist in ambulating a patient who is recovering from a hysterectomy. Two hours later, the patient calls and asked to be walked. According to the patient, she has not seen the nursing assistant. Jerome found the nursing assistant on her phone in the break room. Which of the following should the nurse practitioner do next?

    1. Remind her what Jerome asked her to do.

    2. Demand that the assistant gets off her cell phone right that very minute.

3. Report the nursing assistant to the nursing supervisor.

4. Fill out an incident report right away.

11. Nancy, a nurse practitioner, is caring for a patient in the acute cardiac unit. She is writing her handoff note for the next nurse practitioner. Which of the following is vital information that needs to be communicated to the next shift?

    1. Patient's vital signs and what patient still needs know.

    2. Patient's vital signs, lab work drawn, and nutritional intake.

    3. Any respiratory difficulty, electrocardiogram interpretation results, activity tolerance, and any vital sign instability during his shift.

    4. Patient's physician's name, age and activity tolerance.

12. A male patient with chronic obstructive pulmonary disease (COPD) informs the registered nurse that he did get his annual flu shot this year but has never had his pneumonia vaccination. Which of the following should the registered nurse report to the nurse practitioner?

    1. Blood pressure of 150/85 mmHg.

    2. Respiratory rate of 27 breaths/min.

    3. Heart rate of 93 beats/min.

    4. Oral temperature of 101.2 F (38.4°C).

13. The registered nurse measures the vital signs of an intubated patient after the respiratory therapists perform suctioning. Which vital sign should the nurse report to the nurse practitioner right away?

    1. Respiratory rate of 24 breaths/min.

    2. Heart rate of 98 beats/min.

    3. Blood pressure of 160/90 mmHg.

    4. Tympanic temperature of 101.4°F (38.6°C).

14. During a shift, the team had a reassigned nurse from the postpartum unit. Which of the following patients should be given to the reassigned nurse?

    1. Patient with chronic obstructive pulmonary disease displaying Cheyne–Stokes respiration.

    2. Patient with a head injury and a Glasgow Coma Sale of 5.

    3. Patient with myocardial infarction and complaining of burning on urination.

    4. Patient with a spinal cord injury requiring assistance with his meal.

15. A concerned registered nurse aide approaches the nurse practitioner about a patient's T-tube in the common bile duct. "I'm concerned that it's draining too much. It has drained over 700 mL over the course of our shift!" What would be the nurse practitioner's response?

    1. That is actually a small amount. I had a patient once who drained 2000 mL in one shift.

    2. That is a normal amount of drainage for a T-tube because it is his fifth day after surgery.

    3. That is a normal amount of drainage for a T-tube because it is his first day after surgery.

    4. I will further assess the patient because that is an excessive amount of drainage.

16. The Adult-Gerontology Acute Care Nurse Practitioner (AGACNP) was asked to cover for the NP in the emergency department. For the AGACNP to be more effective, which of the following patients would not be appropriate for the AGACNP to examine and treat?

    1. A 10-year-old patient who has been on pain medications for terminal cancer. Upon initial assessment, she has a relaxed respiratory rate of 12 breaths/min.

    2. A 23-year-old patient who says, "Heaven is near. I can hear the angels singing. You need to give me money for beer since I quit drinking 3 days ago. My arms and legs are jerking."

    3. A 45-year-old patient who says, "My heart is palpitating really fast, like it will jump out of my chest at any minute. It might be due to all the diet pills I took."

    4. A 68-year-old patient who slipped in his bathroom and ended up with a crack on his head.

17. The nurse practitioner was managing five patients during his shift. To lighten his load, he works with the registered nurse. One of his patients was diagnosed with sleep deprivation related to a disrupted sleep cycle. Which action can he delegate to the registered nurse?

    1. Refer the patient to a sleep specialist.

    2. Prescribe a weight-loss medication for the patient to help reduce the chance of sleep apnea.

    3. Remind patient to sleep on his side instead of his back.

    4. Prescribe modafinil (Provigil) to promote daytime wakefulness.

18. The registered nurse informs the nurse practitioner that a patient who is receiving oxygen at a flow rate of 6 L/min by nasal cannula is complaining of nasal passage discomfort. What action would you suggest the registered nurse do to improve the patient's comfort?

    1. A simple face mask be used instead of a nasal cannula.

    2. The patient's oxygen be humidified.

    3. The patient be provided an extra pillow and blanket.

    4. The patient be asked to sit up in a chair at the bedside.

19. The nurse practitioner (NP) is working with an outpatient who is diagnosed with heart failure. Which of the following orders, if written by the physician, should the NP question?

    1. Administer lactated Ringer's solution intravenously (IV) at a rate of 50 mL/hr.

    2. Administer 0.9% normal saline solution IV at a rate of 125 mL/hr.

    3. Administer Potassium 40 mEq tab once daily orally.

    4. Administer Lasix 40 mg twice daily orally.

20. The nurse practitioner is performing a preoperative history and physical on a patient. Which of the following information, when obtained before admitting a patient before arthroscopic knee surgery, should be reported to the surgeon?

    1. Knee pain level of 9 of 10 (0 to 10 pain scale).

    2. Warm, red, and swollen knee.

    3. History of knee surgery on other knee.

    4. Shellfish and iodine allergy.

21. The nurse practitioner (NP) is caring for a patient with acute respiratory syndrome. The patient is receiving oxygen by nonrebreather mask, but the patient's arterial blood gas measurements still show poor oxygenation. As the NP working with the pulmonologist, what order of action would you anticipate from the pulmonologist?

    1. Perform endotracheal intubation and initiate mechanical ventilation.

    2. Administer furosemide (Lasix) 100 mg intravenously push STAT.

    3. Immediately begin continuous positive airway pressure via the patient's nose and mouth.

    4. Call code for respiratory arrest.

22. Which of the following medications for a patient with pulmonary embolism is more important to clarify with the nurse practitioner before administering to the patient?

    1. Morphine sulfate 2 to 4 mg intravenously.

    2. Warfarin (Coumadin) 1.0 mg by mouth (PO).

    3. Cephalexin 250 mg PO.

    4. Heparin infusion at 900 units/hr.

23. A registered nurse is making a home visit to a 51-year-old patient who was recently hospitalized because of right leg deep vein thrombosis and a pulmonary embolism. The patient was ordered enoxaparin (Lovenox) subcutaneously. Which assessment information will the registered nurse need to communicate to the nurse practitioner?

    1. Multiple ecchymotic areas are on the patient's arms.

    2. Patient is unable to remember her husband's first name.

    3. The patient's right calf is warm to the touch and is larger than the left calf.

    4. The patient verbalized that her right leg aches all night.

24. The nurse practitioner just finished thoracentesis for a patient with recurrent left pleural effusion caused by lung cancer. The procedure removed 1800 mL of fluid. On assessment, which of the following side effects would you write as an order to be called to the nurse practitioner if they occur?

    1. The patient's blood pressure is 100/50 mmHg and her heart rate is 100 beats/min.

    2. Patient is complaining of insomnia.

    3. The patient complains of sharp, stabbing chest pain with every deep breath.

    4. The patient's dressing at the procedure site has 1 cm of bloody drainage.

25. Violet, a nurse practitioner, knows that one category of collaboration is nurse practitioner–patient collaboration. It is the nurse practitioner's job to make sure that patients are knowledgeable and have the correct information about their conditions. Before a nurse practitioner can expect cooperation from a patient or any nurse–patient relationship, what is imperative for this relationship to begin?

    1. Information.

    2. Health care plan.

    3. Physician's referral.

    4. Trust.

26. The nurse practitioner is teaching 37-year-old Mr. Gonzales about his newly diagnosed syndrome of inappropriate antidiuretic hormone. Which declaration from the patient best shows that he correctly understands how to manage his condition?

    1. I should drink at least 10 glasses of water every single day.

    2. I should limit my fluid intake. I should drink about four glasses of water daily or about 32 ounces.

    3. I should limit my sodium intake to 2 g every day.

    4. I should report constipation to the doctor.

27. The nurse practitioner has just reviewed instructions with his patient for an oral glucose tolerance test to be performed next week. Which statement made by the patient shows a need for more teaching?

    1. I will eat a light breakfast the morning of the test.

    2. I will take 100 mg of glucose at the start of the test.

    3. I am expecting to have my blood drawn at 30- and 60-minute intervals during the test.

    4. I will report any symptoms of dizziness, sweating, and/or weakness that occur during the test.

28. A patient was just diagnosed with tuberculosis. The nurse practitioner is discussing the management of his condition. Which statement by the patient shows the need for further teaching?

    1. Every member of my family needs to have themselves checked and get tested for tuberculosis.

    2. I will continue taking my isoniazid until I will feel completely well.

    3. I will cover my mouth and nose when I cough or sneeze. I will also put my used tissues in a plastic bag.

    4. I will revise my diet to include more foods that are rich in iron, protein, and vitamin C.

29. The nurse practitioner is making a checklist for a 61-year-old patient who is learning to do self-catherization. Which of the following is most helpful?

    1. Write at a high school reading level.

    2. Use short words and sentences.

    3. Print material in a fun and colorful font.

    4. Include charts and graphs.

30. Bill, the nurse practitioner, is working with a new registered nurse (RN), Jacky. He has observed that Jacky is reluctant to delegate tasks to other members of the health care team. Bill recognizes that this reluctance is most likely due to:

    1. Role modeling behaviors of the preceptor; in this scenario, Bill is the preceptor.

    2. The philosophy of the new RN's school of nursing.

    3. The orientation provided to the new RN.

    4. The RN is still learning to trust the other members of the health care team.

31. Helen, a nurse practitioner, is working with a nursing assistant and a registered nurse (RN). The nursing assistant approaches Helen and informs her that the RN is not assessing a patient with abdominal pain despite multiple requests. Which of the following is best for Helen to do?

    1. Ask the RN if she needs any help.

    2. Assess the patient and inform the RN about what needs to be done.

    3. Ask the patient if he is satisfied with his RN's care.

    4. Contact the nursing supervisor to address the situation.

32. The nurse practitioner has just intubated a patient in acute respiratory distress in the intensive care unit. The registered nurse is verifying placement and positioning of the endotracheal tube. Which action by the registered nurse should cause the nurse practitioner to intervene immediately?

    1. Assessment for bilateral breath sounds and symmetrical chest movements.

    2. Auscultation over the stomach to rule out esophageal intubation.

    3. Marking the tube 1 cm from where it touches the incisor tooth or nares.

    4. Ordering a chest radiograph to confirm placement of tube.

33. A 17-year-old girl is with her mother in the exam room for the girl's school physical. Before asking about the girl's sexual history, which of the following should be stated by the nurse practitioner?

    1. You seem really close as mother and daughter. I will ask questions about your sexual history now.

    2. Mother, I will have to ask you to step out so I can complete the health history.

    3. Mother, do you think your daughter is sexually active?

    4. Do you think your mother should leave the exam room now?

34. A 54-year-old patient is being discharged from the hospital. The nurse practitioner (NP) prescribes lisinopril (Prinivil, Zestril) for him to take at home. The NP should inform the registered nurse to inform the patient about which of the following common side effects?

    1. Hypokalemia.

    2. Constipation.

    3. Hypertension.

    4. Cough.

35. A 28-year-old female patient has type 1 diabetes. She has consulted her endocrinologist because she wants to be pregnant. She is given information about pregnancy and diabetes. What is the first thing a nurse practitioner needs to discuss with the prospective parents?

    1. Education about dietary modifications during pregnancy.

    2. The need for early prenatal medical oversight.

    3. Consider adoption instead of giving birth.

    4. Understanding the health risk to the mother.

36. A 43-year-old male patient visits a urologist inquiring about getting a vasectomy. You are the nurse practitioner assisting the urologist. Which of the following statements should you use during patient education?

    1. If you ever do change your mind, the reversal procedure is simple.

    2. You will need to have annual checkups and sperm count.

    3. You will need to use another type of contraception until your sperm count is zero.

    4. We will not be able to do the vasectomy if you have a history of cardiac disease.

37. The nurse practitioner is working with a patient who is prescribed captopril (Capoten). He realizes that the patient needs further teaching when the patient says:

    1. "I should not stand up too quickly."

    2. "I will take my blood pressure every week."

    3. "I will start using a salt substitute."

    4. "I'll call if I ever get a fever or sore throat."

38. The football coach, together with the school nurse, created a program in which they teach the team about proper hydration, especially during hot weather. The nurse teaches them to avoid dehydration by:

    1. Taking one to two salt tablets before starting practice.

    2. Changing practice times to early morning or evening.

    3. Taking a fluid break every 30 minutes during practice.

    4. Drinking extra water before and after practice.

39. A patient who is combative and mildly confused has an indwelling urinary catheter order. How should the nurse practitioner (NP) proceed?

    1. Gather all equipment for performing the procedure.

    2. Ask a colleague for help because the NP would not be able to do it alone.

    3. Obtain a restraint order before performing the procedure.

    4. Sedate the patient so that the indwelling catheter can be placed.

40. In any health care setting both minor and major errors can occur. Which of the following is considered the most critical in reducing such errors?

    1. Interprofessional collaboration.

    2. Nursing care plan.

    3. Open communication.

    4. Close communication.

41. The nurse practitioner is performing a preoperative history and physical on a patient who is getting ready to undergo an emergent hysterectomy. The patient revealed that she is allergic to latex. To which of the following does the nurse practitioner communicate this information?

    1. Physician.

    2. Dietitian.

    3. OR scrub nurse.

    4. Anesthesiologist.

42. After a discussion with the multidisciplinary team, the team decides to implement behavior modification with a patient. Which of the following actions is of primary importance during this time?

    1. Ensure that the rewards are important to the patient.

    2. Establish a fixed interval schedule for reinforcement.

3. Confirm that all members of the health care team understand and comply with the treatment plan.

4. Establish mutually agreed on, realistic goals.

43. The nurse practitioner is expected to collaborate with all members of the health care team. Which health care team member should the nurse practitioner closely collaborate with?

    1. Physician.

    2. Dietician.

    3. Licensed practical nurse.

    4. Nurse supervisor.

44. With which category of collaboration is health promotion, treatment strategies and options, and end-of-life decision-making discussed?

    1. Nurse–patient.

    2. Nurse–nurse.

    3. Interprofessional.

    4. Interorganizational.

45. Which of the following is the desired outcome when collaboration occurs?

    1. Eliminating patient's disease.

    2. Making patient comfortable in a hospital setting.

    3. Improved health care quality.

    4. More efficient teamwork.

46. Which of the following describes nurse-on-nurse aggression?

    1. Vertical violence.

    2. Lateral violence.

    3. Verbal violence.

    4. Physical violence.

47. The nurse practitioner is managing the care for a patient with pulmonary embolus. Which of the following may be delegated to the licensed practical nurse on your patient care team?

    1. Evaluate the patient's chest pain complaint.

    2. Monitor laboratory values for any changes in oxygenation.

    3. Assess for symptoms of respiratory failure.

    4. Auscultate lungs for crackles.

48. A 16-year-old patient calls your clinic saying that he is concerned he might have a sexually transmitted infection. However, he does not want his parents to know. To appropriately work with the patient, what should be your response?

    1. We can test you, but if it is positive, your parents will be informed.

    2. We apologize, but minors cannot be tested without the presence of a guardian.

    3. We can test and treat you. Records will be kept confidential.

    4. We can test you without parental consent, but if your results are positive, we would have to notify the health department.

49. Your patient has returned to your unit after surgery. The patient is complaining of pain and rates it at a level 9 of 10. You review the chart and saw that the nurse practitioner has an order for 10 mg of morphine sulfate written postoperatively. Before administering the medication, what should be you do first?

    1. Contact the nurse practitioner before proceeding.

    2. Call the pharmacy.

    3. Prepare the medication for administration.

    4. Set up a piggyback infusion system.

50. A 29-year-old, 40-week pregnant woman is about to give birth. Her obstetrician has already been informed and is still on her way and no other obstetrician is available. In this scenario, who is the best to approach?

    1. Nurse practitioner.

    2. Nurse anesthetist.

    3. Nurse midwife.

    4. Clinical nurse specialist.

51. A patient with type 2 diabetes has noticed that her feet have started to swell. She is also experiencing foot pain at rest. Which of the following professionals is the best person to work with to address the patient's concerns?

    1. Nutritionist.

    2. Physical therapist.

    3. Prosthetists.

    4. Podiatrist.

52. A registered nurse is frustrated after working with a very demanding patient. The registered nurse refuses to go back to take care of the patient. What would be the *best* response by the nurse practitioner?

    1. "Ignore him for now and get your work done. We'll have someone else care for him tomorrow."

    2. "Be patient. The patient has a lot of problems."

    3. "The patient is scared and might be taking it out on you. Together, let's figure out what to do."

    4. "I will talk to the patient and will try to figure out what to do."

53. An adult patient with an unstable condition is in the intensive care unit in which visitors are limited to the immediate family. The patient insists on having a visit from a traditional healer that the family visits regularly. How should the nurse practitioner interpret this request to properly work with the patient?

    1. Provision of holistic care requires that the client's belief system is honored.

    2. Traditional healers are not approved by the hospital as legitimate health care providers.

    3. Faith healers do not meet the standards for clergy exemption from the visitation rules.

    4. The principle of justice prohibits giving one client a privilege that other clients are not permitted.

54. As the nurse care coordinator in the mental health clinic, you administer the CAGE-AID alcohol/drug screening questionnaire, and the patient's result is positive. What is the best action the nurse practitioner needs to take next?

    1. Notify the patient's primary care physician for follow-up.

    2. Investigate what substances the patient is taking.

    3. Determine who acts as the patient's support system.

    4. Refer the patient to a rehabilitation program.

55. Your patient who has an ostomy is now home. The nurse practitioner calls her in a few days to see how she is doing. The patient reports that she thinks she is dehydrated. Which of the following is the best response by the nurse practitioner?

    1. "Does your mouth feel dry?"

    2. "You should drink more water. You might not be drinking enough."

    3. "Can you tell me what you have noticed that makes you say so?"

    4. "It's due to your medications."

56. As the nurse practitioner admits a patient who is being evaluated for increased seizures at home, which of the following tasks can you assign to the nursing assistant while you prepare for admission?

    1. Set up the patient's room with the necessary supplies and equipment needed for seizure precautions, which includes a sterile field.

    2. Receive patient report from the emergency department and transport patient to the room.

    3. Set up the patient's room with the necessary supplies and equipment needed for seizure precautions including a vest restraint for emergency use during a possible seizure.

    4. Set up the patient's room with the necessary supplies and equipment needed for seizure precautions.

57. As you call the mother of a patient who has already missed two appointments, she has stated that she is unable to bring her 14-year-old son to the clinic because of transportation issues. Who do you refer the patient to?

    1. Physician.

    2. The clinic social worker.

    3. Her insurance company.

    4. Physical therapist.

58. The nurse practitioner is teaching an immunocompromised patient about a proper diet once discharged. The patient is advised to avoid raw shelled oysters, and he asks why he should avoid them. The nurse practitioner is unsure. Which of the following should she call for more information?

    1. Dietician.

    2. Oncologist.

    3. Cafeteria.

    4. Nutritionist.

59. A nurse practitioner is working with a patient who has been diagnosed with systemic lupus erythematosus (SLE). Your patient has expressed that she wants to have a baby and wants to know what to expect with her condition. What is the best response?

    1. "You should get pregnant. You'll feel so much better."

    2. "How long have you been in remission?"

    3. "It is safer to become pregnant within 6 months of being diagnosed."

    4. "Those with SLE often have longer gestations than normal."

60. Your 65-year-old patient admitted for pneumonia requires nasotracheal suctioning. The patient has an intravenous (IV) infusion of antibiotics. The patient is febrile and asks if he can get a bed bath because of profuse sweating. What can you delegate to the nursing assistant working with you on that shift?

    1. Teach the patient proper use of an incentive spirometer.

    2. Change the IV dressing.

    3. Perform bed bath.

    4. Nasotracheal suctioning.

61. A nursing assistant asks why the patient you are managing needs his blood pressure taken three times per shift. As the nurse practitioner, you explain the purpose of such patient intervention. Your interaction with the nurse assistant is an example of which five rights of delegation?

    1. Right Supervision.

    2. Right Task.

    3. Right Circumstance.

    4. Right Communication.

62. An elderly patient who lives alone is to be discharged in 2 days. He tells the nurse practitioner that it is difficult to prepare to be at home because he lives alone. Who is the proper person to approach?

    1. Registered nurse.

    2. Physician.

    3. Social worker.

    4. Dietician.

63. A patient who underwent surgery is concerned about the adverse effects of his postoperative pain medication. Which of the following members of the interprofessional care team may help the patient understand the medication better?

    1. Nursing assistant.

    2. Nurse practitioner.

    3. Anesthesiologist.

    4. Social worker.

64. A patient informs the nurse practitioner (NP) that he is experiencing a dull ache in his sides that has been ongoing for 4 days now. It happens when he bends over. The NP responds with "Okay, go on." The NP's response is an example of:

    1. Back-channeling.

    2. Open-ended question.

    3. Inference.

    4. Cue.

65. A patient who underwent an excision of a sebaceous cyst was provided specific written and verbal instructions about wound care, signs of infection, and when to follow-up for suture removal. As the nurse practitioner, what is the *best* way to follow up with the patient post procedure?

    1. Calling to evaluate the patient's condition.

    2. Sending a personal message to remind him or her not to drive until the next appointment via Facebook messenger.

    3. Mailing a card reminding him or her to schedule an annual physical.

    4. Texting a survey to assess the facility's performance.

66. Which of the following is the most effective strategy in improving the patient's adherence to a care regimen?

    1. Involve the patient's family in the treatment plan.

    2. Partner with the patient in the teaching/learning process.

    3. Reinforce that the patient must follow the plan of care.

    4. Schedule more frequent follow-up visits.

15 Collaborative Practice Answers & Rationales

1. Answer: 2

Rationale: Interprofessional collaborative practice is defined by the World Health Organization as a situation that occurs "when multiple health workers from different professional backgrounds work together with patients, families, caregivers, and communities to deliver the highest quality of care."

2. Answer: 4

Rationale: The main function of a speech-language pathologist is to assist patients who are communicatively impaired by intervening in speech, language, and/or swallowing disorders.

3. Answer: 1

Rationale: All nurse practitioners or advanced practice nurses make independent decisions. They also work as expert clinicians.

4. Answer: 2

Rationale: When meeting the home care need of a patient, it is the registered nurse that is responsible for the coordination of care.

5. Answer: 4

Rationale: A social worker can contact other agencies and make arrangements to help meet the patient's needs.

6. Answer: 4

Rationale: The best person to collaborate with when the patient is at risk for falls because of impaired gait is a physical therapist. Physical therapists assess, plan, implement, and evaluate interventions related to the patient's functional abilities in terms of gait, strength, mobility, balance, joint range, and coordination.

7. Answer: 1

Rationale: The best person to collaborate with when a patient can benefit from an adaptive device in cutting food would be an occupational therapist. An occupational therapist helps increase a patient's independence in terms of their activities of daily living.

8. Answer: 2

Rationale: Ambulation is one activity with which the nursing assistant can help. The licensed practical nurse may help with the

cerebral palsy patient and may assist with colostomy care. The patient with sepsis needs a registered nurse or a nurse practitioner.

9. Answer: 4

Rationale: The nursing assistant should assist the patient in going to the bathroom. They should walk hand in hand. The main characteristic of Ménière disease is attacks of dizziness, which may cause a fall and injure the patient. The safest way is to assist with ambulation.

10. Answer: 3

Rationale: The chain of command should be utilized in resolving this issue.

11. Answer: 3

Rationale: All the information provided is important, but answer 3 includes vital information that the next shift needs to be aware of. It is the only choice with reports of the patient's overall tolerance to care and cardiac results.

12. Answer: 4

Rationale: By not getting his flu shot and pneumonia vaccine, the patient is at risk for developing pneumonia or influenza. Increased temperature is one indication of infection, which occurs in someone with influenza or pneumonia. All other vital signs, although elevated, are not cause for immediate concern.

13. Answer: 4

Rationale: Increased temperature is a sign of infection. Infections are always a threat for patients that receive mechanical ventilation. The endotracheal tube provides an access route for bacteria or viruses to the lower part of the respiratory system.

14. Answer: 3

Rationale: The reassigned nurse can be assigned to the patient with a urinary tract infection. It is good to remember that reassigned nurses need stable patients.

15. Answer: 3

Rationale: On postoperative day 1, a T-tube can drain from 500 to 1000 mL. After the first day, the amount of drainage decreases. Effective communication from the nurse practitioner is shown in this scenario.

16. Answer: 1

Rationale: Nurse practitioners should only examine and treat those patients who are within their scope of practice.

17. Answer: 3

Rationale: The registered nurse can remind patient about actions and activities that were already taught by the nurse practitioner (NP). Discussing and teaching would require additional education and training and are within the scope of the NP.

18. Answer: 2

Rationale: When the oxygen flow rate is higher than 4 L/min, the mucous membranes can dry out. The best treatment is to add humidification to the oxygen delivery system. None of the other choices will treat the problem.

19. Answer: 2

Rationale: This rate is too high for a patient with heart failure. The patient will not be able to handle such a large amount of fluid with their cardiac system.

20. Answer: 4

Rationale: It is vital to inform the physician of any allergies so the physician can refrain from giving medications that have iodine content. In this way, a safe alternative may be prescribed instead.

21. Answer: 1

Rationale: There is the presence of refractory hypoxemia in this scenario, which is when the oxygenation status of the patient does not improve even with a nonrebreather mask, which delivers nearly 100% oxygen. The patient may go into respiratory arrest unless his health care providers intervene by providing intubation and mechanical ventilation.

22. Answer: 2

Rationale: Based on the patient's diagnosis, the other orders are appropriate. Medication safety guidelines state that using a trailing zero is not appropriate when writing medication orders because the order can easily be mistaken for a larger dose, such as 10 mg.

23. Answer: 2

Rationale: Confusion in a patient this age is unusual and can be an indication of intracerebral bleeding associated with enoxaparin use. The right leg symptoms are consistent with a resolving deep vein thrombosis; the patient may need more

teaching about keeping it elevated above the heart to reduce the pain and swelling. More teaching might also need to be done about injury prevention when taking anticoagulants. This does not indicate a need to call the nurse practitioner.

24. Answer: 1

Rationale: Removal of large amounts of fluid from the pleural space can cause fluid to shift from the circulation into the pleural space. This can cause hypotension and tachycardia. The patient needs to receive intravenous fluids to correct this.

25. Answer: 4

Rationale: Even when the patient is informed about and provided with the health care plan, without trust, the nurse–patient relationship will not be as effective. Cooperation from the patient may not be fully given without trust.

26. Answer: 2

Rationale: In syndrome of inappropriate antidiuretic hormone (SIADH) there is excess secretion of ADH that causes fluid retention, dilutes the plasma causing suppression of aldosterone, and increases renal excretion of sodium. Water then moves into the cells from the plasma and interstitial spaces causing cellular edema.

27. Answer: 1

Rationale: The oral glucose tolerance test is performed fasting. Therefore, the patient needs to be on nothing by mouth after midnight before the test. All other choices are correct responses regarding the test.

28. Answer: 2

Rationale: The patient needs to continuously take the drug for 6 consecutive months.

29. Answer: 2

Rationale: When making written instructions for an elderly client, information should be as simple as possible. Use short words and sentences, and avoid using jargon.

30. Answer: 4

Rationale: Lack of trust is one of the most common reasons for any reluctance in task delegation.

31. Answer: 4

Rationale: The nurse practitioner should use the proper channel of communication. The nursing supervisor is responsible for the actions of the different members of the nursing team.

32. Answer: 3

Rationale: The mark should be at the level where it touches the incisor tooth or nares. This mark is to verify that the tube has not shifted.

33. Answer: 2

Rationale: The nurse practitioner should ask the mother to step out for a couple of minutes to finish the health history. Privacy and confidentially should be observed because it is a critical development for a teenager that needs to be respected.

34. Answer: 4

Rationale: A common side effect of lisinopril (Prinivil, Zestril) is cough. Other side effects include hyperkalemia, proteinuria, and diarrhea. Hypertension is the reason for the prescription.

35. Answer: 2

Rationale: Pregnancy makes metabolic control of type I diabetes more difficult. Clients with type 1 diabetes should start prenatal care early so that potential complications can be avoided, minimized, or controlled.

36. Answer: 3

Rationale: A second method of contraception is necessary until the sperm count is zero. No need for follow-up after that. Reversing a vasectomy is difficult. There is no correlation between the vasectomy and cardiac disease.

37. Answer: 3

Rationale: Patient should not use any salt substitute because angiotensin-converting enzyme inhibitors contain potassium and cause the body to retain potassium. The other responses are appropriate.

38. Answer: 3

Rationale: The combination of physical activity and hot weather accelerates dehydration, especially during hot weather. The body needs regular water and electrolyte replenishment, so a short break every 30 minutes is recommended. Salt tablets need a written approval from each athlete's health care provider. Drinking before and after practice is a good idea but will not provide water and electrolyte balance during strenuous activity.

39. Answer: 2

Rationale: The nurse practitioner should ask a colleague to help because he will not be able to work with the patient alone. The patient needs to be well informed about the procedure before preparing all the materials necessary. Preparing it without informing the patient might increase the patient's anxiety level. Restraint should be the last resort. The procedure is feasible with assistance, and informing the physician otherwise is inappropriate.

40. Answer: 1

Rationale: Interprofessional collaboration is considered to be the most critical instrument in reducing patient care errors. It is widely accepted that interprofessional collaboration may improve communication between all health professionals.

41. Answer: 4

Rationale: Latex allergy is becoming increasingly common but is not usually serious, but it still needs to be communicated to the surgeon or the anesthesiologist.

42. Answer: 3

Rationale: To be able to implement a plan successfully, it is of primary importance that all the members of the health care team understand and will comply with the treatment plan. All other choices are not of primary importance.

43. Answer: 1

Rationale: The health care team member that a nurse practitioner closely collaborates with is the physician to ensure a successful practice.

44. Answer: 1

Rationale: A nurse practitioner collaborates with patients regarding health promotion and disease prevention behaviors, treatment strategies and options, lifestyle changes, and end-of-life decision-making.

45. Answer: 3

Rationale: The desired outcome when collaboration occurs is health care quality. Eliminating patient's disease is not always possible; therefore it can become an unrealistic expectation or outcome. Teamwork occurs when collaboration happens but is not the main goal, and the same goes for answer 2.

46. Answer: 2

Rationale: A nurse-on-nurse aggression and intergroup is a horizontal violence or lateral violence. This may be verbal or physical.

47. Answer: 4

Rationale: A licensed practical nurse who has been trained to auscultate lung sounds may gather data by routine assessment and observation, under the supervision of a registered nurse or nurse practitioner.

48. Answer: 4

Rationale: Some states have a minimum age for seeking treatment for sexually transmitted diseases. Adolescents, however, are able to be seen without parental consent. The Health Insurance Portability and Accountability Act Privacy Rule protects their information and prohibits sharing of this information without the patient's permission. The law does mandate that any positive results are to be reported to public health departments.

49. Answer: 1

Rationale: Because there is no indication about how the medication should be given, the nurse practitioner should be contacted. Keep in mind the rule to prevent medication errors—right patient, right drug, right dose, right route, and the right time. Also, MSO4 may indicate magnesium sulfate as well as morphine. The order needs to be clarified with the nurse practitioner.

50. Answer: 3

Rationale: Nurse midwives are members of the nursing team and the obstetrician team. They are the best to approach in this scenario while waiting for the obstetrician. They are advanced practice registered nurses who work with nonrisk pregnant women during the pregnancy under the supervision of an obstetrician.

51. Answer: 4

Rationale: Podiatrists provide care and services to patients who have foot problems. They often work with diabetic patients to assess the feet to prevent diabetic foot complications. They recommend special footwear, they often clip toenails, and they also treat other nondiabetic patients with disorders of the foot.

52. Answer: 3

Rationale: This response is best because it explains the patient's behavior without belittling the nursing assistant's feelings. The nursing assistant is encouraged to help solve the problem with the nurse practitioner.

53. Answer: 1

Rationale: The patient's spiritual needs must be met within the framework of his personal belief systems, even if those beliefs differ from those of the nurse practitioner. Collaboration includes compromise.

54. Answer: 1

Rationale: The CAGE-AID screening questionnaire, focusing on drug and alcohol, has four questions for the patient. Once the patient answers "yes" to any of the questions, the result is considered a positive screen. The patient needs to be referred to a primary care physician for follow-up regarding drug or alcohol abuse.

55. Answer: 3

Rationale: It is important to make sure that as the nurse practitioner you use effective verbal communication, especially when talking to a patient on the phone. One way of doing that is to get as much detail from the patient as possible.

56. Answer: 4

Rationale: The only thing that you can delegate to the nursing assistant as a nurse practitioner is the indirect aspects of care. This includes setting up the patient's room with supplies and equipment needed for seizure precautions. Sterile fields are not part of seizure precautions, and nursing assistants are not permitted to work with sterile supplies and procedures. Restraints are not used during seizures and are out of scope for a nursing assistant.

57. Answer: 2

Rationale: The clinic social worker knows community resources that can assist the client. These may include a local volunteer agency that provides transportation for medical appointments.

58. Answer: 1

Rationale: Patients with immunosuppression should be taught to avoid raw or undercooked foods including seafood, meat, poultry, and eggs. The following increases risk for bacterial or norovirus infection.

59. Answer: 2

Rationale: Your response needs to be a mix of assessment and implementation. In this situation, it requires assessment because of the patient's condition. The patient needs to be in remission for at least 5 months before conceiving. It is recommended that patients with systemic lupus erythematosus get pregnant at least 2 years from diagnosis.

60. Answer: 3

Rationale: The appropriate task to delegate is a bath. All other choices need a higher level of training and should be done by the nurse practitioner.

61. Answer: 4

Rationale: Effective delegation requires effective communication. Delegation communication is a two-way process; it allows participants to ask questions and to clarify any confusion.

62. Answer: 3

Rationale: A social worker can make arrangements for a meal delivery service to provide nutritious meals daily, or recommend a congregate meal site near the client's home.

63. Answer: 2

Rationale: The nurse practitioner (NP) working with the patient needs to be knowledgeable about the medications the patient is taking, including their actions, effects, and interactions. The anesthesiologist is also knowledgeable, but given that this is symptom is postoperative, the person who is readily available to approach is the NP currently working with the patient.

64. Answer: 1

Rationale: Back-channeling gives positive comments such as "all right," "go on," or "uh-huh" to the speaker, indicating that you heard what the patient is saying and are interested in hearing the full story.

65. Answer: 1

Rationale: As the nurse practitioner who is managing the patient's care, it is best to use direct contact with the patient. Calling the patient is the *best* way to communicate to reduce miscommunication and misunderstandings.

66. Answer: 2

Rationale: One category of collaboration is nurse–patient collaboration. Patients are encouraged for to gain independence, especially for home treatment. It is vital that patients are able to learn how to take care of themselves.

16

Systems Thinking

As a nurse practitioner, you are exploring the systems thinking approach to your practice. Its details and processes are as important as the application itself.

1. As a nurse practitioner, what is one of the major factors that systems thinking pushes you to consider?

    1. Time.

    2. Patient.

    3. Process.

    4. Consequences.

2. Rather than static thinking, what does systems thinking require?

    1. Critical thinking.

    2. Dynamic thinking.

    3. Creative thinking.

    4. Analytical thinking.

3. Rather than "tree-by-tree" thinking, what is utilized in systems thinking?

    1. "Forest" thinking.

    2. "Bush" thinking.

    3. "City" thinking.

    4. "Flower" thinking.

4. What is the very first step in systems thinking?

    1. Specify the problem.

    2. Build hypothesis.

    3. Create conclusion.

    4. Gather details.

5. In systems thinking, what is described as viewing causality as an ongoing process?

1. Systems thinking.

2. Closed-loop thinking.

3. Open-looped thinking.

4. Operational thinking.

6. In systems thinking, what is also known as a mechanistic think?

    1. Scientific thinking.

    2. Closed-loop thinking.

    3. Open-looped thinking.

    4. Operational thinking.

7. In systems thinking, which type of thinking is in relation to hypothesis?

    1. Scientific thinking.

    2. Closed-loop thinking.

    3. Open-looped thinking.

    4. Operational thinking.

8. Which tool of systems thinking believes that everything is reliant on something else for survival?

    1. Interconnectedness.

    2. Synthesis.

    3. Emergence.

    4. Feedback loops.

9. Which tool believes that systems thinking is really about being able to decipher the way things influence each other in a system?

    1. Feedback loops.

    2. Causality.

    3. Systems mapping.

    4. Emergence.

10. Which tool of systems thinking believes that larger things emerge from smaller parts?

    1. Feedback loops.
    2. Causality.
    3. Systems mapping.
    4. Emergence.

11. In systems thinking, what refers to opposed to analysis, which is the dissection of complexity into manageable components?

    1. Interconnectedness.
    2. Synthesis.
    3. Emergence.
    4. Feedback loops.

12. In relation to systems thinking, what is a visual map?

    1. Detailed plans to complete the project.
    2. Organizational chart listing roles and duties for each team member.
    3. Supporting ideas or concepts.
    4. A map for the mind.

13. In mind/visual mapping, what does GTD stand for?

    1. Get to drawing.
    2. Goal too deep.
    3. Got to dig.
    4. Getting things done.

14. Which principle of systems thinking is defined as capturing not only what your product does but understanding why the users do what they do with your product?

    1. Purposefulness.
    2. Composition.
    3. Emergence.
    4. Perspective.

15. In systems thinking, which theory is described as a theory in mathematics to study small changes in the parameters of a nonlinear system?

    1. Chaos theory.
    2. Catastrophe theory.
    3. Cybernetic theory.
    4. General systems theory.

16. In systems thinking, which theory explains why processes can have similar starting points, yet lead to different outcomes?

    1. Chaos theory.
    2. Catastrophe theory.
    3. Path dependency theory.
    4. General systems theory.

17. In systems thinking, which theory is described as where changes occur through fixed rules about changing relationships?

    1. Chaos theory.
    2. Catastrophe theory.
    3. Path dependency theory.
    4. General systems theory.

18. In systems thinking, which theory is synonymous for systems theory?

    1. General systems theory.
    2. Cybernetics theory.
    3. Path dependency theory.
    4. Chaos theory.

19. What is a system context diagram?

    1. High-level map of a system and its surrounding environment.
    2. System that generates diagrams for a company.
    3. Diagram that shows how external entities relate to each other.
    4. Company's in-house method for diagramming systems.

20. Which one of the following is defined as a methodology for mapping and modeling the forces of change in a complex system?

    1. System science.
    2. System dynamics.
    3. System theory.
    4. System investigation.

21. What is the process of knowing how each part of the whole influences the outcome?

    1. Systems thinking.
    2. Global thinking.
    3. Assertive thinking.
    4. Hospitalist thinking.

22. A patient who has shortness of breath benefits from having the head of the bed elevated. This position can result in skin breakdown in the sacral area. The nurse practitioner decides to study the amount of sacral pressure that occurs in other positions. What decision-making process is the nurse engaging in?

    1. Research method.

    2. Trial-and-error method.

    3. Intuition.

    4. The nursing process.

23. In which step of the nursing process does the nurse practitioner analyze data and identify client problems?

    1. Assessment.

    2. Diagnosis.

    3. Planning outcomes.

    4. Evaluation.

24. In which phase of the nursing process does the nurse decide whether her actions have successfully treated the client's health problem?

    1. Assessment.

    2. Diagnosis.

    3. Planning outcomes.

    4. Evaluation.

25. Multiple data are collected every day in the hospital setting. Which of the following data should be validated?

    1. Urinalysis report indicates there are white blood cells in the urine.

    2. Client has clear breath sounds; you count a respiratory rate of 18 breaths/min.

    3. Chest x-ray report indicates the client has pneumonia in the right lower lobe.

    4. Client states she feels feverish; you measure the oral temperature at 97.7°F (36.5°C).

26. While you were doing your rounds, the high-pressure alarm on one of the patient's ventilators goes off. When you enter the room with your staff nurse to check on the patient, who has acute respiratory distress syndrome, the oxygen saturation monitor reads 87% and the patient is struggling to sit up. Which action should be taken next?

    1. Reassure the patient that the ventilator will do the work of breathing for him.

    2. Manually ventilate the patient while assessing possible reasons for the high-pressure alarm.

3. Increase the fraction of inspired oxygen on the ventilator to 100% in preparation for endotracheal suctioning.

4. Insert an oral airway to prevent the patient from biting on the endotracheal tube.

27. A high school student is brought to the emergency department by his friends. He is alert and ambulatory, but his T-shirt is soaked with blood. There is an open wound on his abdomen. His friends tell you that he jumped off the top of a car and landed on a sharp, metal object sticking out of the ground. Which statement should be concerning?

    1. The metal object was very dirty.

    2. His parents are diabetic.

    3. He pulled the metal object out of his abdomen.

    4. His shirt is soaked with blood.

28. A group of people enters the emergency department with complaints of cough, tightness in their throat, and extreme periorbital swelling. They report that someone threw a gas bomb their way. What would be the priority action?

    1. Readily transfer patients and visitors from the area.

    2. Check vital signs and auscultate lung sounds.

    3. Assist patients in the decontamination area.

    4. Direct patients to the cold or clean zone for immediate treatment.

29. The nurse practitioner is counseling patients at a community health fair about the importance of immunizations. Which of the following is most accurate about immunizations?

    1. Risk-free and recommended by all health care providers.

    2. Provide acquired immunity to some serious infectious disease.

    3. Will prevent all infectious diseases.

    4. Will give your body the antibodies to fight infections.

30. A nurse practitioner (NP) is working with disaster relief after a tornado. The NP's goal for the community is to prevent as much injury and death as possible from the uncontrollable event. Finding safe housing for survivors, providing support to families, organizing counseling, and securing physical care when needed are all examples of which type of prevention?

    1. Primary level.

    2. Secondary level.

    3. Tertiary level.

    4. Aggregate.

31. Which of the following is described as "an array of techniques and methods used for the collection and analysis of data gathered in the course of current health care practices in a defined care setting to identify and resolve problems in the system and improve the processes and outcomes of care"?

    1. Quality improvement.

    2. Performance.

    3. Critical pathways.

    4. Systems thinking.

32. As a nurse practitioner using a systems thinking approach, a benchmark should be set. What happens if you are unable to meet the benchmark?

    1. Blame your manager.

    2. Do a root cause analysis.

    3. Have a patient consultation.

    4. Try goal setting.

33. As the nurse practitioner in charge, you are evaluating the infection control procedures on the unit. Which of your findings would indicate a break in technique and the need for education of staff?

    1. The nurse puts on a mask, a gown, and gloves before entering the room of a client in strict isolation.

    2. A patient with active tuberculosis is asked to wear a mask when he leaves his room to go to another department for testing.

    3. A nurse with open, weeping lesions of the hands puts on gloves before giving direct patient care.

    4. The nurse's aide is not wearing gloves when feeding an elderly patient.

34. The nurse practitioner is evaluating whether nonprofessional staff understand how to prevent the transmission of HIV. Which of the following behaviors observed by you indicates correct application of universal precautions?

    1. An assistant puts on a mask and protective eye wear before assisting the nurse to suction a tracheostomy.

    2. A pregnant worker refuses to care for a patient known to have AIDS.

    3. An aide wears gloves to feed a helpless patient.

    4. A lab technician rests his hands on the desk to steady it while recapping the needle after drawing blood.

35. As the nurse practitioner in charge, you are reviewing the critical paths of the patients on the nursing unit. In performing a variance analysis, which of the following would indicate the need for further action and analysis?

    1. A patient's family visiting.

    2. Canceling physical therapy sessions on the weekend.

    3. Normal vital signs and absence of wound infection in a postoperative patient.

    4. A patient demonstrating accurate medication administration following teaching.

36. The nurse practitioner is the head of the Quality Improvement Team in the hospital. You are considering an initiative to prevent falls. Which of the following would be most successful?

    1. Placing all beds in the low position.

    2. Using color-coded wristbands.

    3. Putting a "Fall Risk" sign on patient doors.

    4. Frequent rounds of patient rooms.

37. The nurse practitioner-led Quality Improvement Team has discovered that there is a sudden increase in intravenous (IV) site infiltrations on a surgical unit. The nurse practitioner and team has implemented a Plan-Do-Study-Act initiative. Which step will come first?

    1. Analyze the data.

    2. Implement a new IV insertion policy.

    3. Monitor which IV needle gauges are used.

    4. Perform chart audits.

38. One of your patients in the oncology department is considering participating in a multisite trial of a new cancer medication. According to the "Patient's Bill of Rights," it is important for the patient to know that:

    1. All costs of the research are paid by the patient.

    2. The patient has the right to refuse to participate in research without fear of loss of care.

    3. The physicians will no longer be caring for him if he does not participate in the research.

    4. The research study is his only hope of treatment.

39. The nurse practitioner establishes a physical exercise area in the workplace and encourages all employees to use it. This is an example of which level of health promotion?

    1. Tertiary.

    2. Passive.

    3. Secondary.

    4. Primary.

40. In any approach, safety is of the outmost importance. What does safety in health care settings not provide?

    1. Reduction in the incidence of illness and injury.

    2. Prevention of extended length of treatment.

    3. Resolution of domestic problems the patient will have when they go home.

    4. An increases in patient's sense of well-being.

16 | Systems Thinking Answers & Rationales

1. Answer: 4

Rationale: Systems thinking leaders carefully balance the time needed when making decisions, keeping in mind short-term, long-term, and unintended consequences of actions. Sometimes, decisions need to be made quickly with little time for reflection. In those cases, common sense, instinct, and the importance of safety come into play. There are other times, however, when the consideration of consequences of an important decision becomes a priority. By surfacing and testing assumptions of potential outcomes, systems thinking leaders can carefully weigh the consequences of decisions. They also consider an issue fully and resist the urge to come to a quick conclusion.

2. Answer: 2

Rationale: Dynamic thinking skills enable you to trace your issue or challenge as a trajectory of performance over time. The trajectory should have a historical segment, a current state, and one or more future paths. Dynamic thinking thus puts a current situation in the context of where you came from and where you are going.

3. Answer: 1

Rationale: Forest thinking or pattern-oriented thinking is seeing beyond the details to the context of the relationships in which they are embedded.

4. Answer: 1

Rationale: The systems thinking method begins with specifying the problem situation. The next step would be to build a hypothesis.

5. Answer: 2

Rationale: Closed-loop thinking is viewing causality as an ongoing process, not as a one-time event, with effects feeding back to influence causes, and causes affecting each other.

6. Answer: 4

Rationale: Operational or mechanistic thinking is understanding how a behavior is actually generated.

7. Answer: 1

Rationale: Scientific thinking is knowing how to define testable hypotheses.

8. Answer: 1

Rationale: Systems thinking requires a shift in mindset, away from linear to circular. The fundamental principle of this shift is that everything is interconnected. We talk about interconnectedness not in a spiritual way, but in a biological sciences way. Essentially, everything is reliant on something else for survival. Humans need food, air, and water to sustain our bodies, and trees need carbon dioxide and sunlight to thrive. Everything needs something else, often a complex array of other things, to survive.

9. Answer: 2

Rationale: Causality as a concept in systems thinking is about being able to decipher the way things influence each other in a system. Cause and effect are common concepts in many professions and life in general. Parents try to teach this type of critical life lesson to their young ones, and I am sure you can remember a recent time you were at the mercy of an impact from an unintentional action.

10. Answer: 4

Rationale: From a systems perspective, we know that larger things emerge from smaller parts: emergence is the natural outcome of things coming together. In the most abstract sense, emergence describes the universal concept of how life emerges from individual biological elements in diverse and unique ways. Emergence is the outcome of the synergies of the parts; it is about nonlinearity and self-organization, and we often use the term *emergence* to describe the outcome of things interacting together.

11. Answer: 2

Rationale: In general, synthesis refers to the combining of two or more things to create something new. When it comes to systems thinking, the goal is synthesis, as opposed to analysis, which is the dissection of complexity into manageable components. Analysis fits into the mechanical and reductionist worldview, where the world is broken down into parts.

12. Answer: 3

Rationale: Creating a visual map is like constructing a model that shows those interactions between the different elements. By organizing various separated elements, the map brings coherence and facilitates the emergence of a new order. The use of visual mapping infuses and enforces one to view the information creation and management and exchange flow as process oriented at the base level and systematic at the higher level. This is indeed essential to understanding information and knowledge development.

13. Answer: 4

Rationale: Getting Things Done (GTD), the famous method created by David Allen, uses both the systems thinking approach and visual mapping for organizing tasks. GTD considers our activity as a workflow you can improve by using the right process and understanding it as a system.

14. Answer: 1

Rationale: Purposefulness is capturing not only what your product does or intends to do, but understanding why the users and other stakeholders do what they do with your product within the context of completing their tasks and activities.

15. Answer: 2

Rationale: Catastrophe theory is a theory in mathematics and geometry to study how small changes in parameters of a nonlinear system can lead to sudden and large changes in the behavior of a system.

16. Answer: 3

Rationale: Path dependency theory occurs in economics, social sciences, and physics. It refers to the explanations for why processes can have similar starting points yet lead to different outcomes, even if they follow the same rules, and outcomes are sensitive not only to initial conditions, but also to bifurcations and choices made along the way.

17. Answer: 1

Rationale: Chaos theory is a field of study in mathematics with applications in a wide number of disciplines to explain a dynamic system and that is highly sensitive to the initial conditions produce wildly different results. The changes occur through fixed rules about changing relationships, and without randomness.

18. Answer: 2

Rationale: Historically used as a synonym for systems theory, it is a field of study of the communication and control of regulatory feedback in both living and nonliving systems.

19. Answer: 1

Rationale: The term *system context* refers to the environment of your system. A system to be developed never stands on its own but is connected to its environment.

20. Answer: 2

Rationale: System dynamics is a methodology for mapping and modeling the forces of change in a complex system to better understand their interaction and govern the direction of the system; it enables stakeholders to combine input into a dynamic hypothesis that uses computer simulation to compare various scenarios for achieving change.

21. Answer: 1

Rationale: Systems thinking is an iterative learning process in which one takes a broad, holistic, long-term, perspective of the world and examines the linkages and interactions among its elements.

22. Answer: 1

Rationale: The types of clinical decisions that nurses actually make provide clues about how (and what types of) research information might assist in decision-making. Other authors have examined the clinical decisions of health care professionals (and the clinical questions arising from such decisions) as expressions of potential information need. Thus decisions are an important context for information use.

23. Answer: 1

Rationale: The nurse practitioner uses a systematic, dynamic way to collect and analyze data about a client, which is the first step in delivering nursing care. Assessment includes physiological data and psychological, sociocultural, spiritual, economic, and lifestyle factors.

24. Answer: 4

Rationale: Both the patient's status and the effectiveness of the nursing care must be continuously evaluated, and the care plan modified as needed.

25. Answer: 4

Rationale: Validation should be done when subjective and objective data do not make sense. In answer 4, it is inconsistent data when the patient feels feverish and you obtain a normal temperature. The other distractors do not offer conflicting data. Validation is not usually necessary for laboratory test results.

26. Answer: 2

Rationale: Manual ventilation of the patient will allow you to deliver a big percentage of Fio_2 (up to 100%) to the patient while you attempt to determine the cause of the high-pressure alarm. The first step should be to assess the reason and the resolution of the hypoxemia.

27. Answer: 3

Rationale: An impaled object may be giving a tamponade effect, and removal can result in abrupt hemodynamic decompensation.

28. Answer: 3

Rationale: In this scenario, systems thinking leads to decontamination as the first priority. Many health care facilities have decontamination areas with showers in the nuclear medicine department and/or the emergency departments to use in the case of radiation contamination.

29. Answer: 2

Rationale: The nurse practitioner should understand the mechanism of action, indications, and risks of immunizations as they do for all medications administered. Immunizations work passively providing acquired immunity to specific diseases.

30. Answer: 3

Rationale: Tertiary prevention involves the reduction of the amount and degree of disability, injury, and damage following a crisis. Primary prevention means keeping the crisis from occurring, and secondary prevention focuses on reducing the intensity and duration of a crisis during the crisis itself. There is no known aggregate care prevention level.

31. Answer: 1

Rationale: Quality improvement is an array of techniques and methods used for the collection and analysis of data gathered in the course of current health care practices in a defined care setting to identify and resolve problems in the system and improve the processes and outcomes of care.

32. Answer: 2

Rationale: Root cause analysis usually follows to assess the cause of unsatisfactory performance, and a search for best practices may be used to help address performance problems.

33. Answer: 3

Rationale: Persons with exudative lesions or weeping dermatitis should not give direct patient care or handle patient-care equipment until the condition resolves.

34. Answer: 1

Rationale: Masks and protective eye wear are indicated anytime there is great potential for splashing of body fluids that may be contaminated with blood. Suctioning of a tracheostomy almost always stimulates coughing, which is likely to generate droplets that may splash the health care worker. Patients who are suctioned frequently or have had an invasive procedure like a tracheostomy are likely to have blood in the sputum. It is also important to note that needles that have been used to draw blood should not be recapped. If it is necessary to recap them, an instrument such as a hemostat should be used. The hand should never be used.

35. Answer: 2

Rationale: Health care organizations often use variance analysis to explain variations between planned and actual costs and charges.

36. Answer: 2

Rationale: When staff makes rounds, they can notice current risks and can intervene right away. Rounds also provide the opportunity for teaching patients and families about fall risks.

37. Answer: 3

Rationale: A quality improvement initiative begins with agreeing on what aspect of a problem to study. Plan: In this case, the team suspected that needle gauge was a factor. Do: One chart audit is performed, then the data are analyzed, or studied. The Act phase is the decision to implement a new policy.

38. Answer: 2

Rationale: The right to quality care and treatment is consistent with available resources and generally accepted standards. The patient has the right to refuse treatment to the extent permitted by law and government regulations and to be informed of the consequences of his or her refusal.

39. Answer: 4

Rationale: Primary prevention precedes disease and applies to health patients. Secondary prevention focuses on patients who have health problems and are at risk for developing complications. Tertiary prevention enables patients to gain health from others' activities without doing anything themselves.

40. Answer: 3

Rationale: Patient safety was defined by the Institute of Medicine as "the prevention of harm to patients." Emphasis is placed on the system of care delivery that (1) prevents errors; (2) learns from the errors that do occur; and (3) is built on a culture of safety that involves health care professionals, organizations, and patients. The glossary at the Agency for Healthcare Research and Quality Patient Safety Network website expands on the definition of prevention of harm: "freedom from accidental or preventable injuries produced by medical care." Solving domestic problems that patients may have when they go home is not part of the nurse's responsibility.

17

Response to Diversity

1. Dae-hun is a 34-year-old Asian American and has grown up with an Asian influence. He hands the nurse practitioner (NP) a piece of paper saying he has complaints of being very fatigued, with dry hair and dry skin, and a slow weight gain. The NP suspects he might have a thyroid issue. The NP needs to explain to Dae-hun that he needs a blood test. How does the NP explain the procedure to the patient, who only speaks Korean and barely understands English?

   1. Get a professional translator or interpreter.

   2. Do hand signals.

   3. Speak English because it is the universal language.

   4. Show the patient a picture of the procedure so he knows what will be done.

2. What does the nurse practitioner do when creating a plan of care for a patient with a different cultural background?

   1. Show pictures and speak slowly so patient can understand.

   2. For continuity of tradition and cultural practice, let the family take care of the patient.

   3. Identify cultural variables that may affect the patient's health problems.

   4. Explain to the patient that he or she needs to adjust to the hospital care plan for it to be effective.

3. The nurse practitioner should recognize this when caring for patients with varied cultural backgrounds:

   1. People with the same cultural backgrounds have the same interests.

   2. People from the same cultural backgrounds have the same beliefs.

   3. Not every person who is from the same cultural background has the same beliefs.

   4. Cultural background does not need be considered when basic needs are compromised.

4. Dae-hun is a young Asian American male patient with a normal body mass index (BMI). Which of the following conditions is he more likely to get because of his ethnicity even though he has a low BMI?

   1. Kidney disease.

   2. Gout arthritis.

   3. Schizophrenia.

   4. Diabetes mellitus.

5. The nurse practitioner (NP) is caring for an Asian American patient. As the NP is reviewing the discharge medications and dosages, the patient does not face the NP. What is the most appropriate action?

   1. Continue giving instructions and confirm patient's understanding.

   2. Walk in front of the patient so you can get eye contact.

   3. Increase the volume of your voice so you get the patient's attention.

   4. Just provide a written instruction expecting the patient to understand it.

6. Ichika, a 28-year-old Japanese American female patient, is to undergo surgery the following week. While the nurse practitioner was discussing the preoperative procedures to the patient, Ichika keeps smiling and continuously nods her head. How should this nonverbal behavior be interpreted?

   1. That the patient understood the procedure for his treatment.

   2. Ichika has agreed to the procedure.

   3. It reflects the patient's cultural value.

   4. The patient is doing it so the nurse will stop talking.

7. While the nurse practitioner (NP) was assessing Ichika on the day of the surgery, the NP was telling Ichika about what to expect for the surgery, and the NP maintained eye contact throughout the conversation. The patient suddenly informed the surgeon that she disapproves of the NP's actions. How can the patient's reaction be explained?

   1. In the Japanese culture, small talk is considered rude.

   2. In the Japanese culture, prolonged eye contact is considered rude.

   3. In the Japanese culture, talking about a surgical procedure on the day of the procedure is considered insensitive.

   4. Punctuality is very important in the Japanese culture. Small talk is considered a waste of time and a delaying tactic for the procedure.

8. Yang Yu, a 41-year-old Chinese female patient, is admitted to the hospital with the following vital signs: blood pressure 130/90 mmHg, respiratory rate 26 breaths/min, pulse 76 beats/min, and temperature 101°F. Yang Yu was experiencing pain in her upper back, back of the head, neck, and shoulders. She was also having fever and chills. These symptoms are considered by the Chinese as syndromes of wind. This is considered:

   1. Culture awareness.

   2. Culture biased.

   3. Culture shock.

   4. Culture-bound syndrome.

9. Yang Yu was diagnosed with pneumonia. Based on her Chinese culture, what are the beliefs when it comes to causes of illnesses?

   1. Attributed to stress.

   2. May be passed from one person who can transfer own illness.

   3. Punishment for past sins.

   4. Cast by an enemy.

10. Avraham, a Jewish patient, was admitted to the hospital for surgery. When the nurse practitioner is in the patient's room, the patient asks for a new meal tray because the meal consists of a cheeseburger and whole milk. What is the best action to take?

    1. Ask the dietary department to replace the whole milk with skim milk.

    2. Deliver the tray to the patient.

    3. Ask for a whole new food tray.

    4. Ask that the cheeseburger be replaced with beef wanton soup.

11. The AGACNP knows that Jewish dietary laws expect that people will eat what type of diet?

    1. Vegetarian.

    2. Keto.

    3. Kosher.

    4. Kashrut.

12. What type of Jewish ethnic group, which originated in Europe, has the greatest number of genetic disorders?

    1. Ashkenazi.

    2. Orthodox.

    3. Sephardic.

    4. Hasidic.

13. The nurse practitioner (NP) is caring for Jacob, a 55-year-old Amish patient. Considering the Amish culture, when it comes to decisions, who would the NP need to address?

    1. Husband.

    2. Wife.

    3. Both husband and wife.

    4. Children.

14. Jacob, a 55-year-old Amish patient, needed to ask permission from his church to go to the nurse practitioner. What is the best explanation for such an action by Jacob?

    1. To show respect.

    2. The church will shoulder the cost.

    3. To let everyone know where he is.

    4. Part of their rules and regulations as a culture.

15. Because he is Amish, Jacob does not have health insurance. What is the best explanation for the lack of health insurance?

    1. The Amish community considers it as a "worldly product." Getting health insurance is a sign that one does not have enough faith.

    2. Because the church pays for everything, the Amish community is unable to get every member health insurance.

    3. The Amish community considers it as a "prediction" that one will be sick in the future, so not having health insurance is to avoid attracting sickness.

    4. Jacob has lacked the means to afford insurance.

16. The nurse practitioner is caring for an African American woman in her fifties. The patient keeps asking about each procedure that is going to be done even though it has already been explained. This is a sign of mistrust. How can mistrust in the health care system be best explained?

    1. There is a fear of being experimented on.

    2. They do not trust anybody outside the family.

    3. They are not used to being hospitalized.

    4. African Americans do not feel comfortable being touched, even by health care professionals.

17. The nurse practitioner is caring for an African American woman in her fifties. Based on the patient's culture, what may be her beliefs when it comes to causes of her illness?

    1. Attributed to stress.

    2. May be passed from one person who can "transfer" the illness.

    3. Punishment for past sins.

    4. Cast by an enemy.

18. The nurse practitioner (NP) is caring for a 57-year-old African American female patient. The patient tells the NP that she was once a healer. How is that best interpreted based on her culture?

    1. She was once a physician.

    2. She has the gift of healing others through incantations and prayers.

    3. She used to heal easily.

    4. She is delusional.

19. The nurse practitioner (NP) is caring for a 57-year-old African American female patient. Considering the patient's ethnicity, which of the conditions is she most likely to get?

    1. Vitamin-deficient anemia.

    2. Aplastic anemia.

    3. Hemolytic anemia.

    4. Sickle cell anemia.

20. Malik, a Native American, has been admitted because of a fractured rib. What should the nurse practitioner use as much as possible when educating this patient?

    1. Write all the instructions.

    2. Body language.

    3. Verbalization.

    4. Demonstration.

21. Malik, a Native American, has been admitted because of a fractured rib. As Malik's nurse practitioner, when it comes to pharmacological treatment, Malik will most likely:

    1. Make use of herbal medicines that contains healing properties.

    2. Have a clergy come to the hospital for a treatment consultation.

    3. Get to know his health care providers first before he agrees to any treatment.

    4. Agree with all the treatment as long as it is written and documented.

22. Native Americans believe that everything and everyone is interconnected. What is this belief based on?

    1. Health.

    2. Therapy.

    3. Native American healing.

    4. American Indian healing.

23. Native Americans believe that everything and everyone is interconnected. Keeping this in mind, what modern practice is frowned upon?

    1. Discussion about surgery.

    2. Discussion about amputation.

    3. Discussion about death and dying.

    4. Discussion about dietary preferences.

24. Native Americans believe that everything and everyone is interconnected. Keeping this in mind, the nurse practitioner knows that it is rude to:

    1. Shake hands.

    2. Make direct eye contact.

    3. Stroking the head of the patient.

    4. Hug the patient.

25. Which of the following is a major health problem for Native Americans?

    1. Glaucoma.

    2. Diabetes.

    3. Renal disease.

    4. Arthritis.

26. The process of cultural competency is best defined as:

    1. The ability to provide care that meets the cultural, social, and linguistic needs of the patient.

    2. The provision of equal and the same treatment based on their illness.

    3. A health care provider's exclusion of the cultural background of the patient and give importance to what's best for the patient.

    4. The study of different cultures.

27. Cultural awareness is best defined as:

    1. The knowledge of another's culture.

    2. A person's deep care for people from other cultures.

    3. Recognizing biases and prejudices and a self-examination on one's background.

    4. Being involved in cross-cultural interactions.

28. The nurse practitioner needs to understand that ethnocentrism is:

    1. The understanding of one's culture and other cultures.

    2. The refusal of asking about one's culture.

    3. The assumption that all beliefs are the same.

    4. The belief that one's culture is better than others and is the only right culture to be followed.

29. A male nurse practitioner would be correct if he asks for a female nurse practitioner to take his place in caring for a(an):

    1. Muslim woman.

    2. Muslim man.

    3. Latino woman.

    4. Latino man.

30. As a nurse practitioner, you understand that transcultural nursing is:

    1. Making use of a comparative study of multiple cultures and understanding the similarities and differences.

    2. Combining all the cultures and finding a common ground.

    3. Ignoring cultural preferences and beliefs when it comes to health care because patient safety is a nurse practitioner's responsibility.

    4. To study another culture to understand a patient's culture better.

31. When dealing with patients from different cultures, the nurse practitioner understands that:

    1. When the patient's health is at risk, then cultural considerations must be ignored temporarily.

    2. Generalizations of behaviors and attitudes of a certain culture, ethnicity, or race may be incorrect.

    3. Each person that comes from a certain cultural group will always respond to stress the same way.

    4. One's culture is useless when the nurse practitioner decides the proper treatment for the patient.

32. For a nurse practitioner (NP) to be effective in providing care, the NP must:

    1. Treat all patients the same.

    2. Refrain from asking cultural background.

    3. Be well informed of each patient's cultural background.

    4. Educate the patient how modern medicine is proving their beliefs wrong.

33. The nurse practitioner knows that the most important factor in caring for a patient from a specific cultural group is:

    1. Consideration.

    2. Communication.

    3. Time orientation.

    4. Geographical origin.

34. When one is caring for patients from different backgrounds, one must understand the difference between culture and ethnicity. Culture is one's beliefs, knowledge, attitudes, values, and so forth of one group. Ethnicity is best defined as a certain group's:

    1. Perception of themselves.

    2. Perception of others.

    3. Attitude and way of life.

    4. Beliefs.

17 Respon to Diversity Answers & Rationales

1. Answer: 1

Rationale: The nurse practitioner needs to wait for an interpreter for the patient. It is not advisable to have family members translate because they might be lost in translation when it comes to medical procedures.

2. Answer: 3

Rationale: It is important to identify cultural needs and how this may affect the patient's health to be able to provide proper care.

3. Answer: 3

Rationale: Cultural background does not guarantee that all patients are practicing the same traditions in their culture. Assessment and being informed is very important in planning your health care approach.

4. Answer: 4

Rationale: The body mass index cutoff considered for diabetes is lower in Asians and Asian Americans compared with the overall race or culture. Asians have a different body fat distribution in which fat is usually stored in the waist instead of the limbs. This is a factor that is associated with type 2 diabetes.

5. Answer: 1

Rationale: In the Asian culture, steady eye contact may be deemed inappropriate, especially when talking to someone with higher authority.

6. Answer: 3

Rationale: The Japanese "nodding" means that they are still listening to what one is saying. This is very common in the Japanese culture and is widely practiced.

7. Answer: 2

Rationale: Prolonged eye contact is considered the same as staring, which in the Japanese culture is labeled as rude.

8. Answer: 4

Rationale: Culture-bound syndrome is considered a somatic and psychiatric combination of symptoms. This is common in certain cultural groups.

9. Answer: 3

Rationale: The Chinese community believes that any illness is a punishment for one's sins.

10. Answer: 3

Rationale: In the Jewish religion, they believe that meat should not be eaten with any form of dairy. The Jewish religion has very specific instructions when it comes to their food. In this scenario, the best action is to have the tray fully replaced.

11. Answer: 3

Rationale: Kosher diet/food is observed by some Jewish people. Kashrut is the Jewish dietary laws.

12. Answer: 1

Rationale: One of four Ashkenazi Jews carry a genetic disorder. This has originated from a very small population and has been carried from one generation to the next. This is called the founder's effect.

13. Answer: 3

Rationale: In the Amish community, the husband and wife are considered partners and decide together.

14. Answer: 2

Rationale: When seeking health care, in most Amish churches, you are required to ask permission because the church will shoulder the cost.

15. Answer: 1

Rationale: A lack of faith is frowned on in the Amish culture. One such action would be purchasing a "worldly product," and insurance is considered as such in their community.

16. Answer: 1

Rationale: The African American's distrust in the health care system is well documented and is deeply rooted. This started during slavery when slaves were used for medical experiments.

17. Answer: 3

Rationale: Like other cultures, some African Americans view their illness is a result of their sins.

18. Answer: 2

Rationale: In the African American culture, there are two kinds of healers. One healer is someone who can heal themselves through others. The other type of healer is someone who possesses the gift of healing others through incantations, prayers, and laying of hands.

19. Answer: 4

Rationale: This is not because of their skin color but because of their geographical location. Sickle cell anemia is related to malaria, which has a high prevalence in areas from which African Americans originate.

20. Answer: 4

Rationale: Native Americans are silent people. They do not find power in words unlike other cultures.

21. Answer: 1

Rationale: Native Americans use nature, herbs, and other natural remedies to cure and prevent illnesses in their tribe.

22. Answer: 3

Rationale: Native Americans believe that everything in nature is connected. This helps a person heal from an illness. This is one reason why they rely more on natural healing than modern medicine.

23. Answer: 3

Rationale: Native Americans believe that the body is sacred and should not be disturbed. This makes way for the spirit of the deceased to easily cross over.

24. Answer: 2

Rationale: Eye contact in the Native American culture is considered rude and disrespectful.

25. Answer: 2

Rationale: Native Americans are twice as likely to get diabetes as Caucasians. The correlation between the culture and the health condition has not been discovered. Renal disease is also a major problem as well for Native Americans; however, the renal disease is caused by diabetes. This is why the *best* answer is 2.

26. Answer: 1

Rationale: Cultural competency is when health care providers meet all the needs of the patient including their cultural needs. The study of different cultures is called *cultural anthropology*.

27. Answer: 3

Rationale: Cultural awareness is described as knowing and understanding one's culture and knowing the difference when it comes to values and attitudes from other cultures.

28. Answer: 4

Rationale: Ethnocentrism is defined as the belief that one's culture is the only natural and correct culture.

29. Answer: 1

Rationale: Muslim women are not allowed to see male health providers without a male guardian. They also need to *only* have female health providers.

30. Answer: 1

Rationale: Transcultural nursing is a specialty study by nurses in which the similarities and differences of each culture are identified and studied.

31. Answer: 2

Rationale: The generalization that a certain group has the same attitude or behavior may be incorrect. Differences always exist between individuals, and they are caused by multiple factors.

32. Answer: 3

Rationale: It is the nurse practitioner's responsibility to be aware of a patient's background. It is vital to provide customized and effective care for the patient.

33. Answer: 2

Rationale: Communication is very important in dealing with patients from different cultural groups. It is never safe to assume something. Asking questions is one way of communicating and understanding one's culture so one can provide effective care.

34. Answer: 1

Rationale: Culture is about a group's beliefs and is influenced by multiple factors, whereas ethnicity is how a certain group of people perceives itself; both are interrelated.

18

Clinical Inquiry

1. There are three areas in clinical inquiry. Which area creates projects that are used to improve patient care?

   1. Research.

   2. Quality improvement.

   3. Evidence-based practice.

   4. Patient-based practice.

2. Which area of clinical inquiry is done to generate new knowledge?

   1. Research.

   2. Quality improvement.

   3. Evidence-based practice.

   4. Patient-based practice.

3. In clinical inquiry, how is the problem/patient/population, intervention/indicator, comparison, outcome, or PICO defined?

   1. Framework to identify the practice in question.

   2. Published research.

   3. Asking expert clinicians.

   4. Hospital policy.

4. Clinical inquiry has been part of health care for a long time. In advance practice nursing, what is its purpose?

   1. Questioning the knowledge of others.

   2. Testing your own knowledge.

   3. Curiosity to determine best practice.

   4. It is not important in nursing.

5. Research has different sources. Which of the following is an example of a primary source?

   1. Commentary on findings of a published research study by another researcher.

   2. Book on maternity and child nursing.

   3. Dissertation that critiques all research about autism.

   4. Journal article about a study that used large unpublished databases generated by the United States census.

6. Professional conferences are often done to update the health care professionals. An audio recording of an unpublished research study would have which characteristic?

   1. Database literature.

   2. Not useful since they are unpublished.

   3. More difficult to analyze than written reports.

   4. Secondary sources.

7. In a qualitative research process, which of the following is the first step?

   1. Review of literature.

   2. Study design.

   3. Sample.

   4. Data analysis.

8. In qualitative research, which mode of clinical application is the sharing of qualitative findings with the patient?

   1. Coaching.

   2. Anticipatory guidance.

   3. Empathy.

   4. Assessment of patient's progress.

9. Which of the following is an appropriate qualitative research question?

    1. What is the meaning of health for migrant farmworker women?

    2. Which pain medications decrease the need for sleep medication in elderly patients?

    3. How does frequency of medication administration impact the degree of pain experienced following knee replacement surgery?

    4. Under what conditions does a decubitus ulcer heal most quickly?

10. In a report of a qualitative study, which of the following phrases would you expect?

    1. "The hypothesis of this study is…"

    2. "Perceived pain was measured using the Abbott pain scale…"

    3. "The control group received no instruction…"

    4. "Subjects were asked to relate their perceptions of pain…"

11. In a report of a quantitative study, which of the following phrases would you expect?

    1. "A convenience sample was chosen…"

    2. "The phenomenon studied was…"

    3. "Data were analyzed and interpreted…"

    4. "Researchers sought to explore the meaning of the hospital experience…"

12. Which statement is accurate regarding hypotheses?

    1. Describe the effect of the dependent variable on the independent variable.

    2. Statements about the relationships among variables.

    3. Includes a definition of the treatment or intervention used.

    4. Operationally define the dependent variables.

13. Which of the following is a characteristic of a hypothesis?

    1. Flows from interpretation of the data collected.

    2. Operationally defines the variable to be studied.

    3. Eliminates the need to designate a dependent variable.

    4. Implies a causative or associative relationship.

14. Which research hypothesis is most testable?

    1. There is a relationship between meditation and anxiety disorders.

    2. Teaching one meditation technique to patients with anxiety disorders will be better than teaching multiple techniques.

    3. The ability to meditate causes lower anxiety in patients with anxiety disorder than those who do not meditate.

    4. Patients with anxiety disorders who learn meditation techniques have less anxiety than those who do not.

15. Which of the following is a characteristic of a statistical hypothesis?

    1. Null.

    2. Predicts a positive relationship among variables.

    3. Complex.

    4. Describes data-analysis methods.

16. A null hypothesis can be rejected. When does this occur?

    1. When there is no association among variables.

    2. When there is evidence of significance.

    3. When the independent and dependent variables are related.

    4. When the research hypothesis is rejected.

17. As a nurse practitioner, you encounter different scenarios in your practice and want to know more. You want to research and discover why patients with certain ethnic backgrounds are reluctant to ask for pain medication. Because you only have a very limited source of literature in this topic, you design a study to explore the relationships between cultural systems, the experience of pain, and the effective use of medication to relieve pain. You plan to use your findings of the study to formulate a hypothesis for a future study. Which of the following is a characteristic of your study?

    1. Will lead to level II data.

    2. Is a quasi-experimental study.

    3. Has a directional hypothesis.

    4. Is a hypothesis-generating study.

18. A nurse practitioner has developed the following hypothesis: elderly women receive less aggressive treatment for breast cancer than younger women. Based on the statement, which of the following variables would be a dependent variable?

    1. Degree of treatment received.

    2. Age of the patient.

    3. Type of cancer being treated.

    4. Use of inpatient treatment.

19. A nurse practitioner has developed the following hypothesis: elderly women receive less aggressive treatment for breast cancer than younger women. Based on the statement, which of the following variables would be an independent variable?

    1. Degree of treatment received.

    2. Age of the patient.

    3. Type of cancer being treated.

    4. Use of inpatient treatment.

20. How is "fittingness" of a research study best described?

    1. Truth of findings as judged by the participants.

    2. Appropriateness of the interview questions posed.

    3. Extent to which a project's findings fit into other contexts outside the study setting.

    4. The adequacy of the coding system used.

21. There are often updates in practices, especially in the health care industry. How do nurse practitioners keep up with evidence-based practice?

    1. They read literature that is only 10 years old.

    2. They learn from other health care providers.

    3. They are creatures of habit; they do not change.

    4. They learn from their professional development specialist or education coordinator.

22. Who is responsible for making changes to policy and procedures based on evidence?

    1. Health care leadership mandates change.

    2. Professional development specialist or education coordinator makes the change.

    3. Nurses make the change, discuss it at meetings, and spread the word through classes and in-services.

    4. The nurse who read the literature makes the change.

23. Updates are done time and time again. Why is it so important for nurse practitioners to update their practice with evidence?

    1. What the education coordinator learned has not changed.

    2. Nursing care has not changed since nursing school.

    3. The way intravenous medications are started and equipment in use has not changed.

    4. There are new medications, medical supplies, treatments, and illnesses.

24. When treating pain using evidence-based nursing practice, the best treatment consists of:

    1. Massage.

    2. Pain relief medication.

    3. Sleep.

    4. Combination of treatments.

25. When should a verbal descriptor scale be chosen to evaluate pain?

    1. For pediatric patients.

    2. With adult patients who have the capability to read and understand the written word.

    3. For patients who are unconscious.

    4. It is never used.

26. A nursing student is giving a classroom presentation about evidence-based practice (EBP). Which statement best reflects the student's correct understanding of EBP?

    1. It is the gathering of objective facts and information to advance knowledge about a specific topic.

    2. Involves combining quality research, clinical expertise, and client preferences to achieve the best client outcomes.

    3. Incorporates clinical knowledge, expert opinion, or information resulting from research.

    4. Uses a systematic and strict scientific process to test hypotheses about health-related conditions and nursing care.

27. What should be expected from a meta-analysis study?

    1. Detailed description that is specific to one individual, issue, or event.

    2. Study that uses a control group and an experimental group to illustrate a cause-and-effect relationship.

    3. Study that follows two groups over a period of time that measures the outcomes of an exposure group with those of a nonexposure group.

    4. Examination of a group of studies on a given topic followed by combination and analysis of the results as if they were from one large study.

28. Emily, a nurse practitioner (NP) is attending an in-service about evidence-based practice (EBP). The unit nurse leader, Kyle, asks Emily how she supports the development of EBP. Which response best reflects Emily's misperception about a barrier to implementing EBP?

    1. "I've taken extra patients almost every night for the entire month. I can't handle the thought of adding one more thing to my to-do list."

    2. "I think what we're doing now works just fine; why fix what isn't broken?"

    3. "I've been picking up a lot of extra shifts; I'm too busy to take another work-related responsibility."

    4. "I'm not certified in research and I don't have time to take a course right now. EBP is outside my scope of practice."

29. The nurse practitioner is designing a presentation about evidence-based practice (EBP). Which example best illustrates evidence derived from research?

    1. "A nurse reads studies about the effects of massage on back pain."

    2. "The client may refuse to have back surgery."

    3. "Studies suggest medical massage effectively reduces lower back pain."

    4. "In certain cultures, male clients accept massage treatment only from male therapists."

30. The nurse practitioner is developing a clinical question that explores the etiology of adult respiratory distress syndrome (ARDS). Which of the following is an appropriate clinical question?

    1. What are some potential complications of ARDS?

    2. Which medications lead to best outcomes for clients with ARDS?

    3. What are the causes of ARDS?

    4. How does ARDS affect arterial blood gas values?

31. The nurse practitioner is designing a quantitative research study about the relationship between wellness and yoga. Which research question is most appropriate for this study?

    1. What is the relationship between engaging in yoga and the incidence of hypertension?

    2. How do individuals who engage in yoga perceive the link between exercise and hypertension?

    3. What is the nature of the relationship between engaging in yoga and experiencing wellness?

    4. How do health beliefs about hypertension influence an individual's choice to practice yoga?

32. How can health care quality be improved?

    1. Properly using advance directives.

    2. Following privacy laws.

    3. Striving to reduce errors.

    4. Seeing more patients each day.

33. What do community health centers provide?

    1. High-quality care to uninsured and underinsured.

    2. Low-quality care to uninsured and underinsured.

    3. High-quality care to the insured.

    4. Low-quality care to the insured.

34. According to Maxwell (2002), there are 17 characteristics that effective team members possess. Which of the following is defined as effective and respectful communication and active listening without any judgments are essential to group success.

    1. Superior communication skills.

    2. Dependability.

    3. Adaptability.

    4. Awareness of the mission.

35. Hilda, a nurse practitioner, was called by her nurse supervisor to tell her about the changes in the hospital policy because she was sick during the meeting. Hilda can adapt to the current changes. What characteristic of an effective team member is Hilda exhibiting?

    1. Effective collaboration abilities.

    2. Selflessness.

    3. Adaptability.

    4. Self-discipline.

36. Hilda, a nurse practitioner, has the knowledge, skills, and abilities to perform both clinically and as a group member who has had some formal or informal education relating to groups, group development, and how to function as a group member and group leader. What characteristic of an effective team member is Hilda exhibiting?

    1. Competency.

    2. Ability to be prepared.

    3. Ability to add value.

    4. Commitment.

37. Hilda, a nurse practitioner, just finished her shift and needed to get home to feed her dogs. The nurse practitioner for the next shift called in sick at the last minute. Hilda volunteered to stay for another shift. What characteristic of an effective team member is Hilda exhibiting?

    1. Commitment.

    2. Selflessness.

    3. Enthusiasm.

    4. Ability to add value.

38. Which characteristic of an effective team member by Maxwell (2002) is synonymous with energy and eagerness?

    1. Dependability.

    2. Commitment.

    3. Competency.

    4. Enthusiasm.

39. Vern, the nurse practitioner, has observed that errors are mostly created during patient assessment. He wants to dig deeper to find out what causes the problem. What action should Vern take?

    1. Root cause analysis.

    2. Initiating and implementing the best solution.

    3. Measure the effectiveness of the implemented solution.

    4. Collection of data and information relating to the problem or opportunity for improvement.

40. Which of the following is utilized by health care providers as references for research?

    1. Daily news.

    2. Published articles in the professional literature.

    3. Coworkers reports.

    4. Patient's personal journal.

41. What is the term used for the coding and clustering of data to form categories in the grounded-theory method?

    1. Theoretical sampling.

    2. Constant comparative method.

    3. Emic method.

    4. Metasynthesis.

42. A nurse practitioner organizes a quality improvement team to improve the efficiency of discharging patients from the emergency department. To ensure that the newly designed process is efficiently implemented, who must be part of the team?

    1. Emergency department head nurse.

    2. Chief information officer.

    3. Chief operating officer.

    4. Chief information officer.

43. Which of the following is the most likely root cause of medication errors in health care entities?

    1. Manual medication delivery systems.

    2. Illegible physician handwriting.

    3. Carelessness of nurses.

    4. Systems failure.

44. A nurse practitioner decides to address a quality problem among thoracic surgeons directly with staff. Who should participate in the meetings to address the problem?

    1. Quality assurance committee.

    2. Nurse practitioners only.

    3. Relevant physicians, nurse practitioners, nurses, and nonclinical staff.

    4. Nursing and risk management staff only.

45. You are the lead nurse practitioner for a group of hospital-based nurse practitioners. You discover that one of the nurse practitioners is regularly billing 1-hour appointments but only seeing patients for 20 minutes. Which of the following actions of the lead nurse practitioner is most appropriate?

    1. Documenting the discrepancy in the case notes.

    2. Notifying the patient of the discrepancy.

    3. Reporting the activity to the plan administrator.

    4. Do nothing.

46. Which of the following variables is used to determine which diagnosis-related group is associated with an inpatient admission?

    1. Principal diagnosis.

    2. Prior admission diagnosis.

    3. Secondary diagnosis.

    4. Total number of diagnoses.

47. Which of the following is a major complaint made by nurse practitioners against the use of information obtained from outcomes assessment?

    1. Increased market share will not be realized by cooperating nurse practitioners.

    2. Information about internal costs and processes are not necessary for success.

    3. Information gained cannot be shifted to the point of service.

    4. The information is not statistically valid for individual nurse practitioners.

48. Under which of the following conditions are health care providers permitted to disclose confidential patient information?

    1. Disclosure of the information is not likely to harm the patient.

    2. An insurance company ensures the confidentiality of the information.

    3. A patient authorizes disclosure of the information.

    4. The patient's guardian or proxy permits the disclosure.

49. The National Practitioner Data Bank has been developed under which of the following regulations?

    1. Clinical Laboratory Improvement Act.

    2. Consolidated Omnibus Budget Reconciliation Act.

    3. Health Care Quality Improvement Act.

    4. Tax Equity and Fiscal Responsibility Act.

50. Which of the following reasons for removing a physician from a health maintenance organization provider network requires a report to the National Practitioner Data Bank?

    1. The physician's medical license has been revoked.

    2. The physician hires an associate who has several member complaints and a liability suit pending to provide call coverage.

    3. The physician is an alcoholic and he just received his second ticket for driving under the influence of alcohol.

    4. The physician's provider profile shows that his charges are well in excess of his peers.

51. Which of the following programs was established through the Tax Equity and Fiscal Responsibility Act of 1982 to ensure quality of care to Medicare recipients?

    1. Continuing medical education.

    2. Medicaid.

    3. Civilian Health and Medical Program of the Uniformed Services.

    4. Peer review organizations.

52. Which of the following entities regulates the disposal of infectious waste?

    1. Occupational Safety and Health Administration.

    2. Centers for Disease Control and Prevention.

    3. Food and Drug Administration.

    4. United States Public Health Service.

18 | Clinical Inquiry Answers & Rationales

1. Answer: 2

Rationale: Quality improvement projects are used to improve patient care.

2. Answer: 1

Rationale: Research is used to generate new knowledge, which is often carried into evidence-based practice.

3. Answer: 1

Rationale: The problem/patient/population, intervention/indicator, comparison, outcome (PICO) model is a format to help define your question.

4. Answer: 3

Rationale: A spirit of nursing curiosity drove these projects, and inquiry is the heart of evidence-based practice. The process itself can foster a sense of teamwork, trust, and investment in the care we provide.

5. Answer: 4

Rationale: An original study is an example of a primary source. Unpublished primary sources are original documents and artifacts of all kinds that were created by individuals but not published (that is, made public issued in a format that could be widely distributed) during the period you are studying.

6. Answer: 1

Rationale: Audio and video recordings of research presentations are examples of database literature. Making sense of data in the form of graphics, video, audio, and text requires clear thinking that is aided by theory, models, constructs, and perhaps metaphor.

7. Answer: 1

Rationale: Review of literature is the first step in the qualitative research process. The study design is the second step in the qualitative research process.

8. Answer: 2

Rationale: Qualitative findings can also be applied via anticipatory guidance. This type of application is somewhat interventionist, as nurses share qualitative findings directly with clients, offering a research-based perspective on what patients might be experiencing and how others have described that experience.

9. Answer: 1

Rationale: This question seeks to explore a phenomenon (health) for a specific population. The research question that you ultimately choose guides your inquiry and reflects this stance.

10. Answer: 4

Rationale: Data collected were perceptions of pain, not numeric data. Other options are found in a report of a quantitative study.

11. Answer: 1

Rationale: When a sample of convenience is chosen, the study is a quantitative study. Qualitative studies explore phenomena. Data collected in qualitative studies are "interpreted." Qualitative studies explore the meaning of human experience.

12. Answer: 2

Rationale: Hypotheses are statements about the relationships between two or more variables that suggest an answer to the research question. The independent variable is not affected or changed by the dependent variable. Hypotheses are not concerned with operationally defining the variables involved in the study, including treatments or interventions.

13. Answer: 4

Rationale: A hypothesis implies a causative or associative relationship. A hypothesis guides the research design and collection of data. Operational definitions are not included in the hypothesis. The hypothesis indicates the dependent variable.

14. Answer: 3

Rationale: This hypothesis meets the criteria of testability.

15. Answer: 1

Rationale: Statistical hypotheses, called *null hypotheses*, state that there is no relationship between the independent and dependent variables.

16. Answer: 3

Rationale: Because the null hypothesis states that there is no relationship between the independent and dependent variable, it is rejected if they are related.

17. Answer: 4

Rationale: There is very limited information in this area to formulate a hypothesis, so the researcher will conduct this qualitative study and use the findings to generate hypotheses for future studies. This is a qualitative study, not a quasi-experimental study. Level II evidence is obtained from at least one well-designed randomized, controlled trial. This study has no hypothesis.

18. Answer: 1

Rationale: The degree of treatment received is considered the dependent variable. The dependent variable is the variable experimenters measure in their experiments.

19. Answer: 2

Rationale: The age of the patient would be the independent variable. An independent variable is a variable that stands alone.

20. Answer: 3

Rationale: "Fittingness" is the extent to which the findings of a qualitative study can be of use to other populations or settings. Credibility is the truth of findings as judged by the participants. Auditability assists the reader to judge the appropriateness of the interview questions.

21. Answer: 4

Rationale: Nursing professional development specialists are the keys to successful succession planning, managing competing priorities, and effecting cost avoidance. These practitioners are more than educators. They emphasize safety, quality, efficiency, and effectiveness of practice while rapidly transitioning diverse generations of nurses into practice.

22. Answer: 2

Rationale: The American Nurses Association (2009b) distinguishes Nursing Professional Development as a professional specialty based on the sciences of nursing, technology, research, and evidence-based practice, practice-based evidence, change, communication, leadership, and education.

23. Answer: 4

Rationale: So that all Americans may have access to high-quality, safe health care, federal and state actions are required to update and standardize scope-of-practice regulations to take advantage of the full capacity and education of nurses.

24. Answer: 4

Rationale: Just as experiencing pain is deeply personal, the most effective way to treat it also varies from one individual to the next. Often a combination of approaches will work best.

25. Answer: 2

Rationale: The pain thermometer is used to assess pain intensity is for persons able to self-report. This scale requires either verbal ability or the ability to point to the descriptor on the thermometer most closely representing their pain.

26. Answer: 2

Rationale: It means "integrating individual clinical expertise with the best available external clinical evidence from systematic research." Evidence-based practice is the integration of clinical expertise, patient values, and the best research evidence into the decision-making process for patient care.

27. Answer: 4

Rationale: Meta-analysis is a statistical technique for combining data from multiple studies on a topic. To make a valid decision about using an intervention, ideally, we should not rely on the results obtained from single studies. This is because results can vary from one study to another for various reasons, including confounding factors, and the different study samples used.

28. Answer: 4

Rationale: Evidence-based practice is not outside the scope of practice for nurse practitioners. In fact, it is very much a part of the practice. Today's health care environment demands all advanced practice registered nurses play a role in conducting, translating, integrating, and utilizing research in daily practice.

29. Answer: 3

Rationale: The example is stated as a conclusion to a study or research.

30. Answer: 3

Rationale: A clinical question based on etiology is a question about the causation of the condition. Etiology questions are questions about the harmful effect of an intervention or exposure on a patient.

31. Answer: 2

Rationale: In quantitative research your aim is to determine the relationship between one thing (an independent variable) and another (a dependent or outcome variable) in a population. Quantitative research designs are either descriptive (subjects usually measured once) or experimental (subjects measured before and after a treatment). A descriptive study establishes only associations between variables.

32. Answer: 3

Rationale: An urgent change is needed to address the issue of diagnostic error, which poses a major challenge to health care quality, which means, when errors are minimized, the quality improves.

33. Answer: 1

Rationale: Community health centers are community-based, nonprofit, or public organizations that provide services to people who lack access to other health care, including those without insurance, residents of rural and underserved areas, and some Medicaid patients.

34. Answer: 1

Rationale: Effective and respectful communication and active listening without any judgments are essential to group success.

35. Answer: 3

Rationale: Group members must be flexible, able to adapt to changing situations and circumstances, and achieve the group's goals and fulfill its mission.

36. Answer: 1

Rationale: The person has the knowledge, skills, and abilities to perform both clinically and as a group member who has had some formal or informal education relating to groups, group development, and how to function as a group member and group leader.

37. Answer: 2

Rationale: The team member values and has loyalty to the group and its work even though they have personal goals and interests.

38. Answer: 4

Rationale: Enthusiasm is defined as a feeling of excitement, eager enjoyment, or approval. Effective group members are not only committed to the group and its work, but they are also energized with their participation and enthusiastic about the group and its work.

39. Answer: 1

Rationale: Root cause analysis is used to dig down to the possible causes of the problem.

40. Answer: 2

Rationale: Primary sources are original materials/information on which another research is based. It includes journal articles of original research, conference papers, dissertations, technical reports, and patents. Primary sources are also sets of data, such as health statistics, which have been tabulated, but not interpreted.

41. Answer: 2

Rationale: The purpose of the constant comparative method of joint coding and analysis is to generate theory more systematically than allowed by the second approach by using explicit coding and analytic procedures.

42. Answer: 1

Rationale: For change to be efficiently implemented, the directly involved people should be part of the quality improvement team. "Doing the right thing, at the right time, in the right way, for the right person—and having the best possible results."

43. Answer: 4

Rationale: System failures that result in minor errors can later lead to serious errors. Reporting of errors should be encouraged by creating a blame-free, nonpunitive environment.

44. Answer: 3

Rationale: This scenario would require every single staff member who is involved because a problem is addressed. "Doing the right thing, at the right time, in the right way, for the right person—and having the best possible results."

45. Answer: 3

Rationale: As the lead nurse practitioner, any findings should be reported to the plan administrator. The chain of command needs to be followed.

46. Answer: 1

Rationale: The medical diagnosis codes were divided into medical and surgical categories. Then, the surgical patients were further defined based on the precise surgical procedure performed, whereas the medical patients were further defined based on the precise principal diagnosis for which they were admitted to the hospital.

47. Answer: 4

Rationale: A certain result may be true for one nurse practitioner, but untrue regarding the others. It is not statistically valid for individual physicians. Systematic collection and analysis of outcomes data can add to the complexity of the medical encounter. Yet, if appropriately collected, the information derived can facilitate medical decision-making and enhance the quality of medical care.

48. Answer: 3

Rationale: The Health Insurance Probability and Accountability Act Privacy Rule makes clear that asking a patient for their consent to disclose confidential information demonstrates respect and is part of effective communication with a patient.

49. Answer: 3

Rationale: The Health Care Quality Improvement Act of 1986, as amended, Title IV of Public Law 99-660 (42 U.S.C. §11101 et seq.), led to the establishment of the National Practitioner Data Bank (NPDB). Title IV authorized the NPDB to collect and disclose to authorized queries certain information relating to the professional competence and conduct of physicians, dentists, and other health care practitioners.

50. Answer: 1

Rationale: The National Practitioner Data Bank (NPDB) collects information and maintains reports on the following: medical malpractice payments, federal and state licensure and certification actions, adverse clinical privileges actions, adverse professional society membership actions, negative actions or findings by private accreditation organizations and peer review organizations, health care–related criminal convictions and civil judgments, exclusions from participation in a federal or state health care programs (including Medicare and Medicaid exclusions), and other adjudicated actions or decisions. The reports collected apply to health care practitioners, health care entities, providers, and suppliers based on the laws and regulations that govern the NPDB.

51. Answer: 4

Rationale: An organization was established by the Tax Equity and Fiscal Responsibility Act of 1982 to review quality of care and appropriateness of admissions, readmissions, and discharges for Medicare and Medicaid. These organizations are held responsible for maintaining and lowering admission rates and reducing lengths of stay, while ensuring against inadequate treatment. Peer review organizations (PROs) can conduct a review of medical records and claims to evaluate the appropriateness of care provided. PROs also exist within private carriers and providers. Peer review itself is a process whose confidentiality in private organizations is protected by law. This allows hospitals and groups to conduct internal investigation and monitoring of care decisions and outcomes without the production of related documents in court proceedings. Providers have fought for these protections.

52. Answer: 1

Rationale: In 1991, the Occupational Safety and Health Administration promulgated the Occupational Exposure to Bloodborne Pathogens Standard. This standard is designed to protect approximately 5.6 million workers in the health care and related occupations from the risk of exposure to bloodborne pathogens, such as the HIV and the hepatitis B virus.

19

Facilitation of Learning

1. In what setting are nurse educators typically found?

   1. In the community.

   2. In the hospital.

   3. A university.

   4. All the above.

2. A 45-year-old female patient is transferred to the trauma unit following a car accident. She is unresponsive and was intubated in the field. Her son was called and informed of her condition. The son mentions that his mom has a living will and that she did not want to be kept "alive on machines." The Adult-Gerontology Acute Care Nurse Practitioner tells him that:

   1. He will have to provide a copy of the living will before it can be implemented.

   2. She needs a thorough evaluation to see if her living will is applicable.

   3. The living will is only valid when signed by both patient and legal representative.

   4. You will uphold the patient's wishes and discontinue aggressive actions.

3. The Adult-Gerontology Acute Care Nurse Practitioner is treating a patient with ascites. After a regimen of 200 mg of spironolactone daily, the patient demonstrates a weight loss of 0.75 kg/day. The patient asks, "Is that good?" What is the best answer for this patient?

   1. "Yes. We will continue the current regimen."

   2. "Yes. This is good but you need to lose 0.85 kg/day."

   3. "No. This is too much weight loss too quickly."

   4. "No. How many calories are you eating a day?"

4. A patient presents with a 2-day history of abdominal pain, fever, vomiting, and diarrhea. A surgical abdomen is ruled out, and radiography demonstrates inflammation of the small bowel and colon. Microscopy supports a diagnosis of *Campylobacter jejuni*, and the patient is prepared for discharge from the emergency department. Important patient education includes advising her that:

   1. The disorder should resolve on its own; recurrence is rare but represents a much more serious condition.

   2. The bacteria may be spread for as long as she has diarrhea.

   3. It is important to eat a high-fiber diet.

   4. Eat large meals with high-fat content.

5. The Adult-Gerontology Acute Care Nurse Practitioner is evaluating a 69-year-old female patient in the emergency department. She is extremely anxious and requires significant reassurance that she is not going to die. She is diagnosed with an anterolateral myocardial infarction. Her daughter asks you not to tell the patient the truth. She is afraid that it will worsen her anxiety and her condition. The patient becomes upset and demands to be told precisely what is wrong with her. The most appropriate action would be to:

   1. Have the patient's daughter leave the emergency department.

   2. Lie to the patient and tell her that she is just having a panic attack.

   3. Answer the patient's question truthfully.

   4. Send the patient home so she does not become more agitated.

6. A patient admitted for management of gram-negative sepsis is critically ill and wants to talk with a hospital representative about donating her organs if she dies. Her past medical history includes a traumatic brain injury, ovarian cancer, and dialysis-dependent renal failure. The patient is advised that she is ineligible to donate because of her:

    1. Traumatic brain injury.

    2. Ovarian cancer.

    3. Gram-negative infection.

    4. End-stage renal disease.

7. The Adult-Gerontology Acute Care Nurse Practitioner (AGACNP) is treating a patient who has lung cancer and is receiving chemotherapy. He is eating less because of nausea and anorexia. The AGACNP asks the nurse practitioner student what is recommended for the patient to promote adequate nutrition. The nurse practitioner student is correct when she says:

    1. "Let the patient eat small meals throughout the day."

    2. "Let the patient eat only when hungry."

    3. "Let the patient eat only his favorite foods."

    4. "Let the patient eat large meals but less frequently throughout the day."

8. One of your patients was on a low-residue diet. You asked the student nurse practitioner that you are mentoring to site some examples of food that are appropriate for that kind of diet. The student nurse is correct when she sites which types of food?

    1. Barbeque wings and celery.

    2. Pork chops with peeled white potatoes.

    3. Whole grain pasta with wheat roll.

    4. Cheeseburger, french fries, and milk.

9. A patient asks the Adult-Gerontology Acute Care Nurse Practitioner (AGACNP) to explain to her "why there are weights hanging off the bed." What answer by the AGACNP reflects the best understanding of traction for patient education?

    1. "Traction assists in immobilizing limbs, reducing muscle spasms, and enabling better healing."

    2. "Traction helps you keep your legs still and avoid having muscle spasms. It will also help it to heal straight."

    3. "Traction assists in immobilizing limbs, reducing muscle spasms, and enabling better healing."

    4. "Traction keeps you from moving because you might injure yourself if you move too much."

10. A patient with Cushing disease wants to know her best meal choices. To help increase patient knowledge about meals that she can eat, you provided her a sample meal. Which meal would be correct?

    1. Mexican style beef with guacamole and beans on the side.

    2. Pork chops in cream sauce with mashed potatoes and carrots.

    3. Hamburger with french fries and apple slices.

    4. Roasted chicken with corn and green beans.

11. For the third time in a month, a patient with borderline personality disorder took a handful of pills and was admitted to the emergency department. The Adult-Gerontology Acute Care Nurse Practitioner overhears her student nurse practitioner say, "Here she comes again. If she were serious about committing suicide, she'd have done it by now." You determine that there is a need to teach the student which of the following?

    1. Each suicidal attempt should be taken seriously.

    2. Clients with personality disorders rarely kill themselves.

    3. Exploration of suicidal ideas and intent should be avoided.

    4. The nurse should prepare the client for direct inpatient admission.

12. The Adult-Gerontology Acute Care Nurse Practitioner knows that which percentage of hospitalized patients with acute diverticulitis will require surgical intervention?

    1. 10%.

    2. 5%.

    3. 35%.

    4. 30%.

13. Maxine is being seen in follow-up after removal of an aldosteronoma. The Adult-Gerontology Acute Care Nurse Practitioner expects which of the following aldosterone-related abnormalities will be cured?

    1. Hypernatremia.

    2. Hyperkalemia.

    3. Hypokalemia.

    4. Hyponatremia.

14. Which of the following is *not* a true statement with respect to decision-making for a cognitively impaired patient?

    1. Any patient who is cognitively impaired cannot make his or her own decisions.

    2. A patient can give informed consent if not declared incompetent.

    3. A judge will have to decide whether the patient can make his or her own decisions.

    4. Only the next of kin can declare a person incompetent.

15. Mr. Gibson has a history of chronic ulcerative colitis as well as a family history of colorectal cancer that includes his grandmother and his sister who died at age 50. Genetic testing showed the presence of the adenomatous polyposis coli gene. Today's colonoscopy shows premalignant tissue changes. The Adult-Gerontology Acute Care Nurse Practitioner knows that treatment recommendations for Mr. Gibson likely will include the following:

    1. Colostomy.

    2. Proctocolectomy.

    3. Watching and waiting.

    4. Daily enemas.

16. Misty is a 37-year-old female patient who presents for follow-up after surgical repair of a diaphragmatic hernia. The Adult-Gerontology Acute Care Nurse Practitioner anticipates that patients who have a diaphragmatic hernia repair can expect which of the following?

    1. Recurrence of a smaller hernia.

    2. Excellent recovery.

    3. Recurrence of a larger hernia.

    4. Chronic dyspnea.

17. The Adult-Gerontology Acute Care Nurse Practitioner knows that following bilateral total adrenalectomy, the patient will require which of the following:

    1. Individualized replacement of corticosteroid, mineralocorticoid, and androgen hormones.

    2. A strict diet including a daily sodium intake of only 2 g.

    3. High-dose hydrocortisone for 3 months.

    4. Tapering of intravenous (IV) hydrocortisone, beginning with 100 mg IV every 8 hours on postoperative day 1.

18. Which of the following is NOT a clinical manifestation of cholecystitis?

    1. Fever.

    2. Right upper quadrant pain.

    3. Leukopenia.

    4. Palpable gall bladder.

19. The most important advantage of targeted molecular therapies for cancer, such as monoclonal antibodies (abciximab, nivolumab), is:

    1. They are more toxic but have better long-term outcomes.

    2. They are expressed in vital organs but not in tissues.

    3. The have significantly less toxicity and clinical adverse effect.

    4. They are expressed in cancer cells but not in vital organs and tissues.

20. Variceal bleeding has a mortality rate of up to 70%. According to the Adult-Gerontology Acute Care Nurse Practitioner, which procedure should be performed after the patient becomes hemodynamically stable?

    1. Ultrasound.

    2. Esophagogastroscopy.

    3. Transjugular intrahepatic portosystemic shunt.

    4. Endoscopic variceal ligation.

21. A 48-year-old male patient is being discharged from the hospital today after having gastric bypass surgery. The Adult-Gerontology Acute Care Nurse Practitioner teaches the patient that she will need to take which of the following supplements?

    1. Vitamin D.

    2. Vitamin C.

    3. Folic acid.

    4. Iron.

22. When playing sports, it is not uncommon for people to be exposed to sudden rotation injuries, which lead to an abrupt twisting to the cerebral cortex around the more rigid structures of the midbrain. This can disrupt the flow of blood to and from the reticular activation system and lead to what clinical phenomenon?

    1. Coma.

    2. Cerebral hemorrhage.

    3. Subdural hematoma.

    4. Concussion.

23. When assessing a patient with jaundice, a careful history and physical exam can often help to distinguish prehepatic, hepatic, and posthepatic causes. If the patient reports a dark discoloration of the urine and a light discoloration of the stool, which of the following is the Adult-Gerontology Acute Care Nurse Practitioner most suspicious?

    1. Cirrhosis.

    2. Extrahepatic obstruction.

    3. Cholestasis.

    4. Fatty liver disease.

24. The patient is a 49-year-old man admitted for treatment of an episode of diverticulitis. This is his fifth hospitalization this year, and in previous hospitalizations he has had both abscesses and strictures because of his disease. The discharge summary of his condition should *not* include which of the following:

    1. Drink plenty of water.

    2. Eat a lot of beans.

    3. Exercise regularly.

    4. Follow a low-fat diet.

25. Ian is a 32-year-old patient recovering from an abdominal operation and organ resection after a motorcycle accident. Because of his injuries, a large part of his ileum had to be removed. What discharge education will the Adult-Gerontology Acute Care Nurse Practitioner include?

    1. The patient will need to eat a low-calorie diet to avoid weight gain.

    2. The patient will need to increase his fiber to avoid constipation.

    3. The ileum will be responsible for absorption of vitamins and nutrients.

    4. There is a major risk of vitamin B_1 deficiency.

26. A patient is admitted to the hospital with abdominal pain and significantly elevated serum amylase and lipase; he was diagnosed with pancreatitis and was admitted for pain management. He is feeling better, but he is mad because he knows that "pancreatitis only happens in alcoholics." He makes it clear that he is a religious person and that his religion forbids alcohol. He says he has never drunk alcohol in his life. The Adult-Gerontology Acute Care Nurse Practitioner assures Jack that about 40% of pancreatitis cases are caused by a variety of other issues and which of the following?

    1. Hepatitis.

    2. Gallstone issues.

    3. Opioid abuse.

    4. Genetics.

27. An Adult-Gerontology Acute Care Nurse Practitioner student who just starting his clinical rotation, is watching his mentor during the physical exam of a patient who is admitted to the intensive care unit after a car accident. The student notes that the physical exam includes a rectovaginal exam, an inspection of the urethral duct, and palpation of the pelvic landmarks. The student knows that the patient is being checked for:

    1. Pelvic fracture.

    2. Retroperitoneal bleed.

    3. Ruptured appendix.

    4. Ruptured bladder.

28. Sidney is a 47-year-old man who is receiving radiation for throat cancer. He would like to know what side effects he can expect. The Adult-Gerontology Acute Care Nurse Practitioner tells Sidney that the most common side effects in the acute aftercare period are which of the following:

    1. Constipation and increased appetite.

    2. Halitosis and diarrhea.

    3. Mucositis and yeast superinfections.

    4. Headaches and constipation.

29. The Adult-Gerontology Acute Care Nurse Practitioner (AGACNP) is reading a purified protein derivative (PPD) result for a student nurse practitioner (NP) so she can start her clinical rotation. Forty-eight hours after the injection, there is induration, and the AGACNP comes back in to have it read. The AGACNP knows that:

    1. An induration of 5 mm is considered positive for an immunocompromised person.

    2. As a health care worker, the student should receive prophylactic treatment regardless of induration.

    3. A positive result includes redness and induration.

    4. The NP student should never have received a PPD test.

30. The Adult-Gerontology Acute Care Nurse Practitioner (AGACNP) just admitted a patient to the medical intensive care unit status postsurgical resection for a pheochromocytoma. The AGACNP knows that symptoms of pheochromocytoma include everything *except* the following:

    1. Labile hypertension.

    2. Organ failure.

    3. Hyperthermia.

    4. Confusion.

31. In most cases, what is the first clinical sign of a physiological stress ulcer?

    1. Pain in epigastric area.

    2. Maroon colored bowel movements.

    3. Feeling lightheaded.

    4. Tarry bowel movements.

32. The Adult-Gerontology Acute Care Nurse Practitioner (AGACNP) is going over discharge instructions for hepatic encephalopathy with a patient and his wife. The AGACNP is explaining the signs and symptoms of an elevated ammonia level. All the following are signs or symptoms of an elevated ammonia, *except*:

    1. Confusion.

    2. Disorientation.

    3. Hand tremors.

    4. Insomnia.

33. While reviewing the head computed tomography scan of a 52-year-old African American female patient with a history of hypertension following a bicycle accident, the Adult-Gerontology Acute Care Nurse Practitioner knows that this patient is at a higher risk for which of the following?

    1. Epidural hematoma.

    2. Acute subdural hematoma.

    3. Subarachnoid hemorrhage.

    4. Temporal concussion.

34. The Adult-Gerontology Acute Care Nurse Practitioner (AGACNP) is examining a 59-year-old female patient who presented to the emergency department with complaints of severe abdominal pain. The patient's vital signs are blood pressure 90/50 mmHg, heart rate 142 beats/min, and temperature 100.9°F. She reports that she has constipation. On exam, she has rebound tenderness, abdominal rigidity, and guarding. The AGACNP knows that all of the following diagnostic tests should be ordered *except*:

    1. Complete blood count.

    2. Comprehensive metabolic panel.

    3. 12-lead electrocardiogram.

    4. Abdominal magnetic resonance imaging.

35. The Adult-Gerontology Acute Care Nurse Practitioner knows that the "T" in the TMN tumor staging abbreviation stands for which of the following?

    1. Tumor.

    2. Type.

    3. Telomere.

    4. T cell.

36. What does the ethical principle of nonmaleficence mean?

    1. Doing good and the right thing for the patient.

    2. Being completely truthful with patients.

    3. Doing no harm.

    4. Accepting responsibility for one's own actions.

37. Patient's with an adrenal gland tumor will usually have all the following labs done for diagnosis *except*:

    1. Adrenocorticotropic hormone test.

    2. Cortisol test.

    3. Dexamethasone suppression test.

    4. Complete metabolic panel.

38. The Adult-Gerontology Acute Care Nurse Practitioner knows that a Hgb A1c level higher than _____ indicates a patient is a diabetic.

    1. 5.5%.

    2. 5.8%.

    3. 6.2%.

    4. 6.5%.

39. Jon is a 35-year-old male patient who had a stem cell transplant for leukemia. The Adult-Gerontology Acute Care Nurse Practitioner knows that Jon will need which medication for immunosuppression?

    1. Tacrolimus.

    2. Intravenous immunoglobulin.

    3. Cytarabine.

    4. Ciprofloxacin.

1. Answer: 4

Rationale: Nurse educator positions can often be found in nearly any facility that offers nursing classes. This generally includes some health care facilities, such as hospitals and long-term care facilities, that offer training programs for nurses. Educational institutes that offer nursing degrees or certificate programs also usually will have a need for nurse educators.

2. Answer: 2

Rationale: Living wills come in a variety of forms, but the common aspect is that they are meant to apply when the patient is terminal with no meaningful hope of recovery. In this case, it is too soon to know if that is the case. The living will can only be implemented if the patient is evaluated and deemed applicable.

3. Answer: 1

Rationale: The patient is losing the correct amount of fluid over a safe time frame.

4. Answer: 2

Rationale: The bacteria can still be spread to another person as long as she has diarrhea. *Campylobacter* infection does not resolve on its own. A high-fiber diet is not needed because this will worsen diarrhea, and high-fat meals are not needed because this can cause cramping.

5. Answer: 3

Rationale: Requests for nondisclosure are not rare, but they cause considerable distress for health care providers. It is important to respect the cultural issues of patients and families in a diverse society.

6. Answer: 3

Rationale: Bodies being donated cannot have an infection or contagious disease, such as a gram-negative infection.

7. Answer: 1

Rationale: The patient may not feel hungry because of chemotherapy-induced nausea but should be encouraged to eat even if not hungry. Encouraging the patient to small meals frequently throughout the day can help avoid nutritional deficiencies and improve quality of life. Chemotherapy can cause changes in smell or taste; aversion to favorite foods can result.

8. Answer: 2

Rationale: Low-residue diets include mostly white, carb-heavy foods or simply cooked meats with nothing spicy. Barbeque wings are spicy, cheese is not good, and whole grains will leave residue rather than things made with plain white flour.

9. Answer: 2

Rationale: Use the simplest explanation with the most information available.

10. Answer: 4

Rationale: A patient with Cushing disease needs to eat a low-sodium, high-protein, low-fat diet. Hamburger and french fries, pork chops in cream sauce, and guacamole are all high in fat. Roasted chicken is a high-protein, low-fat choice.

11. Answer: 1

Rationale: The risk of suicide is not reduced because a person makes frequent attempts or threats. Instead, the risk for successful suicide is greater once a single attempt has been carried out. Persons who make verbal threats or attempts are conveying their desperateness and need for assistance in controlling their own impulses for self-harm. Clients with certain personality disorders, including borderline personality disorder, are at higher risk for suicide.

12. Answer: 4

Rationale: 30%. Fifteen to 30% of patients admitted with acute diverticulitis require surgical intervention during admission. Laparoscopic surgery results in a shorter length of stay, fewer complications, and lower in-hospital mortality compared with open colectomy.

13. Answer: 3

Rationale: In patients with an aldosteronoma, medical therapy is used preoperatively to control blood pressure and correct hypokalemia, decreasing surgical risk. Medical therapy is also administered to patients with persistent hypertension postoperatively, poor surgical candidates, and patients who refuse surgery.

14. Answer: 2

Rationale: Capacity is a functional assessment and a clinical determination about a specific decision that can be made by any clinician familiar with a patient's case.

15. Answer: 2

Rationale: Familial adenomatous polyposis is characterized by the development of multiple (greater than 100) colorectal adenomas throughout the colorectum. This disorder can be caused by a germline mutation in the adenomatous polyposis coli gene and can be diagnosed either clinically or genetically. After diagnosis with the condition, patients should undergo prophylactic proctocolectomy with a neoreservoir, usually an ileoanal pouch, at an appropriate time.

16. Answer: 2

Rationale: Because this is a major surgery, a full recovery can take 10 to 12 weeks. Patients can resume normal activities sooner than 10 to 12 weeks, if possible.

17. Answer: 4

Rationale: Management of exogenous hypercortisolism involves optimization of glucocorticoid dose and route. Glucocorticoid-sparing agents are used to minimize the glucocorticoid dose; adjunctive treatments aim to reduce the effect of glucocorticoid treatment.

18. Answer: 3

Rationale: Cholecystitis is inflammation of the gall bladder. It is characterized by symptoms of inflammation, such as fever, pain in the right upper quadrant, and palpable gall bladder due to edema caused by infection. It also causes leukocytosis (not leukopenia).

19. Answer: 4

Rationale: The benefits of monoclonal antibodies are that they are expressed in cancer cells but not in vital organs and tissues.

20. Answer: 2

Rationale: Esophagogastroscopy needs to be performed first to aid in the surveillance and diagnosis of the bleed.

21. Answer: 1

Rationale: Vitamin D deficiency and elevated parathyroid hormone are common following gastric bypass (GBP) and progress over time. There is a significant incidence of secondary hyperparathyroidism in short-limb GBP patients, even those with vitamin D levels greater than or equal to 30 ng/mL, suggesting selective Ca^{2+} malabsorption. Thus calcium malabsorption is inherent to gastric bypass. Careful calcium and vitamin D supplementation and long-term screening are necessary to prevent deficiencies and the sequelae of secondary hyperparathyroidism.

22. Answer: 4

Rationale: A concussion is a type of traumatic brain injury that is caused by a bump, blow, or jolt to the head or by a hit to the body that causes the head and brain to move rapidly back and forth. This sudden movement can cause the brain to bounce around or twist in the skull, creating chemical changes in the brain and sometimes stretching and damaging brain cells.

23. Answer: 2

Rationale: Extrahepatic cholestasis or obstructive cholestasis is caused by excretory block outside of the liver, along with the extrahepatic bile ducts. Clinically, cholestasis leads to retention of the constituents of bile in blood. The two major constituents of bile are bilirubin and bile acids.

24. Answer: 4

Rationale: Education about diverticulitis includes eating a high-fiber diet, drinking lots of water, regular exercise, and considering the addition of a fiber supplement. The amount of fat in your diet does not contribute to flairs of diverticulitis.

25. Answer: 3

Rationale: Short bowel syndrome is a set of symptoms that happen while your remaining bowel adapts after your surgery. People with short bowel syndrome may have gas, cramps, diarrhea, and weight loss. Include enough nutrients in your meals to help you heal. Eat a diet high in protein, low-fiber complex carbohydrates, moderate fats, and low in sugary foods.

26. Answer: 2

Rationale: Many conditions can cause pancreatitis including abdominal surgery; alcoholism; cystic fibrosis; gallstones; high calcium levels in the blood (hypercalcemia), which may be caused by an overactive parathyroid gland (hyperparathyroidism); high triglyceride levels in the blood (hypertriglyceridemia); infection; and obesity.

27. Answer: 2

Rationale: The physical exam of a patient with a suspected retroperitoneal bleed includes a rectovaginal exam, an inspection of the urethral duct, and palpation of the pelvic landmarks.

28. Answer: 3

Rationale: Oral mucositis from chemotherapy or radiation treatment can last from 7 to 98 days. Variables such as the type of therapy and therapy frequency have an impact on oral mucositis symptoms, intensity, and length of time. Other causes of oral mucositis include thrush. Thrush occurs from yeast overgrowth in the mouth and on the tongue. It is also known as oral thrush and oral candidiasis.

29. Answer: 1

Rationale: An induration of 5 mm is considered positive for the following groups: people with suppressed immune systems, HIV-infected people, people with changes seen on chest x-ray that are consistent with previous tuberculosis (TB), recent contact with people with TB, and people who have received organ transplants.

30. Answer: 4

Rationale: Pheochromocytoma (PMC) consists of a constellation of symptoms that can also resemble other life-threatening conditions and can be difficult to diagnose if the patient is not already known to have it. PMC, which consists of hemodynamic instability with either severe hypotension or hypertension, labile hypertension, hyperthermia (greater than or equal to 40°C), encephalopathy, and multiorgan failure, can be confused with other diagnoses such as septic shock, thyroid storm, and malignant hyperthermia.

31. Answer: 1

Rationale: Symptoms of a stress ulcer include pain in the upper stomach, pain that gets better or worse with food, feeling bloated or unusually full, nausea or vomiting, and symptoms of anemia. As ulcers progress, they may bleed and will have red vomit or vomit that resembles coffee grounds; red or maroon bowel movements; very dark, tarry bowel movements; or feeling lightheaded or fainting.

32. Answer: 4

Rationale: Symptoms of elevated ammonia include confusion, excessive sleepiness, disorientation, mood swings, and hand tremors.

33. Answer: 3

Rationale: Subarachnoid hemorrhage is a type of extraaxial intracranial hemorrhage and denotes the presence of blood within the subarachnoid space. Patients tend to be older middle age, typically less than 60 years old. Risk factors include family history; hypertension; heavy alcohol consumption; female gender ~1.5× baseline risk; and African, Japanese, or Finnish descent.

34. Answer: 4

Rationale: Rapid initial diagnosis and treatment of the acute abdomen are crucial. Diagnostic interventions include blood work and imaging. In adults older than 40, a 12-lead electrocardiogram can help exclude myocardial infarction as the cause of apparent severe abdominal pain. Usually, a complete blood count, comprehensive metabolic profile, and lipase are obtained. For sepsis or mesenteric ischemia, a lactate level should be ordered. A urine or serum pregnancy test is needed in the workup of ectopic pregnancy. Diagnostic imaging has advanced rapidly in the past three decades. A bedside ultrasound in the emergency department can diagnose cholecystitis, hydronephrosis, hemoperitoneum, and the presence of an abdominal aortic aneurysm in a less than 5 minutes.

35. Answer: 1

Rationale: The TNM staging system is most often used by doctors to stage cancer. It is maintained by American Joint Committee on Cancer and the Union for International Cancer Control. In this system, the letters T, N, and M describe a different area of cancer growth: T = tumor, N = nodes, and M = metastasis.

36. Answer: 3

Rationale: Nonmaleficence is doing no harm, as stated in the historic Hippocratic Oath. Harm can be intentional or unintentional. Beneficence is doing good and the right thing for the patient. Veracity is being completely truthful with patients. Accountability is accepting responsibility for one's own actions.

37. Answer: 4

Rationale: All incidentalomas should have evaluation with laboratory tests. Dexamethasone suppression test (DST) is used to confirm subclinical adrenal adenoma. If there is an abnormal 1 mg overnight DST, then this should be confirmed with 24-hour urinary free cortisone, serum adrenocorticotropic hormone concentration, dehydroepiandrosterone sulfate, and high-dose (8 mg) overnight DST. If the elevated secretion of glucocorticoids is clinically evident, then this is confirmed when the 8 a.m. DST serum cortisol concentration is greater than 5 mcg/dL (greater than 138 nmol/L).

38. Answer: 4

Rationale: If your A1c level is between 5.7 and less than 6.5%, your levels are in the prediabetes range. If you have an A1c level of 6.5% or higher, your levels are in the diabetes range.

39. Answer: 1

Rationale: Tacrolimus is a macrolide antibiotic extracted from the soil fungus *Streptomyces tsukubaensis*. It is similar to cyclosporine and exhibits a very similar selective immunosuppressive activity. Its mechanism of action is through the inhibition of signaling through the T-cell receptor. Tacrolimus is highly lipophilic. It is generally given intravenously (IV) in the early phases following allogeneic transplantation and then switched to the oral formulation. There is rapid distribution of the drug to the extracellular space after a short IV infusion.

Bibliography

5 ways nurse practitioners can serve as advocates. *Nursing @USC*, (2017). https://nursing.usc.edu/blog/5-ways-nurse-practitioners-can-serve-as-advocates/.

AACN updates scope and standards for Acute Care NPs. *Am Assoc of Crit Care Nurses*, (2017). https://www.aacn.org/newsroom/aacn-updates-scope-and-standards-for-acute-care-nps.

Acaroglu, L. (2017). Tools for Systems Thinkers: The 6 Fundamental Concepts of Systems Thinking. *Disruptive Design*. https://medium.com/disruptive-design/tools-for-systems-thinkers-the-6-fundamental-concepts-of-systems-thinking-379cdac3dc6a.

ACCF/ACG/AHA. (2010). ACCF/ACG/AHA 2010 expert consensus document on the concomitant use of proton pump inhibitors and thienopyridines: A focused update of the ACCF/ACG/AHA. (2008). ACCF/ACG/AHA 2008 expert consensus document on reducing the gastrointestinal risks of antiplatelet therapy and NSAID use. *J Am Coll Cardiol, 56*, 2051–2066.

ACCF/ACG/AHA. (2008). expert consensus document on reducing the gastrointestinal risks of antiplatelet therapy and NSAID use. *Circulation, 118*, 1894–1909.

Acute lymphoblastic leukemia. *Leukemia & Lymphoma Society*, 2016. https://www.sllcanada.org/sites/default/files/National/CANADA/Pdf/InfoBooklets/Acute%20Lymphoblastic%20Leukemia.pdf.

Adams, J. A., Bailey, D. E., Anderson, R. A., & Docherty, S. L. (2011). Nursing roles and strategies in end-of-life decision making in acute care: A systematic review of the literature. *Nurs Res Pract, 2011*, 527834.

Addiction TIP 40. Rockville, MD: U.S. Department of Health and Human Services, 2004.

Advisory Committee on Immunization Practices (ACIP); Centers for Disease Control and Prevention (CDC). (2007). Update: Prevention of hepatitis A after exposure to hepatitis A virus and in international travelers. Updated recommendations of the Advisory Committee on Immunization Practices (ACIP). *MMWR Recomm Rep, 56*, 10804.

Advisory Committee on Immunization Practices; Centers for Disease Control and Prevention (CDC). (2011). Immunization of health-care personnel: Recommendations of the Advisory Committee on Immunization Practices (ACIP). *MMWR Recomm Rep, 60*(RR07), 145.

Afghani, E., Lo S. K., Covington, P. S., et al. (2017). Sphincter of oddi function and risk factors for dysfunction. *Front Nutr, 4*(1).

AGA Institute Guidelines for the Identification, Assessment and Initial Medical Treatment in Crohn's Disease Clinical Decision Support Tool. http://campaigns.gastro.org/algorithms/IBDCarePathway.

Agabegi, S. S., & Agabegi, E. D. (2013). *Step-Up to Medicine* (*3rd ed.*). Philadelphia: Wolters Kluwer Health.

Agrawal, M., & Swartz, R. (2000). Acute renal failure. *American Family Physician, 61*(7), 2077–2088.

Ahern, G. (2019). Communication skills: A guide to practice for healthcare professionals. *Ausmed*. https://www.ausmed.com/cpd/guides/communication-skills.

Ahmed, A., & Keeffe, E. B. (1999). Lamivudine therapy in chemotherapy-induced reactivation of hepatitis B virus infection. *American Journal of Gastroenterology, 94*, 249–251.

Aihara, H., Kumar, N., & Thompson, C. C. (2014). Diagnosis, surveillance, and treatment strategies for familial adenomatous polyposis: Rationale and update. *European Journal of Gastroenterology and Hepatology, 26*(3), 255–262.

Akyol, M., & Ozcelik, S. (2005). Non-acne dermatologic indications for systemic isotretinoin. *American Journal of Clinical Dermatology, 6*(3), 175–184.

Alexander, C. M., Landsman, P. B., Teutsch, S. M., & Haffner, S. M. (2003). NCEP-defined metabolic syndrome, diabetes, and prevalence of coronary heart disease among NHANES III participants age 50 years and older. *Diabetes, 52*(5), 1210–1214.

Alisa, N. Femia (2018). *Dermatomyositis*. https://emedicine.medscape.com/article/332783-overview.

All Nursing Schools. *How to become a nurse educator*. https://www.allnursingschools.com/nurse-educator/.

Almandoz, J. P., & Gharib, H. (2012). Hypothyroidism: Etiology, diagnosis, and management. *Medical Clinics of North America, 96*(2), 203–221.

Al-Mukhtar, R. (2014). Women's visits to hospitals without male guardians banned. *Arab News*. https://www.arabnews.com/news/525696.

Alusik, S., Kalatova, D., & Paluch, Z. (2014). Serotonin syndrome. *Neuroendocrine Letters, 34*(4), 265–273.

American Academy of Dermatology. (2009). *2009 American Academy of Dermatology administrative regulations evidence-based clinical practice guidelines*. http://www.aad.org/Forms/Policies/Uploads/AR/AR%20EvidenceBased%20Clinical%20Practice%20Guidelines.pdf.

American Lung Association. (2020). *Preventing pneumonia*. https://www.lung.org/lung-health-diseases/lung-disease-lookup/pneumonia/preventing-pneumonia.

American Association for the Study of Liver Diseases and Infectious Diseases Society of America. *Recommendations for testing, managing, and treating hepatitis C*. www.hcvguidelines.org/.

American Cancer Society. (2020). *Loss of appetite*. https://www.cancer.org/treatment/treatments-and-side-effects/physical-side-effects/eating-problems/poor-appetite.html.

American College of Gastroenterology (ACG). (2013). Practice guidelines: management of acute pancreatitis. *American Journal of Gastroenterology, 108*, 1400–1401.

American College of Gastroenterology IBS Task Force. (2009). An evidence-based position statement on the management of irritable bowel syndrome. *American Journal of Gastroenterology, 104*, S1–S35.

American College of Obstetrics and Gynecology (ACOG). (2004). Practice bulletin: Nausea and vomiting of pregnancy. *Obstetrics and Gynecology, 103*, 803–814.

American College of Rheumatology. (1997). *The American College of Rheumatology Clinical Guidelines*. Atlanta: GA: American College of Rheumatology.

American College of Rheumatology Ad Hoc Committee on Systemic Lupus Erythematosus Guidelines. (1999). Guidelines for referral and management of systemic lupus erythematosus in adults. *Arthritis Rheumatology, 42*, 1785–1796.

American College of Rheumatology Subcommittee on Rheumatoid Arthritis Guidelines. (2002). Guidelines for the management of rheumatoid arthritis: 2002 update. *Arthritis & Rheumatism, 46*(2), 328–346.

American Diabetes Association (ADA). (2016). Microvascular complications and foot care. *Diabetes Care, 39*(suppl 1), S72–S80.

American Diabetes Association (ADA). (2016). Standards of medical care in diabetes: 2016 summary of revisions. *Diabetes Care, 39*(suppl 1), S4.

American Diabetes Association (ADA). Understanding A1C. https://www.diabetes.org/a1c.

American Gastroenterological Association Institute. (2001). AGA technical review on nausea and vomiting. *Gastroenterology, 120*, 263–286.

American Gastroenterological Association Institute. (2013). Technical review on the use of thiopurines, methotrexate, and anti-TNF-α biologic drugs for the induction and maintenance of remission in Crohn's disease. *Gastroenterology, 145*, 1464–1478.

American Psychiatric Association (APA). (2013). *Diagnostic and Statistical Manual of Mental Disorders* (5th ed.). Washington, DC: APA.

American Psychiatric Association (APA). (2010). *Practice Guideline for the Treatment of Patients with Major Depressive Disorder*.

American Society of Health-System Pharmacists (ASHP). (1999). Therapeutic guidelines on stress ulcer prophylaxis. *American Journal of Health-System Pharmacy, 56*, 347–379.

Amish Studies, The Young Center: Family. https://groups.etown.edu/amishstudies/social-organization/family/.

Ammonia levels. https://medlineplus.gov/lab-tests/ammonia-levels/. Accessed May 9, 2020.

Androus, A. (2020). When should a nurse delegate? https://www.registerednursing.org/answers/when-should-nurse-delegate/.

Angiotensin-converting enzyme (ACE) inhibitors. *Mayo Clinic* (2019). https://www.mayoclinic.org/diseases-conditions/high-blood-pressure/in-depth/ace-inhibitors/art-20047480.

Annane, D., Pastores, S. M., Rochwerg, B., et al. (2017). Guidelines for the diagnosis and management of critical illness-related corticosteroid insufficiency (CIRCI) in critically ill patients (Part I): Society of Critical Care Management (SCCM) and European Society of Intensive Care Medicine (ESICM). *Critical Care Medicine, 45*(12), 2078–2088.

Anonymous. (1972). Acute infectious nonbacterial gastroenteritis: Etiology and pathogenesis. *Ann Intern Med, 76*(6), 993–1008.

Anonymous. (2005). *Understanding transcultural nursing*. https://pubmed.ncbi.nlm.nih.gov/15677986/.

ARDS Definition Task Force, Ranieri, V. M., Rubenfeld G. D., et al. (2012). Acute respiratory distress syndrome: The Berlin Definition. *Journal of the American Medical Association, 307*, 2526.

Areaux, D. (2014). Epistaxis: The common and not-so-common nosebleed. *Clinical Advisor*. https://www.clinicaladvisor.com/home/features/epistaxis-the-common-and-not-so-common-nosebleed/.

Argwala, S., Eley, T., Villegas, C., et al. (2005). Pharmacokinetic interaction between tenofovir and atazanavir coadministered with ritonavir in healthy subjects. In: *6th International Workshop on Clinical Pharmacology of HIV Therapy*, April 28–30, Quebec City, Quebec, Canada.

Aronson, J. K. (2009). Medication errors: What they are, how they happen, and how to avoid them. *QJM: An International Journal of Medicine, 8*(102), 513–521.

Arroyo, V., Ginès, P., Gerbes, A. L., et al. (1996). Definition and diagnostic criteria of refractory ascites and hepatorenal syndrome in cirrhosis. *Hepatology, 23*, 164–176.

ATLS Subcommittee; American College of Surgeons' Committee on Trauma; International ATLS Working group and the International ATLS working group. (2013). Advanced trauma life support (ATLS®): The ninth edition. *Journal of Trauma and Acute Care Surgery, 74*(5), 1363–1366.

Australian Bureau of Statistics. (2013). *Statistical language: Quantitative and qualitative data*. https://www.abs.gov.au/websitedbs/a3121120.nsf/home/statistical+language+quantitative+and+qualitative+data.

Australian Government Department of Health. (2010). Vaccine preventable diseases. https://www1.health.gov.au/internet/main/publishing.nsf/%20content/health-pubhlth-strateg-communic-vpd.htm.

Avanzini, F., Marelli, G., Donzelli, W., et al. (2011). Transition from intravenous to subcutaneous insulin: Effectiveness and safety of a standardized protocol and predictors of outcome in patients with acute coronary syndrome. *Diabetes Care, 34*(7), 1445–1450.

Baddour, L. M., Wilson, W. R., Bayer, A. S., et al. (2015). Infective endocarditis in adults: Diagnosis, antimicrobial therapy and management of complications: A scientific statement for healthcare professionals from the American Heart Association. *Circulation, 132*(5), 1435–1486.

Bagshaw, S. M., Laupland, K. B., Doig, C. J., et al. (2005). Prognosis for long-term survival and renal recovery in critically ill patients with severe acute renal failure: A population-based study. *Critical Care, 9*, R700–R709.

Baker, R. (2015). Adrenal tumors: Anatomy, physiology, diagnosis, and treatment. *International Oncology Nursing*. https://www.interventionaloncology360.com/article/adrenal-tumors-anatomy-physiology-diagnosis-and-treatment.

Ballinger, A. (2011). *Essentials of Kumar and Clark's Clinical Medicine E-Book*. St. Louis: Elsevier Health Sciences.

Ballinger, A. E., Palmer, S. C., Wiggins, K. J., et al. (2014). Treatment for peritoneal dialysis-associated peritonitis. *Cochrane Database of Systematic Reviews, 4*.

Balough, E. P., Miller, B. T., & Ball, J. R. (2015). *Committee on Diagnostic Error in Health Care; Board on Health Care Services; Institute of Medicine; The National Academies of Sciences, Engineering, and Medicine*. Washington (DC): National Academies Press. 2015. https://www.ncbi.nlm.nih.gov/books/NBK338605/.

Bandelow, B., Zohar, J., Hollander, E., et al. (2008). World Federation of Societies of Biological Psychiatry (WFSBP) guidelines for the pharmacological treatment of anxiety, obsessive-compulsive and post-traumatic stress disorders, first revision. *World Journal of Biological Psychiatry, 9*, 248–312.

Barclay, L. (2013). Crystalloids may be best for initial hypovolemia treatment. *Medscape*. https://www.medscape.com/viewarticle/812389.

Bargaining stage. ChangingMinds.org. http://changingminds.org/disciplines/change_management/kubler_ross/bargaining_stage.htm.

Barrow, J. M., & Sharma, S. (2020). Five rights of nursing delegation. *StatPearls[Internet]*. https://www.ncbi.nlm.nih.gov/books/NBK519519/.

Basford, K. (2019). Lisinopril side effects. *ZAVA*. https://www.zavamed.com/uk/side-effects-of-lisinopril.html.

Beal, S.G., & Burton, E.C. (2019). Religions and the autopsy. https://emedicine.medscape.com/article/1705993-overview.

Becher, E.C., & Chassin, M.R. (2001). Improving quality, minimizing error: Making it happen. *Health Affairs, 20*(3), 68–81.

Bell, L. (2014). Collaborative practice and patient safety. *Am J Crit Care, 23*(3), 239.

Bellomo, R., Cass, A., Cole, L., et al. (2009). Intensity of continuous renal replacement therapy in critically ill patients. *New England Journal of Medicine, 361*(17), 1627–1638.

Bellomo, R., Ronco, C., Kellum, J. A., et al. (2004). Acute renal failure—definition, outcome measures, animal models, and information technology needs: The Second International Consensus Conference of the Acute Dialysis Quality Initiative (ADQI) Group. *Critical Care, 8*, R204–R212.

Benson, T. (May 2016). Systems thinking leaders. *Southeast Education Network*. https://www.seenmagazine.us/Articles/Article-Detail/articleid/5610/systems-thinking-leaders.

Berg, K. J. (2000). Nephrotoxicity related to contrast media. *Scandinavian Journal of Urology and Nephrology, 34*(5), 317–322.

Bertsias, G., Ioannidis, J. P., Boletis, J., et al. (2008). EULAR recommendations for the management of systemic lupus erythematosus: Report of a task force of the EULAR standing committee for international clinical studies including therapeutics. *Annals of Rheumatic Diseases, 67*(2), 195–205.

Bharucha, A. E., Pemberton, J. H., & Locke, G. R. (2013). AGA technical review on constipation. *Gastroenterology, 144*, 218–238.

Bielory, L. (2016). Allergic and immunologic eye disease. *Science Direct*. https://www.sciencedirect.com/topics/neuroscience/topical-decongestants.

Blacklow, N. R., & Cukor, G. (1981). Viral gastroenteritis. *N Engl J Med, 304*(7), 397–406.

Bloom, C. I., Palmer, T., Feary, J., et al. (2019). Exacerbation patterns in adults with asthma in England: A population-based study. *American Journal of Respiratory Critical Care Medicine, 199*, 446.

Boden, B. P., & Osbahr, D. C. (2000). High-risk stress fractures: evaluation and treatment. *JAAOS-Journal of the American Academy of Orthopaedic Surgeons, 8*(6), 344–353.

Body Donation at Mayo Clinic. https://www.mayoclinic.org/body-donation/making-donation.

Bogun, M., & Inzucchi, S. E. (2013). Inpatient management of diabetes and hyperglycemia. *Clinical Therapeutics, 35*(5), 724–733.

Born, S. Hydration: What you need to know. *Hammer Nutrition*. https://www.hammernutrition.com/knowledge/advanced-knowledge/hydration-what-you-need-to-know.

Bouglé, A., Harrois, A., & Duranteau, J. (2013). Resuscitative strategies in traumatic hemorrhagic shock. *Annals of Intensive Care, 13*(1), 1–9.

Brakke, R. (2016). What is crepitus. *Arthritis Health*. https://www.arthritis-health.com/types/general/what-crepitus.

Branham, S., DelloSritto, R., & Hilliard, T. (2014). Lost in translation: the acute care nurse practitioners' use of evidence-based practice: a qualitative study. *Journal of Nursing Education and Practice*(4), 53–59.

Bratzler, D. W., Dellinger, E. P., Olsen, K. M., et al. (2013a). Clinical practice guidelines for antimicrobial prophylaxis in surgery. *American Journal of Health-System Pharmacy, 70*, 195–283.

Bratzler, D. W., Dellinger, E. P., Olsen, K. M., et al. (2013b). Clinical practice guidelines for antimicrobial prophylaxis in surgery. *Surg Infect (Larchmt), 14*(1), 73–156.

Brennan, M. G. (2010). Confidentiality in practice; knowing when to keep a secret. *Vital, 7*, 44–46.

Brent, N. J. (2016). Know the law before acting as Good Samaritan. *Nurse.com*. https://www.nurse.com/blog/2016/08/18/know-the-law-before-acting-as-good-samaritan/.

Brigham and Women's Faulkner Hospital. (2020). Understanding Do Not Resuscitate (DNR) orders. https://www.brighamandwomensfaulkner.org/patients-and-families/advance-care-directives/dnr-orders.

Broaddus, C., Mason, R., Ernst, J., et al. (2016). Sarcoidosis. In: *Murray and Nadel's Textbook of Respiratory Medicine* (6th ed.). Pennsylvania: Elsevier, pp. 1188–1206, e7.

Brown, B., & Hough, Falk, L. (2014). 6 steps for implementing successful performance improvement initiatives in healthcare. *Health Catalyst*. https://www.healthcatalyst.com/insights/implementing-healthcare-performance-improvement-initiatives/.

Brubacher, J. W., & Dodds, S. D. (2008). Pediatric supracondylar fractures of the distal humerus. *Current Reviews in Musculoskeletal Medicine*, Dec 1(3–4), 190–196. doi: 10.1007/s12178-008-9027-2.

Brusch, J. L. (2019). *Septic arthritis*. https://emedicine.medscape.com/article/236299-overview.

Brusso, J., *Cushing's Syndrome diet*. https://www.livestrong.com/article/436769-cushings-syndrome-diet/.

Buchanan, R. W., Kreyenbuhl, J. M., Kelly, D. L., et al. (2010). The 2009 schizophrenia PORT psychopharmacological treatment. Recommendations and summary statements. *Schizophrenia Bulletin, 36*, 71–93.

Buddiga, P. (2014). Cardiovascular system anatomy. *Medscape.* https://emedicine.medscape.com/article/1948510-overview.

Bulauitan, C. S. (2018). Fat Embolism. *Medscape.* https://emedicine.medscape.com/article/460524-overview.

Bulauitan, C. S. (2020). Fat Embolism Clinical Presentation. *Medscape.* https://emedicine.medscape.com/article/460524-clinical#b3.

Burke, B. M., & Cunliffe, W. J. (1984). The assessment of acne vulgaris—the Leeds technique. *British Journal of Dermatology, 111*, 83–92.

Burn-Maddoch, R., Fisher, M. A., & Hunt, J. N. (1980). Does lying on the right side increase the rate of gastric emptying. *J Physiol, 302*, 395–398.

Butalia S., Audibert F., Côté A. M., et al. (2018). Hypertension Canada's 2018 guidelines for the management of hypertension in pregnancy. *Canadian Journal of Cardiology, 34*(5), 526–531.

Byrd, R. P. (2019). Respiratory Acidosis. *Medscape.* https://emedicine.medscape.com/article/301574-overview.

California State University Bakersfield. Formatting a testable hypothesis. https://www.csub.edu/~ddodenhoff/Bio100/Bio100sp04/formattingahypothesis.htm.

Camfield, P. R., Bagnell, P., Camfield, C. S., & Tibbles, J. A. R. (1979). Pancreatitis due to valproic acid. *Lancet, 1*, 1198.

Cannon, J. W. (2018). Hemorrhagic shock. *New England Journal of Medicine, 378*(4), 370–379.

Captopril (2019) *Drugs.com.* https://www.drugs.com/cdi/captopril.html.

Captopril (Capoten). (2019). *eMedicine Health.* https://www.emedicinehealth.com/drug-captopril/article_em.htm.

Care coordination and registered nurses' essential role. *ANA Congress on Nursing Practice and Economics.* (2012). https://www.nursingworld.org/~4afbf2/globalassets/practiceandpolicy/health-policy/cnpe-care-coord-position-statement-final–draft-6-12-2012.pdf.

Care of the patient post cardiac catheterization. *The Royal Children's Hospital Melbourne.* https://www.rch.org.au/rchcpg/hospital_clinical_guideline_index/Care_of_the_patient_post_cardiac_catheterisation/.

Carteret, M. (2011). Culturally based beliefs about illness causation. Retrieved from: http://www.dimensionsofculture.com/2011/02/culturally-based-beliefs-about-illness-causation/2011/.

Carvounis, C. P., Nisar, S., & Guro-Rozuman, S. (2002). Significance of the fractional excretion of urea in the differential diagnosis of acute renal failure. *Kidney International*, 2223–2229.

Case di Leonardi, B. (2013). The chain of command protects your patients and you. *RN.com.* https://www.rn.com/nursing-news/chain-of-command-protects-your-patients-and-you/.

Castelino, T., & Mitmaker, E. (2016). Pheochromocytoma crisis. https://www.intechopen.com/books/clinical-management-of-adrenal-tumors/pheochromocytoma-crisis.

Causes of fat embolism syndrome. (2018). *Healthline.* https://www.healthline.com/health/fat-embolism-syndrome#prevention.

Caylor, T. L., & Perkins, A. (2013). Recognition and management of polymyalgia rheumatica and giant cell arteritis. *American Family Physician, 88*(10), 676–684.

Centers for disease control and prevention. (2016). Transmission-based precautions. https://www.cdc.gov/infectioncontrol/basics/transmission-based-precautions.html.

Centers for Disease Control and Prevention. (2019a). *Pneumococcal vaccination: What everyone needs to know.* https://www.cdc.gov/vaccines/vpd/pneumo/public/index.html.

Centers for Disease Control and Prevention. (2019b). *Pneumococcal vaccine.* https://www.cdc.gov/pneumococcal/vaccination.html.

Centers for Disease Control and Prevention. (2020). Oysters and vibriosis). https://www.cdc.gov/foodsafety/communication/oysters-and-vibriosis.html.

Cerebrospinal fluid (CSF). (n.d.). https://www.nationalmssociety.org/Symptoms-Diagnosis/Diagnosing-Tools/Cerebrospinal-Fluid-(CSF).

Cerebrospinal fluid culture). (2016). *Healthline.* https://www.healthline.com/health/cerebrospinal-fluid-culture#next-steps.

Chabot, E., & Nirula, R. (2017). Open abdomen critical care management principles: Resuscitation, fluid balance, nutrition, and ventilator management. *Trauma Surg Acute Care Open, 2*(1), e000063.

Chan, J. (2012). What to do and how to behave in China: 18 practical tips. *Asia Marketing and Management.* http://www.asiamarketingmanagement.com/howtobehaveinchina.html.

Chao, N. (2020). Overview of immunosuppressive agents used for prevention and treatment of graft-versus-host disease. *UpToDate.* https://www.uptodate.com/contents/overview-of-immunosuppressive-agents-used-for-prevention-and-treatment-of-graft-versus-host-disease#H152830127.

Charmandari, E., Nicolaides, N. C., & Chrousos, G. P. (2014). Adrenal insufficiency. *The Lancet, 383*(9935), 2152–2167.

Chen, J., & Wall, M. (2014). Epidemiology and risk factors for idiopathic intracranial hypertension. *Int Ophthalmol Clin, 54*(1), 1–11.

Chey, W. D., Leontiadis, G. I., Howden, C. W., & Moss, S. F. (2017). American College of Gastroenterology Guideline: Treatment of *Helicobacter pylori* infection. *Am J Gastroenterol, 112*, 212–238.

Choi, W. S., Baek, J. H., Seo, Y. B., et al. (2014). Transgovernmental enterprise for pandemic influenza in Korea. Severe influenza treatment guideline. *Korean Journal of Internal Medicine, 29*(1), 132–147.

Chong Y., Han S. J., Rhee Y. J., et al. (2016). Classic peripheral signs of subacute bacterial endocarditis. *Korean J Thorac Cardiovasc Surg, 49*(5), 408–412.

Chou R., Qaseem A., Snow V., et al. (2007). Diagnosis and treatment of low back pain: A joint clinical practice guideline from the American College of Physicians and the American Pain Society. *Annals of Internal Medicine, 147*(7), 478–491.

Chou, S., & Fasano, R. (2016). Management of patients with sickle cell disease using transfusion therapy. *Hematology/Oncology Clinics of North America, 30*(3), 591–608.

Clarke, S. P., Sloane, D. M., & Aiken, L. H. (2002). Effects of hospital staffing and organizational climate on needlestick injuries to nurses. *American Journal of Public Health, 92,* 1115–1119.

Clinical inquiry skills in nursing. *AACN CCRN Certification Exam & Review.* Retrieved from: https://study.com/academy/lesson/clinical-inquiry-skills-in-nursing.html#lesson.

Clinical institute withdrawal assessment for alcohol scale (CIWA-Ar). (1989). *Br J Addict, 84,* 13537.

CMS.gov. National Provider Identifier Standard (NPD). https://www.cms.gov/Regulations-and-Guidance/Administrative-Simplification/NationalProvIdentStand.

Cohen S. H., Gerding D. N., Johnson S., et al. (2010). Clinical practice guidelines for *Clostridium difficile* infection in adults: 2010 update by the Society for Healthcare Epidemiology of America (SHEA) and the Infectious Diseases Society of America (IDSA). *Infection Control & Hospital Epidemiology, 31,* 431–455.

Colorectal cancer: Risk factors and prevention. *Cancer.net.* (2019 Oct). https://www.cancer.net/cancer-types/colorectal-cancer/risk-factors-and-prevention.

Cone, J., & Inaba, K. (2017). Lower extremity compartment syndrome. *Trauma Surg Acute Care Open, 2*(1), e000094.

Confidentiality and disclosure of information. https://www.themdu.com/guidance-and-advice/journals/new-wardround-june-2013/confidentiality-and-disclosure-of-information.

Contrast Materials. *RadiologyInfo.* https://www.radiologyinfo.org/en/info.cfm?pg=safety-contrast.

Cook, D. J., Fuller, H. D., Guyatt, G. H., et al. (1994). Risk factors for gastrointestinal bleeding in critically ill patients [Canadian Critical Care Trials Group]. *New England Journal of Medicine, 330,* 377–381.

Corrêa, T. D., Rocha, L. L., & Pessoa, C. M. S., et al. (2015). Fluid therapy for septic shock resuscitation: Which fluid should be used. *Einstein (São Paulo), 13*(3).

Corticosteroids and diabetes. *Diabetes.co.uk.* (2019). https://www.diabetes.co.uk/diabetes-medication/costicosteroids-and-diabetes.html.

Costa-Bauza, A., Ramis, M., Montesinos, V., et al. (2007). Type of renal calculi: variation with age and sex. *World Journal of Urology, 25*(4), 415–421.

Costedoat-Chalumeau, N., Galicier, L., Aumaître, O., et al. (2013). Hydroxychloroquine in systemic lupus erythematosus: results of a French multicentre controlled trial (PLUS Study). *Annals of Rheumatic Disease, 72,* 1786–1792.

Crismon, M. L., Kattura, R. S., & Buckley, P. F. (2017). Schizophrenia. In: DiPiro, J. T., Talbert, R. L., Yee, G. C., et al. (Eds.), *Pharmacotherapy: A Pathophysiologic Approach* (10th ed.). New York: McGraw-Hill.

Cronenwett, J., & Johnston, K. (2014). *Acute deep venous thrombosis: Pathophysiology and natural history.* In: *Rutherford's Vascular Surgery* (8th ed.): Pennsylvania: Elsevier (pp. 744–761).

Cronenwett L., Sherwood G., Pohl J., et al. (2009). Quality and safety education for advanced nursing practice. *Nursing Outlook, 57*(6), 338–348.

Cuesta, M., & Thompson, C. J. (2016). The syndrome of inappropriate antidiuresis (SIAD). *Best Practice & Research: Clinical Endocrinology & Metabolism, 30*(2), 175–187.

Cullen, G., & O'Donoghue, D. (2007). Constipation and pregnancy. *Best Practice and Research: Clinical Gastroenterology, 21*(5), 807–818.

Cultural Competence. National Prevention Information Network. (2015). https://npin.cdc.gov/pages/cultural-competence.

Cultural competence in health care: Is it important for people with chronic conditions? https://hpi.georgetown.edu/cultural/.

Cultural etiquette: Japan. http://www.ediplomat.com/np/cultural_etiquette/ce_jp.htm.

Cundy, T., & MacKay, J. (2011). Proton pump inhibitors and severe hypomagnesemia. *Current Opinions in Gastroenterology, 27,* 180–185.

Cunha, J. P. (2019). Angiomax side effects. *RXlist.* https://www.rxlist.com/angiomax-side-effects-drug-center.htm.

Cunha, J. P., & Stöppler, M. C. (2019). Collapsed lung (pneumothorax) symptoms, causes, types, treatments, surgery, and outcome. *eMedicine Health.* https://www.emedicinehealth.com/collapsed_lung/article_em.htm.

Cunningham, R. (2006). Proton pump inhibitors and the risk of *Clostridium difficile*-associated disease: Further evidence from the community. *Canadian Medical Association Journal, 175,* 757–758.

Dager W., Halilovic J., et al. (2014). Acute kidney injury. In: J. T. DiPiro, R. L. Talbert, & G. C. Yee et al (Eds.), *Pharmacotherapy: A pathophysiologic approach* (9th ed.) (pp. 611–632). New York: McGraw-Hill.

Danger signs of concussion. (n.d.). *Centers for Disease Control and Prevention.* https://www.cdc.gov/headsup/basics/concussion_danger_signs.html.

Dassopoulos, T., Sultan, S., Falck-Ytter, Y. T., Inadomi, J. M., & Hanauer, S. B. (2013). American Gastroenterological Association Institute technical review on the use of thiopurines, methotrexate, and anti-TNF-α biologic drugs for the induction and maintenance of remission in inflammatory Crohn's disease. *Gastroenterology, 145,* 1464–1478.

Dastidar, J. G., & Odden, A. (2011). How do I determine if my patient has decision-making capacity. *The Hospitalist.* https://www.the-hospitalist.org/hospitalist/article/124731/how-do-i-determine-if-my-patient-has-decision-making-capacity.

Dealing with challenging patients. (2020). https://www.themdu.com/guidance-and-advice/guides/guide-to-dealing-with-challenging-patients.

Dealing with the loss of a loved one. (2011). *Mayo Clinic Proceedings.* https://www.myhealth.va.gov/mhv-portal-web/dealing-with-the-loss-of-a-loved-one/-/journal_content/56_INSTANCE_TZBICHAuVEtk/12612/206054?p_p_state=pop_up&_56_INSTANCE_TZBICHAuVEtk_page=1&_56_INSTANCE_TZBICHAuVEtk_viewMode=print.

Della Rocca, G. J., & Crist, B. D. (2013). Hip fracture protocols: What have we changed. *Orthopedic Clinics, 44*(2), 163–182.

Developing cultural awareness. (2019). https://www.notredameonline.com/resources/intercultural-management/developing-your-cultural-awareness/#.W3VGFSQzbMw.

de Vries, F. M., Denig, P., Pouwels, K. B., Postma, M. J., & Hak, E. (2012). Primary prevention of major cardiovascular and cerebrovascular events with statins in diabetic patients. *Drugs, 72*(18), 2365–2373.

DeWitt, D. (2019). All about the L4-L5 spinal segment. https://www.spine-health.com/conditions/spine-anatomy/all-about-l4-l5-spinal-segment.

Dhikav, V. (2001). Aspirin misconceptions. *Drugs News and Views, 6*(1), 64–65.

Diabetes and American Indians/Alaska Natives. https://minorityhealth.hhs.gov/omh/browse.aspx?lvl=4&lvlid=33.

Dill, T. (2008). Contraindications to magnetic resonance imaging. *Heart, 94,* 943–948. https://doi.org/10.1136/hrt.2007.125039.

Divakaran, S., & Loscalzo, J. (2017). The role of nitroglycerin and other nitrogen oxides in cardiovascular therapeutics. *Journal of the American College of Cardiology, 70*(19), 2393–2410.

Dodds, S. (2017). The how-to for type 2: An overview of diagnosis and management of type 2 diabetes mellitus. *Nursing Clinics of North America, 52*(4), 513–522.

Doering, P., & Li, R.M. (2017). Substance-related disorders II: Alcohol, nicotine, and caffeine. In: DiPiro, J. T., Talbert, R. L., Yee, G. C., et al. (Eds). *Pharmacotherapy: A Pathophysiologic Approach* (10th ed.). New York: McGraw-Hill.

Doherty, M. (2020). *Clinical manifestations and diagnosis of osteoarthritis.* Retrieved from https://www.uptodate.com/contents/clinical-manifestations-and-diagnosis-of-osteoarthritis.

Do-not-resuscitate order. *MedlinePlus.* (2020). https://medlineplus.gov/ency/patientinstructions/000473.htm.

Dove, H. G., & Forthman, T. (1995). Helping financial analysts communicate variance analysis. *Healthcare Finance Management, 49*(4), 52–54.

Dreno, B., Thiboutot, D., Gollnick, H., et al. (2014). Antibiotic stewardship in dermatology: Limiting antibiotic use in acne. *European Journal of Dermatology, 24,* 330–334.

Drent, M. L., Larsson, I., William-Olsson, T., et al. (1995). Orlistat, a lipase inhibitor, in the treatment of human obesity: A multiple dose study. *Int J Obes Relat Metab Disord, 19,* 221–226.

Duck, A. (2009). Does oxygen need humidification? *Nursing Times.* https://www.nursingtimes.net/clinical-archive/respiratory-clinical-archive/does-oxygen-need-humidification-14-12-2009/.

Duke University Medical Center Library & Archives. (2019). Evidence-based tutorial. https://guides.mclibrary.duke.edu/ebptutorial.

Durán, K., Hsu, B. B., & Ma, H (2008). Endotracheal Tube Position Monitoring Device. *Semantic Scholar.* https://www.semanticscholar.org/paper/Endotracheal-Tube-Position-Monitoring-Device-Dur%C3%A1n-Hsu/9e5e2addc35cc6ae350b54a35f33640f748e3c0f?p2df.

Durning, M. (2011). HIPAA privacy rule & patient confidentiality. *Nursing Link.*

Eke, S. (2019 Dec). Heparin-induced thrombocytopenia. *Medscape.* https://emedicine.medscape.com/article/1357846-overview.

Emens L, Ascierto P., Darcy P., et al. (2017). Cancer immunotherapy: Opportunities and challenges in the rapidly evolving clinical landscape. *European Journal of Cancer, 81,* 116–129.

Endocarditis. *Mayo Clinic.* (2017). https://www.mayoclinic.org/diseases-conditions/endocarditis/symptoms-causes/syc-20352576.

English, A., & Ford, C.A. The HIPAA privacy rule and adolescents: Legal questions and clinical challenges. *Perspectives on Sexual and Reproductive Health.* https://www.guttmacher.org/sites/default/files/pdfs/pubs/psrh/full/3608004.pdf.

Enoxaparin. *Medscape,* https://reference.medscape.com/drug/lovenox-enoxaparin-342174.

Epstein, M., McGrath, S., & Law, F. (2006). Proton-pump inhibitors and hypomagnesemic hypoparathyroidism. *New England Journal of Medicine, 355,* 1834–1836.

Estimated glomerular infiltration rate (eGFR). *National Kidney Foundation.* (2020). https://www.kidney.org/atoz/content/gfr.

Estimating glomerular filtration rate. *National Institute of Diabetes and Digestive and Kidney Diseases.* https://www.niddk.nih.gov/health-information/communication-programs/nkdep/laboratory-evaluation/glomerular-filtration-rate/estimating.

Ethnocentrism. *Lumen Cultural Anthropology.* https://courses.lumenlearning.com/culturalanthropology/chapter/ethnocentrism/.

Everts, H. B. (2012). Endogenous retinoids in the hair follicle and sebaceous gland. *Biochimica et Biophysica Acta, 1821*(1), 222–229.

Evidence-based medicine: What is the PICO model? *University of Illinois Library.* (2020). https://researchguides.uic.edu/c.php?g=252338&p=3954402.

Evidence-based practice in health. *University of Canberra.* (2019). https://canberra.libguides.com/c.php?g=599346&p=4149723.

Exercise & Type 1. *American Diabetes Association.* https://www.diabetes.org/fitness/get-and-stay-fit/exercise-and-type-1.

Exposure therapies for specific phobias. *Society of Clinical Psychology.* (2016). https://div12.org/treatment/exposure-therapies-for-specific-phobias/.

Fagan, S. P., Bilodeau, M. L., & Goverman, J. (2014). Burn intensive care. *Surgical Clinics of North America, 94*(4), 765–779.

Family visitation in the adult intensive care unit. (2016). *Crit Care Nurse, 36*(1), e15–e18. https://doi.org/10.4037/ccn2016677.

Farkas, J. (2014). Large volume thoracentesis: How much can safely be removed. *Pulm Crit.* https://emcrit.org/pulmcrit/large-volume-thoracentesis-how-much-can-safely-be-removed/.

Farmer, L., & Lundy, A. (2017). Informed consent: Ethical and legal considerations for advanced practice nurses. *The Journal for Nurse Practitioners, 13*(2), 124–130.

Fauci, A. S., Kasper, D. L., Hauser, S. L., Jameson, J. L., & Loscalzo, J. (2012). In D. L. Longo (Ed.), New York: McGraw-Hill.

Fawcett, R. S., Linford, S., & Stulberg, D. S. (2004). Nail abnormalities: Clues to systemic disease. *Am Fam Physician, 69*(6), 1417–1424.

Fayfman, M. M., Pasquel, F. J., & Umpierrez, G. E. (2017). Management of hyperglycemic crises: Diabetic ketoacidosis and hyperglycemic hyperosmolar state. *Medical Clinics of North America, 101*(3), 587–606.

Federal government. (2016 Aug). ADA emphasize importance of flossing and interdental cleaners. *American Dental Association.* https://www.ada.org/en/press-room/news-releases/2016-archive/august/statement-from-the-american-dental-association-about-interdental-cleaners.

Feldman, S., Careccia, R. E., Barham, K. L., et al. (2004). Diagnosis and treatment of acne. *American Family Physician, 69,* 2123–2130.

Feng, Q. Z., Cheng, L. Q., & Li, Y. F. (2012). Progressive deterioration of left ventricular function in a patient with a normal coronary angiogram. *World J Cardiol, 4*(4), 130–134.

Ferri, F. (2018). Acquired immunodeficiency syndrome. In: *Ferri's Clinical Advisor* (pp. 17–24). Philadelphia: Elsevier.

Ferri, F. (2018). Kaposi's sarcoma. In: *Ferri's Clinical Advisor* (p. 735). Philadelphia: Elsevier.

Ferrone, M., Raimondo, M., & Scolapio, J. S. (2007). Pancreatic enzyme pharmacotherapy. *Pharmacotherapy, 27,* 910–920.

Ferwerda, J. (2016). How to care for patients from different cultures. *Nurse.org.* https://nurse.org/articles/how-to-deal-with-patients-with-different-cultures/.

Fihn, S. D., Blankenship, J. C., Alexander, K. P., et al. (2014). 2014 ACC/AHA/AATS/PCNA/SCAI/STS focused update of the guideline for the diagnosis and management of patients with stable ischemic heart disease: A report of the American College of Cardiology/American Heart Association Task Force on Practice Guidelines, and the American Association for Thoracic Surgery, Preventive Cardiovascular Nurses Association, Society for Cardiovascular Angiography and Interventions, and Society of Thoracic Surgeons. *Journal of the American College of Cardiology, 64*(18), 1929–1949.

Finlay, A. Y., & Ortonne, J. P. (2004). Patient satisfaction with psoriasis therapies: An update and introduction to biologic therapy. *Journal of Cutaneous Medicine and Surgery, 8,* 310–320.

First aid for tonic-clonic seizures. (2017). *Epilepsy Foundation.* https://www.epilepsy.com/learn/seizure-first-aid-and-safety/adapting-first-aid-plans/first-aid-tonic-clonic-seizures.

Flake, Z. A., Scalley, R. D., & Bailey, A. G. (2004). Practical selection of antiemetics. *American Family Physician, 69,* 1169–1174.

Fliers, E. E. (2015). Thyroid function in critically ill patients. *The Lancet, Diabetes & Endocrinology, 3*(10), 816–825.

Ford, A. C., Moayyedi, P., Lacy, B. E., et al. (2014). American College of Gastroenterology monograph on the management of irritable bowel syndrome and chronic idiopathic constipation. *American Journal of Gastroenterology, 109,* S2–S26.

Fosco, C. (2013). Understanding the four stages of pressure ulcers. *Wound Rounds.* https://woundrounds.com/understanding-the-four-stages-of-pressure-ulcers/.

Fouere, S., Adjadj, L., & Pawin, H. (2005). How patients experience psoriasis: Results from a European survey. *Journal of the European Academy of Dermatology and Venereology*(19), 2–6.

Frendl, G., Sodickson, A. C., Chung, M. K., et al. (2014). 2014 AATS guidelines for the prevention and management of perioperative atrial fibrillation and flutter for thoracic surgical procedures. *Journal of Thoracic Cardiovascular Surgery, 148*(3), e153.

Frink, M., Hildebrand, F., Krettek, C., Brand, J., & Hankemeier, S. (2010). Compartment syndrome of the lower leg and foot. *Clinical Orthopaedics and Related Research, 468*(4), 940–950.

Frost A., Badesch D., Gibbs J. S. R., et al. (2019). Diagnosis of pulmonary hypertension. *European Respiratory Journal, 53.*

Fu, P. P., Xia, Q., Boudreau, M. D., et al. (2007). Physiological role of retinyl palmitate in the skin. *Vitamins and Hormones, 75,* 223–256.

Fuster, V., Alexander, R. W., O'Rourke, R. A., et al. (2004). *Hurst's The Heart* (11th ed.). New York: McGraw-Hill.

Gabriel, S. E., Jaakkimainen, L., & Bombardier, C. (1991). Risk for serious gastrointestinal complications related to use of nonsteroidal anti-inflammatory drugs: A meta-analysis. *Ann Intern Med, 115,* 787–796.

Gaieski, D. F., O'Brien, N. F., & Hernandez, R. (2017). Emergency neurologic life support: Meningitis and encephalitis. *Neurocritical Care, 27*(Suppl 1), 124–133.

Galanti, G. A. (2000). An introduction to cultural differences. *Western Journal of Medicine*(5), 172.

García-De La Torre, I., & Nava-Zavala, A. (2009). Gonococcal and nongonococcal arthritis. *Rheumatic Disease Clinics, 35*(1), 63–73.

Garcia-Tsao, G., Abraldes, J. G., Berzigotti, A., & Bosch, J. (2017). Portal hypertensive bleeding in cirrhosis: risk stratification, diagnosis, and management: 2016 practice guidance by the American Association for the Study of Liver Diseases. *Hepatology, 65,* 310–335.

Garcia-Tsao, G., Groszmann, R. J., Fisher, R. L., Conn, H. O., Atterbury, C. E., & Glickman, M. (1985). Portal pressure, presence of gastroesophageal varices and variceal bleeding. *Hepatology, 5,* 419–424.

Gastrointestinal bleeding. *MedlinePlus.* (2020). https://medlineplus.gov/gastrointestinalbleeding.html.

Gastrointestinal bleeding. Wake Gastroenterology. https://wakegastro.com/patient-info/patient-education/gastrointestinal-bleeding/.

Geeraerts, T., Velly, L., Abdennour, L., Asehnoune, K., Audibert, G., & Bouzat, P. (2018). Association des anesthesistes-reanimateurs pediatriques d'expression. Management of traumatic brain injury (first 24 hours). *Anaesthesiol Critical Care Pain Medicine, 37*(2), 80–87.

Gender and Ageism. Available at http://faculty.webster.edu/woolflm/ageismgender.html.

Get informed about informed consent. *Nursing Made Incredibly Easy!.* (2008), *6*(1), 56. https://doi.org/10.1097/01.NME.0000304929.48056.6f.

Ghosh, S., Cowen, S., Hannan, W. J., & Ferguson, A. (1994). Low bone mineral density in Crohn's disease, but not in ulcerative colitis, at diagnosis (see comments). *Gastroenterology, 107,* 1031–1039.

Gibbons, S., Robinson, L., Dickinson, L., et al. (2004). Therapeutic drug monitoring of atazanavir in routine clinical settings in the UK. In: *7th International Congress of Drug Therapy in HIV Infection. Glasgow* [P274].

Gilkes, M. (2018). Peplau's Theory: A nurse/patient collaboration. *ASUMed.* https://www.ausmed.com/cpd/articles/peplaus-theory.

Gillis, J. C., & Brogden, R. N. (1997). Ketorolac: A reappraisal of its pharmacodynamic and pharmacokinetic properties and therapeutic use in pain management. *Drugs, 53,* 139–188.

Gines, P., Angeli, P., Lenz, K., Moller, S., Moore, K., & Moreau, R. (2010). EASL clinical practice guidelines on the management of ascites, spontaneous bacterial peritonitis and hepatorenal syndrome in cirrhosis. *J Hepatol, 53*(3), 397–417.

Glaser, B. G. (2008). The constant comparative method of qualitative analysis. *Grounded Theory Review: An International Journal.* http://groundedtheoryreview.com/2008/11/29/the-constant-comparative-method-of-qualitative-analysis-1/.

Global Initiative for Chronic Obstructive Lung Disease (GOLD). Global strategy for the diagnosis, management and prevention of chronic obstructive pulmonary disease: 2019 Report. www.goldcopd.org.

Glomerular filtration rate. *MedlinePlus.* (2020). https://medlineplus.gov/ency/article/007305.htm.

Goldman, L., & Schafer, A. (2016a). Approach to anemias. In *Goldman-Cecil Medicine* (25th ed., pp. 1059–1068). Philadelphia: Elsevier.

Goldman, L., & Schafer, A. (2016b). Autoimmune and intravascular hemolytic anemias. In *Goldman-Cecil Medicine* (25th ed., pp. 1073–1080. Philadelphia: Elsevier.

Goldman, L., & Schafer, A. (2016c). *Rheumatoid arthritis.* In: *Goldman-Cecil Medicine* (25th ed., pp. 1754–1762). Philadelphia: Elsevier.

Goldman, L., & Schafer, A. (2016d). The spondyloarthropathie. *Goldman-Cecil Medicine* (25th ed., pp. 1762–1769). Philadelphia: Elsevier.

Goldsmith, D. R., Wagstaff, A. J., Ibbotson, T., & Perry, C. M. (2004). Spotlight on lamotrigine in bipolar disorder. *CNS Drugs, 18,* 63–67.

Gordon, K. A., Beach, M. L., Biedenbach, D. J., et al. (2002). Antimicrobial susceptibility patterns of β-hemolytic and viridans group streptococci: Report from the SENTRY Antimicrobial Surveillance Program (1997–2000). *Diagnostic Microbiology and Infections Disease, 432,* 157–162.

Gotthardt D., Riediger C., Heinze Weiss K., et al. (2007). Fulminant hepatic failure: Etiology and indications for liver transplantation. *Nephrology Dialysis Transplantation, 22*(8), viii5–viii8.

Grannis, Jr., F. W., Cullinane, C. A., & Lai, L. (2007). Fluid complications. *Cancer Network.* https://www.cancernetwork.com/view/fluid-complications.

Gray, R., Robson, D., & Bressington, D. (2002). Medication management for people with a diagnosis of schizophrenia. *Nursing Times, 98*(47), 38. https://www.nursingtimes.net/roles/mental-health-nurses/medication-management-for-people-with-a-diagnosis-of-schizophrenia-19-11-2002/.

Gregory, J. R. (2019). Osgood-Schlatter Disease. *Medscape.* https://emedicine.medscape.com/article/1993268-overview.

Griffiths, A. M., Ohlsson, A., Sherman, P. M., & Sutherland, L. R. (1995). Meta-analysis of enteral nutrition as a primary treatment of active Crohn's disease. *Gastroenterology, 108,* 1056–1067.

Haag, S., Andrews, J. M., Katelaris, P. H., et al. (2009). Management of reflux symptoms with over-the counter proton pump inhibitors: Issues and proposed guidelines. *Digestion, 80,* 226–234.

Haavisto, M., & Jarva, S. (2018). Developing trust in a nurse-patient relationship. *JAMK University of Applied Science.* https://www.theseus.fi/bitstream/handle/10024/146659/Developing%20Trust%20in%20a%20Nurse-Patient%20Relationship% 20-%20Haavisto%20and%20Jarva%20-%20May%202018.pdf?sequence=1.

Hall, J. (Ed.) (2009). *Handbook of critical care.* London: Springer.

Hall, L. L. (2016). Plan-Do-Study-Act (PDSA). *AMA EdHub.* https://edhub.ama-assn.org/steps-forward/module/2702507#resource.

Haloperidol. WebMD. https://www.webmd.com/drugs/2/drug-8661/haloperidol-oral/details.

Haloperidol (Haldol). eMedicine Health. https://www.emedicinehealth.com/drug-haloperidol/article_em.htm.

Hamdy, O. (2019 May). Diabetic ketoacidosis (DKA) treatment & management. *Medscape.* https://emedicine.medscape.com/article/118361-treatment.

Hanks, R. G., Starnes-Ott, K., & Stafford, L. (2017). Patient advocacy at the APRN level: A direction for the future. *Nursing Forum.* https://doi.org/10.1111/nuf.12209.

Haq, I., & Isenberg, D. A. (2002). How does one assess and monitor patients with systemic lupus erythematosus in daily clinical practice. *Best Practice & Research: Clinical Rheumatology, 16,* 181–194.

Harman, E. M. (2020). Acute respiratory distress syndrome (ARDS) treatment & management. *Medscape.* https://emedicine.medscape.com/article/165139-treatment.

Harris, S. K., Bone, R. C., & Ruth, W. E. (1977). Gastrointestinal hemorrhage in patients in a respiratory intensive care unit. *Chest, 72,* 301–304.

Haugeberg, G., Ørstavik, R. E., Uhlig, T., Falch, J. A., Halse, J. I., & Kvien, T. K. (2002). Clinical decision rules in rheumatoid arthritis: Do they identify patients at high risk for osteoporosis? Testing clinical criteria in a population-based cohort of patients with rheumatoid arthritis recruited from the Oslo Rheumatoid Arthritis Register. *Annals of Rheumatic Diseases, 61*(12), 1085–1089.

Haupel, H., Bynum, G. D., Zamora, E., & El-Serag, H. B. (2001). Risk factors for the development of renal dysfunction in hospitalized patients with cirrhosis. *Am J Gastroenterol, 96,* 2206–2210.

Hayes, A. (2020). Null hypothesis. https://www.investopedia.com/terms/n/null_hypothesis.asp.

Heaf, J. (2014). Metformin in chronic kidney disease: Time for a rethink. *Peritoneal Dialysis International, 34*(4), 353–357.

Healthcare settings: Preventing the spread of MRSA. *Centers for Disease Control and Prevention.* (2019). https://www.cdc.gov/mrsa/healthcare/index.html?CDC_AA_refVal=https%3A%2F%2Fwww.cdc.gov%2Fmrsa%2Fhealthcare%2Fclinicians%2Fprecautions.html.

Health literacy universal toolkit. *Consider culture, customs, and beliefs: Tool #10.* (2nd ed.). (2015). https://www.ahrq.gov/health-literacy/quality-resources/tools/literacy-toolkit/healthlittoolkit2-tool10.html.

Healthline (n.d.). *About oral mucositis.* Accessed May 1, 2020. https://www.healthline.com/health/oral-mucositis.

Healthline. What is traction? https://www.healthline.com/health/traction.

Heart Protection Study Collaborative Group. (2002). MRC/BHF heart protection study of cholesterol lowering with simvastatin in 20,536 high-risk individuals: A randomized placebo-controlled trial. *Lancet, 360,* 7–22.

Hedayati, S. S., Elsayed, E. F., & Reilly, R. F. (2011). Non-pharmacological aspects of blood pressure management: What are the data. *Kidney International, 79*(10), 1061–1070.

Helmenstein, A.M. (2019). What is a testable hypothesis? https://www.thoughtco.com/testable-hypothesis-explanation-and-examples-609100.

Henrich, W. L. (1986). Hemodynamic instability during hemodialysis. *Kidney International, 30,* 605–612.

Heparin. *RXlist.* (2018). https://www.rxlist.com/heparin-drug.htm#description.

Hess, E. P., Knoedler, M. A., Shah, N. D., et al. (2012). The chest pain choice decision aid: A randomized trial. *Circulation: Cardiovascular Quality and Outcomes, 5*(3), 251–259.

High, W. A. (2019). Stevens-Johnson syndrome and toxic epidermal necrolysis: Management, prognosis, and long-term sequelae. https://www-uptodate-com./contents/stevens-johnson-syndrome-and-toxic-epidermal-necrolysis-management-prognosis-and-long-term-sequelae?search=steven%20johnson%20syndrome%20treatment&source=search_result&selectedTitle=1~150&usage_type=default&display_rank=1#H3644514009.

HIPAA Privacy Rule. (2002). https://www.hhs.gov/hipaa/for-professionals/privacy/index.html.

HIV, other health conditions and opportunistic infections. *Avert.* (Feb. 2020), https://www.avert.org/living-with-hiv/health-wellbeing/health-conditions.

HIV transmission: Centers for Disease Control and Prevention. (2019). https://www.cdc.gov/hiv/basics/transmission.html.

Hochman, J. S. (2003). Cardiogenic shock complicating acute myocardial infarction. *Circulation, 107*(24), 2998–3002.

Hoffman, R., Benz, E. J., Silberstein, L. E., et al. (2018a). The antiphospholipid syndrome. In *Hematology: Basic principles and practice* (7th ed., pp. 2088–2101). Philadelphia: Elsevier.

Hoffman, R., Benz, E. J., Silberstein, L. E., et al. (2018). Clinical considerations in platelet transfusion therapy. In *Hematology: Basic principles and practice* (7th ed., pp. 1715–1720). Philadelphia: Elsevier.

Hoffman, R., Benz, E. J., Silberstein, L. E., et al. (2018c). Chronic myeloid leukemia. In *Hematology: Basic Principles and Practice* (7th ed., pp. 1055–1070). Philadelphia: Elsevier.

Hoffman, R., Benz, E. J., & Silberstein, L. E. (2018d). Clinical manifestations and treatment of acute myeloid leukemia. In *Hematology: basic principles and practice* (7th ed.). Philadelphia: Elsevier.

Hoffman, R., Benz, E. J., Silberstein, L. E., et al. (2018e). Hemophilia A and B. In *Hematology: Basic principles and practice* (7th ed., pp. 2001–2022). Philadelphia: Elsevier.

Hoffman, R., Benz, E. J., Silberstein, L. E., et al. (2018f). Human blood group antigens and antibodies. In *Hematology: Basic principles and practice* (7th ed., pp. 1687–1701). Philadelphia: Elsevier.

Hoffman, R., Benz, E. J., Silberstein, L. E., et al. (2018g). Principles of red blood cell transfusion. In *Hematology: Basic principles and practice* (7th ed., pp. 1702–1714). Philadelphia: Elsevier.

Holter monitor. Mayo Clinic (n.d.). https://www.mayoclinic.org/tests-procedures/holter-monitor/about/pac-20385039.

Hopkins, W. G. (2008). Qualitative research design. *Sportscience* (4), 1.

Horst, G. R. (2019). Care of the body after death. *Canadian Virtual Hospice.* https://www.virtualhospice.ca/en_US/Main+Site+Navigation/Home/Topics/Topics/Final+Days/Care+of+the+Body+After+Death.aspx.

How to take an adolescent sexual history. (n.d.). *TN Dept of Health HIV/STD Program.* https://www.tn.gov/content/dam/tn/health/documents/Adolescent_Sexual_History.pdf.

Howlet, J. G. Cor pulmonale. (2020). *MSD Manual: Professional Version.* https://www.msdmanuals.com/professional/cardiovascular-disorders/heart-failure/cor-pulmonale.

Huber, C (2009). Safety monitor: Safety after cardiac catheterization. *AJN: American Journal of Nursing, 109*(8), 57–58. https://www.nursingcenter.com/journalarticle?Article_ID=927655&Journal_ID=54030&Issue_ID=927565.

Hudson, J. Q., & Wazny, L. D. (1999). Chronic kidney disease: Management of complications. In DiPiro, J. T., & Hunt, R. H. (Eds.), Importance of pH control in the management of GERD. *Arch Intern Med, 159,* 649–657.

Hughes, R. G., & Blegen, M. A. (2008). Medication administration safety. In Hughes, R. G. (Ed.), *Patient safety and quality: An evidence-based handbook for nurses.* Rockville, MD: Agency for Healthcare Research and Quality. https://www.ncbi.nlm.nih.gov/books/NBK2656/.

Hypothesis testing summary. (2002). http://www.indiana.edu/~educy520/sec5982/week_12/hypothesis_test_summary011109.pdf.

Hypothesis testing. Laerd statistics. https://statistics.laerd.com/statistical-guides/hypothesis-testing.php.

Importance of communication in nursing. *University of New Mexico.* (2016). https://rnbsnonline.unm.edu/articles/importance-of-communication-in-nursing.aspx.

Immunization Action Coalition. (2015). Pneumococcal vaccines: IAC answers your questions. https://www.immunize.org/catg.d/p2015.pdf.

Informed consent to medical treatment. *Australian Government.* (2014). https://www.alrc.gov.au/publication/equality-capacity-and-disability-in-commonwealth-laws-dp-81/10-review-of-state-and-territory-legislation/informed-consent-to-medical-treatment/.

Inker, L. A., Astor, B. C., Fox, C. H., et al. (2014). KDOQI commentary on the 2012 Clinical Practice Guideline for the evaluation and management of CKD. *Am J Kidney Dis, 63,* 713–735.

Institute for Safe Medical Practices. (2008). *Strong safety signal seen for Chantix (varenicline).* https://www.ismp.org/quarterwatchtm/strong-safety-signal-seen-chantix-varenicline.

Institute for Safe Medican Practices. (2014). *Strengthen warnings for varenicline (Chantix).* https://www.ismp.org/quarterwatch/warnings-varenicline-chanti.x.

Institute of Medicine. (2010). *Bridging the evidence gap in obesity prevention: A framework to inform decision making.* Washington, DC: The National Academies Press. https://doi.org/10.17226/12847.

Internal bleeding: Causes, treatments, and more. *Healthline.* (2019). https://www.healthline.com/health/internal-bleeding#outlook.

Iodine allergy. (2018). *Healthline.* https://www.healthline.com/health/allergies/iodine#outlook.

Institute of Medicine; Committee on the Robert Wood Johnson Foundation Initiative on the Future of Nursing, at the Institute of Medicine, (2011). *The future of nursing: Leading change, advancing health.* Washington, DC: National Academies Press. https://www.ncbi.nlm.nih.gov/books/NBK209880/.

Inzucchi, S. E. (2014). Metformin in patients with type 2 diabetes and kidney disease: A systematic review. *Journal of the American Medical Association, 312*(24), 2668–2675.

Iron deficiency anemia secondary to inadequate dietary iron intake. *Healthline.* (2016). https://www.healthline.com/health/iron-deficiency-inadequate-dietary-iron#treatment-and-prevention.

Ismail, A. (2016). Meta-analysis: What, why, and how. https://www.students4bestevidence.net/blog/2016/12/02/meta-analysis-what-why-and-how/.

Issa, M., & Wasan, A. D. (2014). Cage questionnaire. *Science Direct.* https://www.sciencedirect.com/topics/medicine-and-dentistry/cage-questionnaire.

Jaffe, E., Arber, D., Campo, E., Harris, N., & Quintanilla-Martinez, L. (2017). Reactive lymphadenopathies. In *Hematopathology* (2nd ed., pp. 153–177). Philadelphia: Elsevier.

Jaïs X., Olsson K. M., Barbera J. A., et al. (2012). Pregnancy outcomes in pulmonary arterial hypertension in the modern management era. *European Respiratory Journal, 40*, 881.

Jameson, L., De Groot, L., Kretser, D., et al. (2016a). Autoimmune endocrine disorders. In *Endocrinology: Adult and pediatric* (7th ed., pp. 2549–2565). Philadelphia: Saunders e5.

Jameson, L., De Groot, L., Kretser, D., et al. (2016b). Chronic (Hashimoto's) thyroiditis. In *Endocrinology: Adult and pediatric* (7th ed., pp. 1515–1527). Philadelphia: Saunders.

Jannot-Lamotte, M. F., & Raccah, D. (2000). Management of diabetes during corticosteroid therapy. *Presse Med, 29*(5), 263–266. https://pubmed.ncbi.nlm.nih.gov/10701409/.

Janz, D. R., & Ware, L. B. (2014). Approach to the patient with the acute respiratory distress syndrome. *Clin Chest Med, 35*(4), 685–696. https://doi.org/10.1016/j.ccm.2014.08.007.

JNC. (2014). 8 Guidelines for the management of hypertension in adults. *American Family Physician, 90*(7), 503–504.

Johannsson, G. (2015). Adrenal insufficiency: Review of clinical outcomes with current glucocorticoid replacement therapy. *Clinical Endocrinology (Oxford), 82*(1), 2–11.

Johns Hopkins Hospital, Hughes, H., & Kahl, L. (2018). Hematology. In *The Harriet Lane handbook*, pp. 364–394. Philadelphia: Elsevier.

Johnson, J. M., Maher, J. W., DeMaria, E. J., et al. (2006). The long-term effects of gastric bypass on Vitamin D metabolism. *Annals of Surgery, 243*(5), 701–705.

Johnson, R., Feehally, J., & Floege, J. (2015). Anemia in chronic kidney disease. In *Comprehensive Clinical Nephrology* (5th ed., pp. 967–974). Philadelphia: Saunders.

Johnson, T. C. (2019). Pregnancy and lupus. *WebMD.* https://www.webmd.com/lupus/guide/pregnancy-lupus#1.

Johnson, V. A. (1994). Combination therapy: More effective control of HIV type 1. *AIDS Res Hum Retroviruses, 10*(8), 907–912. https://doi.org/10.1089/aid.1994.10.907.

Joint Task Force on Practice Parameters. (2000). The diagnosis and management of urticaria: a practice parameter. Part I: Acute urticaria/angioedema. Part II: Chronic urticaria/angioedema. *Annals of Allergy, Asthma & Immunology, 85*, 521–544.

Jolles, S., Sewell, W. A., & Leighton, C. (2000). Drug-induced aseptic meningitis: Diagnosis and management. *Drug Safety, 22*, 215–226.

Jordan, R. S., & Burns, J. L (2013). Understanding stoma complications. *Wound Advisor, 2*(4). https://woundcareadvisor.com/understanding-stoma-complications_vol2-no4/.

Jun, M., Heerspink, H. J., Ninomiya, T., et al. (2010). Intensities of renal replacement therapy in acute kidney injury: A systematic review and meta-analysis. *Clinical Journal of the American Society of Nephrology, 5*(6), 956–963.

Kalil, A. (2019 Jan). Septic shock. *Medscape.* https://emedicine.medscape.com/article/168402-overview.

Kalil, A. (2019). Septic shock treatment & management. *Medscape.* https://emedicine.medscape.com/article/168402-treatment.

Kalil, A. C., Metersky, M. L., Klompas, M., et al. (2016). Management of adults with hospital-acquired and ventilator-associated pneumonia: 2016 clinical practice guidelines by the Infectious Diseases Society of America and the American Thoracic Society. *Clinical Infectious Diseases, 63*(5), e61–e111.

Kam-Tao Li, P., Szeto, C. C., Piraino, B., et al. (2010). Peritoneal dialysis-related infections recommendations: 2010 update. *Peritoneal Dialysis International, 30*, 393–423.

Kappel, J., & Calissi, P. (2002). Nephrology: 3. Safe drug prescribing for patients with renal insufficiency. *Canadian Medical Association Journal, 166*, 473–477.

Kapur, V. K., Auckley, D. H., Chowdhuri, S., et al. (2017). Clinical practice guideline for diagnostic testing for adult obstructive sleep apnea: An American Academy of Sleep Medicine Clinical Practice Guideline. *Journal of Clinical of Sleep Medicine, 13*(3), 479.

Kasper, D. L., Braunwald, E., Fauci, A. S., et al. (2005). *Harrison's principles of internal medicine* (16th ed). New York: McGraw-Hill.

Kasper, D. L., Fauci, A. S., Hauser, S. L., Longo, D. L., Jameson, J. L., & Loscalzo, J. (2009). *Harrison's manual of medicine.* New York: McGraw Hill.

Katz, P. O., Gerson, L. B., & Vela, M. F. (2013). Guideline for the diagnosis and management and diagnosis of gastroesophageal reflux disease. *American Journal of Gastroenterology, 108*, 308–328.

Kaw, D., & Malhotra, D. (2006). Platelet dysfunction and end-stage renal disease. *Semin Dial, 19*(4), 317–322. https://doi.org/10.1111/j.1525-139X.2006.00179.x.

Keisler, B., & Carter, C. (2015). Abdominal aortic aneurysm. *Am Fam Physician, 15;91*(8), 538–543.

Kellerman, R., & Bope, E. (2018a). Hemophilia and related conditions. In *Conn's current therapy*, pp. 392–399. Philadelphia: Elsevier.

Kellerman, R., & Bope, E. (2018b). Hemolytic anemia. In *Conn's current therapy*, pp. 387–392). Philadelphia: Elsevier.

Kelly, D. A. (2002). Managing liver failure. *Postgraduate Medical Journal, 78*, 660–667.

Kellum, J. A. (2008). Acute kidney injury. *Critical Care Medicine, 36*, S141–S145.

Kerkar, P. Treatment & exercises for collapsed lung or pneumothorax. Pain Assist. https://www.epainassist.com/chest-pain/lungs/treatment-and-exercises-for-collapsed-lung-or-pneumothorax.

Khalid, S., Seepana, J., Sundhu, M., & Maroo, P. (2017). Left ventricular free wall rupture in transmural myocardial infarction. *Cureus, 9*(8).

Khosal, S., Ahmed, A., Siddiqui, M., et al. (2006). Safety of angiotensin-converting enzyme inhibitors in patients with bilateral renal artery stenosis following successful renal artery stent revascularization. *Am J Ther, 13*(4), 306–308. https://doi.org/10.1097/00045391-200607000-00005.

Khurana, V. G., & Kaye, A. H. (2012). An overview of concussion in sport. *Journal of Clinical Neuroscience, 19*(1), 1–11.

Kibbe, D. C., Phillips, R. L., & Green, L. A. (2004). The continuity of care record. *Am Fam Physician, 70*(7), 1220–1223.

Kidney Disease: Improving Global Outcomes (KDIGO) Anemia Work Group. (2012). KDIGO clinical practice guideline for anemia in chronic kidney disease. *Kidney International Supplements, 2*, 279–335.

Kidney Disease: Improving Global Outcomes (KDIGO) CKD-MBD Work Group. (2009). KDIGO clinical practice guideline for the diagnosis, evaluation, prevention, and treatment of chronic kidney disease–mineral and bone disorder (CKD-MBD). *Kidney International Supplements, 76*(suppl 113), S1–S130.

Kidney Disease: Improving Global Outcomes (KDIGO) CKD Work Group. (2013). KDIGO 2012 clinical practice guideline for the evaluation and management of chronic kidney disease. *Kidney International Supplements, 3*, 1–150.

Kidney Disease: Improving Global Outcomes (KDIGO) CKD-MBD Update Work Group. (2017). KDIGO 2017 clinical practice guideline update for the diagnosis, evaluation, prevention, and treatment of chronic kidney disease–mineral and bone disorder (CKD-MBD). *Kidney International Supplements, 7*, 1–59.

Kidney Disease: Improving Global Outcomes (KDIGO) CKD-MBD Update Work Group. (2017). KDIGO 2017 clinical practice guideline update for the diagnosis, evaluation, prevention, and treatment of chronic kidney disease–mineral and bone disorder (CKD-MBD). *Kidney International Supplements, 7*, 1–59.

Kidney Disease: Improving Global Outcomes (KDIGO). http://kdigo.org/home/guidelines/.

Kim, J., Ochoa, M. T., Krutzik, S. R., et al. (2002). Activation of toll-like receptor 2 in acne triggers inflammatory cytokine responses. *Journal of Immunology, 169*, 1535.

King, E. G., Bauzá, G. J., Mella, J. R., & Remick, D. G. (2017). Pathophysiologic mechanisms in septic shock. *Lab Invest, 94*(1), 4–12. https://doi.org/10.1038/labinvest.2013.110.

King, J. R., Acosta, E. P., Chadwick, E., et al. (2003). Evaluation of multiple drug therapy in human immunodeficiency virus-infected pediatric patients. *Pediatr Infect Dis J, 22*(3), 239–244. https://doi.org/10.1097/01.inf.0000055093.42130.40.

Kirkwood, C. K., Melton, S. T., Wells, B. G., et al. (2017). Anxiety disorders II: Posttraumatic stress disorder and obsessive-compulsive disorder. In J. T. DiPiro, R. L. Talbert, & G. C. Yee et al (Eds.), *Pharmacotherapy: A Pathophysiologic Approach* (10th ed.). New York: McGraw-Hill.

Kisvetrová, H., Vévodová, S., & Školoudík, D. (2017). Comfort-supporting nursing activities for end-of-life patients in an institutionalized environment. *Journal of Nursing Scholarship, 50*, 126–133. https://doi.org/10.1111/jnu.12341.

Kitchens, C., Kessler, C., & Konkle, B. (2013). Disseminated intravascular coagulation. In *Consultative Hemostasis and Thrombosis*, 174–189.

Kjekshus, J., & Pedersen, T. R. (1995). Reducing the risk of coronary events: Evidence from the Scandinavian Simvastatin Survival Study (4S). *American Journal of Cardiology, 76*, 64C–68C.

Kliegman, R., Stanton, B., St Geme, J., & Schor, N. (2018). Hemostasis. In *Nelson Textbook of Pediatrics* (20th ed., pp. 2379–2384). Philadelphia: Elsevier.

Kliger, A. S., Foley, R. N., Goldfarb, D. S., et al. (2013). KDOQI U.S. Commentary on the 2012 KDIGO clinical practice guideline for anemia in CKD. *American Journal of Kidney Disease, 62*, 849–859.

Knee noise: Crepitus and popping explained. (2020). *Healthline.* https://www.healthline.com/health/osteoarthritis/crepitus#takeaway.

Know the Signs and Symptoms of Infection. (2019). *Centers for Disease Control and Infection.* https://www.cdc.gov/cancer/preventinfections/symptoms.htm.

Knowler, W. C., Barrett-Connor, E., Fowler, S. E., et al. (2002). Diabetes Prevention Program Research Group: Reduction in the incidence of type 2 diabetes with lifestyle intervention or metformin. *New England Journal of Medicine, 346*, 393–403.

Koch, K. A. (1992). Patient self-determination act. *J Fla Med Assoc, 79*(4), 240–243. https://pubmed.ncbi.nlm.nih.gov/1588296/.

Koithan, M., & Farrell, C. (2010). Indigenous Native American healing traditions. *Journal of Nursing Practice, 6*, 477–478.

Kornbluth, A., & Sachar, D. B. (2010). Ulcerative practice guidelines in adults: American College of Gastroenterology, Practice Parameters Committee. *American Journal of Gastroenterology, 105*, 501–523.

Kornum J. B., Thomsen R. W., Riis A., et al. (2007). Type 2 diabetes and pneumonia outcomes: A population-based cohort study. *Diabetes Care, 30*(9), 2251–2257. https://doi.org/10.2337/dc06-2417.

Kotby, A. A., Habeeb, N. M., & Elarab, S. E. (2012). Antistreptolysin O titer in health and disease: Levels and significance. *Pediatr Rep, 2;4*(1), e8. https://doi.org/10.4081/pr.2012.e8.

Kroeger, R. J., & Groszmann, R. J. (1985). Increased portal venous resistance hinders portal pressure reduction during the administration of beta-adrenergic blocking agents in a portal hypertensive model. *Hepatology, 5*, 97–101.

Krousel-Wood, M. A. (1999). Practical considerations in the measurement of outcomes in healthcare. *The Ochsner, 4*(1).

Kufe, D. W., Pollock, R. E., Weichselbaum, R. R., et al. (2003). Manifestations of cachexia. In *Holland Frei Cancer Medicine*, (6th ed.). Hamilton, Ontario: BC Decker.

Kumar, P. (2016). *Kumar and Clark's Clinical Medicine* (9th ed.). St. Louis, MO: Elsevier.

Kwon, J. (2018). Screen at 23–type 2 diabetes risk at lower BMI for Asians and Asian Americans. https://diatribe.org/screen23.

Laine, L., & Jensen, D. M. (2012). Management of patients with ulcer bleeding. *American Journal of Gastroenterology, 107*, 345–360.

Landau, P. (2019). 12 Resource allocation tips for managers. https://www.projectmanager.com/blog/resource-allocation.

Lange, J., & Mager, D. (2012). ELDER Project: Cultural diversity: African American culture. Retrieved from: https://www.pogoe.org/productid/21115.

Langer-Gould, A., Atlas, S. W., Green, A. J., Bollen, A. W., & Pelletier, D. (2005). Progressive multifocal leukoencephalopathy in a patient treated with natalizumab. *New England Journal of Medicine, 353*, 375–381.

Lansang, M. C. (2016). Inpatient hyperglycemia management: a practical review for primary medical and surgical teams. *Cleveland Clinic Journal of Medicine, 83*(5 suppl 1), S34–S43.

Lasky, M. R., Metzler, M. H., & Phillips, J. O. (1998). A prospective study of omeprazole suspension to prevent clinically significant gastrointestinal bleeding from stress ulcers in mechanically ventilated trauma patients. *Journal of Trauma, 44*, 527–533.

Latha, K. S., & Phil, M. (2010). The noncompliant patient in psychiatry: The case for and against covert/surreptitious medication. *Mens Sana Monogr, 8*(1), 96–121. https://www.ncbi.nlm.nih.gov/pmc/articles/PMC3031933/.

Lee, K. M., Jeen, Y. T., Cho, J. Y., et al. (2013). Efficacy, safety, and predictors of response to infliximab therapy for ulcerative colitis: a Korean multicenter retrospective study. *Journal of Gastroenterology and Hepatology, 28*, 1829–1833.

Lee, M., & Geelhoed, E. (2011). Teaching resource allocation— and why it matters. *Virtual Mentor, 13*(4), 224–227.

Lee, S. H., Yang, M. S., Kim, T., et al. (2007). Lamotrigine-induced hypersensitivity syndrome accompanied with aseptic meningitis. *Korean Journal of Asthma Allergy and Clinical Immunology, 27*(2), 140–142.

Lee, S. S., & Farwell, A. P. (2016). Euthyroid sick syndrome. *Comprehensive Physiology, 6*(2), 1071–1080.

Leighton, E., Sainsbury, C. A., & Jones, G. C. (2017). A practical review of C-peptide testing in diabetes. *Diabetes Therapy, 8*(3), 475–487.

Lerner, N. (2016). The anemias. In *Nelson textbook of pediatrics* (20th ed., pp. 2309–2312). Philadelphia: Elsevier.

Levine, G. N., Bates, E. R., Bittl, J. A., et al. (2016). 2016 ACC/AHA guideline focused update on duration of dual antiplatelet therapy in patients with coronary artery disease: A report of the American College of Cardiology/American Heart Association Task Force on Clinical Practice Guidelines: An update of the 2011 ACCF/AHA/SCAI guideline for percutaneous coronary intervention, 2011 ACCF/AHA guideline for coronary artery bypass graft surgery, 2012 ACC/AHA/ACP/AATS/PCNA/SCAI/STS guideline for the diagnosis and management of patients with stable ischemic heart. *Circulation, 134*(10), e123–e155.

Levine, G. N., Bates, E. R., Blankenship, J. C., et al. (2016). 2015 ACC/AHA/SCAI focused update on primary percutaneous coronary intervention for patients with ST-elevation myocardial infarction: An update of the 2011 ACCF/AHA/SCAI guideline for percutaneous coronary intervention and the 2013 ACCF/AHA guideline for the management of ST-elevation myocardial infarction. *Journal of the American College of Cardiology, 67*(10), 1235–1250.

Levine, R. E., & Gaw, A. C. (1995). Culture-bound syndromes. *Psychiatr Clin North Am, 18*(3), 523–536. https://pubmed.ncbi.nlm.nih.gov/8545265/.

Lew, D. P., & Waldvogel, F. A. (2004). Osteomyelitis. *The Lancet, 364*(9431), 369–379.

Leyon, J. J., Jaiveer, S., Connolly, D. L., & Babu, S. (2010). Statin prescription is essential in peripheral vascular disease. *Journal of Vascular and Interventional Radiology: JVIR, 21*(2), 175–177.

Li, P. K., Szeto, C. C., Piraino, B., et al. (2010). Peritoneal dialysis–related infections recommendations. *Peritoneal Dialysis International, 30*(4), 393–423.

Liamis, G., Filippatos, T. D., & Elisaf, M. S. (2015). Correction of hypovolemia with crystalloid fluids: Individualizing infusion therapy. *Postgraduate Medicine, 127*(4), 405–412.

Library research for undergraduate history students: An introduction. http://guides.library.illinois.edu/historicalresearch/primary.

Lieberman, D. A., Rex, D. K., Winawer, S. J, et al. (2012). Guidelines for colonoscopy surveillance after screening and polypectomy: A consensus update by the US Multi-Society Task Force on Colorectal Cancer. *Gastroenterology, 143*, 844–857.

Lilitsis, E., Xenaki, S., Athanasakis, E., et al. (2018). Guiding management in severe trauma: Reviewing factors predicting outcome in vastly injured patients. *Journal of Emergencies, Trauma, and Shock, 11*(2), 80–87.

Lim, W., Le Gal, G, Bates, S. M., et al. (2018). American Society of Hematology 2018 guidelines for management of venous thromboembolism: Diagnosis of venous thromboembolism. *Blood Advances* (2), 3226.

Living with your pacemaker: A patient's guide to understanding cardiac pacemakers. *St. Jude Medical* 2015. https://www.accessdata.fda.gov/cdrh_docs/pdf14/P140033D.pdf.

Logemann, J. (1986). Treatment for aspiration related to dysphagia: An overview. *Dysphagia, 1*, 34–38.

Lollar, P. (1991). The association of factor VIII with von Willebrand factor. *Mayo Clin Proc, 66*(5), 524–534. https://doi.org/10.1016/s0025-6196(12)62395-7.

Long, L. O., & Park, S. (2007). Update on nephrolithiasis management. *Minerva Urologica a Nefrologica, 59*(3), 317–325.

Longo, S. A., Moore, R. C., Canzoneri, B. J., & Robichaux, A. (2010). Gastrointestinal conditions during pregnancy. *Clin Colon Rectal Surg, 23*(2), 80–89.

Lovenox prescribing information. *Sanofi-Aventis* 2009. https://www.accessdata.fda.gov/drugsatfda_docs/label/2009/020164s083lbl.pdf.

Low blood cell counts: Side effect of cancer treatment. *Mayo Clinic* (2019). https://www.mayoclinic.org/diseases-conditions/cancer/in-depth/cancer-treatment/art-20046192.

Lozada, C. J. (2020). *Osteoarthritis*. https://emedicine.medscape.com/article/330487-overview.

Lu, H. A. J. (2017). Diabetes insipidus. *Advances in Experimental Medicine and Biology, 969*, 213.

Lupus Foundation of America. (2013). *Planning a pregnancy when you have lupus*. https://www.lupus.org/resources/planning-a-pregnancy-when-you-have-lupus#.

Ma, Y., Yuan, J., Hu, J., Gao, W., Zou, Y., & Ge, J. (2019). ACE inhibitor suppresses cardiac remodeling after myocardial infarction by regulating dendritic cells and AT2 receptor-mediated mechanism in mice. *Biomedicine & Pharmacotherapy, 114*, 108660.

Mabuchi, N., Tsutamoto, T., & Kinoshita, M. (2000). Therapeutic use of dopamine and beta-blockers modulates plasma interleukin-6 levels in patients with congestive heart failure. *J Cardiovasc Pharmacol, 36*(Suppl 2), S87–S91. https://doi.org/10.1097/00005344-200000006-00019.

Macleod, J., Edwards, C., & Bouchier, I. (1977). *Davidson's principles and practice of medicine: A textbook for students and doctors*. London: Churchill Livingstone.

Maddox, T. G. (2002). Adverse reactions to contrast material: Recognition, prevention, and treatment. *American Family Physician, 66*(7), 1229–1235.

Madhok, R., & Wu, O. (2007). Systemic lupus erythematosus. *American Family Physician, 76*, 1351–1353.

Mallory, A., & Kern, F. (1980). Drug-induced pancreatitis: A critical review. *Gastroenterology, 78*, 813.

Mandell, L. A., Wunderdrink, R. G., Anzueto, A., et al. (2017). Infectious Diseases Society of America/American Thoracic Society consensus guidelines on the management of community-acquired pneumonia in adults. *Clinical Infectious Diseases, 44*(suppl 2), S27–S72.

Manual Ventilation. *Nurse Key* 2016. https://nursekey.com/manual-ventilation/.

Marino, P. L. (2014). *The ICU book* (4th ed). Philadelphia: Wolters Kluwer Health.

Markman, M (2020). Colorectal cancer risk factors. *Cancer Treatment Centers of America*. https://www.cancercenter.com/cancer-types/colorectal-cancer/risk-factors.

Marmor, M. F., Carr, R. E., Easterbrook, M., et al. (2002). Recommendations on screening for chloroquine and hydroxychloroquine retinopathy: A report by the American Academy of Ophthalmology. *Ophthalmology, 109*, 1377–1382.

Martin, J. F. (2014). Privacy and confidentiality. In H. A. M. J. ten Have & B. Gordijin (Eds.), *Handbook of global bioethics* (p. 119): Springer.

Mayo Clinic. (2020). Nitroglycerin (oral route, sublingual route). https://www.mayoclinic.org/drugs-supplements/nitroglycerin-oral-route-sublingual-route/proper-use/drg-20072863.

Mayo Clinic (n.d.). Pancreatitis. https://www.mayoclinic.org/diseases-conditions/pancreatitis/symptoms-causes/syc-20360227.

McCabe, M. S., & Wood, W. A. (2010). When the family requests withholding the diagnosis: Who owns the truth. *Journal of Oncology Practice, 6*(2), 94–96.

McColl, K. E. L, El-Nujumi, A., Murray, L., et al. (1997). The *Helicobacter pylori* breath test: A surrogate marker for peptic ulcer disease in dyspeptic patients. *Gut, 40*, 302–306.

McCormick, A., Fleming, D., Charlton, J. (1995) Morbidity statistics from general practice. Fourth National Study 1991–1992. Office of Population Censuses and Statistics. Series MB5 No. 3. London, UK: Her Majesty's Stationery Office.

McCrea, D. L. (2017). A primer on insulin pump therapy for health care providers. *Nursing Clinics of North America, 52*(4), 553–564.

McDonald, L. C., Gerding, D. N., Johnson, S., et al. (2018). Clinical practice guidelines for *Clostridium difficile* infection in adults and children: 2017 updated by the Infectious Diseases Society of America (IDSA) and Society for Healthcare Epidemiology of America (SHEA). *Clinical Infectious Diseases, 66*(7), e1–e48.

McDonnell, G. Systems Thinking Method. https://insightmaker.com/article/30513/Systems-%20Thinking-Method.

McFarlane, S., & Lavorato, A. (1984). The use of video endoscopy in the evaluation and treatment of dysphonia. *Journal of Communication Disorders, 9*(8), 117–126.

McGrattan, J. (2020). Hypothyroidism: Underactive thyroid causes, symptoms and treatment. *NetDoctor*. https://www.netdoctor.co.uk/conditions/a4459/hypothyroidism/.

McLeod, S. (2020). Maslow's hierarchy of needs. *Simply Psychology*. https://www.simplypsychology.org/maslow.html.

McLeod, S. (2019). What are independent and dependent variables. *Simple Psychology*. https://www.simplypsychology.org/variables.html.

McNicholas, L. Clinical guidelines for the use of buprenorphine in the treatment of opioid addiction. U.S. Department of Health and Human Services: Substance Abuse and Mental Health Services Administration Center for Substance Abuse Treatment. https://www.naabt.org/documents/TIP40.pdf.

McPherson, R., & Pincus, M. (2017a). Antithrombotic therapy. In *Henry's clinical diagnosis and management by laboratory methods* (23rd ed., pp. 842–853). St. Louis, MO: Elsevier).

McPherson, R., & Pincus, M. (2017b). Erythrocyte disorders. In *Henry's clinical diagnosis and management by laboratory methods* (23rd ed. pp. 559–605). St. Louis, MO: Elsevier.

McPherson, R., & Pincus, M. (2017c). Interpreting laboratory results. In *Henry's clinical diagnosis and management by laboratory methods* (23rd ed., pp. 84–101). St. Louis, MO: Elsevier.

McPherson, R., & Pincus, M. (2017d). Transfusion medicine. In *Henry's clinical diagnosis and management by laboratory methods* (23rd ed., pp. 735–750). St. Louis, MO: Elsevier.

Medication administration: Why it's important to take drugs the right way. (2019). *Healthline*. https://www.healthline.com/health/administration-of-medication#takeaway.

Medication errors: Best practices. (2010). *American Nurse*. https://www.myamericannurse.com/medication-errors-best-practices/.

Meeting your patient's spiritual needs. *American Nurse*. (2007). https://www.myamericannurse.com/meeting-your-patients-spiritual-needs/.

Mehta, C., & Mehta, Y. (2016). Management of refractory hypoxemia. *Ann Card Anaesth, 19*(1), 89–96.

Mehta, R. L., Kellum, J. A., Shah, S. V., et al. (2007). Acute Kidney Injury Network: report of an initiative to improve outcomes in acute kidney injury. *Critical Care, 11*, R31.

Melton, S. T., Kirkwood, C. K., et al. (2017). Anxiety disorders I: Generalized anxiety, panic, and social anxiety disorders. In J. T. DiPiro, R. L. Talbert, & G. C. Yee et al (Eds.), *Pharmacotherapy: A pathophysiologic approach* (10th ed.). New York: McGraw-Hill .

Memorial Sloan Kettering (n.d.). *Nutrition Guidelines for People with Short Bowel Syndrome.* Retrieved from: https://www.mskcc.org/cancer-care/patient-education/nutrition-guidelines-patients-short-bowel-syndrome.

Meta-analysis: Definition. https://himmelfarb.gwu.edu/tutorials/studydesign101/metaanalyses.cfm.

Metnitz, P. G., Krenn, C. G., Steltzer, H., et al. (2002). Effect of acute renal failure requiring renal replacement therapy on outcome in critically ill patients. *Critical Care Medicine, 30*, 2051–2058.

Mikstas, C. (2018). Iron-rich foods. *Nourish WebMD.* https://www.webmd.com/diet/iron-rich-foods#1.

Miller, W. R. (2010). Qualitative research findings as evidence: Utility in nursing practice. *Clinical Nurse Specialist, 24*(4), 191–193.

Misra, S., & Oliver, N. S. (2015). Diabetic ketoacidosis in adults. *British Medical Journal, 351*, h5660.

Mitchell, P. H. (2008). Defining patient safety and quality care editor. In Hughes, R. G. (Ed.), *Patient safety and quality: An evidence-based handbook for nurses.* Rockville, MD: Agency for Healthcare Research and Quality. https://www.ncbi.nlm.nih.gov/books/NBK2681/.

Moayyedi, P. M., Lacy, B. E., Andrews, C. N., et al. (2017). ACG and CAG clinical guideline: Management of dyspepsia. *Am J Gastroenterol, 112*(7), 988–1013.

Morley, L., & Cashell, A. (2017). Collaboration in health care. *Journal of Medical Imaging and Radiation Sciences, 48*, 207–216.

Mount Sinai. (2013). Topical vasoconstrictors for epistaxis. https://sinaiem.org/topical-vasoconstrictors-for-epistaxis/.

Moz, T. (2004). Wound dehiscence and evisceration. *Nursing, 34*(5), 88.

Mullur, R., Liu, Y., & Brent, G. A. (2014). Thyroid hormone regulation of metabolism. *Physiol Rev, 94*(2), 355–382. https://doi.org/10.1152/physrev.00030.2013.

Multidisciplinary team working: From theory to practice. *Mental Health Commission Discussion Paper.* (2006). https://www.mhcirl.ie/file/discusspapmultiteam.pdf.

Multistate Reimbursement Alliance: Enhancing NP support for insurance credentialing, contracting, and reimbursement. American Association of Nurse Practitioners (n.d.). https://www.aanp.org/practice/practice-management/business-resources-for-nurse-practitioners/multistate-reimbursement-alliance-msra.

Munoz, A., & Katerndahl, D. A. (2000). Diagnosis and management of acute pancreatitis. *American Family Physician, 62*(1), 164–174.

Nabili, S. N., & Balentine, J. R. (2018). Advance directives. *eMedicine Health.* https://www.emedicinehealth.com/advance_directives/article_em.htm.

Naci, H., Brugts, J. J., Fleurence, R., Tsoi, B., Toor, H., & Ades, A. E. (2013). Comparative benefits of statins in the primary and secondary prevention of major coronary events and all-cause mortality: A network meta-analysis of placebo-controlled and active-comparator trials. *European Journal of Preventive Cardiology, 20*(4), 641–657.

Nadeau, M., Rosas-Arellano, M. P., Gurr, K. R., et al. (2013). The reliability of differentiating neurogenic claudication from vascular claudication based on symptomatic presentation. *Canadian Journal of Surgery, 56*(6), 372.

Nail abnormalities. *MedlinePlus 2020.* https://medlineplus.gov/ency/article/003247.htm.

National Asthma Education and Prevention Program. (2007). Expert panel report III: Guidelines for the diagnosis and management of asthma. *National Heart, Lung, and Blood Institute.* Bethesda, MD: NIH publication. 08-4051. www.nhlbi.nih.gov/guidelines/asthma/asthgdln.htm.

National Center for Education Statistics. What are independent and dependent variables? https://nces.ed.gov/nceskids/help/user_guide/graph/variables.asp.

National Clinical Guideline Centre for Acute and Chronic Conditions (UK). (2010 Mar). *Chest Pain of Recent Onset: Assessment and Diagnosis of Recent Onset Chest Pain or Discomfort of Suspected Cardiac Origin [Internet].* London: Royal College of Physicians (UK) PMID: 22420013.

National Comprehensive Cancer Network (NCCN). Cancer staging guide. https://www.nccn.org/patients/resources/diagnosis/staging.aspx.

National Hemophilia Foundation. (n.d.). Von Willebrand disease. https://www.hemophilia.org/Bleeding-Disorders/Types-of-Bleeding-Disorders/Von-Willebrand-Disease.

National Institute of Aging. (2017). *Tips for communicating with a confused patient.* https://www.nia.nih.gov/health/tips-communicating-confused-patient.

National Institute of Diabetes and Digestive and Kidney Diseases. (2017). *Pregnancy if you have diabetes).* https://www.niddk.nih.gov/health-information/diabetes/diabetes-pregnancy.

National Institute of Diabetes and Digestive and Kidney Diseases. (2017). Talking with patients about weight loss: Tips for primary care providers. https://www.niddk.nih.gov/health-information/professionals/clinical-tools-patient-management/weight-management/talking-adult-patients-tips-primary-care-clinicians.

National Kidney Disease Education Program (NKDEP). www.nkdep.nih.gov/.

National Kidney Disease Education Program. (April 2015). Chronic kidney disease and drug dosing: information for providers. *Revised.* https://www.niddk.nih.gov/health-information/professionals/clinical-tools-patient-educationoutreach/ckd-drug-dosing-providers.

National Kidney Foundation (NKF). (2012). KDOQI clinical practice guideline for diabetes and CKD: 2012 update. *American Journal of Kidney Disease, 60*, 850–886.

National Kidney Foundation (NKF). (2004). KDOQI clinical practice guidelines on hypertension and antihypertensive agents in chronic kidney disease. *American journal of kidney disease, 43*(suppl 5), S1.

National Kidney Foundation (NKF). (206). KDOQI clinical practice guidelines and recommendations for anemia of chronic kidney disease. *American Journal of Kidney Disease, 47*(suppl 3), S1-S146.

National Research Council. (2005). *Measuring performance and benchmarking project management at the department of energy*. Washington, DC: The National Academies Press. https://doi.org/10.17226/11344.

Native Americans with diabetes. https://www.cdc.gov/vitalsigns/aian-diabetes/index.html.

Nelson, D. (2018). All 12 cranial nerves and their function. *Science Trends*. https://sciencetrends.com/12-cranial-nerves-function/.

Nelson, H. D., Haney, E. M., Dana, T., Bougatsos, C., & Chou, R. (2010). Screening for osteoporosis: An update for the US Preventive Services Task Force. *Annals of Internal Medicine, 153*(2), 99–111.

Neo, S. Strategies for effective cross-cultural communication within the workplace. *Training Industry*. https://trainingindustry.com/blog/performance-management/strategies-for-effective-cross-cultural-communication-within-the-workplace/.

Nguyen, Q. A. (2020). Epistaxis. *Medscape*. https://emedicine.medscape.com/article/863220-overview.

NICE Clinical Knowledge Summaries. *Lipid modification—CVD prevention*. (2020). https://webcache.googleusercontent.com/search?q=cache:MFJY3qHDy-4J:https://cks.nice.org.uk/topics/lipid-modification-cvd-prevention/+&cd=2&hl=en&ct=clnk&gl=us.

Nichols, W. L., Hulton, M. B., James, A. H., et al. (2008). von Willebrand disease (VWD): Evidence-based diagnosis and management guidelines, the National Heart, Lung, and Blood Institute (NHLBI) Expert Panel report (USA). *Hemophilia, 14*, 171–232.

Niederhuber, J., Armitage, J., Doroshow, J., Kastan, M., & Tepper, J. (2014). Tumor lysis syndrome. In *Abeloff's clinical oncology* (5th ed., pp. 591–596). Philadelphia: Elsevier.

Niederhuber, J., Armitage, J., Doroshow, J., et al. (2014). Superior vena cava syndrome. In *Abeloff's clinical oncology* (5th ed.). Philadelphia: Elsevier.

Nolin, T. D., & Himmelfarb, J. (2014). *Drug-induced kidney disease*. In DiPiro, J. T., Talbert, R. L., Yee, G. C., et al. (Eds.), *Pharmacotherapy: A pathophysiologic approach* (9th ed., pp. 687–704). New York: McGraw-Hill.

Nowicka, J., & Mróz, E. (1989). Bacterial urinary infections in acute leukemia. *Pol Tyg Lek, 44*(25-26), 607–610. https://pubmed.ncbi.nlm.nih.gov/2637431/.

NPDB Research statistics. https://www.npdb.hrsa.gov/resources/methods.jsp.

Nurse practice act. (n.d.). *Medical Dictionary for the Health Professions and Nursing*. (2012). https://medical-dictionary.thefreedictionary.com/nurse+practice+act.

O'Brien, M. E., Ciuleanu, T. E., Tsekov, H., et al. (2006). Phase III trial comparing supportive care alone with supportive care with oral topotecan in patients with relapsed small-cell lung cancer. *Journal of Clinical Oncology, 24*(34), 5441.

O'Donovan, K. (2010). Continuing education – Cardiology – Nursing care of acute and chronic heart failure. *WIN, 19*(1). https://www.inmo.ie/tempDocs/CardioWINFeb_33.pdf.

O'Gara, P. T., Kushner, F. G., Ascheim, D. D., et al. (2013). 2013 ACCF/AHA guideline for the management of ST-elevation myocardial infarction: A report of the American College of Cardiology Foundation/American Heart Association Task Force on Practice Guidelines. *Journal of the American College of Cardiology, 61*(4), e78–e140.

Olausson, J., & Ferrer, B. (2013). Care of the body after death. *Clinical Journal of Oncology Nuring, 17*(6), 647–651.

O'Mara, N. B., (2014). Management of patients on dialysis. In Murphy, J. E., & Lee, M. W. (Eds.), *Pharmacotherapy self-assessment program, 2014 Book 2. Chronic illnesses*, pp. 203–207. Lenexa, KS: American College of Clinical Pharmacy.

Onuki, Y., Ikegami-Kawai, M., Ishitsuka, K., et al. (2012). A 5% glucose infusion fluid provokes significant precipitation of phenytoin sodium injection via interruption of the cosolvent effect of propylene glycol. *Chem Pharm Bull (Tokyo), 60*(1), 86–93.

Ortho Bullets (2020a). *Proximal Humerus Fractures*. https://www.orthobullets.com/trauma/1015/proximal-humerus-fractures.

Ortho Bullets. (2020b). *Supracondylar fracture—pediatric*. https://www.orthobullets.com/pediatrics/4007/supracondylar-fracture–pediatric.

Osgood-Schlatter disease. *Mayo Clinic* 2019. https://www.mayoclinic.org/diseases-conditions/osgood-schlatter-disease/symptoms-causes/syc-20354864.

OSHA standards for bloodborne pathogens. http://www.hercenter.org/rmw/osha-bps.php.

Overstreet, L. (n.d.). Bereavement and grief. *ERServices*. https://courses.lumenlearning.com/suny-hccc-ss-152-1/chapter/bereavement-and-grief/.

Pacchiarotti, I., Bond, D. J., Baldessarini, R. J., et al. (2013). The International Society for Bipolar Disorders (ISBD) task force report on antidepressant use in bipolar disorders. *Am J Psychiatry, 170*, 1249–1262.

Park, E. (2014). Altered mental status and endocrine diseases. *Emergency Medicine Clinics of North America, 32*(2), 367–378.

Pascal, J. P., & Cales, P. (1987). Propranolol in the prevention of first upper gastrointestinal tract hemorrhage in patients with cirrhosis of the liver and esophageal varices. *N Engl J Med, 317*, 856–861.

Pascual, E., Sivera, F., & Andrés, M. (2011). Synovial fluid analysis for crystals. *Current Opinion in Rheumatology, 23*(2), 161–169.

Pasquel, F. J., Spiegelman, R., McCauley, M., et al. (2010). *Diabetes Care, 33*(4), 739–741.

Patel, B. K. (2020). Acute hypoxemic respiratory failure (AHRF, ARDS). *MDS Manual: Professional Version*. https://www.msdmanuals.com/professional/critical-care-medicine/respiratory-failure-and-mechanical-ventilation/acute-hypoxemic-respiratory-failure-ahrf,-ards.

Patient documents and confidentiality of information. *Helsinki University Hospital*. https://www.hus.fi/en/patients/patients-rights/patient-documents-confidentiality/Pages/default.aspx.

Patient Self Determination Act of 1990 Law and Legal Definition. *USLegal.com*. https://definitions.uslegal.com/p/patient-self-determination-act-of-1990/.

Patterson, J. W., & Dominique, E. (2019). Acute abdomen. *Stat-Pearls*. https://www.ncbi.nlm.nih.gov/books/NBK459328/.

Peer Review Organization (PRO). https://www.plexishealth.com/glossary/peer-review-organization-pro/.

Pellicori, P., Kaur, K., & Clark, A. L. (2015). Fluid management in patients with chronic heart failure. *Cardiac Failure Review, 1*(2), 2015. https://www.cfrjournal.com/articles/fluid-management-chronic-HF.

Peppard, P. E., Young, T., Barnet, J. H., et al. (2013). Increased prevalence of sleep-disordered breathing in adults. *American Journal of Epidemiology, 177*(9).

Peppercorn, M.A., & Kane, S.V. (2019). *Patient education: Ulcerative colitis.* https://www.uptodate.com/contents/ulcerative-colitis-beyond-the-basics#H10.

Performance improvement & risk management: NCLEX-RN. https://www.registerednursing.org/nclex/performance-improvement-risk-management/.

Peters, D. H. (2014). The application of systems thinking in health: Why use systems thinking. *Health Research Policy and Systems, 12*(51). https://doi.org/10.1186/1478-4505-12-51.

Phillips, J. O., Metzler, M. H., Palmieri, T. L., Huckfeldt, R. E., & Dahl, N. G. (1996). A prospective study of simplified omeprazole suspension for the prophylaxis of stress-related mucosal damage. *Critical Care Medicine, 24*, 1793–1800.

Phillips, T. G., Reibach, A., & Slomiany, W. P. (2004). Diagnosis and management of scaphoid fractures. *American Family Physician, 70*(5), 879–884.

Physical therapy for gait and balance. (2015). *ProFhysio Physical Therapy*. https://www.profysionj.com/blog/2015/march/physical-therapy-for-gait-and-balance-impairment/.

Practice guidelines and interpretive guidelines. *Texas Board of Nursing*. https://www.bon.texas.gov/practice_guidelines.asp.

Prichard, P. J., Yeomans, N. D., Mihaly, G. W., et al. (1985). Omeprazole: A study of its inhibition of gastric pH and oral pharmacokinetics after morning or evening dosage. *Gastroenterology, 88*, 64–69.

Quality and performance improvement concepts. Case Management. https://casemanagementstudyguide.com/ccm-%20knowledge-domains/case-management-%20concepts/quality-and-performance-improvement-%20concepts/.

Quon, M. J., Behlouli, H., & Pilote, L. (2018). Anticoagulant use and risk of ischemic stroke and bleeding in patients with secondary atrial fibrillation associated with acute coronary syndromes, acute pulmonary disease, or sepsis. *JACC: Clinical Electrophysiology, 4*(3).

Rahimi, R. S., Singal, A. G., Cuthbert, J. A., & Rockey, D. C. (2014). Lactulose vs polyethylene glycol 3350 electrolyte solution for treatment of overt hepatic encephalopathy: The HELP randomized clinical trial. *JAMA Internal Medicine, 174*, 1727–1733.

Rahimi, S. A. (2019). Abdominal aortic aneurysm clinical presentation. *Medscape*. https://emedicine.medscape.com/article/1979501-clinical.

Rakieh, C., & Conaghan, P. G. (2011). Diagnosis and treatment of gout in primary care. *The Practitioner, 255*(1746), 17–21.

Ramkumar, D., & Rao, S. S. C. (2005). Efficacy and safety of traditional medical therapies for chronic constipation: Systematic review. *American Journal of Gastroenterology, 100*, 936–971.

Rao, J. V., & Chandraiah, K. (2012). Occupational stress, mental health and coping among information technology professionals. *Indian J Occup Environ Med, 16*(1), 22–26.

Raskin, J. B. (1999). Gastrointestinal effects of NSAID therapy. *American Journal of Medicine, 106*(S 5B), 3–12.

Raychaudhuri, S. K., Maverakis, E., & Raychaudhuri, S. P. (2014). Diagnosis and classification of psoriasis. *Autoimmunity Reviews, 13*(4–5), 490–495.

Reed, D. (2019). Resources for primary, secondary, and tertiary sources in the health sciences. https://libguides.umn.edu/c.php?g=986651.

Reporting abuse and neglect. Mandatory Reporter 2018. http://www.rn.org/courses/coursematerial-10011.pdf.

Respiratory acidosis. (2017). *Healthline*. https://www.healthline.com/health/respiratory-acidosis#prevention.

Revord, J. (2005). Typical symptoms of a herniated disc. *Spine-health*. https://www.spine-health.com/conditions/herniated-disc/typical-symptoms-a-herniated-disc.

Rhodes, A., Evans, L. E., Alhazzani, W., et al. (2017). Surviving sepsis campaign: International guidelines for management of sepsis and septic shock: 2016. *Critical Care Medicine, 45*(3), 486–552.

Rice, M. Differences in communication. https://unioncollegenativeamericans.weebly.com/cultural-differences-in-communication.html.

Rich, T.R. (2011). Kashrut: Jewish dietary laws. http://www.jewfaq.org/kashrut.htm.

Richardson, W.J. (2012). Cultural awareness to help while serving native veterans. https://www.ruralhealth.va.gov/docs/webinars/richardson-cultural-sensitivity-062712.pdf.

Riddell, M. C., Gallen, I. W., Smart, C. E., et al. (2017). Exercise management in type 1 diabetes: A consensus statement. *The Lancet Diabetes & Endocrinology, 5*(5), 377–390.

Rifai, N. (2018). Blood groups, pretransfusion testing, and red blood cell transfusion.). In *Tietz textbook of clinical chemistry and molecular diagnostics* (6th ed., pp. 17–43). St. Louis, MO: Elsevier.

Riley, J. (2015). The key roles for the nurse in acute heart failure management. *Card Fail Rev, 1*(2), 123–127. doi: 10.15420/cfr.2015.1.2.123.

Rucker, M. (2016). Qualitative research question examples. https://unstick.me/qualitative-research-question-examples/.

Runyon, B. A. (2013). Management of adult patients with ascites due to cirrhosis: An update. *Hepatology, 57*, 1651–1653.

Rutgeerts, P., Sandborn, W. J., Feagan, B. G., et al. (2005). Infliximab for induction and maintenance therapy for ulcerative colitis. *New England Journal of Medicine, 353*, 2462–2476.

Safer sex guidelines. *The Body: The HIV/AIDS resource.* (2013 Nov.) https://www.thebody.com/content/art6098.html.

Saha, S., Beach, M. C., & Cooper, L. A. (2008). Patient centeredness, cultural competence and healthcare quality. *J Natl Med Assoc, 100*(11), 1275–1285. doi: 10.1016/s0027-9684(15)31505-4.

Sahu, P. K., Giri, D. D., Singh, R., et al. (2013). Therapeutic and medicinal uses of aloe vera: A review. *Pharmacology & Pharmacy, 4*, 599–610.

Salters-Pedneault, K. (2020). *Suicidality in borderline personality disorder.* https://www.verywellmind.com/suicidality-in-borderline-personality-disorder-425485.

Sanderlin, B. W., & Raspa, R. F. (2003). Common stress fractures. *American Family Physician, 68*(8), 1527–1532.

Sateia, M. J., Buysse, D. J., Krystal, A. D., et al. (2017). Clinical practice guideline for the pharmacologic treatment of chronic insomnia in adults: An American Academy of Sleep Medicine Clinical Practice Guideline. *Journal of Clinical Sleep Medicine, 13*, 307–349.

Sateia, M., & Nowell, P. (2004). Insomnia. *Lancet, 364*, 1959–1973.

Schenzel, H. A., & Tracy, M. E. (n.d.). *An Acute Care Nurse Practitioner Model of Care for Stroke Patients.* Unpublished manuscript. https://dspace2.creighton.edu/xmlui/bitstream/handle/10504/43046/Schenzel_Manuscript_05182013.pdf?sequence=1&isAllowed=y.

Schmidt, A. H. (2017). Acute compartment syndrome. *Injury, 48*(suppl 1), S22–S25.

Schortgen, F. (2003) Hypotension during intermittent hemodialysis: New insights into an old problem. *Applied Physiology in Intensive Care Medicine.* Berlin: Springer Heidelberg. https://doi.org/10.1007/3-540-37363-2_20.

Schweiger, M. J., Chambers, C. E., Davidson, C. J., et al. (2007). Prevention of contrast induced nephropathy: Recommendations for the high-risk patient undergoing cardiovascular procedures. *Catheterization and Cardiovascular Interventions, 69*, 135–140.

Scott, L. J. (2017). Sitagliptin: A review in type 2 diabetes. *Drugs, 77*(2), 209–224.

Seeger, D. M. (2015). Muslim women and United States healthcare: challenges to access and nation. *The Cupola: Scholarship at Gettysburg College.* https://cupola.gettysburg.edu/cgi/viewcontent.cgi?referer=https://www.google.com.ph/&httpsredir=1&article=1002&context=islamandwomen.

Sertkaya, A., Eyraud, J., Sands, M., Moore, K., Berlind, A., & Salcedo, G. (2011). Food and feed import practices of foreign governments to improve food safety. *U.S. Food and Drug Administration.* https://www.fda.gov/media/85837/download.

Shah, R., & John, S. (2019). Cholestatic jaundice (cholestasis, cholestatic hepatitis). *Stat Pearls.* https://www.ncbi.nlm.nih.gov/books/NBK482279/.

Shah, S. M. (2020). Vasectomy and vasectomy reversal. *Penn State Hershey Medical Center.* http://pennstatehershey.adam.com/content.aspx?productId=114&pid=10&gid=000037.

Shaw, J., Whitbread, M., & Fothergill, R. T. (2016). A clinical audit examining the use of furosemide by the London ambulance service. *American Journal of Education, 4*(6), 491–495.

Shiel, W. C. (n.d.). Hospice care. *eMedicineHealth.* https://www.emedicinehealth.com/hospice/article_em.htm#hospice_facts.

Shiel, W. C. (2017). *Medical definition of patient autonomy.* https://www.medicinenet.com/script/main/art.asp?articlekey=13551.

Shprecher, D., Schwalb, J., & Kurlan, R. (2008). Normal pressure hydrocephalus: Diagnosis and treatment. *Current Neurology and Neuroscience Reports, 8*(5), 371–376.

Sider, L., Mintzen, R., Deschler, T., Kim, K., & Weinberg, P. (1983). Control of swallowing by use of topical anesthesia during digital subtraction angiography. *Radiology, 148*, 563–564.

Silvester, W., Bellomo, R., & Cole, L. (2001). Epidemiology, management, and outcome of severe acute renal failure of critical illness in Australia. *Critical Care Medicine, 29*, 1910–1915.

Singer, M., Deutschmann, C. S., Seymour, C. W., et al. (2016). The Third International Consensus Definitions for Sepsis and Septic Shock (Sepsis-3). *Journal of the American Medical Association, 315*(8), 801–810.

Singh, J., Saag, K. G., Bridges, S. L., Jr., et al. (2016). 2015 American College of Rheumatology Guideline for the Treatment of Rheumatoid Arthritis. *Arthritis Rheumatol, 68*(1), 1–26.

Skilled hospice providers offer compassionate end-of-life care. Hope Hospice & Health Services. https://hopehospice.com/services/hospice-care/.

Sleight, P., Yusuf, S., Pogue, J., Tsuyuki, R., Diaz, R., & Probstfield, J. (2001). Blood-pressure reduction and cardiovascular risk in HOPE study. *The Lancet, 358*(9299), 2130–2131.

Smith, D., & Gaillard, F. (n.d.). Subarachnoid hemorrhage. https://radiopaedia.org/articles/subarachnoid-haemorrhage?lang=us.

Smith, P., Hanks, L., Salomone, L., & Hanks, J. (2017). Thyroid. In *Sabiston textbook of surgery*, (pp. 880–922). Philadelphia: Elsevier.

SOAS University of London. Unit 1: Introduction to research. https://www.soas.ac.uk/cedep-demos/000_P506_RM_3736-Demo/unit1/page_25.htm.

Sørensen, D., Frederiksen, K., Groefte, T., & Lomborg, K. (2013). Nurse–patient collaboration: A grounded theory study of patients with chronic obstructive pulmonary disease on non-invasive ventilation. *International Journal of Nursing Studies, 50*, 26–33.

Sowinski, K. M., Churchwell, M. D., Decker, B. S., et al. (2014). Hemodialysis and peritoneal dialysis. In J. T. DiPiro, R. L. Talbert, & G. C. Yee et al. (Eds.), *Pharmacotherapy: A pathophysiologic approach* (9th ed., pp. 665–685). New York: McGraw-Hill.

Sports nutrition and type 1 diabetes. (n.d.). https://www.diabetes.org.uk/guide-to-diabetes/enjoy-food/eating-with-diabetes/out-and-about/sports-nutrition-and-type-1-diabetes.

Stamatakis, M. K. (2010). Acute kidney injury. In M. A. Chisholm-Burns, B. G. Wells, & T. L. Schwinghammer et al. (Eds.), *Pharmacotherapy: Principles and practice* (2nd ed., pp. 431–444). New York: McGraw-Hill.

Stanley, K. M. (2010). Lateral and vertical violence in nursing. *South Carolina Nurse.* https://cdn.ymaws.com/www.scnurses.org/resource/resmgr/imported/LateralandVerticalViolenceinNursing.pdf.

Stein, R.L., & Bodager, P. What is cultural anthropology? https://culturalanthropology.duke.edu/undergraduate.

Stephenson, R. O. (2020, March). Autonomic dysreflexia in spinal cord injury. *Medscape.* https://emedicine.medscape.com/article/322809-overview.

Stone, N. J., Robinson, J. G., Lichtenstein, A. H., et al. (2014). 2013 ACC/AHA guideline on the treatment of blood cholesterol to reduce atherosclerotic cardiovascular risk in adults: a report of the American College of Cardiology/American Heart Association Task Force on Practice Guidelines. *Journal of the American College of Cardiology, 63*(25 Part B), 2889–2934.

Stöppler, M.C. (2019a). *Glucose Tolerance Test.* https://www.medicinenet.com/glucose_tolerance_test/article.htm.

Stöppler, M.C. (2019b). *Tuberculosis Skin Test (PPD Skin Test).* https://www.medicinenet.com/tuberculosis_skin_test_ppd_skin_test/article.htm.

Strait, J. B., & Lakatta, E. G. (2013). Aging-associated cardiovascular changes and their relationship to heart failure. *Heart Fail Clin, 8*(1), 143–164.

Sullivan, J. T., Sykora, K., Schneiderman, J., Naranjo, C. A., & Sellers, E. M. (1989). Assessment of alcohol withdrawal: The revised clinical institute withdrawal assessment for alcohol scale (CIWA-Ar). *British Journal of Addiction, 84*(11), 1353–1357.

Suter, W. N. (2012). *Introduction to educational research: A critical thinking approach* (2nd ed.). https://www.sagepub.com/sites/default/files/upm-binaries/43144_12.pdf.

Swihart, D. (2009). Nursing professional development: Roles and accountabilities. Retrieved from: https://www.medscape.com/viewarticle/705515.

Syed, I. (2004). Revision boxes of cardiovascular medicine. In A. Hingorani (Ed.), *EMQs in Clinical Medicine* (pp. 22–25). London: The Hodder Headline Group.

Symptoms and stages of HIV infections. *Avert: Information on HIV* 2020. Available at: https://www.avert.org/about-hiv-aids/symptoms-stages.

Takahashi, R., Akamoto, S., Nagao, M., et al. (2016). Follow-up of asymptomatic adult diaphragmatic hernia: Should patients with this condition undergo immediate operation? A report of two cases. *Surgical Case Reports, 2*(1), 95.

Takhar, S., & Chin, R. (2018a). HIV infection and AIDS. In *Rosen's emergency medicine: Concepts and clinical practice* (9th ed., pp. 1626–1638). Philadelphia: Elsevier.

Takhar, S., & Chin, R. (2018b). Pulmonary embolism and deep venous thrombosis. In *Rosen's emergency medicine: Concepts and clinical practice* (10th ed., pp. 1051–1066). Philadelphia: Elsevier.

Talbert, R. L., Yee, G. C., et al. (2014). *Pharmacotherapy: A pathophysiologic approach* (9th ed., pp. 633–663). New York: McGraw-Hill.

Talbert, R. L., Yee, G. C., et al. (2017). *Pharmacotherapy: A pathophysiologic approach* (10th ed.), New York: McGraw-Hill.

Taler, S. J., Agarwal, R., Bakris, G. L., et al. (2013). KDOQI U.S. commentary on the 2012 KDIGO clinical practice guideline for management of blood pressure in CKD. *American Journal of Kidney Disease, 62*, 201–213.

Talley, N. J., Abreu, M. T., Anchkar, J. P., et al. (2011). An evidence-based systematic review on medical therapies for inflammatory bowel disease. *American Journal of Gastroenterology, 106*, S2–S25.

Talley, N. J., O'Keefe, E. A., Zinsmeister, A. R., & Melton, L. J., III (1992). Prevalence of gastrointestinal symptoms in the elderly: A population-based study. *Gastroenterology, 102*, 895–901.

Tamblyn, R., Berkson, L., Dauphinee, L. L., et al. (1997). Unnecessary prescribing of NSAIDs and the management of NSAID-related gastropathy in medical practice. *Ann Intern Med, 127*, 429–438.

Taylor, B. J. (2006). *Research in nursing and health care: Evidence for practice.* Stamford, CT: Thomson Publishing.

Taylor, K. (2020). Back channeling. *ESL Base.* https://www.esl-base.com/tefl-a-z/back-channelling.

Tejada, T., Fornoni, A., Lenz, O., & Materson, B. J. (2006). Non-pharmacologic therapy for hypertension: Does it really work. *Current Cardiology Reports, 8*(6), 418–424.

Terdiman, J. P., Gruss, C. B., Heidelbaugh, J. J., et al. (2013). American Gastroenterological Association Institute technical review on the use of thiopurines, methotrexate, and anti-TNF-biologic drugs for the induction and maintenance of remission in Crohn's disease. *Gastroenterology, 145*, 1459–1463.

Teter, C. J., Kando, J. C., Wells, B. G., et al. (2017). Major depressive disorder. In J. T. DiPiro, R. L. Talbert, & G. C. Yee et al. (Eds.), *Pharmacotherapy: A pathophysiologic approach* (10th ed.), New York: McGraw-Hill.

Thakral, B., Anastasi, J., & Wang, S. A. (2018). Myeloproliferative and "overlap" myelodysplastic/myeloproliferative neoplasms. In E. D. Hsi (Ed.), *Hematopathology*, (pp. 488–538). Elsevier.

The 12 cranial nerves. (2019). *Healthline.* https://www.healthline.com/health/12-cranial-nerves.

The five stages of grief. (n.d.). https://grief.com/the-five-stages-of-grief/.

The goals of hospice care. (n.d.). *Center for Hospice Care.* https://www.hospicesect.org/hospice-and-palliative-care/the-goals-of-hospice-care.

The impaired nurse: Would you know what to do if you suspected substance abuse. *American Nurse.* (2011). https://www.myamericannurse.com/the-impaired-nurse-would-you-know-what-to-do-if-you-suspected-substance-abuse/.

The Mayo Clinic. (2019). Treating pain: Overview. https://www.mayoclinic.org/treating-pain-overview/art-20208633.

The role of safe prescribing in the prevention of medication errors. *Shands Jacksonville Drug Update.* http://hscj.ufl.edu/resman/manualpdfs/safe_prescribing.pdf.

Thomas, C. P. (2019). Syndrome of Inappropriate Antidiuretic Hormone Secretion (SIADH). *Medscape.* https://emedicine.medscape.com/article/246650-overview.

Thompson, C., Cullum, N., McCaughan, D., Sheldon, T., et al. (2004). Nurses, information use, and clinical decision making—the real world potential for evidence-based decisions in nursing. *BMJ Journals: Evidence-Based Nursing, 7*, 68–72. https://ebn.bmj.com/content/7/3/68.

Thrive, A. P. (XXXX). Licensing guide for new grads. https://thriveap.com/blog/free-ebook-licensing-guide-new-grad-nps.

Thursz, M. R., Richardson, P., Allison, M., et al. (2015). Prednisolone or pentoxifylline for alcoholic hepatitis. *New England Journal of Medicine, 372*, 1619–1628.

Tidy, C. (2016). Cor pulmonale. *Patient Info.* https://patient.info/doctor/cor-pulmonale.

Tinker, A., & Hough Falk, L. (2016). The top five essentials for outcomes improvement. https://www.healthcatalyst.com/Outcomes-Improvement-Five-Essentials.

Todd, B. (2015). Evidence-based practice and the curiosity of nurses. *American Journal of Nursing.* https://ajnoffthecharts.com/evidence-based-practice-and-the-curiosity-of-nurses/.

Tomajan, K. (2012). Advocating for nurses and nursing. *OJIN: Online J Issues Nurs, 17*(1), p. 4.

Tomesko, J. (2018). Total parenteral nutrition & blood glucose levels. *SFGate.* https://healthyeating.sfgate.com/total-parenteral-nutrition-blood-glucose-levels-6235.html.

Tommy's. (2018). *Planning a pregnancy with type 1 or 2 diabetes.* https://www.tommys.org/pregnancy-information/planning-pregnancy/are-you-ready-conceive/planning-pregnancy-type-1-or-2-diabetes.

Tornøe, K. A., Danbolt, L. J., Kvigne, K., & Sørlie, V. (2014). The power of consoling presence: Hospice nurses' lived experience with spiritual and existential care for the dying. *BMC Nurs, 13,* 25.

Trivedi, A. (2019). Case-based learning: Meningitis. https://www.pharmaceutical-journal.com/cpd-and-learning/learning-article/case-based-learning-meningitis/20206581.article?firstPass=false.

Trivedi, C. D., & Pitchumoni, C. S. (2005). Drug-induced pancreatitis. *J Clin Gastroenterol, 39,* 709–716.

Turvey, B. E., Sovino, J. O., & Coronado Mares, A. (2018). Mandated reporter *False Allegations*: Academic Press. https://doi.org/10.1016/B978-0-12-801250-5.12001-4.

Uhlig, K., Berns, J. S., Kestenbaum, B., et al. (2010). KDOQI U.S. commentary on the 2009 KDIGO clinical practice guideline for the diagnosis, evaluation, and treatment of CKD–mineral and bone disorder (CKD-MBD). *American Journal of Kidney Disease, 55,* 773–799.

University of Wisconsin. (2017). *What works for health: Policies and programs to improve Wisconsin's health.* http://whatworksforhealth.wisc.edu/program.php?t1=2%202&t2=17&t3=90&id=386.

Umoh, N. J., Fan, E., Mendez-Tellez, P. A., et al. (2008). Patient and intensive care unit organizational factors associated with low tidal volume ventilation in acute lung injury. *Critical Care Medicine, 36,* 1463.

University of West Florida. (2019). Literature review: Conducting & writing. https://libguides.uwf.edu/c.php?g=215199&p=1420520.

Updates to the Guidelines for the Prevention and Treatment of Opportunistic Infections in Adults and Adolescents with HIV. *AIDS Info, National Institute of Health* 2020. https://aidsinfo.nih.gov/guidelines/html/4/adult-and-adolescent-opportunistic-infection/392/whats-new.

U.S. Department of Justice, Drug Enforcement Administration. https://www.deadiversion.usdoj.gov/online_forms_apps.html.

U.S. Public Health Service. (2001). Updated U.S. Public Health Service guidelines for the management of occupational exposures to HBV, HCV, and HIV and recommendations for postexposure prophylaxis. *MMWR Recomm Rep, 50*(RR11), 1–52.

Uwaifo, G.I. (2020). *Primary aldosteronism.* https://emedicine.medscape.com/article/127080-overview.

Vahlquist, A. (2010). *Carotenoids and the skin: An overview, retinoids and carotenoids in dermatology.* Boca Raton, FL: CRC Press.

van Aerde, J. (2001). Guidelines for health care professionals supporting families experiencing a perinatal loss. *Paediatr Child Health, 6*(7), 469–477.

Vann, M. R. (2009). Holter monitors: A tool to detect heart disease. *EveryDayHealth.* https://www.everydayhealth.com/heart-health/holter-monitor.aspx.

van Ramshorst, G. H., Nieuwenhuizen, J., Hop, W. C., et al. (2010). Abdominal wound dehiscence in adults: Development and validation of a risk model. *World J Surg, 34*(1), 20–27.

Varela-Roman, A., Grigorian, L., Barge, E., et al. (2005). Heart failure in patients with preserved and deteriorated left ventricular ejection fraction. *Heart, 91,* 489–494.

Varghese, S., & Ohlow, M. A. (2019). Left ventricular free wall rupture in myocardial infarction: A retrospective analysis from a single tertiary center. *JRSM Cardiovasc Dis, 8,* 2048004019896692.

Varshney, M., Sharma, K., Kumar, R., & Varshney, P. G. (2011). Appropriate depth of placement of oral endotracheal tube and its possible determinants in Indian adult patients. *Indian J Anaesth, 55*(5), 488–493.

Vega, C. P., & Bernard, A. (2016). Interprofessional collaboration to improve health care: An introduction. *Medscape.* https://www.medscape.org/viewarticle/857823.

Victoria State Government. (2018). Tuberculosis treatment. https://www.betterhealth.vic.gov.au/health/conditionsandtreatments/tuberculosis-treatment.

Von Hebra, F. (2009). *On diseases of the skin including the exanthemata (translated by Fagge, C. H.).* London: New Sydenham Society.

Wale, J. (2016). Physicians' responsibility to obtain informed consent. *Medical News.* https://www.medicalnews.md/physicians-responsibility-to-obtain-informed-consent/.

Waljee, A. K., Dimagno, M. J., Wu, B. U., et al. (2009). Systematic review: Pancreatic enzyme treatment of malabsorption associated with chronic pancreatitis. *Alimentary Pharmacology & Therapeutics, 29,* 235–246.

Walker, B., College, N., Ralston, S., & Penman, I. (2014). Blood disease. In *Davidson's principles and practice of medicine* (22nd ed., pp. 989–1056). Philadelphia: Elsevier.

Walls, R., Hockberger, R., & Gausche-Hill, M. (2018). *Rosen's emergency medicine: Concepts and clinical practice* (9th ed.). Philadelphia: Elsevier.

Wan, L., Bellomo, R., Di Giantomasso, D., & Ronco, C. (2003). The pathogenesis of septic acute renal failure. *Curr Opin Crit Care, 9*(6), 496–502.

Wanner, C., & Tonelli, M. (2014). KDIGO clinical practice guideline for lipid management in CKD: Summary of recommendation statements and clinical approach to the patient. *Kidney International, 85,* 1303–1309.

Weber, S. (n.d.). 5 side effects of chemotherapy and how to deal with them. *DailyHealthWire.* https://www.trihealth.com/dailyhealthwire/cancer/5-side-effects-of-chemotherapy-and-how-to-deal-with-them/.

WebMD. *Should you try a low-residue diet?* https://www.webmd.com/ibd-crohns-disease/low-residue-diet-foods#1-3.

Weinbaum, C. M., Williams, I., Mast, E. E., et al. (2008). Recommendations for identification and public health management of persons with chronic hepatitis B virus infection. *MMWR Recomm Rep, 57*(RR08), 1–20.

Weinberger, S. E., Cockrill, B. A., & Mandel, J. (2019). *Principles of pulmonary medicine.* Philadelphia: Elsevier.

Weiser, K. (2020). Native American medicine. https://www.legendsofamerica.com/na-medicine/.

Welsh, A. (1982). The practical and economic value of flexible system laryngoscopy. *J Laryngol Otol, 96,* 1125–1129.

Weston, W. L., & Howe, W. (2019). *Treatment of atopic dermatitis (eczema).* https://www-uptodate-com./contents/treatment-of-atopic-dermatitis-eczema?search=eczema%20treatment&source=search_result&selectedTitle=1~150&usage_type=default&display_rank=1#H7.

What is palliative care? Get Palliative Care. https://getpalliative-care.org/whatis/.

What is the window period for an HIV test? *I-base Info.* https://i-base.info/guides/testing/what-is-the-window-period.

What to expect at your first HIV care visit. (2017). *HIV.gov.* https://www.hiv.gov/hiv-basics/starting-hiv-care/getting-ready-for-your-first-visit/what-to-expect-at-your-first-hiv-care-visit.

What to know about hypovolemic shock. (n.d.). *Medical News Today.* https://www.medicalnewstoday.com/articles/312348.

What to know about stress ulcers. (n.d.). *Medical News Today.* https://www.medicalnewstoday.com/articles/324990#prevention.

What you must report to the NPDB. https://www.npdb.hrsa.gov/hcorg/whatYouMustReportToTheDataBank.jsp.

What you need to know about Ashkenazi genetic diseases. (2014). https://forward.com/culture/203580/what-you-need-to-know-about-ashkenazi-genetic-dise/.

When patients don't speak English: A guide to the why and how of a quality language access program. https://www.indemandinterpreting.com/wp-content/uploads/2014/12/indemand-when-patients-dont-speak-english.pdf.

Who are speech-language pathologists, and what do they do? *Am Sp Lang Hear Assoc.* https://www.asha.org/public/Who-Are-Speech-Language-Pathologists/.

Wilkins, T., Embry, K., & George, R. (2013). Diagnosis and management of acute diverticulitis. https://www.aafp.org/afp/2013/0501/p612.html.

Williams, B., Mancia, G., Spiering, W., et al. (2018). 2018 ESC/ESH guidelines for the management of arterial hypertension: The Task Force for the management of arterial hypertension of the European Society of Cardiology (ESC) and the European Society of Hypertension (ESH). *European Heart Journal, 39*(33), 3021–3104.

Williams, J. C. (2017). Black Americans don't trust our healthcare system – here's why. https://thehill.com/blogs/pundits-blog/healthcare/347780-black-americans-dont-have-trust-in-our-healthcare-system.

Witkowski, J. A., & Parish, L. C. (2004). The assessment of acne: An evaluation of grading and lesion counting in the measurement of acne. *Clinical Dermatology, 22,* 394–397.

Witt, H., Apte, M. V., Kiem, V., et al. (2007). Chronic pancreatitis: challenges and advances in pathogenesis, genetics, diagnosis, and therapy. *Gastroenterology, 132,* 1557–1573.

Wolf, D. C. (2020). Hepatic encephalopathy. *Medscape.* https://emedicine.medscape.com/article/186101-overview#a1.

Wolfe, F., Zhao, S., & Lane, N. (2000). Preference for nonsteroidal anti-inflammatory drugs over acetaminophen by rheumatic disease patients: a survey of 1799 patients with osteoarthritis, rheumatoid arthritis, and fibromyalgia. *Arthritis & Rheumatology, 43,* 378–385.

World Health Organization. (2018). Latent TB infection: Updated and consolidated guidelines for programmatic management. (2018). http://www.who.int/tb/publications/2018/latent-tuberculosis-infection/en/.

Wright, J. M., Musini, V. M., & Gill, R. (2018). First-line drugs for hypertension. *Cochrane Database of Systematic Reviews, 4*(4), CD001841.

Yatham, L. N., Kennedy, S. H., Parikh, S. V., et al. (2013). Canadian Network for Mood and Anxiety Treatments (CANMAT) and International Society for Bipolar Disorders (ISBD) collaborative update of CANMAT guidelines for the management of patients with bipolar disorder: Update 2013. *Bipolar Disorder, 15,* 1–44.

Ympa, Y. P., Sakr, Y., Reinhart, K., et al. (2005). Has mortality from acute kidney injury decreased? A systematic review of the literature. *American Journal of Medicine, 118,* 827–832.

Yoshida, T., & Delafontaine, P. (2015). Mechanisms of cachexia in chronic disease states. *Am J Med Sci, 350*(4), 250–256.

Yousefi, H., & Abedi, H. A. (2011). Spiritual care in hospitalized patients. *Iran J Nurs Midwifery Res, 16*(1), 125–132.

Zarbock, A., Gomez, H., & Kellum, J. A. (2014). Sepsis-induced AKI revisited: Pathophysiology, prevention and future therapies. *Curr Opin Crit Care, 20*(6), 588–595.

Zilberstein, J., McCurdy, M. T., & Winters, M. E. (2014). Anaphylaxis. *Journal of Emergency Medicine, 47*(2), 182–187.